Essential Radiology

Clinical Presentation • Pathophysiology • Imaging

Second Edition

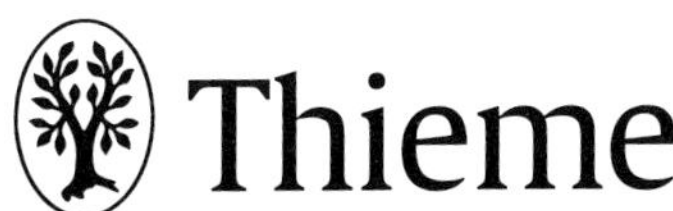

Essential Radiology

Clinical Presentation • Pathophysiology • Imaging

Second Edition

Richard B. Gunderman, M.D., Ph.D., M.P.H.
Associate Professor
Radiology, Pediatrics, Medical Education
Vice Chair, Radiology (Education)
Indiana University School of Medicine
Director, Pediatric Radiology
Riley Hospital for Children of Indiana
Indianapolis, Indiana

Thieme
New York • Stuttgart

Thieme Medical Publishers, Inc.
333 Seventh Ave.
New York, NY 10001

Editor: Timothy Hiscock
Associate Editor: Birgitta Brandenburg
Vice President, Production and Electronic Publishing: Anne T. Vinnicombe
Production Editor: Print Matters, Inc.
Sales Manager: Ross Lumpkin
Associate Marketing Manager: Verena Diem
Chief Financial Officer: Peter van Woerden
President: Brian D. Scanlan
Compositor: Thomson Digital
Printer: Edwards Brothers

Library of Congress Cataloging-in-Publication Data

Gunderman, Richard B.
Essential radiology : clinical presentation, pathophysiology, imaging / Richard B. Gunderman. — 2nd ed.
p. ; cm.
Includes bibliographical references and index.
ISBN 1-58890-082-7 (TMP : softcover) — ISBN 3-13-110472-4 (GTV : softcover)
1. Radiography, Medical—Handbooks, manuals, etc. I. Title.
[DNLM: 1. Radiography—Handbooks. 2. Diagnostic Imaging—Handbooks. WN 39 G975 2006]
RC78.G85 2006
616.07′572–dc22 2005056853

Important note: Medical knowledge is ever-changing. As new research and clinical experience broaden our knowledge, changes in treatment and drug therapy may be required. The authors and editors of the material herein have consulted sources believed to be reliable in their efforts to provide information that is complete and in accord with the standards accepted at the time of publication. However, in view of the possibility of human error by the authors, editors, or publisher of the work herein or changes in medical knowledge, neither the authors, editors, or publisher, nor any other party who has been involved in the preparation of this work, warrants that the information contained herein is in every respect accurate or complete, and they are not responsible for any errors or omissions or for the results obtained from use of such information. Readers are encouraged to confirm the information contained herein with other sources. For example, readers are advised to check the product information sheet included in the package of each drug they plan to administer to be certain that the information contained in this publication is accurate and that changes have not been made in the recommended dose or in the contraindications for administration. This recommendation is of particular importance in connection with new or infrequently used drugs.

Some of the product names, patents, and registered designs referred to in this book are in fact registered trademarks or proprietary names even though specific reference to this fact is not always made in the text. Therefore, the appearance of a name without designation as proprietary is not to be construed as a representation by the publisher that it is in the public domain.

Printed in the United States of America

5 4 3 2

TMP ISBN 1-58890-082-7

GTV ISBN 3-13-110472-4

For Laura

Contents

Foreword

No specialty of medicine has advanced more rapidly over the past 35 years than radiology. Those of us who have practiced medicine during that period have witnessed the clinical implementation of such extraordinary innovations as ultrasonography, x-ray computed tomography, magnetic resonance imaging, positron emission tomography, and an inventive array of image-guided treatment modalities, to name just a few. While it is possible to carp about how modern radiology has increased the cost of care, it is also inarguably the case that without the advances of medical imaging, modern medicine would be nowhere near so effective and safe as it is today.

Despite how remarkable the past third of a century has been, I believe that medical imaging now stands on the cusp of a new era that will make everything that has come before seem pale by comparison. Innovation in medical imaging is being both pulled along by the drive toward "molecular medicine" and is pushing forward molecular diagnosis and treatment. The digitizing of medical images means that advanced imaging and expert interpretation are nearly instantly available to physicians in their offices and clinics–indeed, anywhere in the world. Thus, it is imperative that future physicians become well-versed in how imaging is properly employed in the care of their patients.

Understanding the proper uses of imaging, the meaning of important imaging signs, and how to apply these principles to excel as a physician are the goals of this excellent book. True to these goals, the book is directed at learners (primarily medical students and trainees in non-radiological specialties), who are looking for insight into how medical imaging can help integrate the diverse aspects of anatomy and pathophysiology of disease processes. This is the role of imaging in modern medicine. Nearly every medical specialty depends on imaging as a (if not *the*) primary diagnostic method. Yet education in how images are employed by various specialties tends to be fragmented; much of the teaching is performed by physicians for whom medical imaging is only a sidelight to their principal interests. This book seeks to–and succeeds in–making sense of imaging by integrating imaging knowledge for the edification of learners wishing a more coherent understanding. The organization of the text by organ system, the elegant, well-described images, and the sensitivity of the author to the interests of his learners all work to help achieve the desired end.

This book is an enjoyable and instructive work that fills an important need in radiological education. The author has expanded on his previous edition, updating it to accommodate progress in radiology. With pleasure, I extend congratulations to the author on an important achievement.

Bruce J. Hillman, M.D.
Theodore E. Keats Professor of Radiology
The University of Virginia
Charlottesville, Virginia

Preface

The need for radiology in medical education has never been greater. Each year, over 16,000 students graduate from US medical schools, and more than 24,000 physicians begin training in over 8,000 residency programs across the country. Another 30,000 US residents and fellows complete their training annually. It is vital that these new physicians understand radiology and the role it should play in patient care. The benefits that flow from expanding radiology's role in our undergraduate and graduate medical curricula are numerous, and the better we understand what it has to offer, the more effectively we can integrate it in practice.

Radiology is the context in which contemporary physicians most often encounter the internal anatomy of our patients, and provides great opportunities for anatomical study and review. When we need to see what is going on beneath the skin, it is to the radiology department that we usually turn. Moreover, the internal structures are visualized in life, when the anatomy of the heart, brain, intestines, and other organs differs radically from post-mortem morphology.

Radiology opens up some of the most striking vistas in all of medicine, making visible not only normal anatomy but pathologic anatomy and even pathophysiology. Through its images, radiology enables students to visualize the biological signatures of disease processes in tissues and organs. It illustrates for the imagination and anchors in the visual memory difficult anatomic and pathophysiological concepts. These can be correlated with patients' histories, physical examination findings, and laboratory results to produce a richer, more accurate picture of health and disease.

Radiology also has a crucial integrative role to play in contemporary medical education. As medicine has become more and more specialized, the educational experiences of medical students and residents have tended to become increasingly fragmented. Radiology is a natural integrator in part because no other medical specialty regularly interacts with a wider range of clinical disciplines than radiology. It is not uncommon for multiple specialists to gather around radiological images to plan patient management.

What medicine's students need most is not a greater number of trees with which to populate their educational forest. What they need above all is an opportunity to step back and see the forest as a whole. Radiology's integrative role enables it to provide learners with a comprehensive overview of how the various pieces of the puzzle of contemporary medical practice fit together. It often enjoys a more encompassing view of these domains than any other department in the hospital.

The ubiquity of radiology's role in contemporary medical practice is reflected in the 400 million radiological examinations performed each year in the United States, a number that exceeds the nation's population. It is difficult to imagine the practice of neurology, neurosurgery, otolaryngology, cardiology, pulmonology, gastroenterology, orthopedic surgery, urology, obstetrics and gynecology, and a host of other pediatric and adult specialties without the input of radiology. Radiology has become the department that provides answers to some of medicine's most vital questions: Is my patient sick? What is the diagnosis? How extensive is the injury or disease? What are the treatment options? Is the patient responding to treatment? Has the disease recurred? And so on.

Thanks to cross-sectional imaging, it is much less common for emergency department patients to be admitted to the hospital for observation, to see how their conditions evolve. Many patients can be sent home sooner, lowering hospitalization rates, hospital-related morbidity, and healthcare costs. Exploratory laparotomies have become largely a relic of the past. It is now rare that we need to operate on patients to find out whether they really need surgery. In many medical centers, it is becoming common for cross-sectional imaging to be ordered before consulting specialists even see the patient, because imaging plays so pivotal a role in clinical decision making.

The purpose of providing first-rate radiology education to all medical students is not to lure them into radiological careers, but to prepare them to make effective use of radiology in the care of their patients. In this day and age, it is impossible to excel as a clinician without thoroughly understanding radiology's role.

Medical student and resident education should focus on several key missions. First, our graduates need to understand what imaging tests to order in key clinical situations. What is the role of plain skull radiographs in head trauma? What imaging examination is most appropriate in patients who present with an acute abdomen? When should intravenous contrast material be administered? Failing to order the appropriate imaging test, or ordering the wrong one, can jeopardize patients.

Students and residents also need to develop basic image interpretation skills. It is both embarrassing to us and hazardous to patients if we are not able to recognize such common and urgent imaging findings as a malpositioned endotracheal tube, pneumothorax, pneumoperitoneum, hip fracture, and subarachnoid hemorrhage. How can any of our medical schools presume to be doing a good job of educating the next generation of physicians if learners cannot recognize at least readily apparent examples of such abnormalities?

Radiology also demonstrates great promise as a forum in which to educate learners in basic principles of medical reasoning. Consider the example of disease screening. In detecting early breast and lung cancers, what is the sensitivity, specificity, and accuracy of common imaging techniques? What is the effect on false positive rates of the pretest probability of disease, including the presence or absence of risk factors? What are the costs of screening examinations, and how can we weigh them against the benefits? In other words, what sorts of considerations enter into a comprehensive assessment of the effectiveness and efficiency of a screening regimen? These are educationally important questions that radiology is especially well situated to address.

Radiology can also help future physicians become more effective communicators. When a referring physician orders an imaging study, what sort of clinical information should be provided? What information is relevant in helping the radiologist determine what study to perform, how to perform it, and how to interpret it? What sort of report should the referring physician expect to receive, and how should that information be implemented in patient management? By seeing what can go wrong when communication is poor and the many advantages that flow from effective communication, we can better prepare ourselves to excel as physicians.

Finally, radiology occupies a position of honor in the history of medicine. At the turn of the 21st century, Victor Fuchs of Stanford University and Harold Sox of Dartmouth University conducted a survey of 225 senior US general internists, asking them to rank the most important innovations in medicine during their career. In a field that included ACE inhibitors, balloon angioplasty, statins, mammography, coronary artery bypassing grafting, H2 blockers, new types of antidepressants, cataract extraction and lens implantation, and hip and knee replacement, the most highly rated innovations were, by a substantial margin, CT and MRI. No innovations in the lifetimes of our students have more transformed the practice of medicine than cross-sectional imaging. In an even broader historical context, x-ray imaging is invariably ranked among the most important innovations in the history of modern medicine.

In spite of these and other arguments for integrating radiology into our curricula, many medical school and residency programs need to improve the quality of radiology education we provide. In many cases, radiology plays little or no role in the formal curriculum. In some programs, even elective opportunities in radiology are scarce or non-existent.

This book is intended to answer this challenge, by providing a comprehensive overview of radiology and its role in contemporary medicine, one that can work effectively for independent study or as a textbook in a required course. The goal is not to produce radiologists, but to provide future physicians with a basic understanding of the imaging modalities, characteristic imaging findings of illustrative disease processes, and strategies for making optimal use of radiology in caring for patients.

To achieve these purposes, it is not necessary to cover every disease process or to provide countless examples of every imaging technique. Instead it is sufficient to focus on the underlying principles of diagnostic imaging, and to situate those principles in the larger context of patients' clinical presentations and the pathophysiologies of their disorders.Only if we study radiology in this larger medical context will we truly understand how to make effective use of radiology in caring for our patients.

Acknowledgments

If this book provides students a richer and more comprehensive understanding of radiology, it is largely because its author worked from a perch on the shoulders of giants. I would like to thank my former colleagues at the University of Chicago. Ruth Ramsey, M.D., suggested the first edition of this book. Arunas Gasparaitis, M.D., contributed many of the gastrointestinal images retained in this second edition. Thanks also to my other teachers at Chicago, especially John Fennessy, M.D., who first taught me this craft, and who supported me in the development of new radiology courses for medical students during my training there.

Upon my arrival at Indiana University, I was fortunate to step into a thriving medical student education program, thanks in large measure to the efforts of Stan Alexander, M.D., Ruth Patterson, and Aslam Siddiqui, M.D.. I am grateful for the School of Medicine's continuing strong support of this program, under the leadership of Deans Robert Holden, M.D. and Craig Brater, M.D. I owe an immense debt to two individuals who have served as Chair of the Department of Radiology during my tenure at Indiana, Drs. Mervyn Cohen and Valerie Jackson, whose unwavering support for educational excellence helped to make this project possible.

Most of the images for this second edition were gleaned from the Department of Radiology's digital teaching file at Indiana, which runs on Edactic software created by Mark Frank, M.D. I drew many of the images from the digital collections of current and former colleagues including Drs. Stan Alexander, Donald Hawes, Kenyon Kopecky, Vince Matthews, and Robert Tarver, as well as other faculty members, residents, and fellows too numerous to mention. I am indebted to the authors of several other Thieme radiology texts, from which additional images have been borrowed.

I want to thank my colleagues in pediatric radiology at Riley Hospital for Children, Drs. Kimberly Applegate, Mervyn Cohen, Donald Corea, Mary Edwards-Brown, Boaz Karmazyn, Eugene Klatte, Francis Marshalleck, and Aslam Siddiqui, whose clinical acumen and dedication have been very helpful. Special thanks are due to our wonderful administrative assistants, Ruth Patterson and Rhonda Gerding, who cheerfully devoted many hours to the preparation of this manuscript.

Several programs have fostered my professional development as an educator, including a two-year General Electric-Association of University Radiologists Radiology Research Academic Fellowship, as well as a two-year award from the Radiological Society of North America's Educational Scholar Program. These helped to support my studies in Public Health at Indiana's School of Medicine, where I first enjoyed an opportunity to explore medical education from a professional educator's point of view.

The text itself would have lacked in both need and quality were it not for my ongoing opportunity to help educate the next generation of physicians at Indiana University, whose School of Medicine and Diagnostic Radiology Residency Program rank among the largest in the United States. I am very grateful to our wonderful medical students and residents for all they have taught me, as well as their enthusiasm for learning.

Finally, I would like to express my deepest appreciation to my wife, Laura, and our three children, Rebecca, Peter, and David, whose patience and encouragement made this book possible, and in whose love life itself is such a joy.

1

Introduction to Radiology

◆ History

The foundations of the medical specialty of radiology were laid when German physics professor Wilhelm Roentgen presented his preliminary report, "On a New Kind of Rays," to the secretary of the Wurzburg Physico-Medical Society in Germany on December 28, 1895, announcing the discovery of x-rays, for which he would later receive the first Nobel Prize in physics. Within weeks, newspapers around the world trumpeted the story of his "marvelous triumph of science," noting that Roentgen was "already using his discovery to photograph broken limbs and bullets in human bodies." A new age was dawning, in which humans would for the first time peer into the hidden reaches of the body without the use of a scalpel (**Fig. 1–1**).

Roentgen had achieved his great discovery 7 weeks earlier, late on the afternoon of November 8, 1895. While experimenting with cathode ray tubes in his darkened laboratory, Roentgen discovered quite by accident that its discharges produced shimmers of light on a nearby fluorescent screen. Repeating the experiment multiple times, he proved to himself that the emissions were invisible to his own eyes, yet able to penetrate the walls of the cardboard box in which the tube was enclosed. After investigating the phenomenon further, he concluded that only one explanation was possible: the cathode ray tube was producing a new kind of ray.

Roentgen's discovery was so revolutionary that, rather than accept that the great physicists of the day had repeatedly failed to detect such a momentous new phenomenon throughout 10 years of experimentation with cathode rays, Lord Kelvin initially speculated that x-rays were a hoax. Yet the phenomenon was undeniable. The Prussian Academy of Sciences later wrote to Roentgen: "Probably never has a new truth from the quiet laboratory of a scientist made triumphal progress so quickly and universally as has your epoch-making discovery of those wonderful rays." In the history of medicine, only the microscope could boast of a comparable technological contribution to medical vision.

Roentgen himself was a remarkable man (**Fig. 1–2**). Although he lived another 27 years after his discovery, which he made at age 50, he declined nearly all of the great honors and invitations to speak accorded him, and donated the entire sum of his Nobel Prize money (50,000 Swedish kroner) to the University of Wurzburg, to be used for scientific research. He resisted all suggestions that he profit by his discovery, saying, "I am of the opinion that . . . discoveries and inventions belong to humanity," thereby establishing a tradition of altruism that continues among radiologists to the present day. Sadly, despite his extraordinary eminence, Roentgen's last years were difficult. Shortly after the death of his wife following a long and painful illness, Roentgen's personal property was consumed by postwar inflation. He died in 1923.

Along with microscopy, epidemiology, inhalation anesthesia, asepsis, antibiotics, and deoxyribonucleic acid (DNA), x-rays constituted one of the half dozen greatest discoveries in the history of modern medicine. Over the course of the

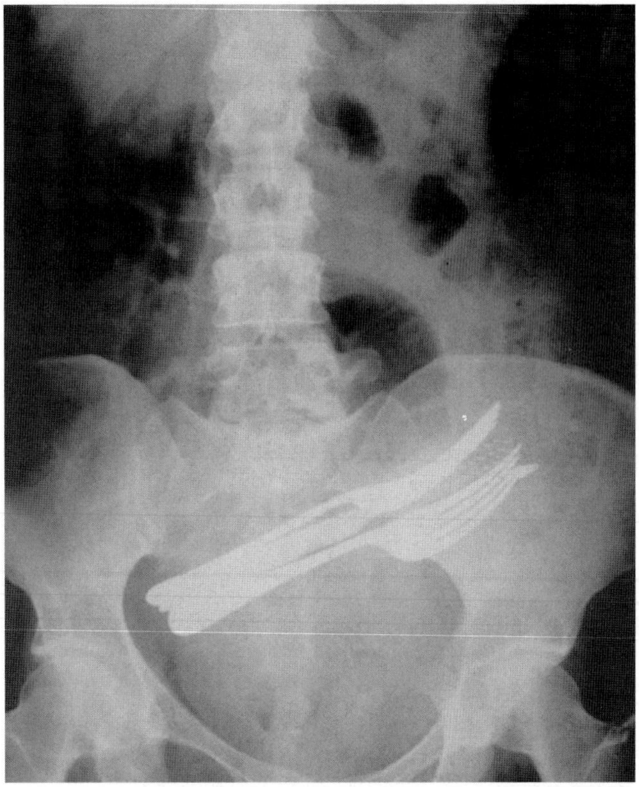

Figure 1–1 What is wrong with this picture? This plain radiograph of the abdomen demonstrates four metallic or partly metallic foreign bodies superimposed over the patient's pelvis. Can you identify them? Two are forks. One is a plastic hairbrush, the bristles of which are radiopaque (block x-rays sufficiently to be visible on radiographs). The last is a plastic pen, of which only the metal tip is radiopaque. Because they could be in front of or behind the patient, a lateral radiograph was obtained to prove that they were in fact inside the patient—in this case, in the gastrointestinal tract.

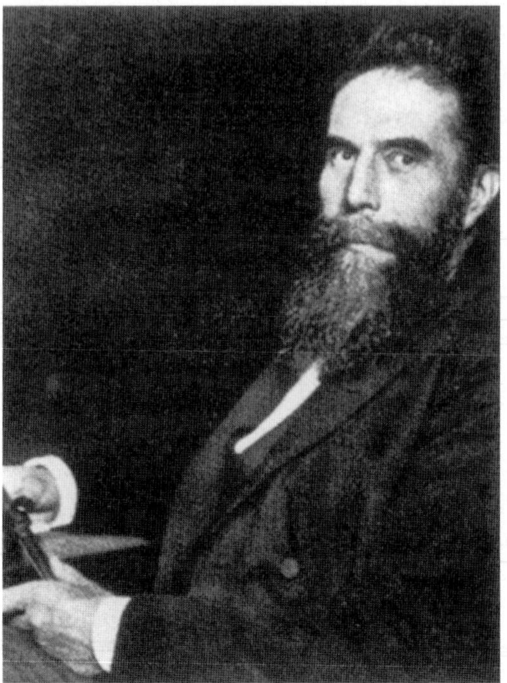

Figure 1–2 Wilhelm Roentgen.

20th century, the medical specialty of radiology was born, and to Roentgen's plain x-ray were added other modalities such as fluoroscopy, contrast studies of the gastrointestinal (GI) tract and blood vessels, nuclear medicine, ultrasound, computed tomography, and magnetic resonance imaging. Because the discovery of x-rays was the work of a physicist, it is fitting that a discussion of medical imaging should begin with a discussion of imaging physics.

◆ Visual Characteristics of Images

Contrast and Detail

From a physical point of view, an image exhibits two crucial characteristics, contrast and detail. The level of contrast between a structure and its background must be at least several percent if it is to be detected by the human eye. Through image postprocessing, rendered possible by computed radiography and digital radiography, it is often possible to adjust and optimize the level of contrast in an image and to perform such manipulations as edge enhancement. The maximum detail detectable by the unaided human eye is ~10 line pairs per millimeter. Each radiologic modality has a characteristic range of detail or spatial resolution. In decreasing order, they are plain radiography, fluoroscopy, computed tomography (CT), magnetic resonance imaging (MRI), ultrasound, and nuclear medicine (**Fig. 1–3**). Under ideal conditions, the detail captured by plain radiography is so high that magnification enhances detail, as in the detection of microcalcifications in mammography.

Noise

The term *noise* refers to a variety of factors that detract from the information contained in an image. Some amount of noise is inherent in every modality, but additional noise may be added by the techniques used to generate or view the image. For example, ambient light in the viewing room decreases the signal-to-noise ratio; when the overhead lights in the viewing room are turned on, many of the photons striking the observer's retina no longer carry diagnostic information. In contrast, when the overhead lights are dimmed and the only source of light is a computer monitor or the viewbox on which a film is mounted, the signal-to-noise ratio is maximized. Radiologists work in darkened rooms not because they fear the sun, but because they are attempting to maximize the signal-to-noise ratio.

◆ Three Modes of Image Production

There are three basic means by which radiologic images are produced: transmission of energy, reflection of energy, and emission of energy.

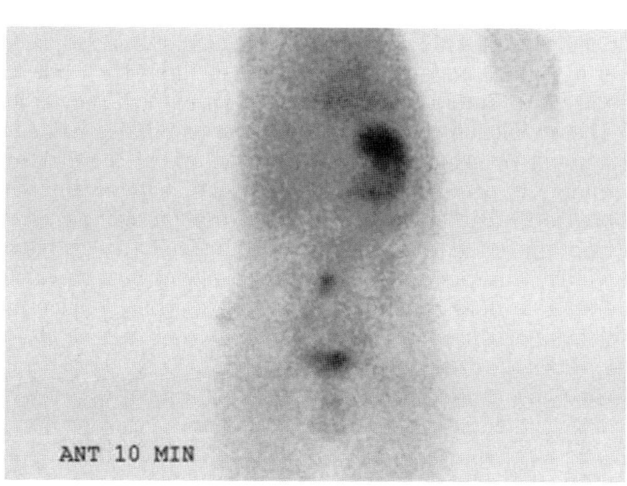

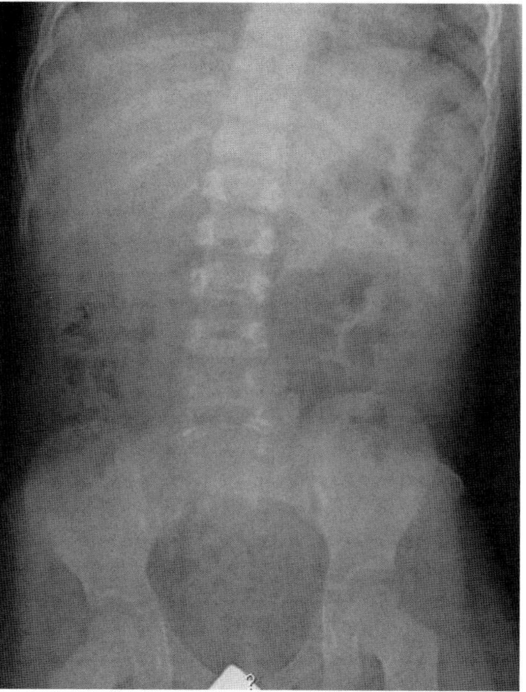

Figure 1–3 **(A)** This child presented with unexplained hematochezia—blood in the stool. An image from a nuclear medicine technetium (Tc) 99m pertechnetate scan demonstrates an abnormal focus of radiotracer uptake in the midabdomen, representing a Meckel's diverticulum. The anatomic detail and spatial resolution of this study are relatively poor, but its functional imaging capability reveals a diagnosis that had eluded endoscopists, who cannot visualize much of the small bowel. The radiotracer is taken up by gastric mucosa, which is often found in Meckel's diverticula. **(B)** A plain abdominal radiograph, by contrast, provides much better spatial resolution but does not reveal the diagnosis.

Transmission Imaging

The so-called x-ray or radiograph is produced by the transmission of energy. A beam of high-energy photons is passed through the body, some of which are attenuated or blocked when they strike subatomic particles. The higher the atomic weight of the substance through which the photons are passing, the "denser" it appears to photons, and the more likely they are to be blocked, or attenuated. In decreasing order of density, the principal densities visible in a radiograph are metal, bone, water (including soft tissues such as muscle), fat, and air (**Fig. 1–4**). Of course, even though muscle is denser than fat, the x-ray beam would be more attenuated by passing through a meter of fat than a centimeter of muscle. Both density and thickness, then, are factors to take into account in assessing the degree of opacification noted on a radiograph (**Fig. 1–5**). Radiographs were initially referred to as "skiagraphs," from the Greek for "shadow pictures," because they represent recordings of the shadows cast by anatomic structures as photons pass through the body.

The principal transmission modalities include plain radiography, such as chest radiographs and abdominal radiographs, fluoroscopy, and CT. Plain radiography may be conceptualized as a snapshot: it provides a static view of anatomic structure obtained in a fraction of a second. Fluoroscopy represents a kind of "movie," or moving picture, in which continuous detection and display of the pattern of photon transmission enables the visualization of dynamic processes in real time (**Fig. 1–6**). CT gathers transmission data from multiple perspectives and employs a mathematical algorithm (the Fourier transform) to reconstruct an image of the slice of tissue through which the x-ray beams passed (**Fig. 1–7**). The multidetector CT scanners being manufactured now make it possible to acquire multiple "slices" at once in a continuous fashion. In each case, the contrast in the image is a reflection of the attenuation of the x-ray beam by the tissues through which it passes.

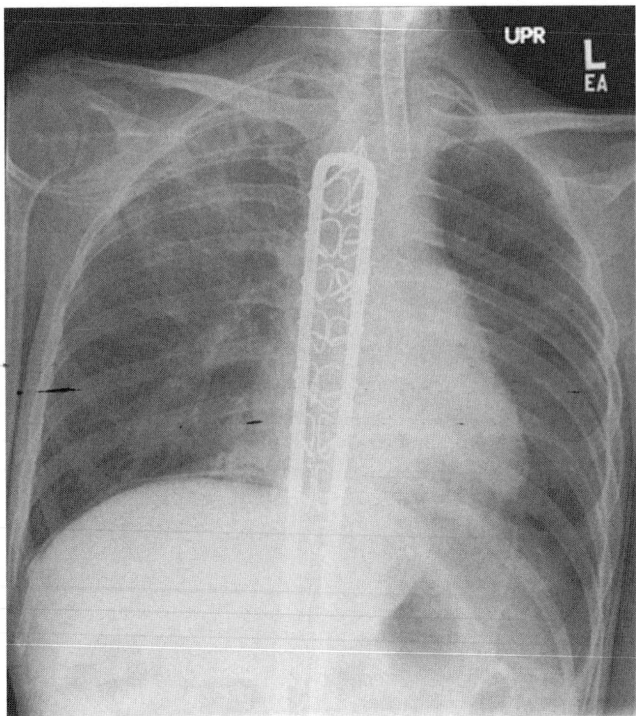

Figure 1–4 This young man suffers from advanced Duchenne's muscular dystrophy. This chest radiograph shows numerous different densities. Overlying the spine are metallic wires and rods that were placed to correct scoliosis (curvature of the spine). Note that the patient's tracheostomy tube is radiopaque, which enables its position to be confirmed with radiographs. Many medical appliances are made to be radiopaque for this reason. Note that the patient is virtually devoid of skeletal musculature. There are pulmonary opacities in the right upper lobe and both lung bases, likely reflecting atelectasis or aspiration. The most urgent diagnostic finding is a crescent of lucency underneath the right hemidiaphragm, indicating pneumoperitoneum. This suggests a perforated abdominal viscus and may represent a surgical emergency.

Throughout most of radiology's history, detection and display of photon shadows were combined in a single step: the film. As radiology makes the transition to the digital age, these two functions can be separated, permitting the optimization of each. Computer monitors are replacing radiographs and lightboxes as the preferred way to view images. Using picture archiving and communication systems (PACS), images are acquired, stored, and retrieved electronically, making images available anytime and anywhere. The display function can be further subdivided into image production and image processing. For example, when a CT examination is performed, the initial data acquired bear no resemblance whatsoever to a medical image. The image acquired with CT results from the ability of a powerful computer to perform countless computations necessary to assemble the data into a CT image. Once an image is produced, however, further processing is possible to optimize desired image characteristics, such as the contrast between soft tissue structures. This accounts for the difference between so-called soft tissue windows, bone windows, and lung windows on a chest CT examination. Through postimaging processing, it is also possible to "reconstruct" the data acquired in one plane (in CT, generally the axial plane) in other planes (e.g., the coronal or sagittal planes) (**Fig. 1–8**).

Penetrating Light

X-rays are a form of electromagnetic radiation (**Fig. 1–9**). In medicine, they are produced when electrons boiled off from a tungsten cathode filament are accelerated by a potential difference into a tungsten anode, with which they collide. These collisions result in the production of a considerable amount of heat, but a small percentage of the electronic energy is converted into x-ray radiation (generally ~1%). Hence, the cathode functions in electron production, and the rotating anode functions in converting electron energy into x-rays. The anode rotates to spread out the heat production over its surface, so that it is less likely to melt. The quantity of x-rays produced is proportional to the current flowing through the cathode (in milliamperes, mA), and the energy of the x-rays produced is proportional to the kinetic energy with which the electrons strike the anode (in kilovolts, kV, potential) (**Fig. 1–10**).

What enables the x-ray to penetrate the entire human body? The answer lies in the fact that the photon, which can be thought of as a mobile electromagnetic field with no mass and no charge, is incredibly small. Moreover, the atoms of which we are composed are, relatively speaking, incredibly

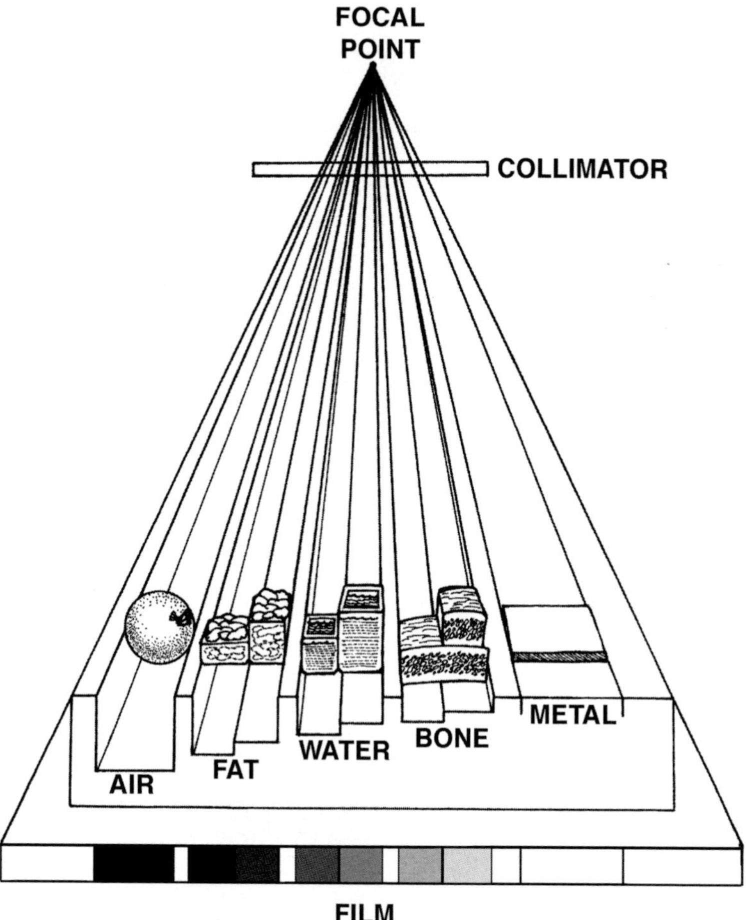

Figure 1–5 The effects of density and thickness on the exposure of x-ray film, using commonly imaged substances. Note that air blocks virtually none of the beam, whereas metal blocks virtually all of it.

big and have an incredibly low density, meaning that their volume is almost entirely composed of "empty space." For example, the diameter of an atom is about one million times the diameter of its nucleus, where almost all of its mass is found. If the nucleus were 1 mm in diameter, the atom would be 1000 m wide, or about the length of 10 football fields. Hence, the chance that a photon would strike any particular atom in the body is very low. Even so, only about 1 in 100 photons in a medical x-ray actually passes completely through the patient and strikes the detector (**Fig. 1–11**).

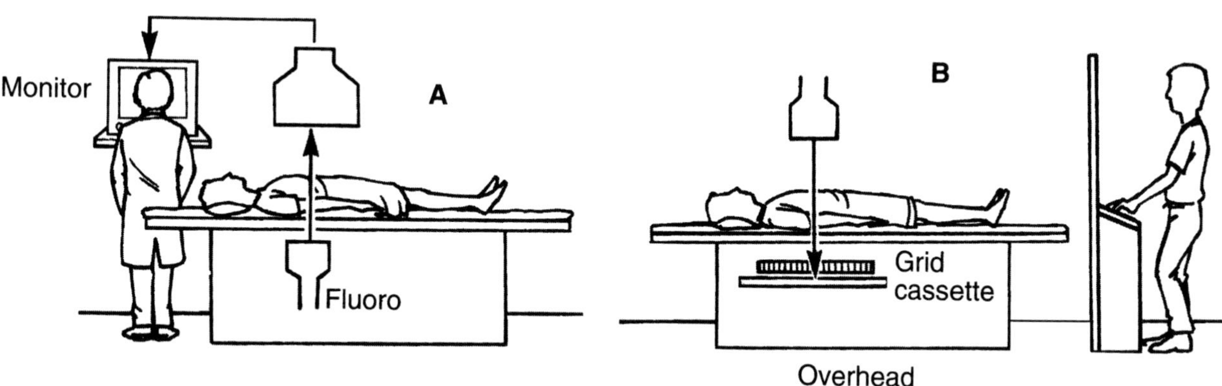

Figure 1–6 The contrast between **(A)** fluoroscopy and **(B)** plain radiography. In fluoroscopy, the x-ray tube sends x-rays up through the patient from below, where the transmitted photons are captured by an image intensifier and projected onto a television screen in real time. In plain radiography, in contrast, the beam passes from the tube above through the patient and exposes the film or detector below. In **(B)**, the exposure cannot be obtained at a precise moment based on the position of contrast material because its position is not known.

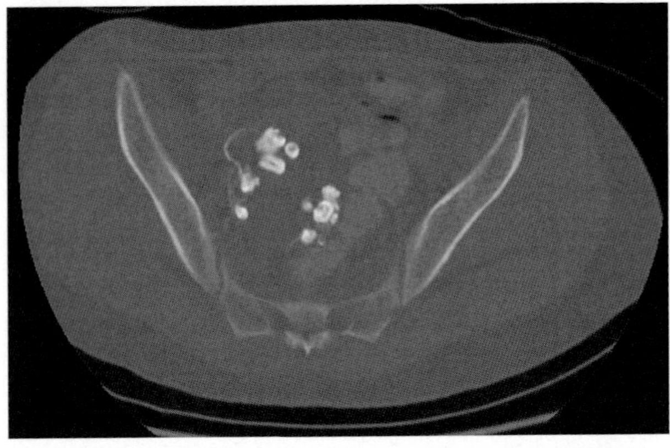

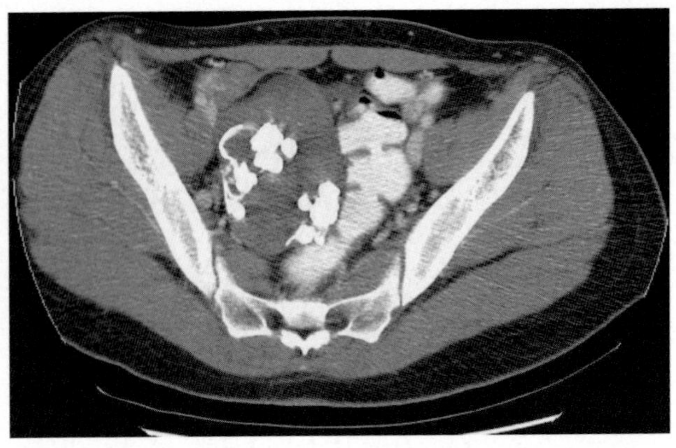

Figure 1–7 This young woman presented with a 2-week history of right lower quadrant pain. **(A)** This "bone window" image of the pelvis, so called because it optimizes visualization of dense structures while sacrificing soft tissue detail, demonstrates multiple toothlike calcifications in a right adnexal mass. **(B)** This "soft tissue" window image demonstrates that the lesion also contains muscle-density and fat-density tissue. This appearance is characteristic of an ovarian dermoid cyst (containing both ectodermal and mesodermal tissues) or teratoma (containing ectoderm, mesoderm, and endoderm).

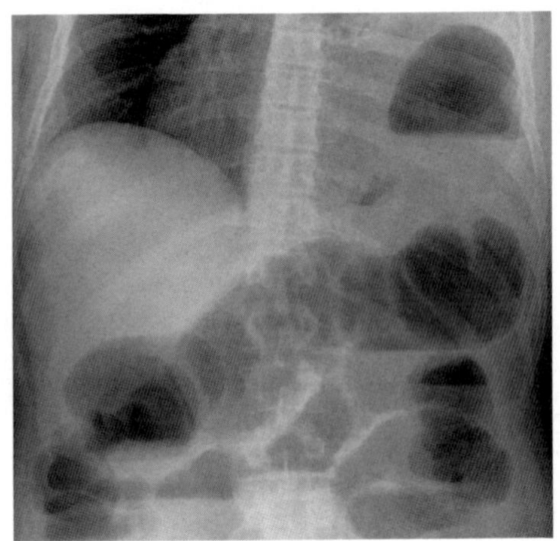

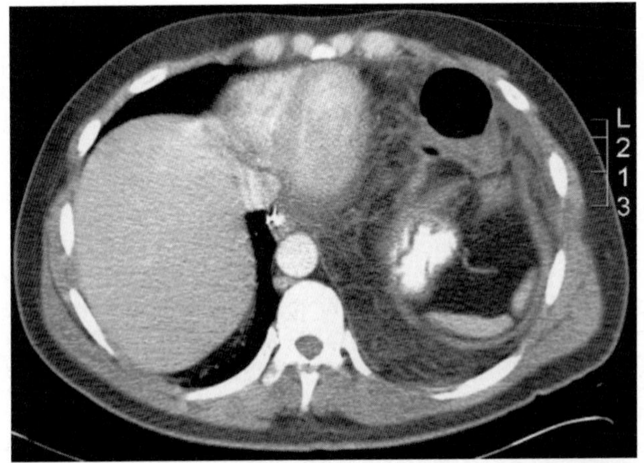

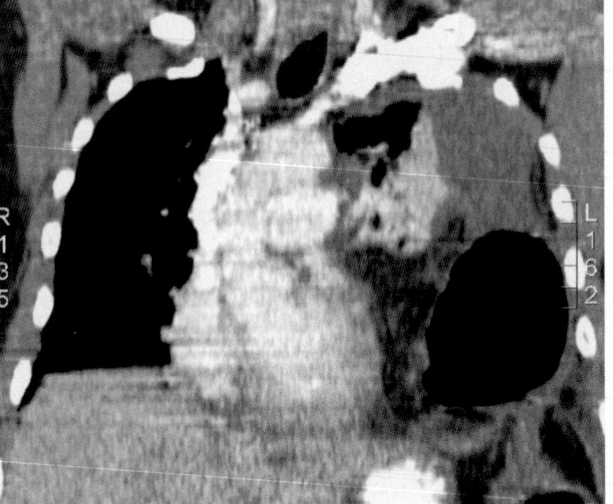

Figure 1–8 This young man presented with abdominal pain years after being stabbed. **(A)** The upright radiograph of the upper abdomen demonstrates an air–fluid level containing mass in the left lower thorax. **(B)** An axial CT image of the lower thorax demonstrates air-containing bowel, the contrast-containing stomach, and abdominal fat at the level of the heart, where the left lung base should be. **(C)** A coronal reconstruction of the axially acquired data shows the splenic flexure of the colon herniating through a diaphragmatic defect. This was a post-traumatic diaphragmatic hernia.

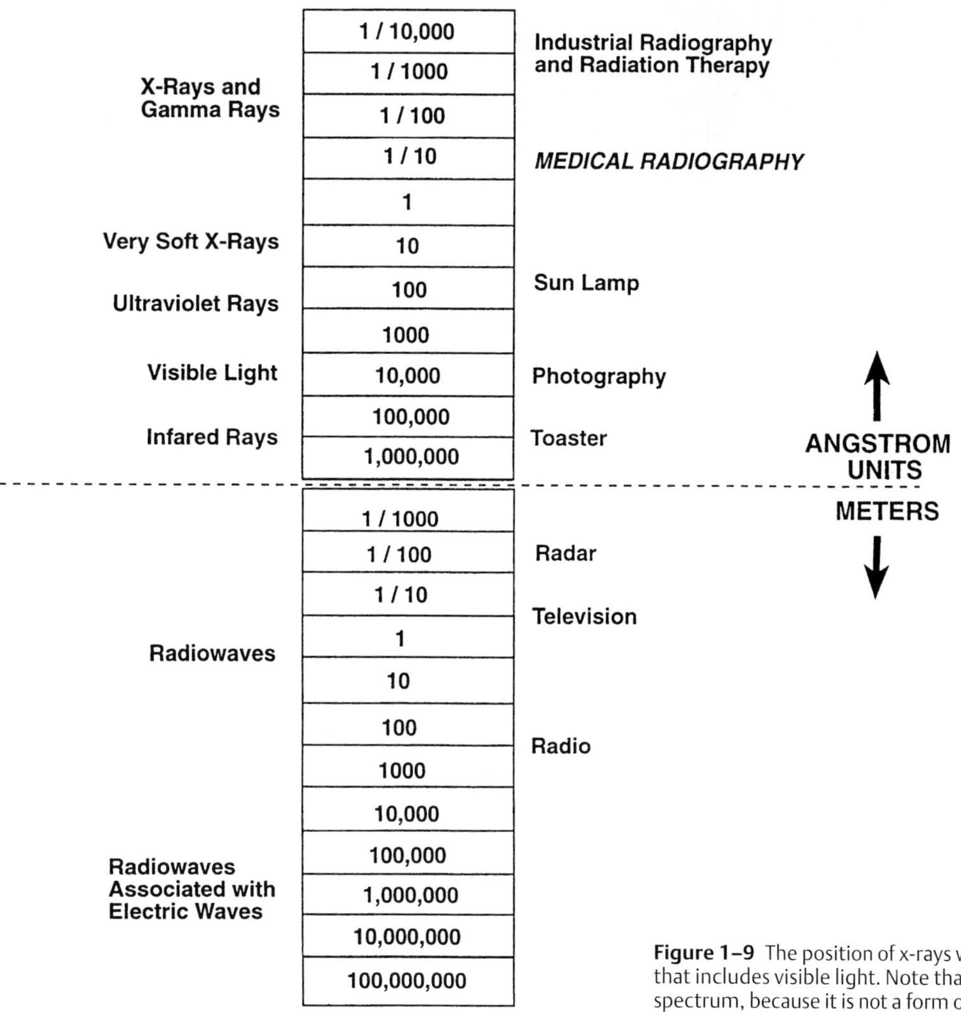

Figure 1–9 The position of x-rays within the electromagnetic spectrum that includes visible light. Note that ultrasound does not appear on this spectrum, because it is not a form of electromagnetic radiation.

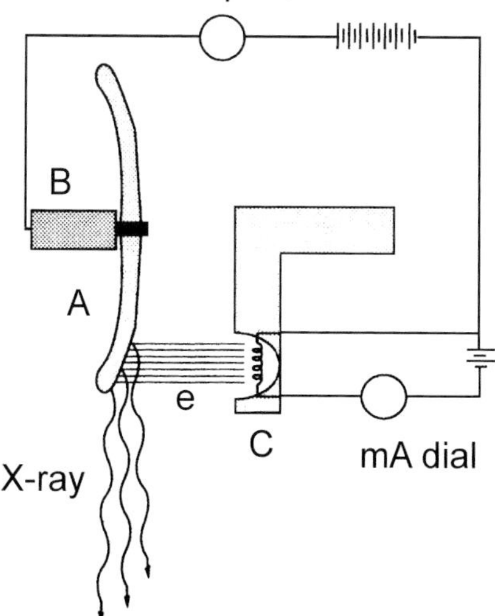

Figure 1–10 X-ray tube. **(A)** Rotating anode. **(B)** Rotor. **(C)** Cathode filament. "Boiled off" electrons (e) are accelerated in a vacuum and collide with the anode, producing x-rays.

As photons pass through the patient, they may be scattered. In the case of a scattered photon, the place on the detector that is exposed does not correspond to the location of an anatomic structure in the patient. Hence scattered photons degrade the signal-to-noise ratio. Grids are commonly employed to screen out scattered photons, which emerge at an angle, although at the cost of some increase in patient radiation exposure (**Fig. 1–12**).

Hazards of Ionizing Radiation

Each of the transmission imaging modalities utilizes x-rays, and therefore subjects the patient to ionizing radiation. Ionizing radiation refers to electromagnetic emissions of sufficient energy that, when they strike molecules in the human body such as hydrocarbons, they may disrupt their structure. They do so by colliding with atoms and causing the removal of one of their electrons, which causes the atom to become positively charged and highly reactive. Because most of the human body is water,

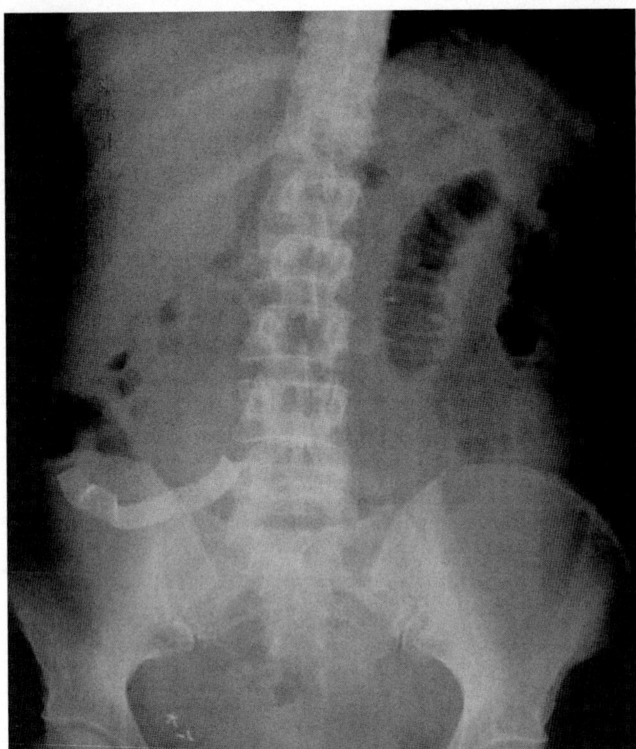

Figure 1–11 This woman suffered unexplained fevers after pelvic surgery. Note the surgical clips in the right side of the pelvis. What is the etiology of her fevers? The answer is probably a retained surgical sponge, to which is sewn a radiopaque marker, visible over the right ilium. Because surgical applicances that are not naturally radiopaque are so marked, it is possible to check for their presence by simply taking a radiograph, rather than reexploring the patient surgically.

most of the photons absorbed ionize water, resulting in the formation of highly reactive free radical molecules, which may in turn react chemically with such molecules as DNA and proteins, damaging them. Every person receives a daily dose of ionizing radiation from cosmic sources (e.g., the sun) and radioisotopes in both the environment (e.g., radon) and the body itself (e.g., potassium 40 and carbon 14) (**Fig. 1–13**). Happily, sophisticated protective and reparative physiologic systems are in place that are capable of softening the blow; however, these repair mechanisms are not 100% effective.

The hazards of ionizing radiation were recognized soon after the discovery of the x-ray by Roentgen in 1895. A famous example is that of Antoine-Henri Becquerel, the professor of eventual two-time Nobel laureate Marie Curie, one of the discoverers (along with her husband, Pierre) of radium. In 1902, Marie Curie had painstakingly extracted a tenth of a gram of the new metal from large quantities of pitchblend, in which it was contained at a concentration of one part per million. The professor was so proud of his pupil's discovery that he carried a vial containing the first sample of radium ever produced in his vest pocket. Soon he noticed that he had developed a severe burn on the skin of his abdomen underneath the vial. The causative role of the radium in the production of the burn was verified when other researchers intentionally taped pieces of the new metal to their skin, producing similar burns. Experiments on animals by the Curies and others led to the development of therapeutic uses of radium emissions, known at the time as Curie therapy. That the same invisible rays used to diagnose diseases such as cancer could also both cause and cure the disease astonished early x-ray researchers.

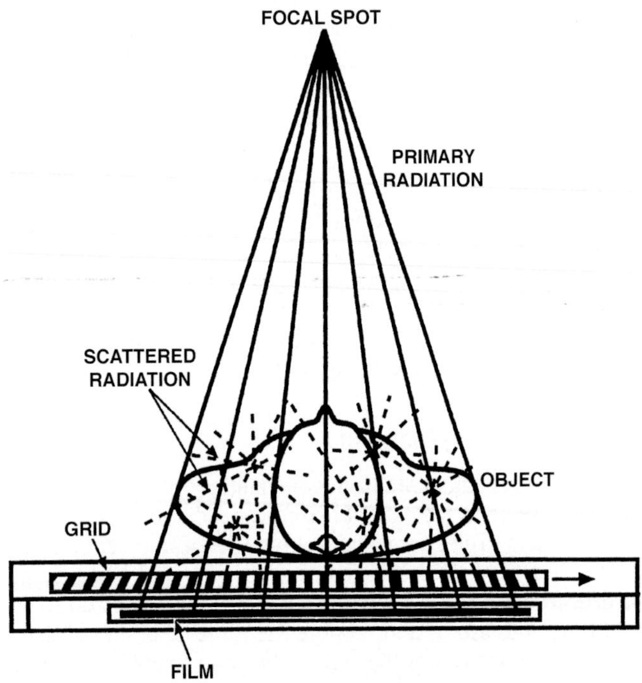

Figure 1–12 Illustration of how grids help to prevent radiation scattered within the patient from reaching the x-ray film and degrading the signal-to-noise ratio.

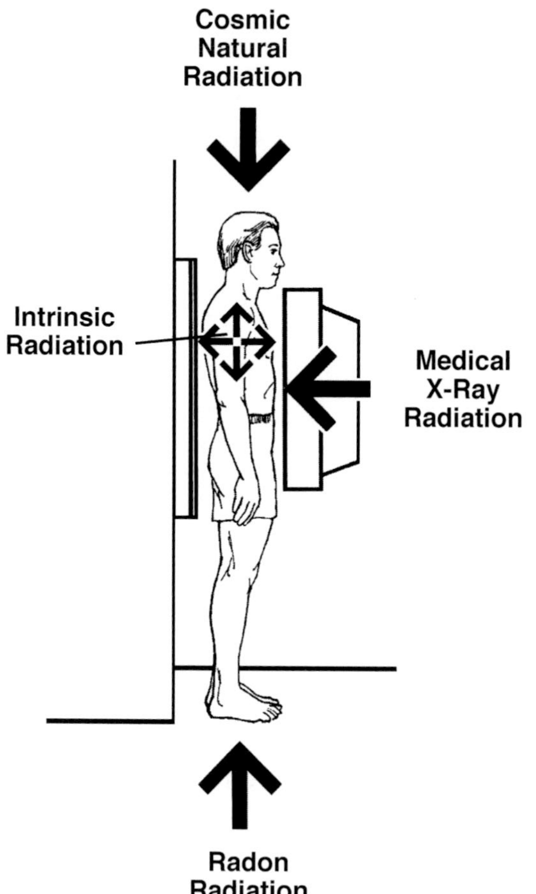

Figure 1–13 The common sources of background radiation, as well as the contribution of medical x-rays.

Thanks in part to the lessons learned from such early experiences, the risks of contemporary radiological techniques are extremely low. They are so low, in fact, that an investigation to quantify them precisely would require intervention and control groups numbering in the millions and followed for decades. Hence, estimates of risk are typically based on extrapolations from data on survivors of atomic bombs. For example, based on such data, it is estimated that the lifetime risk of breast cancer from a single mammogram in a woman in her 50s is less than one in a million. By contrast, the risk of death from spontaneous breast cancer is at least 1000 times that great. Against the small theoretical risks of ionizing radiation must be weighed the increased anxiety, length of hospital stay, morbidity, mortality, and costs of treating patients without the diagnostic benefits of x-rays. In the case of cancer, radiology makes it possible to detect lesions sooner, stage disease more accurately, direct therapy more precisely, and monitor response to therapy more closely. Moreover, radiology puts the minds of many more patients at ease by proving that they do not have cancer to begin with.

Likewise, image-guided therapy, such as percutaneous abscess drainage, provides huge benefits over open surgical laparotomy because of its minimally invasive nature. Again, many patients in whom an abscess is suspected are spared such treatment altogether when their imaging studies are negative, and those who do undergo image-guided percutaneous drainage enjoy a quicker procedure, no general anesthesia, shorter recovery time and length of stay, and dramatically reduced cost. They leave the hospital not with a long incision covered with a surgical dressing, but with a small skin nick less than a centimeter in length, covered with a Band-Aid.

Radiation Protection

A patient's exposure to ionizing radiation often can be dramatically decreased by following a few relatively simple steps. First, diagnostic examinations should be performed only when they are truly indicated. By avoiding radiography where it is unnecessary, the dose can be reduced 100%. One way of avoiding the use of x-rays where imaging is needed is to substitute another modality that does not employ ionizing radiation, such as ultrasound or magnetic resonance imaging. A second approach is to limit the dose received by the patient during the examination. By optimizing technical factors such as the x-ray source and the detector, avoiding repeat exposures due to factors such as patient motion, and reducing the duration of fluoroscopic procedures, patient doses can be lowered dramatically. These steps also reduce the radiation doses to healthcare workers, who can further reduce their exposure by using lead shielding such as lead aprons, keeping their body out of the path of the x-ray beam, and increasing the distance between themselves and the patient from whom scatter radiation emerges (**Fig. 1–14**). Because of the inverse-square law, doubling the distance between patient and health-care worker decreases the healthcare worker's dose by 75%.

Computed Tomography

The first clinical CT scanners were introduced in 1972. They drew on the work of two investigators who shared the Nobel Prize for their work in this area in 1979. The first was the South African, Allen Cormack, who devised a means of displaying the varying attenuation coefficients found in the various portions of a section of body tissue as a gray-scale image. The second was Godfrey Hounsfield, who worked in the 1960s and 1970s at Electronic Music Industries (EMI) in London, England. EMI, flush with cash thanks to the success of recording groups such as the Beatles, was able to finance Hounsfield's offbeat but pioneering work.

CT markedly increases the radiologist's sensitivity to differences in tissue contrast. Because many lesions exhibit a degree of x-ray attenuation different from that of normal tissues, even a slight increase in contrast sensitivity pays huge dividends in lesion detection. In fact, whereas plain radiography requires about a 10% difference in x-ray attenuation to detect an abnormality, CT can detect differences smaller than 0.5%.

To understand how this huge increase in contrast resolution is achieved, it is necessary to explore the differences between plain radiography and CT. The conventional x-ray beam, though in many respects virtually miraculous, exhibited several imaging shortcomings. First, the information contained in a radiograph is presented in two dimensions, such that the information contained in the depth dimension

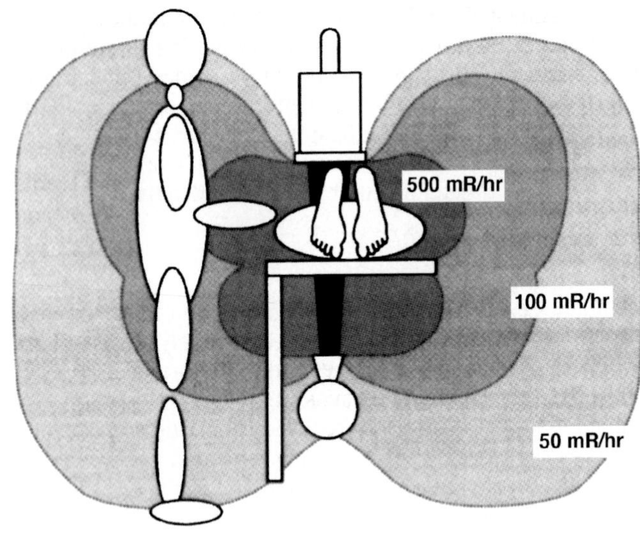

Figure 1–14 Scatter distribution during fluoroscopy. A leaded glass shield between the operator and the patient, as well as a leaded shield strategically placed at the patient's side and at the top of the table, will dramatically reduce the radiation dose to the operator.

is superimposed. Obtaining a second radiograph in the orthogonal (right-angled) projection only compensates for this to a minor degree. Second, soft tissue resolution by conventional radiography is very poor. We can distinguish to some degree between air, fat, water (or soft tissue), bone, iodinated contrast agents, and metal, but further differentiation is very difficult or impossible. Third, the conventional radiograph is unable to distinguish between the differing densities of the tissues through which the beam has passed. Once it passes through a very dense substance, conventional radiographs make the entire thickness through which a portion of the beam has passed appear quite dense, or white, regardless of the density of the tissue on either side of the dense structure.

CT, on the other hand, is able to measure and display the varying x-ray attenuations of the tissues in a section of the body by passing x-rays through the section from many different angles. It then utilizes reconstruction algorithms and the computational capacities of a computer to display the differing densities in a gray-scale image. In contemporary CT scanners, a circular array of detectors around the patient acquires data as the x-ray tube rotates around the patient (**Fig. 1–15**). Sufficient data to image a single "slice" of the body can be acquired in fractions of a second, and multiple "slices" can be obtained at once.

Hounsfield's contributions are memorialized in the Hounsfield scale, which is used to measure the x-ray attenuation values in CT scanning. Water is arbitrarily assigned a value of 0 Hounsfield units (HU), air is –1000 HU, and dense cortical bone is 1000 HU. Also known as CT numbers, the respective attenuation values of many volume units within the patient are measured and used to construct the two-dimensional image. Measurements of attenuation values can also be used to determine the density of a lesion. For example, a cystic structure with a homogenous attenuation value of 0 HU represents a simple water-filled cyst. A solid lesion with an attenuation value of –100 HU represents a fat-containing lesion such as a lipoma. In both cases, such lesions could be dismissed as benign and would not require biopsy. Furthermore, we can optimize contrast in an area of interest by altering the window width and window level settings at which the image data are displayed. Typically, the window level is set at 35 HU when examining the abdomen, above 100 when examining bone, and at –700 when examining the air-filled lungs. In each case, a window width is then selected that optimizes contrast resolution of the type of structures being examined (**Fig. 1–16**).

Reflection Imaging

The radiologic modality that exemplifies reflection imaging is ultrasound. As we shall see, ultrasound creates images not according to the density differences between various tissues, but by their acoustic differences. A very low-density structure such as fat, which appears black on a radiograph, may be very "echogenic" acoustically, and hence appear bright on a sonogram.

Ultrasound

◇ Auditory Diagnosis

The use of sound as a means of "visualization" far predated the evolution of the human species. Its most widely known example is the highly developed ultrasonic system of airborne navigation employed by bats, which enables them to maneuver with precision even in the dark. The use of sound waves as a medium of medical diagnosis extends at least back to the time of the ancient Hippocratics, who recognized the importance of the sound of air and fluid sloshing about in the thorax, which we today call the "succussion splash." The medical production of sound for diagnostic purposes began in earnest when the 18th-century German physician Leopold Auenbrugger, the son of a brewer, realized that the percussion used to assess the amount of beer remaining in barrels could also be applied to patients, with various disease processes producing characteristic percussive findings (compare the tympanitic sound of a gas-distended abdomen to the dullness to percussion of the chest overlying consolidated lung).

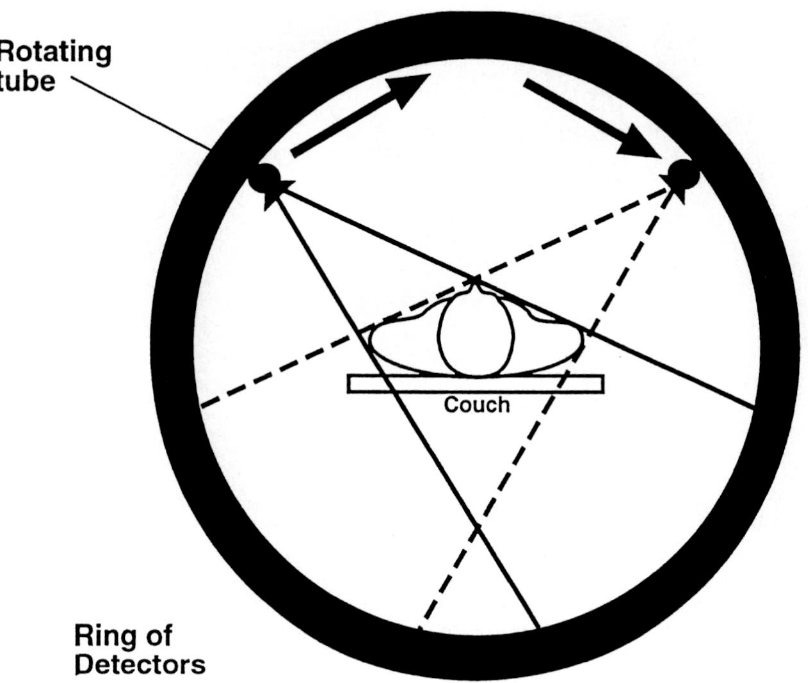

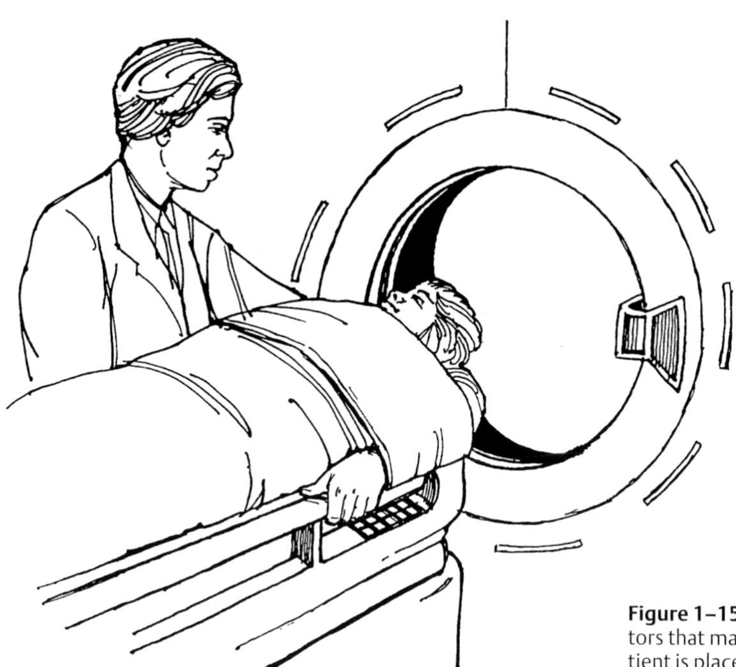

Figure 1–15 **(A)** The rotating x-ray tube and the circular array of detectors that make up a typical computed tomography scanner. **(B)** The patient is placed on a table that moves through the donut-shaped gantry as shown.

◇ Technical Developments

From a medical point of view, the use of sound as a means of visualizing human structures required a dramatic technological innovation, specifically, some means of producing sounds and receiving echoes that would permit the construction of a two- or three-dimensional picture (**Fig. 1–17**). The first crucial development occurred in the 19th century, when Pierre and Jacques Curie discovered the piezoelectric effect, by which passing an alternating electric current through certain ceramics causes them to contract and expand, producing sound waves (sound production). The process also works in reverse, meaning that sound waves striking the crystal produce electrical currents (echo detection). The transducer, the "probe" placed on or inside the patient's body during an ultrasonographic examination, contains many such piezoelectric crystals. Recall that a transducer converts energy

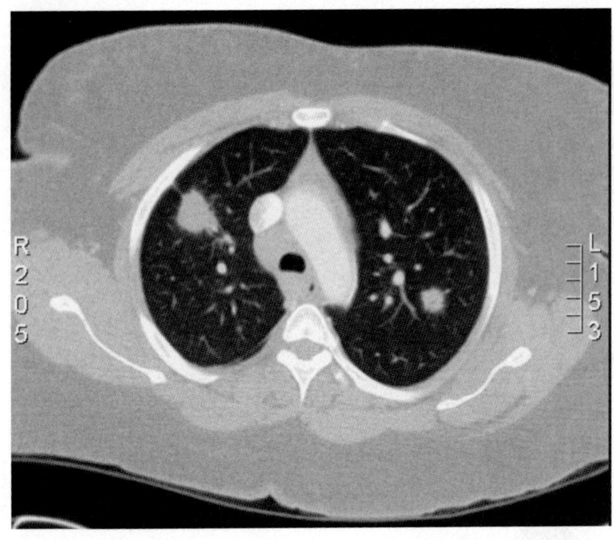

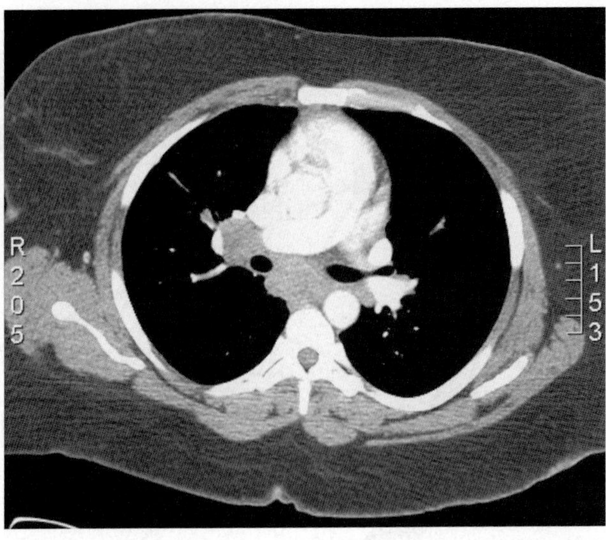

Figure 1–16 **(A)** This lung-window chest CT image beautifully demonstrates the pulmonary paranchyma but offers relatively poor visualization of the mediastinum and other soft tissues. This patient with alveolar sarcoidosis has bilateral irregular pulmonary nodules, with air bronchograms in the one on the left. **(B)** This soft tissue (mediastinal) window image shows mediastinal anatomy well but visualizes lung parenchyma poorly. Note the right hilar and subcarinal adenopathy, which does not enhance with intravenous contrast, as do the great vessels. Thus contrast helps to differentiate lymph nodes from blood vessels.

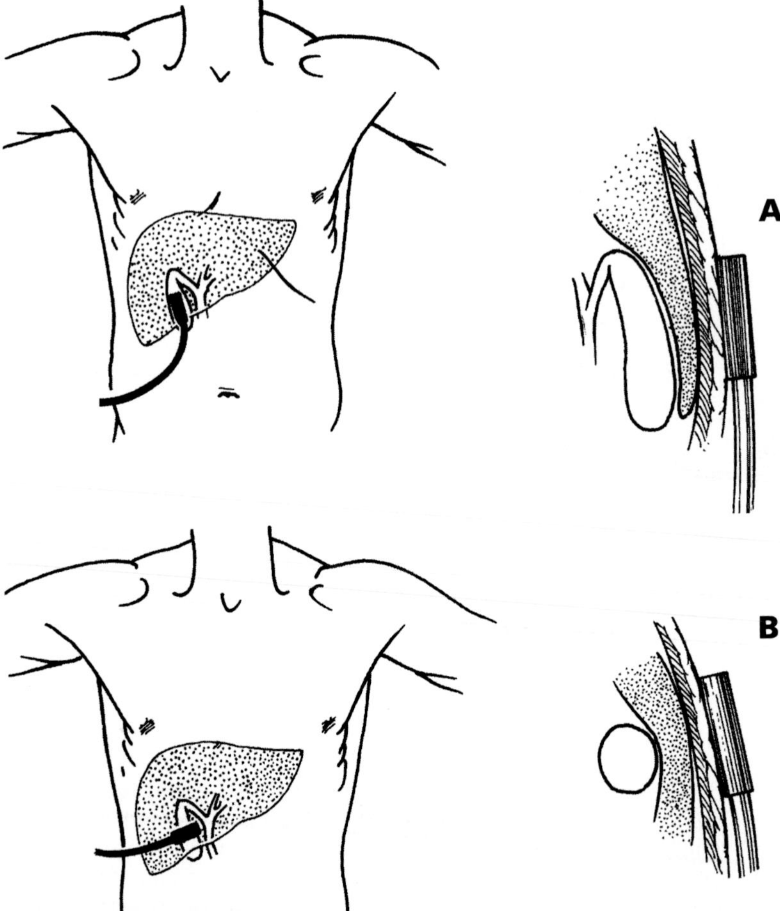

Figure 1–17 How the ultrasound probe can be positioned to obtain images of the gallbladder in both **(A)** longitudinal and **(B)** transverse planes. The orientation of the transducer can be varied with instant image feedback to determine which position provides the best images.

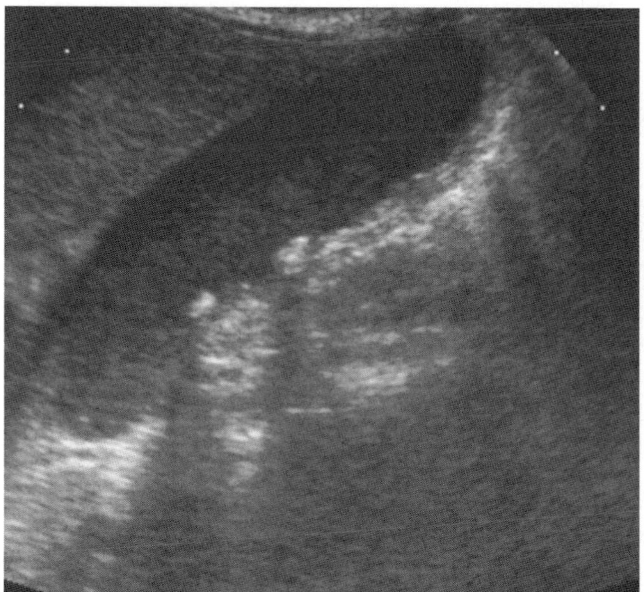

Figure 1–18 This young patient has spherocytosis, a hemolytic anemia. This longitudinal image of the gallbladder demonstrates anechoic (black-appearing) bile along the anterior portion of the gallbladder lumen. Just below it, forming a fluid–fluid level, is somewhat echogenic (gray-appearing) sludge. Within the sludge are several very echogenic (white-appearing) foci that cast acoustic shadows. These moved when the patient changed position, representing gallstones. Patients with hemolytic anemias are at increased risk for the formation of bilirubin stones, which on gross inspection tend to appear much darker than the more common cholesterol stones.

from one form to another, just as the inner ear converts mechanical energy to electrical energy.

During World War II, naval powers made extensive use of ultrasound, then known as SONAR (*so*und *na*vigation and *r*anging), to track the movements of enemy submarines. Ultrasound is widely used today in industry, where echoes help to detect a variety of flaws in materials and construction. One of the best known examples occurs in the airline industry, where tiny, imperceptible cracks in the wings of an airplane can be sonographically identified prior to catastrophic failure.

Although ultrasound now enjoys many medical applications, its most common uses include the evaluation of the structure and function of the heart via echocardiography, obstetrical ultrasound, and abdominal imaging (such as the detection of gallstones) (**Fig. 1–18**). The fact that it employs no ionizing radiation makes it especially good for imaging the pelvis of a patient who is or might be pregnant.

◇ Physics

Sound waves can be thought of as alternating bands of compression and rarefaction within the medium through which they are transmitted. A critical element in the preceding sentence is the fact that sound waves require a medium for their transmission; unlike visible light and x-rays, there is no sound in a vacuum. Because some media are denser than others, meaning that molecules are more tightly packed together, the speed of sound transmission varies by medium. Sound travels through air at a velocity of ~330 m/s, whereas sound in the soft tissues of the body travels at ~1540 m/s. Hence the distance between the ultrasound transducer and a structure within tissue can be computed by multiplying 1540 m/s by the time it takes for the sound wave to return to the transducer, then dividing by 2 (because the sound wave first travels out from and then back to the transducer).

◇ Frequency

The frequency (often called pitch) of sound is measured in hertz (Hz) or cycles per second. The range of frequencies audible to the human ear extends from ~20 to 20,000 Hz, with the greatest hearing acuity in the area of 4000 Hz, the approximate frequency of the human voice. Medical ultrasonic frequencies, by contrast, are measured in millions of hertz, or megahertz (MHz), and most equipment uses frequencies in the range of 2 to 15 MHz. The higher the frequency, the shorter the wavelength and the higher the energy of the sound.

◇ Attenuation

Fortunately, the sound beam is not transmitted with 100% efficiency through tissues. Factors that cause the beam to be attenuated include reflection, scattering, and absorption. In imaging, reflection is the critical factor, because it allows us to create images by collecting the echoes that return to the transducer. The reflections themselves result from differences in acoustic impedance between tissues (**Fig. 1–19**). In some cases, the difference in acoustic impedance between two tissues is so great that the entire ultrasound beam is reflected from their interface, rendering it impossible to image structures. Examples of such interfaces include the interface between the chest wall and the lung (air) and the interface between muscle and bone cortex. This explains why ultrasound cannot be used to image aerated lung and bone. In contrast, the difference in acoustic impedance between

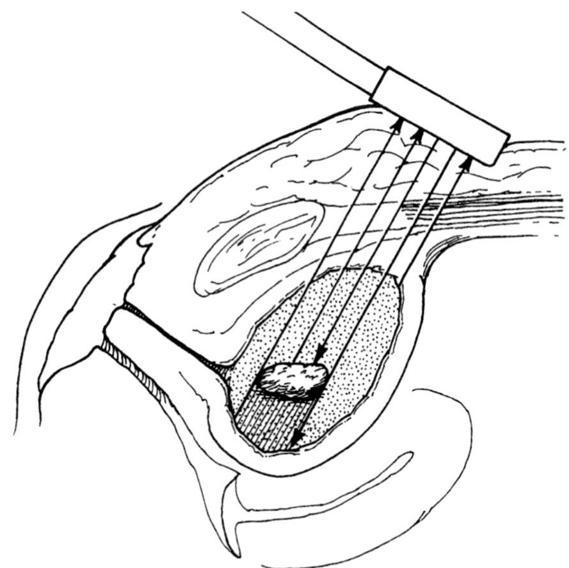

Figure 1–19 An ultrasound examination of the bladder shows how a stone within the urine-filled bladder may reflect nearly all of the beam, which would produce the appearance of a highly echogenic, shadowing interface.

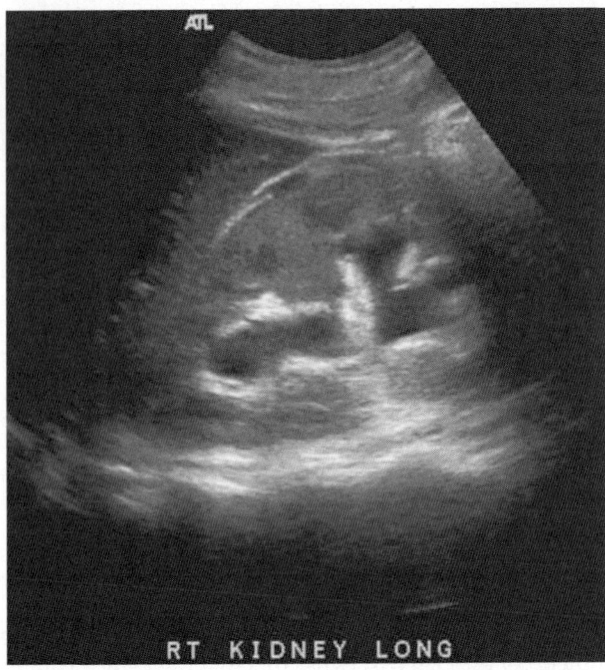

Figure 1–20 **(A)** This longitudinal ultrasound image of the right upper quadrant demonstrates the edge of the liver to the left of the image and the right kidney in the center of the image. Note that the renal collecting system is dilated with anechoic fluid, representing hydronephrosis. **(B)** A similar image on another patient demonstrates markers at the upper and lower tips of the right kidney (placed to measure its length), with the liver again anterior and cephalad to the kidney. Why is there anechoic space between the kidney and liver? This patient has ascites, which commonly collects in the hepatorenal space (Morrison's pouch).

most soft tissue structures is very small, causing only ~1% of the beam to be reflected (which causes enough echoes to form an image), but allowing most of the beam to be transmitted to deeper structures, where additional echoes can produce an image of structures 10 to 20 cm deep, or even deeper. The tiny differences in acoustic impedance within the parenchyma of organs such as the kidney or liver are responsible for its gray-scale echotexture, or characteristic parenchymal appearance (**Fig. 1–20**).

◇ Frequency and Attenuation

The frequency of sound used affects both the resolution and penetrating power of the beam. The higher the frequency, the better the resolution, meaning that finer details in the structure being inspected can be imaged. Higher frequency also entails less penetration power, meaning that only superficial structures can be imaged. These principles are exemplified in the selection of ultrasound transducers. Clinically, this means that when imaging superficial structures such as the carotid arteries or the testes, a high-frequency transducer should be used, in the range of 10 MHz or even higher. When imaging deep structures such as the liver or the kidneys, especially in large patients, lower frequency transducers must be used, such as 3 or 5 MHz.

◇ Imaging

As we have seen, the critical scientific breakthrough that made the development of clinical ultrasound instruments possible was the discovery of the piezoelectric crystal, which can be made to vibrate by an electric current and will generate an electric current in response to mechanical vibrations to which it is subjected. By first passing a current through the crystal, we can send out sound waves into tissue, and then by turning off the current and allowing the crystal to receive echoes generated by the tissues, thereby generating electrical impulses, we can create a "picture" of the tissues. Most contemporary scanners are composed of arrays of 64 to 200 transducers, which create an equal number of separate beam components that can be used to focus and steer the beam as a whole (**Fig. 1–21**). In real-time ultrasound, the piezoelectric crystals can be alternated back and forth between the transmit and receive modes with sufficient frequency to generate 10 to 15 images per second, enabling almost instant feedback as the examiner adjusts the direction and other characteristics of the beam.

◇ Doppler Ultrasound

The so-called Doppler effect, named after Johann Doppler, the Austrian physicist who described it, refers to the change in frequency of sound waves as their source moves toward or away from the observer. Doppler ultrasound exploits the fact that the frequency of a reflected sound wave is affected by the velocity of the object generating the echo, producing a frequency shift (**Fig. 1–22**). An object moving toward the transducer will cause an increase in the frequency of the reflected sound, whereas an object moving away from the transducer will produce a decrease in the received frequency. This is familiar to anyone who has ever stood at an intersection as a train whistles past; just as the train passes by, the pitch of its whistle drops, due to the Doppler effect. In vascular Doppler imaging, the most important moving

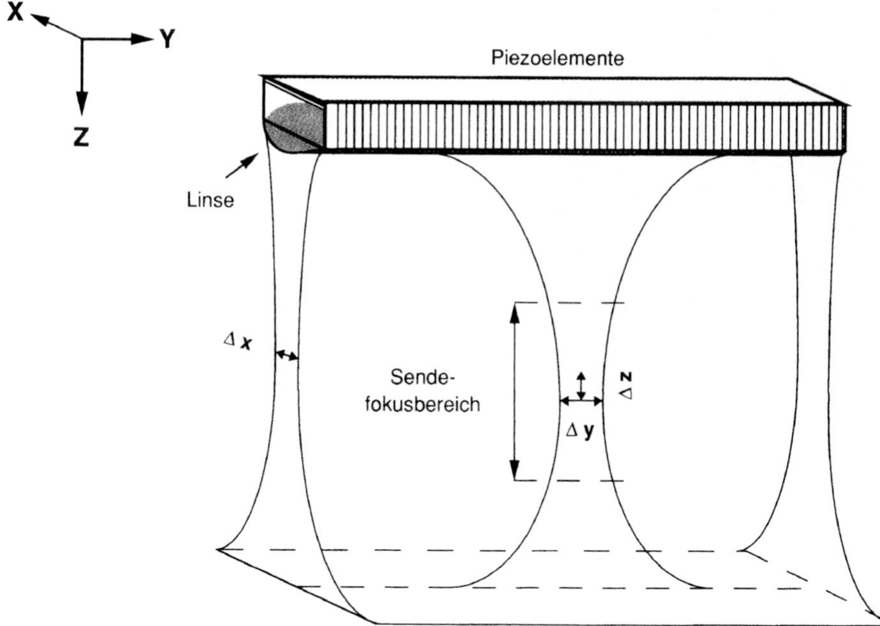

Figure 1–21 How the array of piezoelectric crystals that make up a transducer can be used to produce a focused beam, thereby optimizing spatial resolution.

reflector of sound is the red blood cell, which enables us to determine the velocity of flow of blood within a vessel. Of course, the frequency shift also depends on the angle at which the beam strikes its moving target. At an angle of 90 degrees, no shift will occur, because the blood is moving neither toward nor away from the transducer. A good angle of incidence is somewhere between 0 and 60 degrees, which allows a reasonably accurate assessment of velocity.

Several refinements of the Doppler technique are widely used in clinical imaging. Duplex Doppler ultrasound employs a combination of gray-scale and Doppler imaging by using two different transducers within the probe, which usually operate at different frequencies. Using duplex, one can simultaneously view a gray-scale image of a vessel and a waveform being generated by flow within it (**Fig. 1–23**). In color flow Doppler, velocity measurements are assigned color values, with red used to represent blood flowing toward the transducer and blue, blood flowing away. In contrast to duplex Doppler, which measures the maximal velocity of reflected sound, color flow Doppler measures the mean velocity. Color Doppler allows assessment of flow within larger fields of view, although it is associated with poorer temporal resolu-

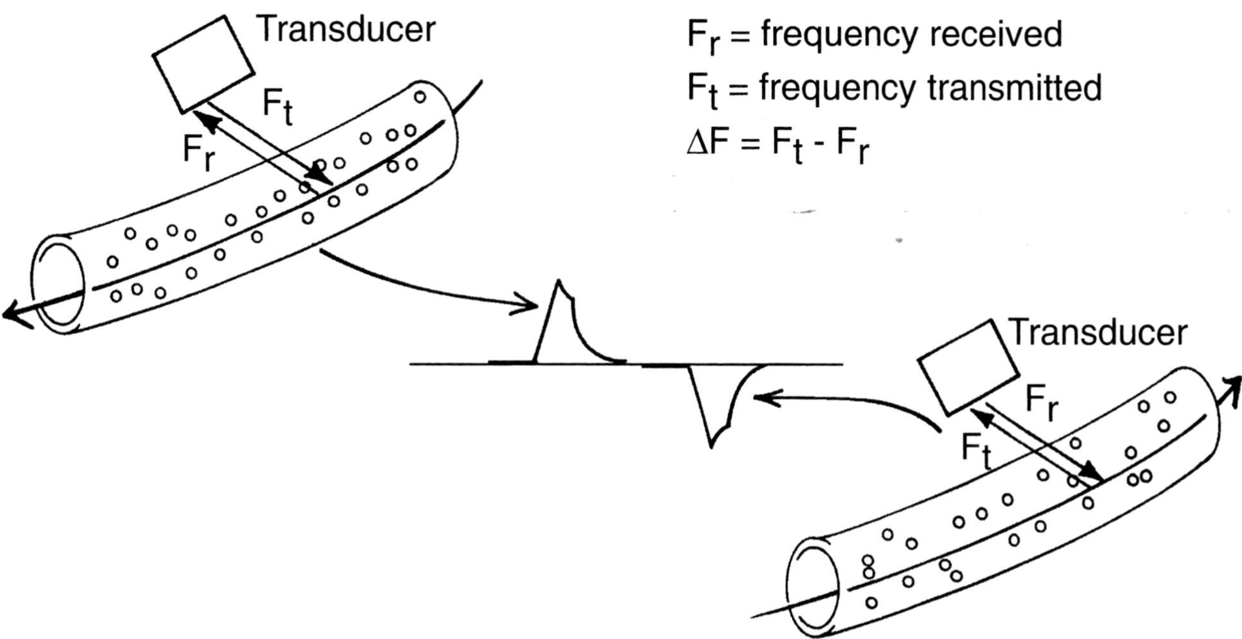

Figure 1–22 The Doppler frequency shift, in which the frequency of echoes returning from reflectors moving toward the transducer is increased (and above the baseline), while the frequency of echoes returning from reflectors moving away from the transducer is decreased (and below the baseline).

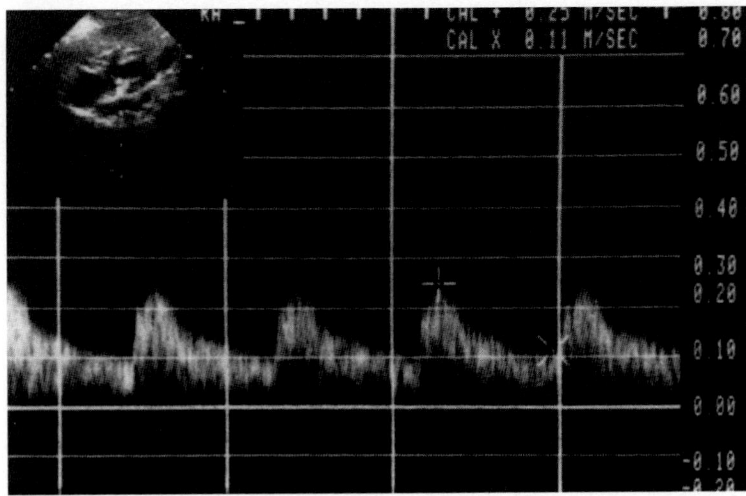

Figure 1–23 This duplex Doppler image provides a spectral display of the frequency shift produced by the motion of red blood cells in an artery over time. Peak systolic (+) and diastolic (x) velocities are displayed in m/s. The shape of the resultant curve is influenced by factors such as the resistance to flow in the vessel being interrogated and the resistance in the distal vascular bed.

tion (due to the lower associated rate of sampling). One way of minimizing the latter drawback is to limit the area of Doppler sampling.

As expected, different organs in the body exhibit varying normal flow resistance patterns, producing different characteristic duplex Doppler waveforms. For example, the brain and kidneys are low-resistance vascular beds, which demonstrate forward flow throughout the cardiac cycle. Arteries supplying resting skeletal muscles typically demonstrate a high-resistance flow pattern, with a reversal of flow during diastole. In disease states, organs may exhibit alterations in their normal flow patterns; for example, the finding of reversed diastolic flow in the renal artery of a transplant kidney would suggest rejection or vascular obstruction. Of course, these resistance patterns are not always static and may vary under normal circumstances. For example, a muscle at rest will exhibit a high-resistance flow pattern but convert to a low-resistance pattern with exercise (**Fig. 1–24**).

Emission Imaging

The emission modalities include MRI and nuclear medicine. MRI creates images by distinguishing between the nuclear magnetic properties of various tissues, a property very different from simple atomic density. This ability is crucial to MRI's superior soft tissue differentiation capabilities, as compared with transmission modalities. MRI also utilizes no ionizing radiation, generating images using a magnetic field and radio waves. The other emission modality, nuclear medicine, creates images by introducing radioisotopes into the human body and then detecting their emission of gamma rays (like x-rays, except from a different source). Nuclear medicine adds a dimension to medical imaging, by depicting not only static or dynamic anatomy, but also physiology. This is accomplished by attaching the radioisotope to molecules that enter into a physiologic pathway, which causes them to accumulate in particular locations, from which their photon emissions can then be detected. Exploiting the different magnetic properties of substances such as oxygenated and deoxygenated hemoglobin, MRI can also be used to provide functional information about tissues. In contrast to MRI, nuclear medicine involves ionizing radiation.

Magnetic Resonance Imaging

Although MRI only came into wide clinical use in the 1980s, the physics behind it had been worked out in the 1940s, by two independent researchers, Felix Bloch at Stanford University and Edward Purcell at Harvard University. Both knew that many atomic nuclei behave like tiny bar magnets, tending to align their axes with an externally applied magnetic field, around which they precess, or spin like a top. The frequency of a proton's precession, which depends in part on the strength of the magnetic field it is in, is called the Larmor frequency, and is measured in MHz (millions of cycles per second). Bloch and Purcell discovered that this axis of precession could be displaced by electromagnetic radiation in the radiofrequency range, and that once the radio signal was withdrawn, the nuclei would gradually return to their previous orientation, during which time they would become radiofrequency emitters (**Fig. 1–25**). The phenomenon was called nuclear magnetic resonance (NMR), and Bloch and Purcell shared the Nobel Prize in physics for their discovery in 1952.

◇ Applications in Chemistry

During the first few decades after this discovery, NMR was employed primarily by chemists, who could exploit a phenomenon called the chemical shift artifact to characterize different chemical compounds. The chemical shift referred to the fact that the resonant frequency (the frequency at which the nuclear magnetic moments precess) varies according to the chemical environment in which the nuclei find themselves. NMR spectroscopy remains today an invaluable tool in chemical research. For some time, NMR was regarded as a strictly chemical tool, and its potential in bio-

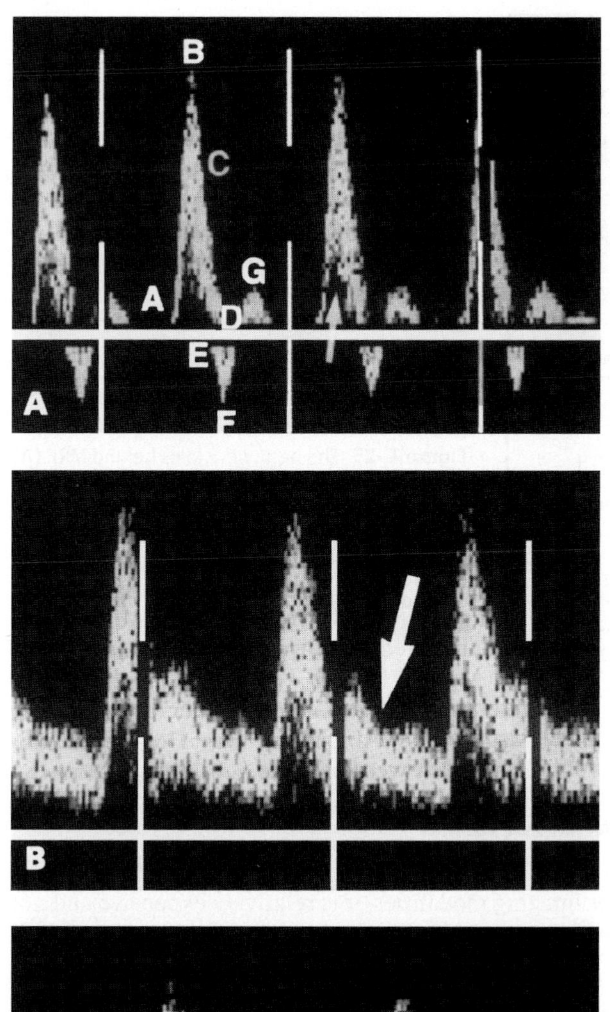

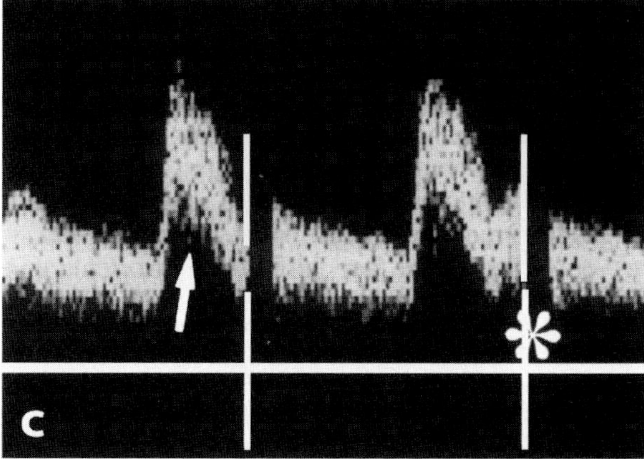

Figure 1–24 **(A)** A duplex sonogram of the brachial artery in a normal subject at rest demonstrates a high-resistance, triphasic waveform. This is characterized by a sharp systolic velocity increase (A,B), a rapid drop in velocity late in systole (C,D), diastolic flow reversal (E,F), and late diastolic forward flow (G). **(B)** After exercise consisting of 10 fist clenchings, the waveform shifts to a low-resistance pattern, with a pronounced forward flow in diastole (arrow). **(C)** An image of the normal internal carotid artery, which supplies the brain, demonstrates a very low resistance waveform, with less pulsatility and very high forward flow in diastole.

logical and medical research was largely unrecognized. This had to do with the fact that a key characteristic of NMR from an imaging point of view was regarded by chemists largely as a flaw or impurity. This characteristic was the inhomogeneity of the magnetic field. Because of field nonuniformity, protons in different locations tended to precess at slightly different frequencies, which "contaminated" the purity of the received radiofrequency signal. The larger the specimen, the greater the potential effect of these nonuniformities.

◇ Medical Imaging

In the 1970s, Paul Lauterbur at the State University of New York realized that these nonuniformities in the magnetic field could be exploited for imaging purposes. The nonuniformities could be regarded not as a contaminant, but as a means of encoding the spatial location of the protons whose radiofrequency emissions were being received. This could be accomplished by intentionally superimposing a spatially graded magnetic field over the specimen (a portion of a patient's body). Because this external magnetic field varies in strength across a specimen, the Larmor frequency will also vary, and these variations in the frequency of radiofrequency emissions will "encode" the location from which they emanate. In combination with the phase-encoding gradient (which causes some protons to be at 1:00 o'clock in their precession, others at 2:00 o'clock, and so on), frequency encoding permits the determination of the point of origin within a slice of the patient of a particular radiofrequency emission in both the x- and y-axes.

The first two-dimensional image of a section of the human body was produced in 1977, and in the early 1980s, researchers were demonstrating the superior sensitivity of NMR as compared with CT in the differentiation of benign and malignant tissues and in the detection of lesions in disorders such as multiple sclerosis (**Fig. 1–26**). More powerful magnets were introduced, exploiting the phenomenon of superconductivity (using liquid helium at a temperature of −269°C), which enabled the commercial production of magnets with strengths of several tesla (by comparison, the earth's magnetic field is less than 1/10,000th of a tesla, T). By the early 1980s, NMR was rapidly gaining wide acceptance, and it soon became the imaging modality of choice for the central nervous system (CNS). In the mid-1980s, however, concern was voiced about the public's reaction to the term *nuclear* in the modality's name, and it was changed to *magnetic resonance imaging.* In 2003, Paul Lauterbur and Peter Mansfield shared the Nobel Prize in medicine for the development of clinical MRI.

◇ Strengths of MRI

The advantages of MRI over the other cross-sectional imaging modalities—CT, ultrasound, and positron emission tomography—are numerous. First, like ultrasound, it employs no ionizing radiation and poses no known human health risks. Unlike ultrasound, it can produce images through an entire section of the body, and the images are not degraded by the presence of bone or air in the imaging plane. MRI provides soft tissue contrast superior to that of the other modalities and is able to image in multiple planes, including sagittal, coronal, axial, and various obliquities, although reconstruction of axial data now allows CT to provide multiplanar imaging as well (**Fig. 1–27**). Its sensitivity to

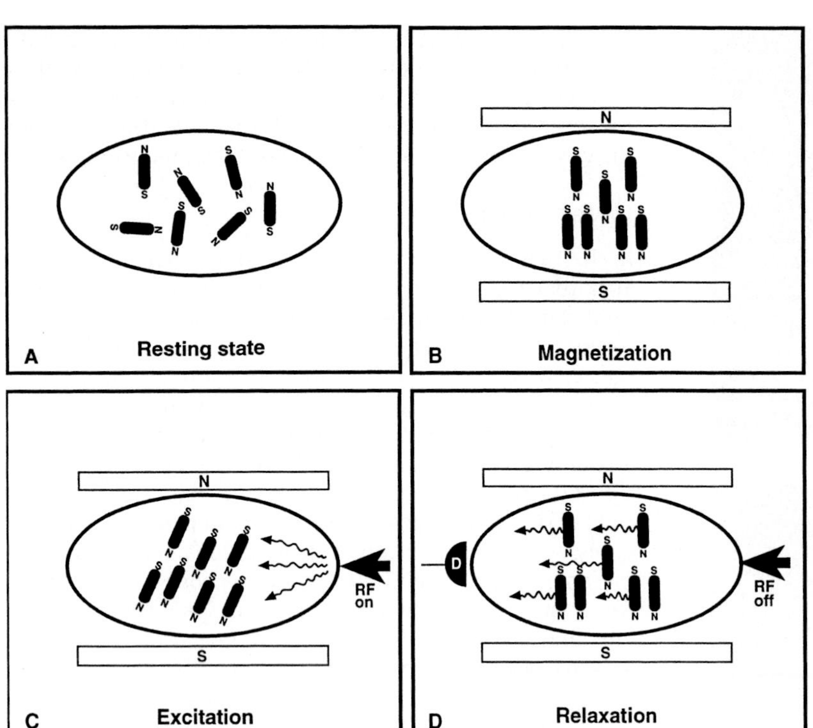

Figure 1–25 The basic principles behind MRI. **(A)** The magnetic moments of the protons are randomly oriented. **(B)** The protons have acquired a net magnetic moment due to their presence in the powerful magnet of the MR scanner. **(C)** A radiofrequency (RF) pulse has tipped the protons' axis, around which they precess, or spin like a top. **(D)** The radio pulse emitter has been turned off, and the radiofrequency signals emitted by the protons as they return to their state in **(B)** are measured and used to produce an image. N, north; S, south; D, detector.

motion enables the visualization of vascular structures with or without the administration of contrast material. MRI spectroscopy provides important clinical benefits through the in vivo characterization of chemical composition and metabolic activity.

◇ Weaknesses of MRI

MRI has certain weaknesses as well. As compared with the other imaging modalities, it is relatively expensive and not as widely available. Some patients cannot undergo MRI

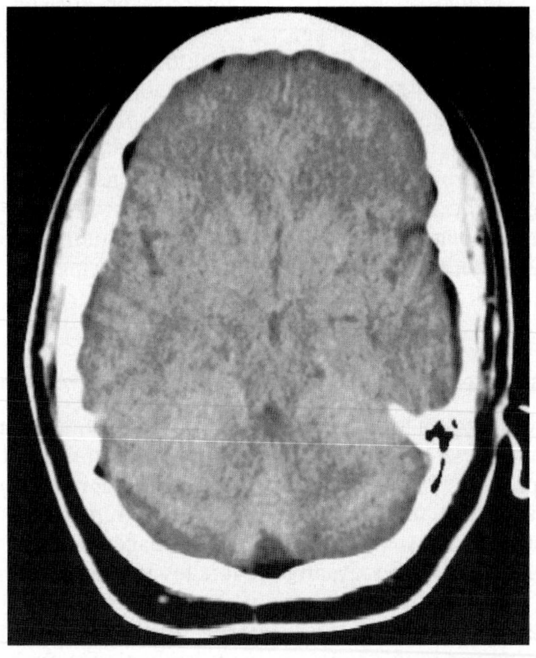

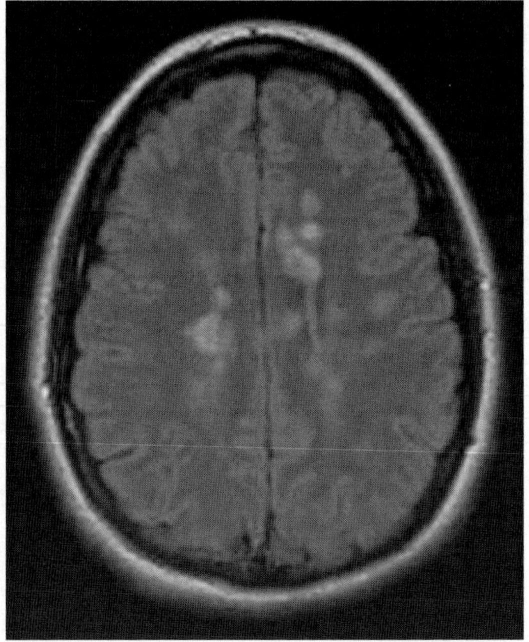

Figure 1–26 This young woman presented with blurry vision and leg weakness. **(A)** An axial head CT image demonstrates a small arachnoid cyst in the posterior fossa but appears otherwise fairly unremarkable. **(B)** In contrast, a T2-weighted MR image demonstrates multiple bilateral foci of increased signal (bright) in the white matter. The fact that the cerebrospinal fluid appears bright suggests that the image is T2-weighted. This patient suffers from multiple sclerosis.

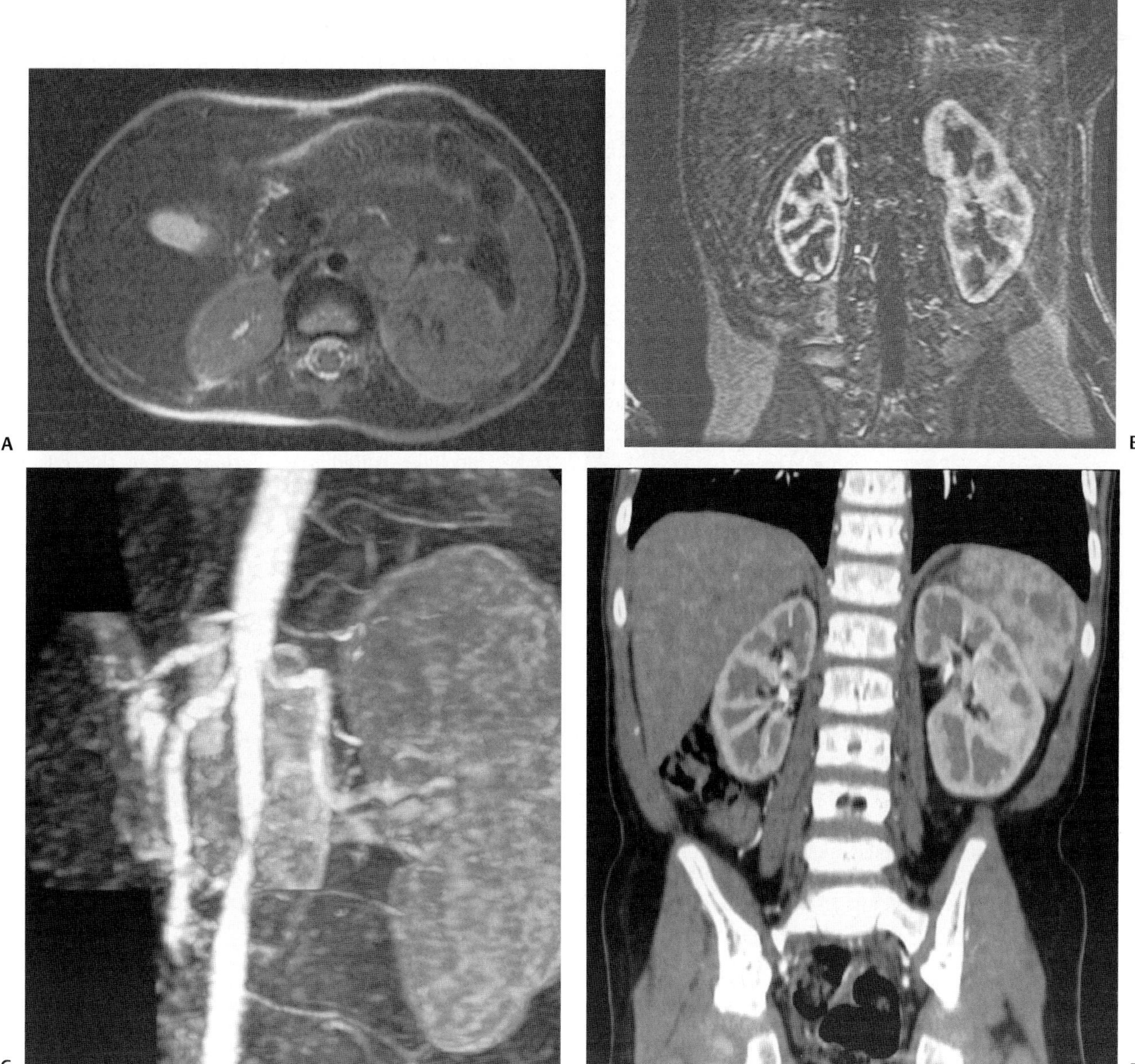

Figure 1–27 This young girl with neurofibromatosis type I presented with hypertension. **(A)** This axial MR image demonstrates asymmetry of the kidneys, with the right kidney abnormally small. **(B)** A coronal image again demonstrates the renal asymmetry, an important finding in a patient with hypertension because it may indicate renal scarring. Note that the right renal cortex is thinned, confirming scarring. **(C)** A magnetic resonance angiogram in oblique projection demonstrates focal narrowing of the infrarenal abdominal aorta, an abdominal aortic coarctation, which is associated with neurofibromatosis. Other images also demonstrated to better advantage right renal artery stenosis, which was responsible for the scarring and hypertension. **(D)** A coronal reconstruction of axially acquired data from a CT angiogram also demonstrates the right renal scarring.

evaluation, including those who are too large to fit in the bore of the magnet (although this is not an issue with "open bore" scanners), those who are too claustrophobic (although this problem can often be alleviated with sedation), patients with cardiac pacemakers or other electrical devices in which the magnet would create currents, and patients with certain ferromagnetic foreign bodies, such as cerebral aneurysm clips. Surgical staples and prosthetic joints create imaging artifact but do not generally constitute contraindications to MRI. Another hazard of MRI is the strength of the magnetic field itself, which not only can erase virtually any magnetic storage device (e.g., a cassette tape or credit card) but also can turn ferromagnetic objects into high-velocity projectiles (**Fig. 1–28**). For this reason, patients and staff must remove such objects from their person before entering the MRI suite, and special monitoring

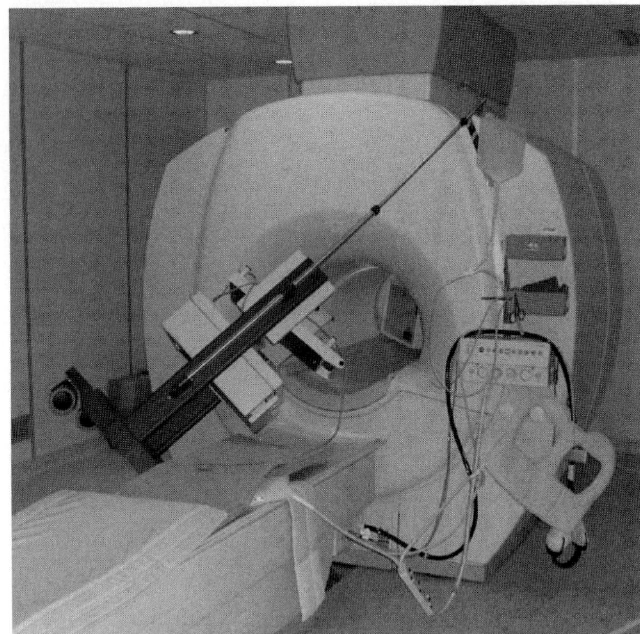

Figure 1–28 What is wrong with this picture? This photograph depicts an IV pole that has been pulled across the floor of the MR suite, lifted up, and slammed into the MR scanner gantry by the powerful MR magnet. A careless nurse had pushed the pole across the threshold of this room. Luckily, there was no patient in the scanner. It is important to recall that the very powerful MR magnet is always "on," whether scanning is under way or not.

and support devices, including the "crash cart" used for resuscitation, must be available.

◇ T1- and T2-Weighting

Many pulse-sequence techniques are used in MRI, but the most classic are T1- and T2-weighted images. What do these terms mean? T1- and T2-weighted images provide different assessments of the molecular environment surrounding the protons of the tissues imaged. T1 measures the ability of protons within a tissue to exchange energy with the surrounding environment, or how quickly the tissue can become magnetized, and T2 measures how quickly it loses its magnetization. So-called proton density images are neither T1- nor T2-weighted and measure exactly what one would expect, namely, the density of protons within the tissue. Fat appears relatively bright and water relatively dark on T1-weighted images, whereas the reverse is true on T2-weighted images. As a general rule, T1-weighted images are good for viewing anatomy, and T2-weighted images are good for detecting pathology (**Fig. 1–29**).

Nuclear Medicine

Nuclear medicine relies on the use of radioactive materials to evaluate the functional status of various organs and tissues. Generally speaking, x-ray imaging modalities provide excellent imaging of anatomy, from which function can often be inferred. By contrast, nuclear medicine typically images functional activity, from which anatomy can be inferred. The spatial resolution of nuclear medicine images is relatively poor, but the opportunity to directly visualize function more than makes up for this deficiency in numerous clinical and research contexts.

◇ Nuclear Radiation

The ionizing radiation employed in most diagnostic nuclear medicine imaging is no different from that employed in x-ray imaging, in the sense that both types of imaging involve the detection of photons emerging from the patient's body; however, the photons employed are of two types. X-rays are high-energy photons that originate in an extranuclear source, most often produced by bombarding an atom (usually tungsten) with electrons. By contrast, the gamma rays used in nuclear medicine are produced by the decay of unstable atomic nuclei.

◇ Scintillations

The foundations of nuclear medicine were laid in the first decades of the 20th century, when chemist Ernest Rutherford discovered that the emissions of certain radioactive elements could be detected using a zinc sulfide screen, producing tiny flashes of light called scintillations. Over the ensuing decades, several researchers pursued the medical implications of this observation and soon were able to demonstrate that various isotopes could be introduced into the body of a patient, the photons emitted could be identified by newer scintillation detectors, and an image could be produced of the distribution of the isotope within the body. When isotopes were coupled with other chemical compounds that are handled by the body in various stereotypical ways, the radiopharmaceutical (or radiotracer) was born (**Fig. 1–30**).

◇ Diagnosis and Therapy

Radiopharmaceuticals fall into one of two fundamental categories, diagnostic or therapeutic. The ideal diagnostic radiopharmaceutical is a pure gamma (photon) emitter, has an energy in the range of 100 to 250 kilo-electron volts (keV) and a half-life in the body of 1 to 2 times the duration of the test, exhibits a high target–nontarget ratio (meaning that it is especially concentrated by the organ or tissue of interest), involves a minimal radiation dose to the patient, and can be inexpensively and safely produced and handled. Far and away the most commonly employed radiolabel in diagnostic nuclear medicine studies is technetium (Tc) 99m, which has a half-life of 6 hours, has principal imaging photons with an energy of 140 keV, and is inexpensive, safe, and easy to produce on site from commercially available generators.

The ideal therapeutic radiopharmaceutical should be a pure beta (β) particle (electron) emitter, because β particles, in contrast to gamma rays, transfer a considerable amount of energy to tissue as they pass through it, resulting in tissue destruction. In addition, it should have a moderately long half-life (days), a high target–nontarget ratio (decreasing the dose to nontarget organs), and, like diagnostic agents, should be inexpensive and safe. A commonly used therapeutic radiopharmaceutical is iodine 131 in the form of sodium iodide, which is heavily concentrated in the thyroid gland, and whose β particle emissions destroy thyroid cells in diseases such as thyroid carcinoma and the hyperthyroidism of Graves' disease.

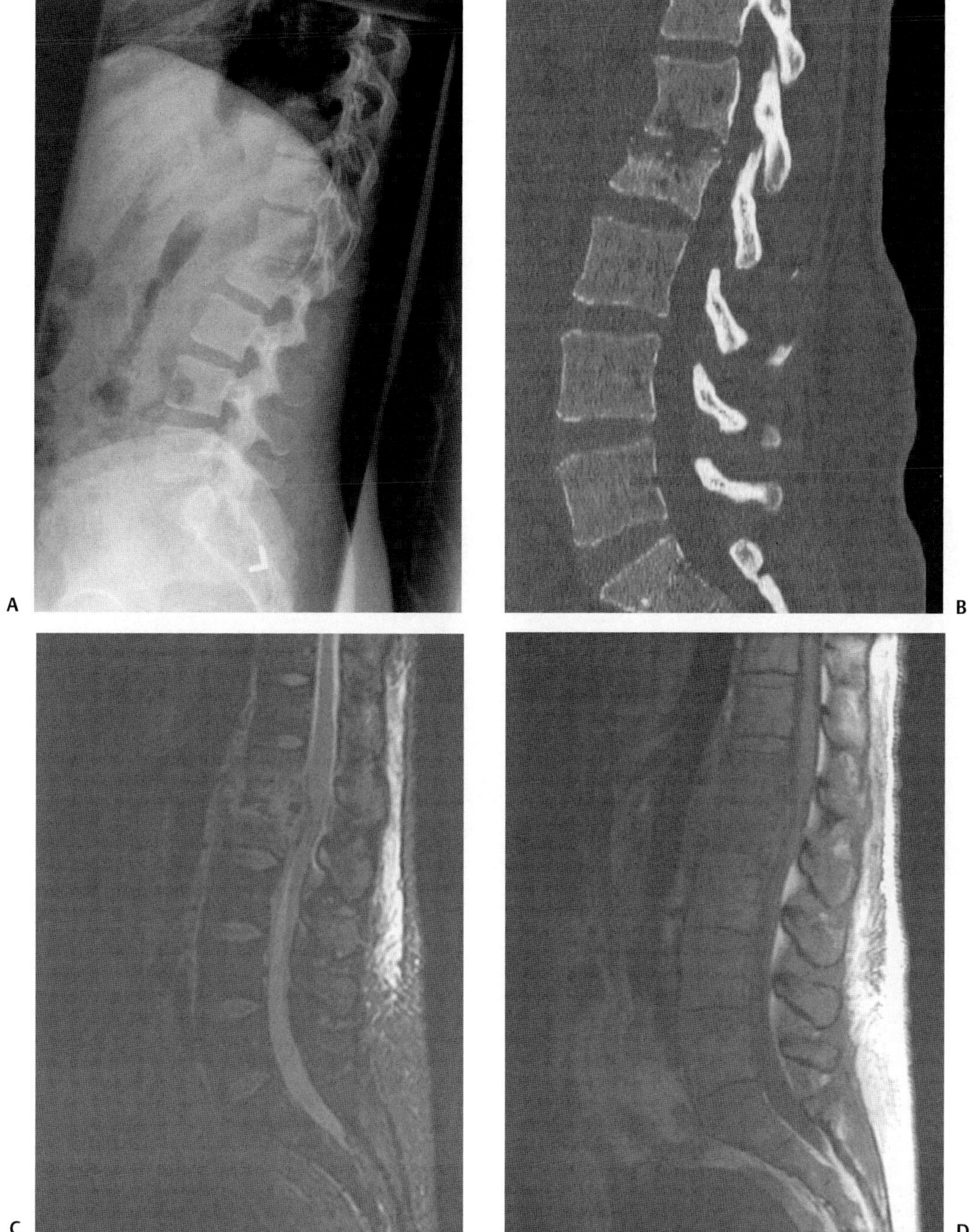

Figure 1–29 This middle-aged intravenous drug abuser presented with several weeks of low back pain radiating into the lower extremity. **(A)** This lateral spine radiograph demonstrates destruction and collapse of the upper portion of the second lumbar vertebral body and obliteration of the L1–L2 intervertebral disk space. **(B)** This sagittal reconstruction of axially acquired CT data displayed at bone windows demonstrates these abnormalities, as well as destruction of a portion of the first lumbar vertebral body. **(C)** A sagittal STIR MR image demonstrates high signal in the vertebral bodies and intervertebral disk at this level, as well as an epidural abscess compressing the spinal cord. STIR imaging is like T2 weighting, in that abnormalities such as infection and neoplasm tend to appear bright, due to their increased water content (edema). **(D)** Note that on this sagittal T1-weighted image the areas of abnormality, as well as the cerebrospinal fluid around the spinal cord, now appear dark, whereas the subcutaneous fat now appears bright. On T1, water (and edema) appears dark and fat appears bright, whereas on T2 water appears bright and fat is relatively dark.

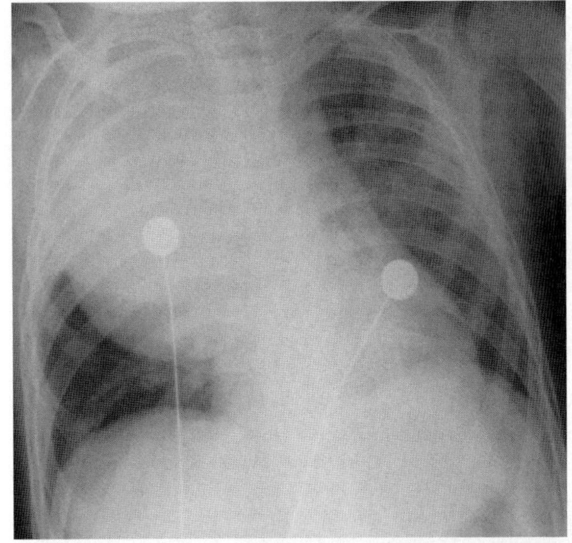

Figure 1–30 This 5-year-old boy presented with severe bilateral leg pain. **(A)** A frontal chest radiograph demonstrates a large right posterior mediastinal mass that is eroding the posterior segments of multiple ribs (compare with the ribs on the left). **(B)** A nuclear medicine bone scan, in which radiotracer accumulates in areas of increased bone metabolic activity, demonstrates multiple abnormal foci of increased uptake involving the skull, spine, sternum, ribs, pelvis, and both humeri, femurs, and tibias. **(C)** Images of the abdomen and lower extremities from a nuclear medicine iodine-131 meta-iodobenzylguanidine (MIBG) scan, in which the radiotracer localizes in catecholamine-secreting tissue, demonstrate abnormal uptake in the distal femurs and proximal tibias. This represented metastatic neuroblastoma.

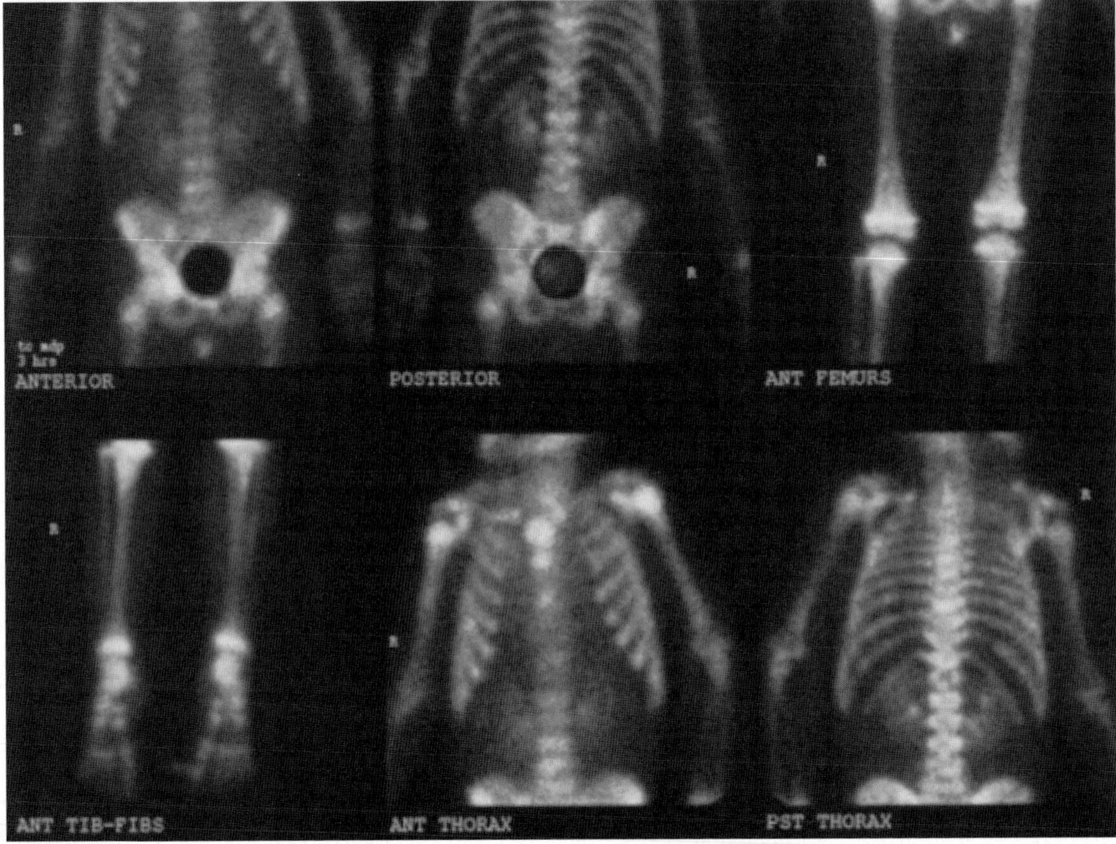

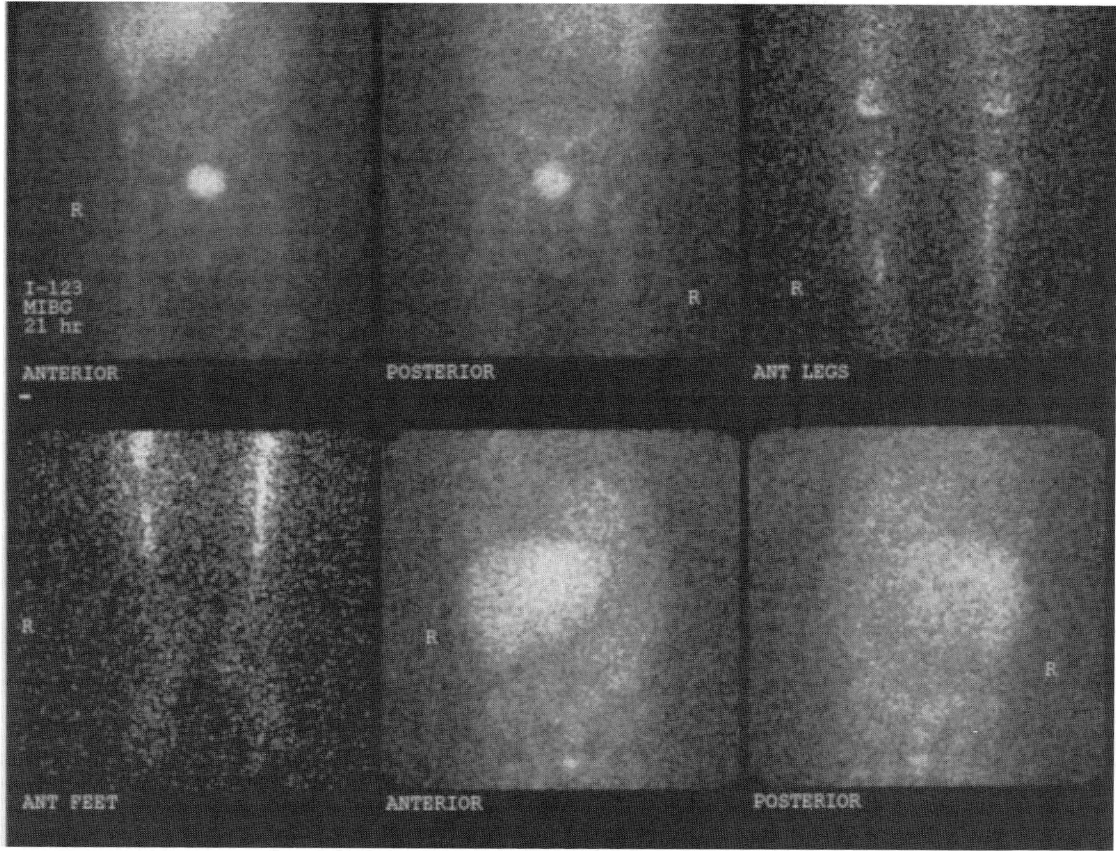

C

Figure 1–30 (*Continued*)

◇ Mechanisms of Localization

Radiopharmaceuticals localize in the body by a variety of mechanisms. One such mechanism is capillary blockade, in which injected radiotracer embolizes capillaries. The most important example of capillary blockade is pulmonary perfusion imaging, in which tiny particles of Tc-99m-labeled macroaggregated human albumin injected into a systemic vein embolize the pulmonary capillary bed. This produces an image of the perfusion of each lung, with more radiopharmaceutical accumulating in more heavily perfused areas, and none accumulating in lung tissue devoid of perfusion (as in pulmonary embolism).

The phagocytic activity of Kupffer's cells can be exploited to image the reticuloendothelial system, with phagocytosis the mechanism of localization. For example, micron-sized particles of Tc-99m-sulfur colloid are avidly phagocytized by the reticuloendothelial system, with the biodistribution of the radiopharmaceutical providing an image of normal tissue in the liver, spleen, and bone marrow. Such a scan can be used to determine whether a patient who has undergone splenectomy has any residual functional splenic tissue.

Compartmental localization is the mechanism used in such studies as pulmonary ventilation imaging, GI bleeding scans, and cystograms. In these studies, a radiopharmaceutical is injected into a fluid space, into which it quickly diffuses (**Fig. 1–31**). Images are then obtained of the compartment in question. In the case of lung scans, inhaled xenon-133 gas provides an image of ventilated portions of the lung. In the GI bleeding study, Tc-99m-labeled erythrocytes accumulate within the bowel lumen at the point where bleeding is occurring. In the voiding cystogram, vesicoureteral reflux is detected as scintillations from radiotracer that has flowed retrograde up into the ureter.

Thyroid scans use the mechanism of active transport, in which the radiopharmaceutical substitutes for iodine in the energy-requiring process of thyroxin synthesis within the thyroid gland (**Fig. 1–32**). Thyroid tumors, which often carry out this process less efficiently, tend to appear as "cold" areas within the normally "hot" tissue of the thyroid gland. In Graves' disease, however, the entire overstimulated gland tends to appear diffusely enlarged and "hot." Another example of active transport is the use of thallium 201 in myocardial perfusion studies, where the radiopharmaceutical is transported across the myocardial cell membrane as though it were a potassium ion. Tc-99m-MAG-3 is actively secreted by the renal tubules, making it very useful in renal imaging.

The localization of Tc-99m-HDP in skeletal imaging occurs by the process of physicochemical adsorption. The phosphate groups in the bone agent are avidly bound to the hydroxyapatite element of bone mineral. Areas of active bone metabolism, such as the epiphyseal growth plate, most metastatic bone lesions, and osteomyelitis are imaged as "hot" spots. Conversely, multiple myeloma and certain other tumors that replace bone without exciting a metabolic response from it may appear as "cold" areas against the normally "warm" surrounding bone.

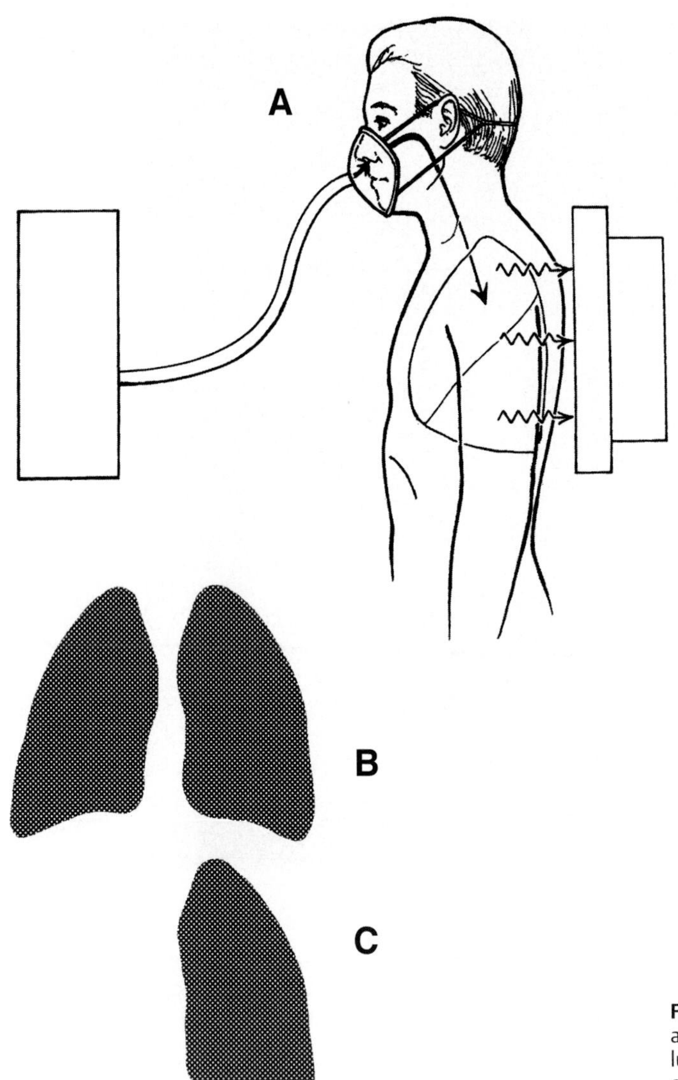

Figure 1–31 **(A)** How radioactive xenon-133 gas can be administered to a patient through a mask. **(B)** There is normal radiotracer activity in both lungs, producing images of each lung when the patient is placed in front of a scintillation detector. **(C)** One lung is blocked by a mucus plug, and no radiotracer activity is detected in it.

Certain newer radiopharmaceuticals exploit other mechanisms of localization, such as binding to specific hormone receptors (e.g., the receptors for somatostatin in several endocrine tumors) and antigen-antibody binding, as in the use of monoclonal antibodies to image recurrent or metastatic colorectal and ovarian carcinomas.

◆ Contrast Agents

Enhancement

Enhancement is a term frequently used by radiologists to describe the effect of contrast agents on the conspicuity of anatomic or pathologic structures.

Barium

One of the most common types of enhancement seen in radiology is that produced by introducing radiopaque substances into the GI tract, typically using barium sulfate suspensions (hereafter referred to as barium). For example, the colon is normally visible on plain radiographs only if it contains air, and even then, the ability to discern structural details of colonic anatomy and pathology is severely limited; however, by filling the colon with barium, many of its structural features, including pathologic lesions, become apparent, because of the impression they make on the barium column. This so-called single-contrast type of examination is excellent for discerning large masses, strictures, or leaks, but is somewhat limited in the detection of smaller mucosal lesions. For the latter purpose, the double-contrast technique is superior. This involves coating the luminal surface of the colon with a relatively small amount of barium and then insufflating air, which distends its walls.

Iodinated Compounds

A similar rationale underlies the use of iodine-containing contrast agents in settings such as angiography. Although the

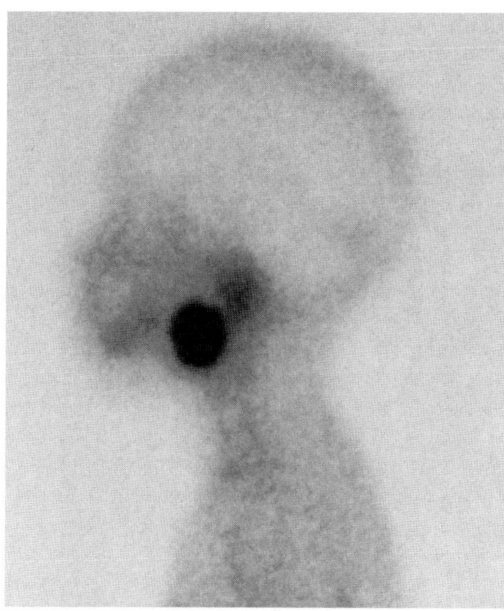

Figure 1–32 This young woman with a history of hypothyroidism presented with a mass at the base of her tongue that was producing worsening dysphagia. An iodine-123 scan was performed. This lateral view demonstrates no uptake of radiopharmaceutical in the thyroid gland's usual location, the base of the neck. There is, however, intense uptake more cephalad at the base of the tongue. This represented a sublingual thyroid gland. Such ectopic thyroid tissue is often nonfunctioning or hypofunctioning.

aorta is normally visible on posteroanterior (PA) and lateral chest radiographs, only portions of its outline are typically seen. With the exception of portions of the aorta and the superior and inferior vena cavae, the arteries and veins of the body are not normally visible on plain radiographs at all, the exception being patients whose arteries are calcified, most often secondary to arteriosclerosis. When contrast is injected into a vessel, however, its lumen is opacified in the same way that barium opacifies the mucosa of the colon (**Fig. 1–33**). Of course, when contrast is injected into a blood vessel, it moves with the blood, and imagir.g of any vessel is possible only during the seconds during which the contrast is injected. When contrast is injected into the vasculature of an organ such as the lung, both arterial and venous phases can be distinguished, the arterial phase beginning as soon as the contrast reaches the pulmonary artery. Once contrast passes through the capillary bed, it begins to appear in the pulmonary veins, which is the venous phase. Similar principles apply to the angiographic examination of any organ.

Radiologists inject iodinated contrast media into many other spaces as well. In a cystogram, for example, contrast is usually infused through a urethral catheter into the bladder, and multiple x-ray images are obtained in different projections to outline the bladder mucosa. A voiding cystourethrogram extends the examination to include views of the ureters, bladder, and urethra, which are useful to assess for vesicoureteral reflux, urethral morphology, and the dynamic character of the voiding process. Contrast is injected into the subarachnoid space (utilizing a technique similar to that employed for routine lumbar puncture) to assess for a variety of CNS and spinal pathologies, such as an extradural tumor pressing on the thecal sac. With the advent of CT and MRI, many traditional contrast examinations are performed much less frequently. For example, high-resolution CT and bronchoscopy have virtually eliminated bronchography, which was performed by introducing contrast into the tracheobronchial tree. Pneumoencephalography, which utilized air as a contrast medium to examine the cerebral ventricles, has likewise become a thing of the past.

Enhancement in CT and MRI

The term *enhancement* is most often employed in the context of CT and MRI studies, and an understanding of its meaning is vital to understanding these two types of examinations. A crucial point to be made about the difference between the enhancement that takes place with contrast administration in CT and MRI is the fact that they rely on completely different physical principles. The contrast material used in CT is the same as that employed in angiography and urography, namely, iodinated molecules based on a benzene ring. These agents diffuse rapidly into the extracellular space and are excreted primarily via glomerular filtration. The enhancement of vessels or tissues in CT is due to the presence of iodine-containing molecules within them, which attenuate the x-ray beam. The more iodine present, the more the beam is attenuated.

The contrast agent used in MRI, often referred to as gadolinium, is a rare-earth paramagnetic substance. What we call gadolinium is actually gadolinium-labeled diethylenetri-

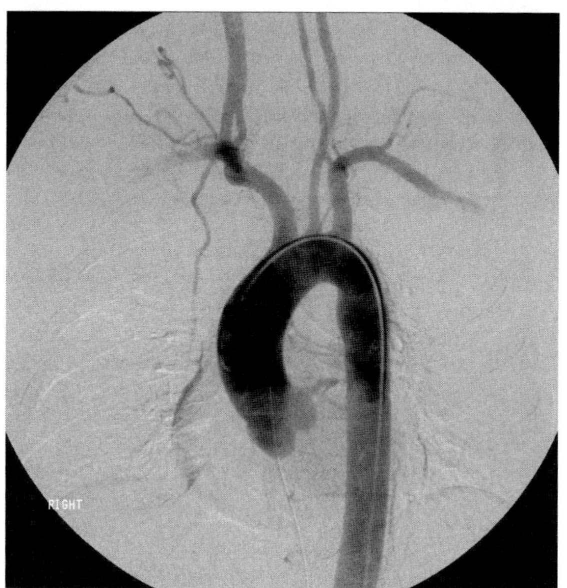

Figure 1–33 This digital subtraction angiogram of the aorta was performed by catheterizing the common femoral artery, then passing a pigtail catheter up the iliac artery, abdominal and thoracic aorta, and around the aortic arch, so that the catheter tip lies in the ascending aorta. Iodinated contrast material was then injected. Structures such as ribs that were visible in both pre- and postinjection images have been subtracted. There is excellent visualization of the aortic arch and its major branches, including the brachiocephalic artery on the right and the carotid and subclavian arteries on the left.

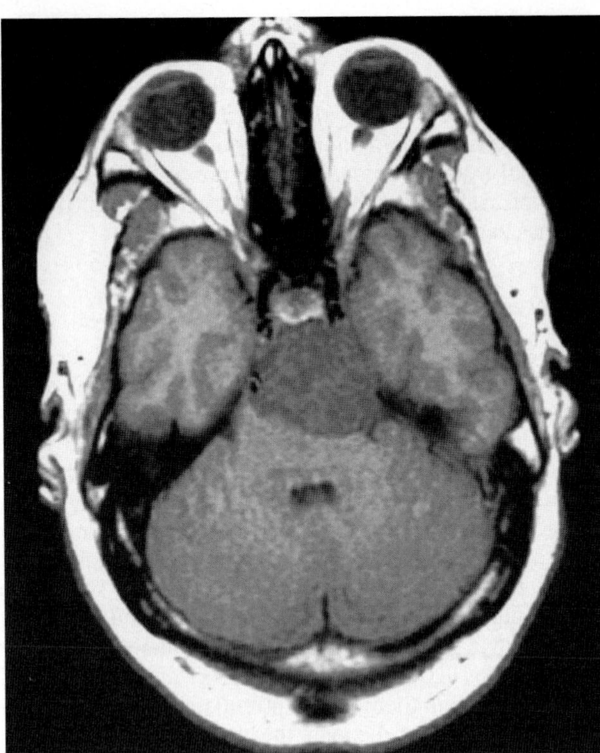

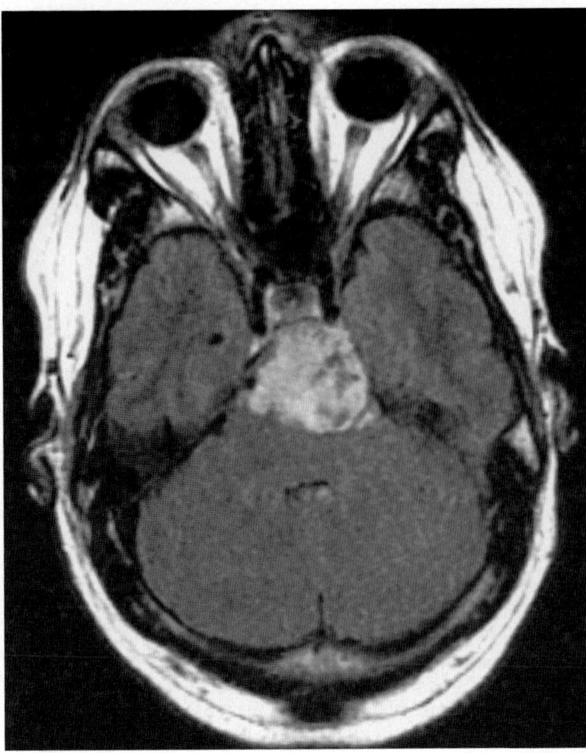

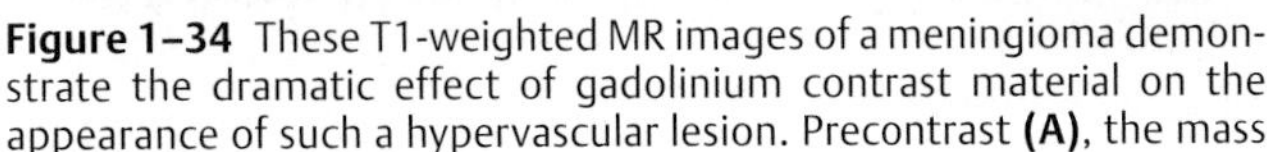

Figure 1–34 These T1-weighted MR images of a meningioma demonstrate the dramatic effect of gadolinium contrast material on the appearance of such a hypervascular lesion. Precontrast **(A)**, the mass appears relatively dark, but postcontrast **(B)**, it becomes dramatically brighter, thereby qualifying it as a strongly enhancing lesion.

amine pentaacetic acid (DTPA). Like the iodinated contrast agents used in x-ray imaging, gadolinium diffuses rapidly into the extracellular space and is excreted primarily via glomerular filtration. In MRI, enhancement is due to the shortening effect of gadolinium on the T1-relaxation times of protons within its local magnetic field, which increases their signal, making them appear bright (**Fig. 1–34**).

◇ Risks of Intravascular Contrast

The use of intravascular contrast agents is associated with a small but important risk of adverse reactions. Reactions to gadolinium are rare and tend to be mild, though pregnancy and lactation are considered contraindications. By contrast, reactions to iodinated contrast media in angiography and CT are more frequent and can be severe. Mild reactions include nausea and vomiting, hives, and bronchospasm; severe reactions include hypotension, shock, and even death. Mild reactions occur in ~1 in 20 patients, and death may result in as many as 1 in every 40,000 patients. Patients at highest risk include those with a history of previous contrast reaction, as well as patients with heart disease, diabetes, and impaired renal function. Patients at increased risk can be premedicated using agents such as prednisone and diphenhydramine.

The higher osmolality iodinated contrast agents used for decades have an osmolality ~6 times that of serum, whereas newer low-osmolality agents have an osmolality only twice that of serum. Though more expensive, these agents demonstrate a decreased risk of both minor and major adverse reactions.

Because of the risk of acute renal failure associated with iodinated contrast agents, the serum creatinine is often checked in patients whose renal function might be impaired. Unlike the other adverse reactions, contrast nephrotoxicity is dose-related, and a second contrast examination should be postponed for a day or two in a patient who has already received a standard dose of 2 mL/kg. So long as a patient with renal failure will be dialyzed within 24 hours, most radiologists regard the administration of iodinated contrast as safe.

When more severe adverse reactions occur, they are treated in the usual fashion: inhalers and, if necessary, epinephrine for bronchospasm; Trendelenburg's position and fluid resuscitation for bradycardia and hypotension; and aggressive fluid resuscitation and epinephrine for anaphylactoid circulatory collapse. In some cases, the use of iodinated contrast media can be avoided altogether, through the substitution of other modalities such as ultrasound and MRI. In any case, it is important to bear in mind that the use of iodinated contrast material has been regarded as safe and effective for many decades.

◆ Angiography

Though not a distinct imaging modality in the sense of ultrasound or MRI, angiography (literally, "vessel picturing") plays a major role in contemporary medical imaging. Whereas multiple angiographic imaging procedures are discussed in detail in the following chapters, it is helpful to undertake a brief systematic overview of angiography at this point, to cover some of the general principles that apply in every angiographic context. Broadly speaking, angiography employs intravascular injection of contrast agents to characterize both vascular and parenchymal pathologic processes, using fluoroscopic monitoring and digital or conventional radiographic recording (**Fig. 1–35**). Common examples include the diagnosis of vascular disorders such as atherosclerosis and vasculitis, evaluation of trauma, characterization of tumor vascularity, and preoperative assessment in organ transplantation (where the vascular supply of the transplanted organ is critical). Moreover, various therapeutic endovascular procedures may be undertaken, as described later.

It should be noted that many angiographic procedures can now be performed using CT or MRI; for example, instead of advancing a catheter into the abdominal aorta to perform renal arteriography, a peripheral IV and precise timing of the contrast bolus can be used to obtain a diagnostically adequate CT renal arteriogram. MR angiography can produce superb images as well. Of course, there are certain roles that CT and MRI cannot play, such as renal vein sampling for renin levels, and angioplasty to open up a focal renal artery stenosis.

Preprocedure Assessment

The preprocedure assessment of the patient is vital to good angiographic practice. Aside from the risk factors for contrast

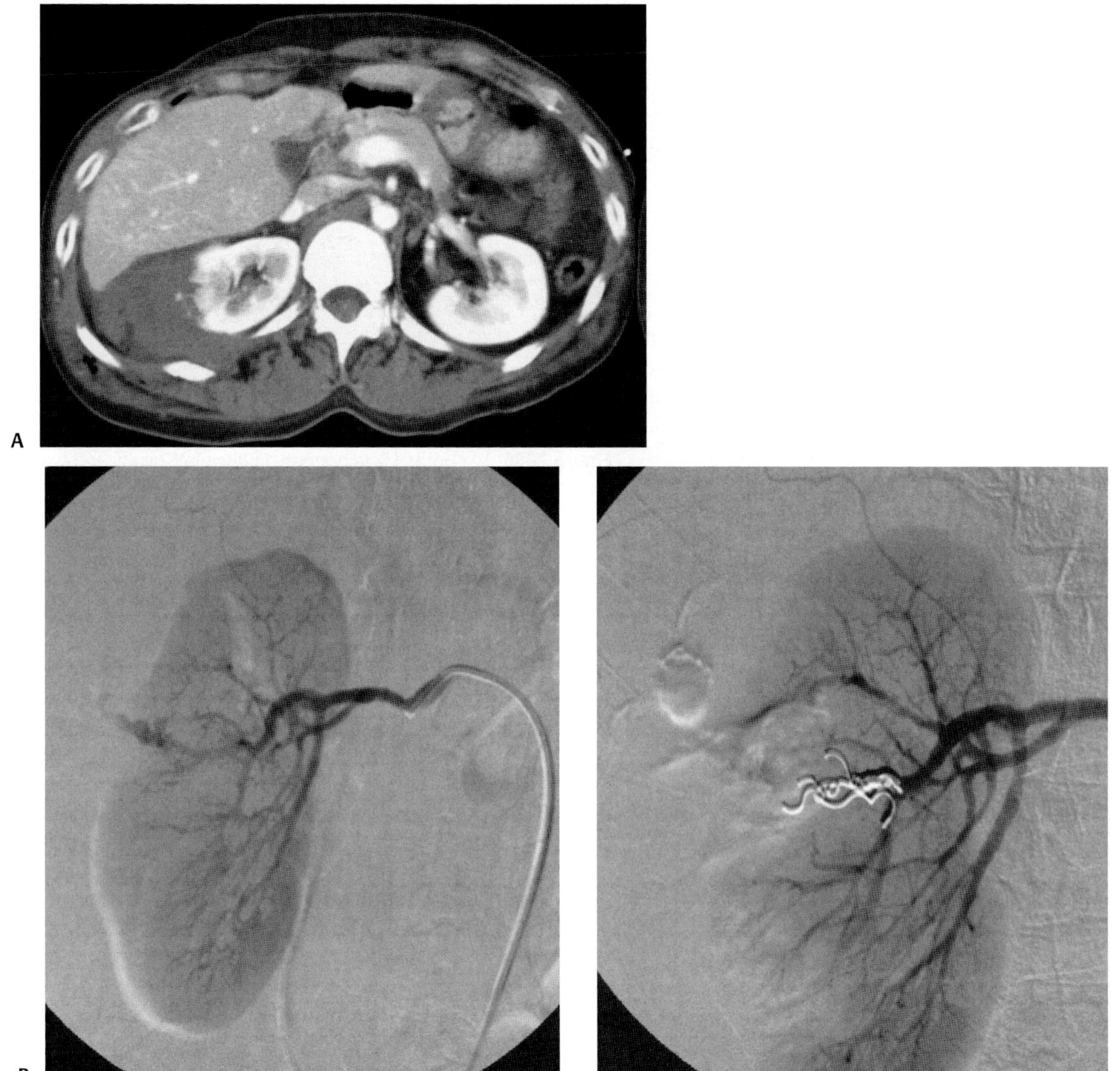

Figure 1–35 This middle-aged woman was struck by an automobile. An abdominal CT scan with IV contrast material was performed. **(A)** This axial image demonstrates a laceration of the right kidney with a large hypodense perinepheric hematoma and a focus of hyperdensity representing active extravasation of contrast-opacified blood. Why is the hematoma hypodense (dark) relative to the liver and kidney? Because the blood was extravasated before contrast was administered, and a fresh hematoma has no blood supply and therefore cannot enhance. **(B)** This digital subtraction right renal arteriogram demonstrates the bleeding as an area of contrast pooling in the midportion of the kidney. **(C)** Metallic embolization coils were injected into the bleeding vessel, which halted the extravasation.

reaction, additional points to be assessed are the patient's bleeding profile, the patient's ability to lie still on the angiographic table, and the presence of residual contrast material from a previous examination such as a barium enema. Coumadin should be discontinued several days prior to the procedure, but more rapid reversal can be accomplished by the administration of fresh frozen plasma or vitamin K. Heparin should be discontinued 4 hours prior to the procedure, but protamine sulfate can be administered in more acute situations.

Informed Consent

Angiographic procedures involve risks of bleeding, infection, vessel injury, and adverse contrast reaction, as well as specific risks of individual procedures; therefore, except in emergent situations, informed consent must be obtained. The goal of informed consent is not to obtain the patient's signature as quickly and effortlessly as possible, but to explain the procedure, its benefits and risks, as well as any alternatives, in terms that the patient can understand. Although medicolegal risk was a driving consideration in the evolution of the informed consent forms now found in every hospital, in reality physician–patient communication and the partnership that it implies are simply good medicine.

Vascular Access

The most common technique for obtaining vascular access is the Seldinger technique, usually employed at the common femoral artery or common femoral vein (**Fig. 1–36**). Both are located at the level of the femoral head, just below the inguinal ligament. Position can be verified fluoroscopically using a radiopaque marker. Puncture is performed at this level because the femoral head provides a firm structure against which to compress the artery or vein after the procedure, when hemostasis is critical. The arterial pulse is palpated, recalling that the vein is located ~1 cm medial to the artery. Lidocaine is infiltrated at the planned puncture site, a needle is advanced through the vessel to the bone at a 45-degree angle to the skin, the center stylet is withdrawn, and the needle is gradually pulled back until blood flow is seen. In the case of the artery, there is pulsatile flow of bright blood, whereas the vein generally produces a trickle of dark blood. A guidewire is then inserted into the vessel through the needle, the needle is withdrawn, and a catheter is passed over the guidewire. When the subsequent procedure is completed and the catheter withdrawn, pressure is held at the puncture site for 10 to 15 minutes, and the patient is given strict instructions not to move at the hip for 6 to 8 hours, to ensure hemostasis.

Specific diagnostic angiographic procedures, such as coronary angiography, pulmonary angiography, and cerebral angiography, are discussed in subsequent chapters. In addition to diagnosis, angiographic techniques may also be applied to therapy. Following are brief discussions of several interventional angiographic procedures.

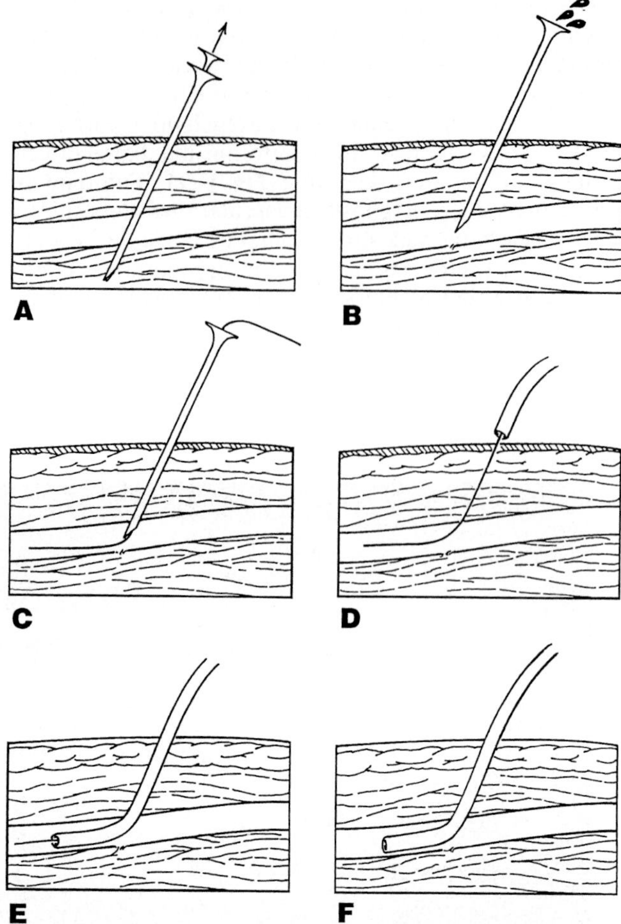

Figure 1–36 The normal Seldinger technique of obtaining intravascular access. **(A)** A needle is advanced at an angle through the vessel. **(B)** The needle is withdrawn until blood return is seen, which indicates that the needle tip is in the lumen. **(C)** A wire is advanced through the needle. **(D)** The needle is withdrawn, and the wire is left in place. **(E)** A catheter is advanced over the wire into the vessel. **(F)** The wire is withdrawn, and the catheter is left in place in the vessel.

Angioplasty

Transluminal angioplasty (literally, "vessel molding") is commonly used to treat atherosclerotic stenoses of the coronary and iliofemoral arteries, and has applications elsewhere as well. A balloon catheter is placed into vascular stenosis under fluoroscopic guidance, and the balloon is then inflated (**Fig. 1–37**). Circumferential increased intraluminal pressure fractures the intima and media of the vessel, stretching the adventitia, and expanding the luminal orifice. Examples of indications for angioplasty include angina pectoris in coronary disease, as well as claudication, rest pain, and tissue loss in the lower extremities. Angioplasty may be augmented by the placement of intravascular stents, which help to prevent restenosis (**Fig. 1–38**). The stents are usually composed of a metallic mesh, which expands when released from the catheter sheath and can be further dilated using a balloon catheter.

Embolization

Transcatheter embolization is used primarily to halt uncontrolled bleeding, to obliterate arteriovenous malformations or tumors, and, in the presurgical setting, to decrease operative

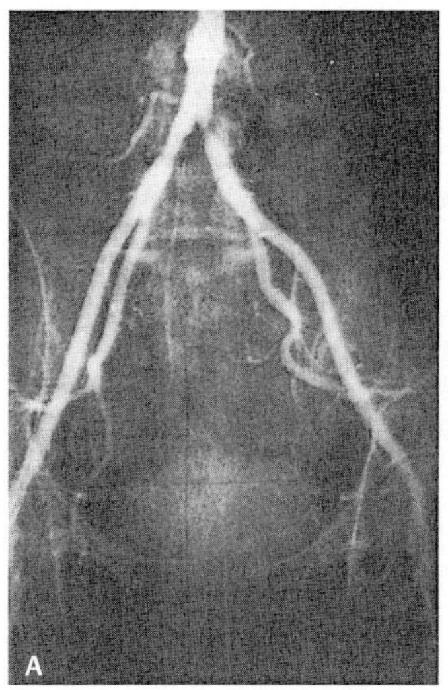

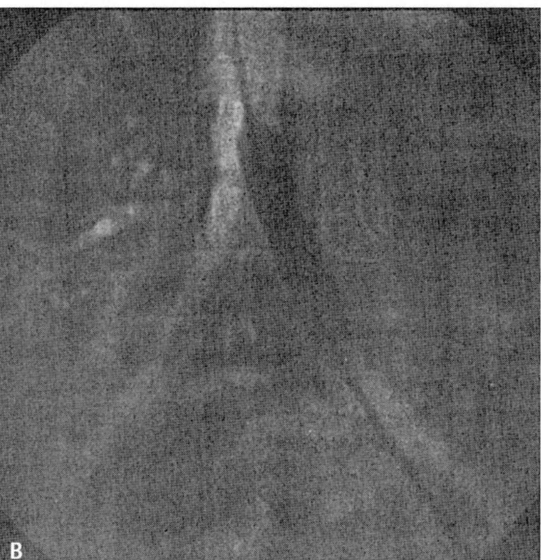

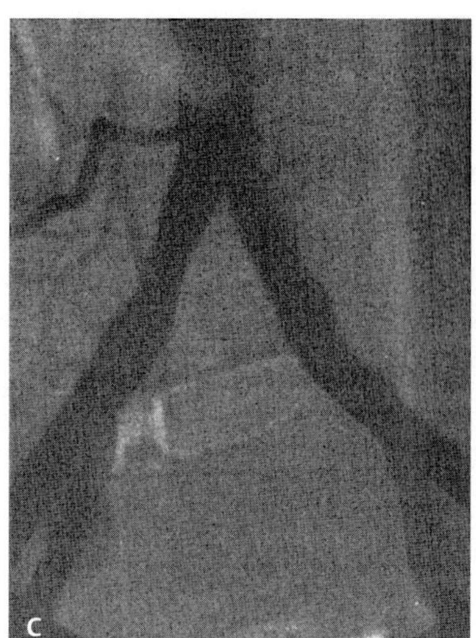

Figure 1–37 A 45-year-old man, a smoker, presented with claudication on the left. **(A)** Angiogram via the right common femoral artery demonstrates a focal moderate to severe stenosis at the origin of the left common iliac arty. A left common femoral artery puncture is performed, and pressures obtained above and below the lesion demonstrate a 40-mm mercury gradient. **(B)** Percutaneous angioplasty is performed with an 8 mm × 4 cm balloon via the left common femoral artery approach. **(C)** Postpercutaneous transluminal angiography demonstrates a residual defect with persistent pressure gradient. (From Hoppenfeld BM, Cynamon J. Vascular recanalization techniques. In: Bakal CW et al. Vascular and Interventional Radiology: Principles and Practices. New York: Thieme Medical Publishers; 2002:72. Used with permission.)

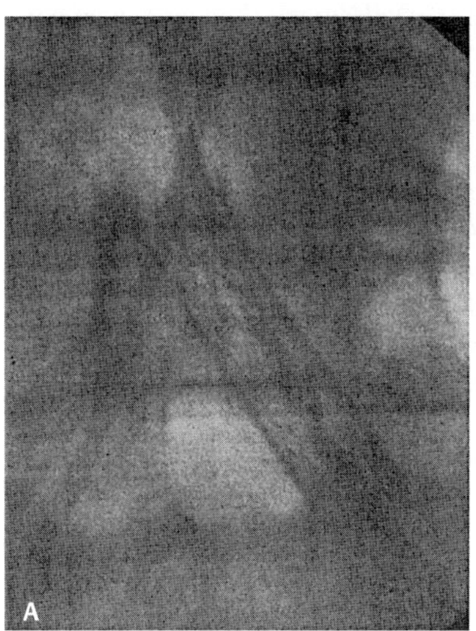

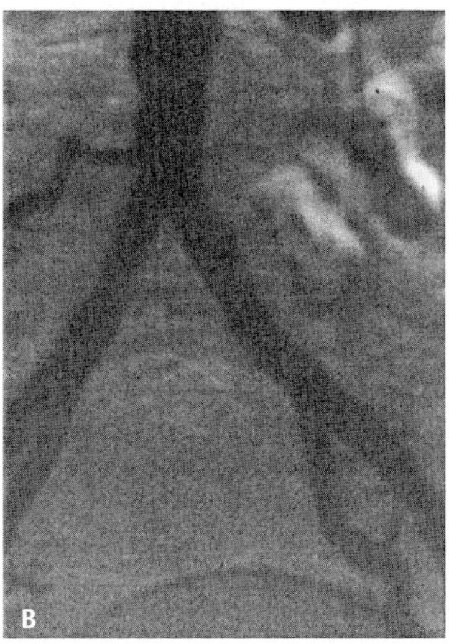

Figure 1–38 (*Continued from Fig. 1-37*) **(A)** A metallic stent is deployed across the lesion. **(B)** Poststenting angiogram demonstrates resolution of the stenosis. No further pressure gradient is observed. (From Hoppenfeld BM, Cynamon J. Vascular recanalization techniques. In: Bakal CW et al. Vascular and Interventional Radiology: Principles and Practices. New York: Thieme Medical Publishers; 2002:72. Used with permission.)

blood loss, such as prior to nephrectomy. A more recent application is uterine artery embolization, used to treat dysfunctional uterine bleeding and other problems in patients with leiomyomas ("fibroid" tumors). A variety of techniques are employed. Vasopressin may be selectively infused into an artery supplying a bleeding lesion, almost always in the GI tract, relying on its potent arteriolar vasoconstrictive activity to stop the hemorrhage. Gelfoam may be placed into the arteries supplying a bleeding lesion, which causes temporary occlusion that will become recanalized in a period of weeks. Permanent occlusive agents include alcohol, glue, coils, and balloons. The closer to the site of extravasation the vessel is occluded, the less likely infarction will result due to the presence of collaterals; the presence of collaterals, however, decreases the probability of completely halting bleeding.

Thrombolysis

Thrombolytics (literally, "clot dissolvers") such as tissue plasminogen activator (TPA) are used to declot dialysis grafts and, in some cases, to treat acute myocardial or cerebral ischemia. Contraindications include active bleeding, recent CNS surgery or cerebrovascular accident, and intracranial neoplasms. Potential complications include bleeding and the formation of emboli due to the distal migration of a partially lysed clot.

◆ Interventional Radiology

Like angiography, interventional radiology is not a distinct imaging modality, but it too plays a major role in contemporary medical and surgical therapeutics. Interventional radiology involves the use of various imaging modalities, including fluoroscopy, CT, ultrasound, and even MRI, in conjunction with equipment such as wires, catheters, needles, and endoluminal stents, to perform a variety of therapeutic procedures that were formerly either impossible or required more laborious, hazardous, and costly techniques. It should be noted that angiography and interventional radiology are closely related fields, and both are often practiced by the same subspecialists. To develop a general sense of what interventional radiology does, let us briefly review one very common interventional procedure, percutaneous abscess drainage. Other interventional procedures are reviewed in the appropriate chapters.

Abscess Drainage

Along with herniorrhaphy, incision and drainage of abscesses constitutes one of the most commonly performed surgical procedures in the world. For millennia, surgeons have recognized that drainage of pus is critical to the treatment of localized infection. In the days prior to bacteriology and aseptic technique, the flow of pus from a traumatic or surgical wound was welcomed, as it meant that the wound was beginning to heal. Absent the flow of pus, a loculus of infection had most likely developed, which in many cases would prove fatal, if not adequately drained. In contemporary medicine, abdominal abscesses and fluid collections remain a major clinical challenge. Untreated, many abscesses continue to cause death, and even in this era of effective antibiosis, drainage of such collections remains a critical component of therapy.

Surgical versus Catheter Drainage

Before such abdominal collections could be reached percutaneously, open laparotomy was the mainstay of surgical treatment, and was often necessary not only for treatment but for diagnosis. With the advent of CT scanning and ultrasound, it became possible to accurately localize and characterize such collections. Imaging made it possible to determine with a high degree of confidence whether a mass represented a solid tumor or a fluid collection, and further ascertain whether fluid collections were likely to be abscesses, based on the presence of surrounding inflammation, the thickness and contrast enhancement of the wall, and other criteria.

It soon became apparent that these imaging modalities could be used not only to find the lesions, but to guide aspiration of them as well. Percutaneous aspiration is considerably simpler, less invasive, less hazardous, and less costly than open laparotomy. A patient undergoing laparotomy for drainage of an abdominal abscess requires general anesthesia, hospitalization, a relatively long period of postoperative recovery, and a relatively expensive course of care. By contrast, percutaneous aspiration can be performed on an outpatient basis, with only local anesthesia, and the patient requires less time to recover at a fraction of the cost. If the aspiration yields pus, a percutaneous drainage catheter may be left in place to prevent or treat sepsis and allow the infectious process to resolve.

Risks of Percutaneous Drainage

The principal contraindication to percutaneous drainage is the lack of a safe route, such as the presence of major blood vessels or solid organs such as the spleen or bowel between the skin and the abscess. Transgressing the bowel and potentially seeding the abdomen with enteric contents is associated with an increased risk of peritonitis, and puncturing a major blood vessel or a vascular organ increases the risk of hemorrhage. Fortunately, the risks of both are decreased when a skinny needle, such as a 21-gauge needle, can be used. As with angiographic procedures, coagulopathies must be corrected and the usual preangiographic considerations obtain.

Procedure

The procedure is performed by positioning the patient, setting up a sterile field, using ultrasound or CT guidance to mark the skin entry point, administering local anesthesia, and then advancing the appropriate needle into the collection, using imaging to verify position. Fluid is withdrawn for Gram stain, culture and sensitivity, and special chemistry tests (e.g., amylase in a pancreatic pseudocyst). Often, the fluid is frankly purulent, and the interventionalist may proceed directly to therapeutic drainage. Using the diagnostic needle already in place, a wire is advanced through the needle, which can then be used to guide the placement of a suitable catheter, typically a 10 to 14 French catheter with multiple side holes for adequate drainage. The cavity is then aspirated, followed by irrigation with normal saline until the return is clear. It is usually desirable to evacuate the cavity completely, but the catheter is typically left to gravity drainage for routine irrigation (**Fig. 1–39**). Typically, drainage results in rapid resolution of sepsis and fevers. The persistence or recurrence of fevers after this period suggests inadequate drainage or the presence of another source of infection.

◆ Principles of Medical Imaging

Clinical Context of Medical Imaging

Uncertain or Low Probability of Pathology

Medical imaging studies are obtained for a variety of reasons. One common reason is the search for unspecified pathology. In this case, the clinician is unable to formulate a solid diagnostic hypothesis, and the imaging study is obtained in the hopes that it will uncover an anatomic or physiologic explanation for the patient's symptoms and signs. On occasion, such studies may amount to "fishing expeditions," the yield of which is often relatively low. Many cases of trauma are similar, in that the clinical suspicion of significant injury is low, but the adverse consequences of a missed diagnosis are so grave that an imaging study is obtained "just in case." Certain types of studies are less suited to this role than others. For example, ultrasound performs better as a means of testing specific diagnostic hypotheses regarding specific anatomic areas or organs, such as the right upper quadrant or the kidneys, than as a general screening test for abdominal

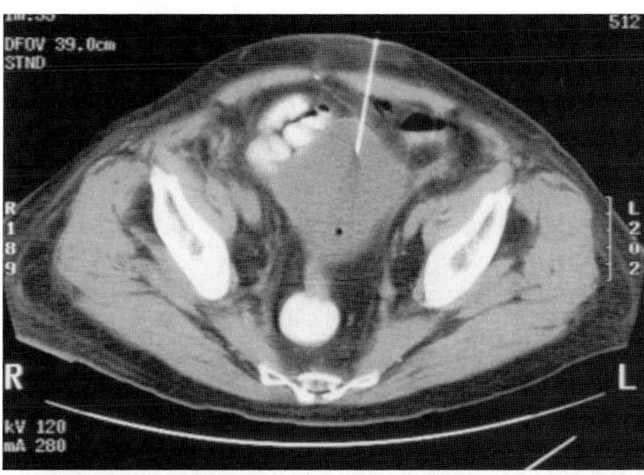

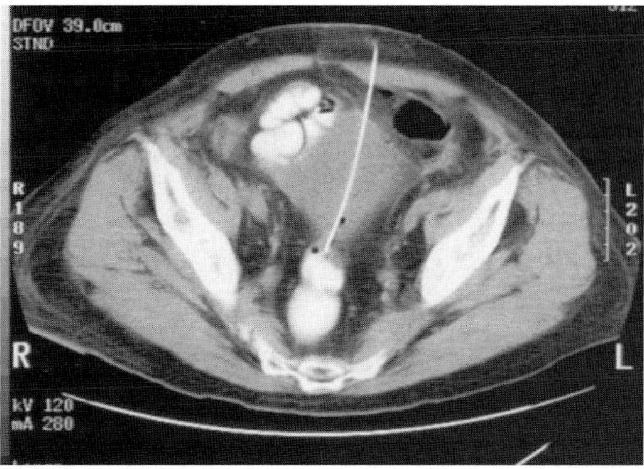

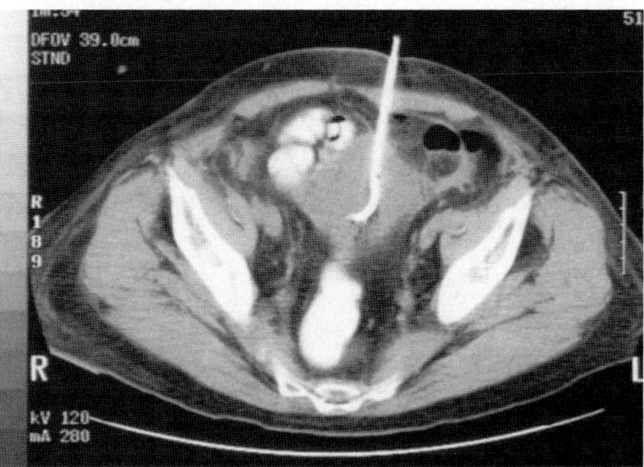

Figure 1–39 CT was used to guide biopsy of this patient's pelvic abscess. **(A)** Under CT guidance, a needle has been advanced from the anterior abdominal wall into the fluid collection. **(B)** A wire has now been advanced through the needle, and the needle is withdrawn. **(C)** A catheter with multiple side holes has been advanced over the wire, and the wire withdrawn. Pus was aspirated through the catheter, which was left in place to drain over several days. It is important to send a sample of the aspirate for microbiological analysis including Gram stain and culture and sensitivity so that appropriate antibiotic therapy can be administered.

pathology. This is true in part because the ultrasound beam can only be directed at a relatively small portion of the patient's anatomy at a time, and surveying the entire abdomen is a time-consuming and laborious process. CT, on the other hand, which naturally images the entire abdomen in a relatively short period of time, is usually better suited to the search for unspecified abdominal pathology (**Fig. 1–40**).

Known Diagnosis

Imaging studies play an important role even in cases where the diagnosis is known. From a surgeon's point of view, imaging studies may prove immensely useful in surgical planning. For example, the surgeon planning to perform laparoscopic cholecystectomy may wish to obtain a CT, ultrasound, or MRI to visualize the anatomy of the biliary tree and rule out anomalies, such as aberrant ductal anatomy, that could produce postoperative complications. Similarly, angiographic studies are often obtained as part of a routine presurgical workup in patients being evaluated as potential organ donors, to assess such factors as vascular and ductal anatomy.

Another important role of imaging in known diagnoses is the staging of malignant neoplasms (**Fig. 1–41**). Prognosis and therapeutic protocols are powerfully affected by radiologic staging of such neoplasms as lung cancer and Hodgkin's disease. Imaging also plays a major role in evaluating response to therapy. A chemotherapy protocol may be abandoned if imaging studies demonstrate continued growth of a patient's tumor; a significant reduction in tumor burden, in contrast, generally indicates that the current regimen should be continued. In the case of interventional radiology, imaging studies constitute an integral part of therapy, as when ultrasound is used to guide percutaneous abscess drainage.

Confirming or Disconfirming a Hypothesis

Perhaps the two most important reasons to obtain an imaging study are to confirm or disconfirm a diagnostic hypothesis. Consider the cases of two patients who present to the emergency room with lower extremity swelling. Each may receive a lower extremity ultrasound examination to rule out the presence of deep venous thrombosis (DVT), a potentially life-threatening condition associated with pulmonary embolism, but the reasoning behind the test in each case may be radically different. In the case of a chronically ill patient with a history of previous DVT who has recently stopped taking his or her anticoagulant medication, clinical suspicion of DVT may be very high. In this case, the study would likely be obtained primarily to confirm and localize recurrent thrombosis before an inferior vena caval

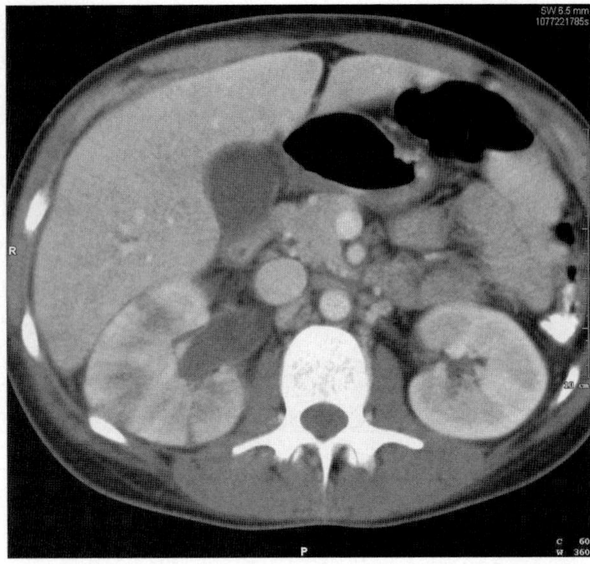

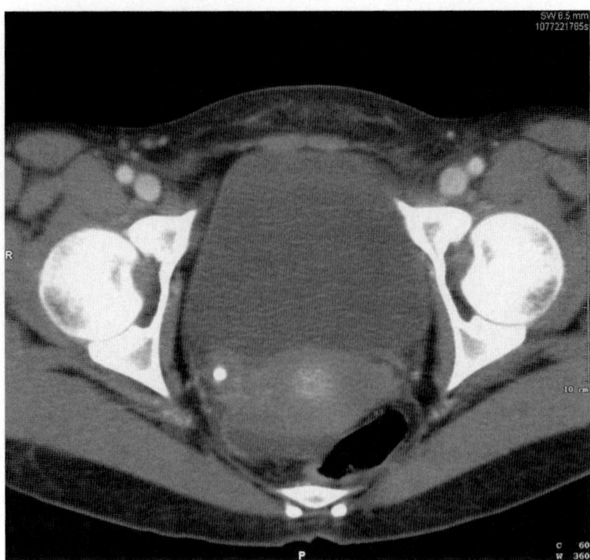

Figure 1–40 This patient presented with fever and vague abdominal pain. An abdominal CT scan with oral and IV contrast was performed. **(A)** This axial image at the level of kidneys demonstrates a swollen right kidney with multiple areas of decreased parenchymal enhancement, a so-called striated nephogram. Also, there is mild hydronephrosis. **(B)** An image at the level of the urinary bladder reveals the culprit: a kidney stone lodged in the distal right ureter, which was causing obstruction. Had the diagnosis of nephrolithiasis been clinically suspected, the exam would have been performed without IV contrast, because contrast material in the urinary tract can obscure a stone.

filter is placed (**Fig. 1–42**). In another case, that of a previously healthy patient with clinical signs of cellulitis, clinical suspicion may be quite low. In this scenario, the study is obtained to verify that no life-threatening pathology (DVT that could result in pulmonary embolism) is present before the patient is sent home on antibiotics. In the former case, the imaging study confirms a diagnostic impression before invasive therapy is instituted, whereas in the latter its purpose is to “rule out” an unlikely but life-threatening pathology. In both cases, important clinical management decisions hang in the balance.

This raises an important issue in radiology and the broader arena of diagnostic reasoning. Except in the case of medical research or teaching, imaging studies should be performed only if they are likely to affect clinical management. Both clinicians and radiologists should always remember that (1) no imaging study should be ordered unless it is likely to influence clinical management; that is, if clinical management is the same whether the test is “positive” or “negative,” then the test should not be performed; and (2) every imaging study should be performed and reported in such a way that its clinical utility is maximized. The clinician’s job is to supply the radiologist with

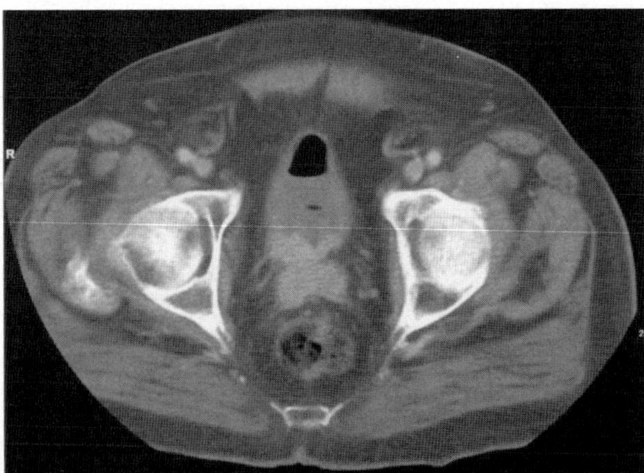

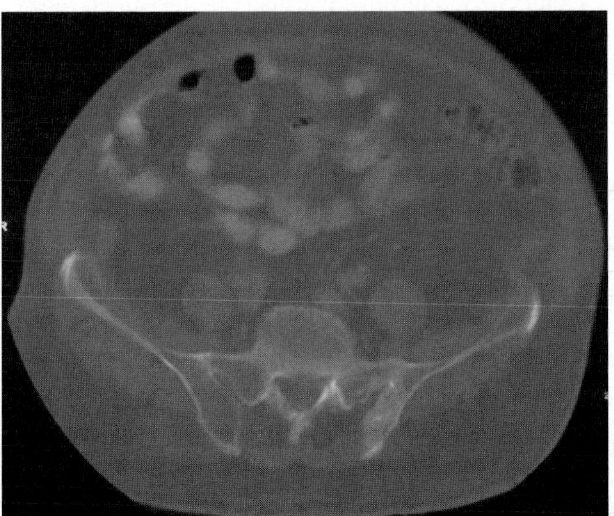

Figure 1–41 This elderly man presented with lower abdominal pain. **(A)** This soft tissue window pelvic CT image demonstrates irregular enlargement of the prostate gland and irregular thickening of the posterior wall of the urinary bladder. This was locally invasive adenocarcinoma of the prostate. **(B)** This bone-window image demonstrates an osteoblastic metastasis in the left ileum adjacent to the sacroiliac joint.

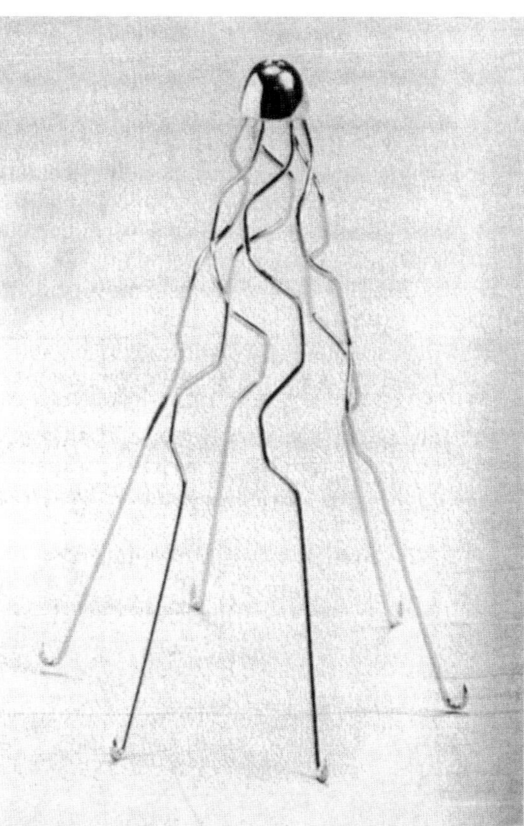

Figure 1–42 Photograph of the metallic inferior cava filter, used to prevent deep venous thrombosis from giving rise to pulmonary embolism in patients with contraindication to anticoagulation. (From Savader SJ, Trerotola SO. Venous Interventional Radiology with Clinical Perspectives, 2nd ed. p. 518, Fig. 39–8.)

the necessary information to determine whether an imaging study is indicated, which study is best suited to the circumstances, how the study should be performed (for example, with or without intravenous contrast material), and what question(s) the study is expected to answer. The radiologist's job is not to produce laundry lists of differential diagnostic possibilities, nor is it to recommend "clinical correlation" for every possible finding. Wherever possible, the radiologist's report should be clear and concise, and should answer as definitively as possible the clinical question at hand.

The Radiologic Thought Process

The radiologic thought process can be divided into three components. Students of diagnostic imaging should be familiar with each. For one thing, nonradiologists may at times need to interpret an imaging study without the immediate assistance of a radiologist. Moreover, all physicians who order imaging studies need to understand how they are performed, their different strengths and limitations, their roles in various diagnostic algorithms, and the important role of clinical information in optimizing radiologic diagnosis. By understanding these three components of the radiologic thought process, all physicians can make better use of radiology in the care of their patients.

Detection

The first component of the radiologic thought process is the detection of lesions. This is the component on which novices usually focus their attention, although detection is only a small part of radiologic diagnosis. To detect lesions, knowledge of normal anatomy and the imaging characteristics of pathologic lesions is critical (**Fig. 1–43**). Radiologists excel at lesion detection not because their eyes are better than nonradiologists', but because they understand normal anatomy and how it can be altered by various pathologic processes. It is possible to train medical students and even nonmedical personnel to detect a single lesion such as a pneumothorax just as well as radiologists, but the radiologist is able to detect dozens or hundreds of such pathologies with equal facility.

It should be emphasized that clinical information often plays a crucial role in the detection of lesions. For example, suppose a patient presents to the emergency room complaining of severe pain in a digit following a fall. It is vital that the referring physician furnish relevant information to the radiologist regarding the patient's clinical presentation. For one thing, the radiologist may suggest a different study based on this information. The clinician may reason that hand

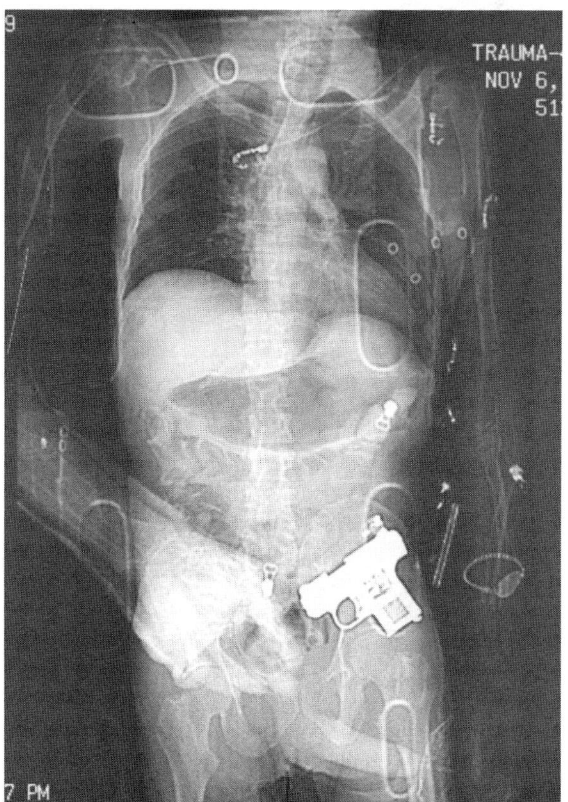

Figure 1–43 In some cases, the detection of abnormalities on radiologic images requires no special expertise. This man was injured in an automobile accident and was brought to the radiology department for an abdomen/pelvis CT scan. A "scout" CT image demonstrates an obvious and somewhat alarming finding: a handgun in the patient's left hip pocket. Hospital security staff was summoned to the CT suite before any additional imaging was performed.

radiographs would be the best examination, because they not only show the digit in question, but also help to rule out other unsuspected fractures, thus "killing two birds with one stone." However, a hand radiograph is less sensitive than a finger radiograph in detecting a finger fracture. Moreover, additional views of the digit may need to be obtained. The clinician's mission is not to "stump" the radiologist, because failure to detect a lesion reflects unfavorably on both the clinician and the radiologist. Rather, the radiologist and the clinician should work together, enhancing one another's performance to optimize patient care. What would be an inadequate history in this situation? Examples include "Rule out fracture" or "Pain after fall." By contrast, a good history would be "Point tenderness in middle phalanx of fourth digit after fall."

Description

The second component of the radiologic thought process is the description of the finding. An accurate description is vital to good radiologic practice, because it is often not possible to make a definitive diagnosis based solely on the radiologic findings, and the correct differential diagnosis hinges on accurate characterization of the lesion. Only when the finding is accurately described is it clear which differential diagnostic possibilities warrant strongest consideration. For example, determining whether pulmonary opacities seen on high-resolution CT are "ground glass," reticulonodular, or nodular in character powerfully influences the appropriate differential diagnosis. This is true not only in radiology but throughout medicine, as when an accurate description of a patient's chest pain determines whether such diverse possibilities as myocardial ischemia or esophageal spasm is the more likely explanation.

Several key elements should be present in most descriptions of radiologic findings. These include the location of the lesion, its extent or size, and its general imaging characteristics (**Fig. 1–44**). The latter includes general descriptors such as the clarity of its borders and its general morphology (round, stellate, cavitary), as well as more specific radiologic descriptors such as density (CT), echogenicity (ultrasound), signal intensity (MRI), and its enhancement after the administration of contrast material.

One of the cardinal signs of a first-rate physician is the ability accurately to describe a patient's problem. Not only should the description be precise, it should also be pertinent, in the sense that it highlights the most salient aspects of the lesion. Once an accurate description is in hand, it provides a benchmark against which to weigh diagnostic hypotheses, to determine which provides a better fit.

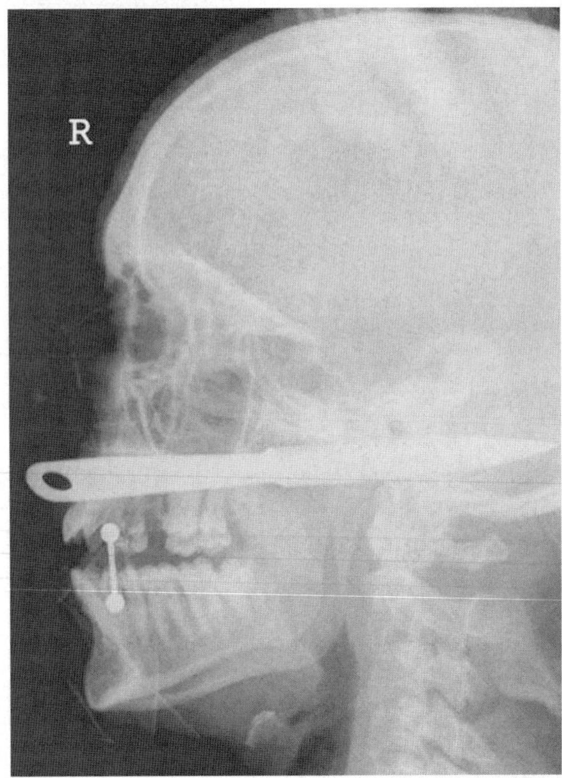

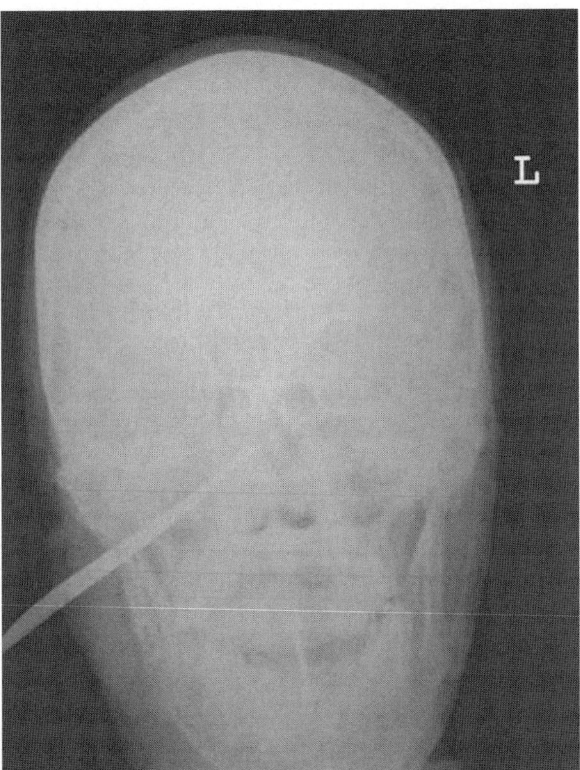

Figure 1–44 **(A)** This lateral skull radiograph demonstrates two foreign bodies that are brighter (and therefore denser) than bone. The first is dumbbell shaped and appears to span the teeth of the upper and lower jaw. The second more cephalad foreign body has an ovoid lucency at its left end and comes to a point on the right. Two critical questions come to mind. First, are these objects inside the patient or merely beside the patient? Second, what are they? **(B)** This frontal radiograph proves both are in the patient, because they overlap the head on two orthogonal (right-angle) projections. The first object is a tongue ring. The second is a knife, embedded in the patient's posterior fossa.

Differential Diagnosis

The third and final component of the radiologic thought process is the production of a differential diagnosis (**Fig. 1–45**). One crucial factor in differential diagnosis that can hardly be overemphasized is clinical history. Only a minority of radiologic findings are pathognomonic (from Greek roots for "disease" and "to know"), meaning that the imaging findings alone indicate the diagnosis. In most cases, the radiologist can at best generate an ordered list of likely explanations for a particular radiologic finding, which will be powerfully influenced by clinical factors. In the case of a segmental opacity on a chest radiograph, such clinical clues as whether the patient is febrile, whether the illness is acute or chronic, and whether the patient is immunologically compromised will exert a powerful effect on the differential diagnosis the radiologist constructs.

There is no single magic formula for producing an adequate differential diagnosis for the myriad radiologic findings that may arise in a dozen or more organ systems; however, it is possible to outline a general approach to differential diagnosis by which to order one's thoughts, thereby ensuring that major pathologic categories are at least considered. The mnemonic acronym is CITIMITV.

◇ Congenital

This category is especially important in pediatrics, but it should be considered in adults as well. It includes heritable disorders, developmental anomalies, and anatomic variants that can be mistaken for pathology. Examples include cystic fibrosis, developmental dysplasia of the hip, and a bicuspid aortic valve. Approximately 3% of newborns have a major malformation, accounting for about one quarter of deaths in the neonatal period, but many congenital malformations, such as a bicuspid aortic valve, are not detected until adulthood, and many patients with heritable disorders such as cystic fibrosis now survive well into their adult years. The remainder of the items on this list consist of acquired disorders (**Fig. 1–46**).

◇ Inflammation

Some degree of inflammatory response is associated with all forms of cell and tissue injury, helping to isolate the injurious agent and setting into motion the healing process; however, this category is meant to include noninfectious disorders that manifest themselves primarily through an inflammatory response, either acute or chronic. An example of an inflammatory disorder in the musculoskeletal system is rheumatoid arthritis, in which the underlying pathology is

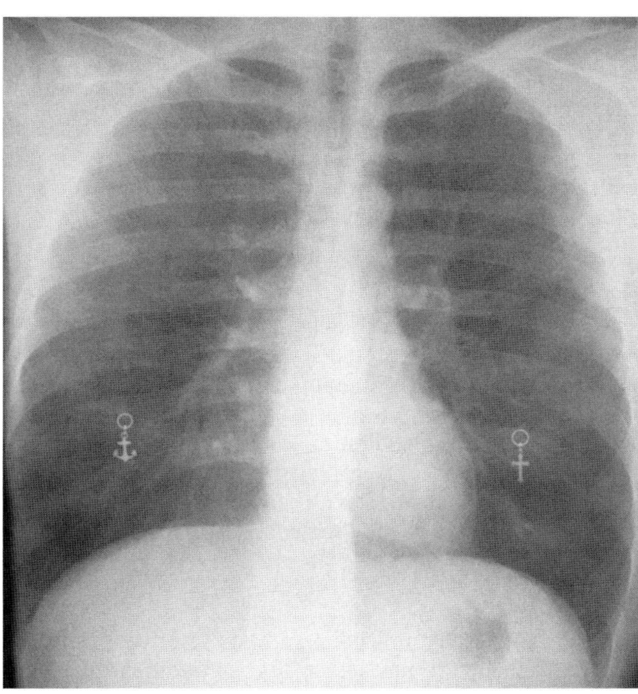

Figure 1–45 What, if anything, can we infer about the patient based on the findings on this frontal chest radiograph? First, the absence of breast shadows suggests the patient is probably male. Overlying both midlungs are metallic artifacts composed of circular rings connected to what appears to be a replica of a ship's anchor on the right and a cross on the left. These represent nipple rings. Is the patient a Christian sailor, or is he expressing his distaste for evangelicals and maritime commerce? Unfortunately, no additional clinical information was available. The lungs were, however, interpreted as clear.

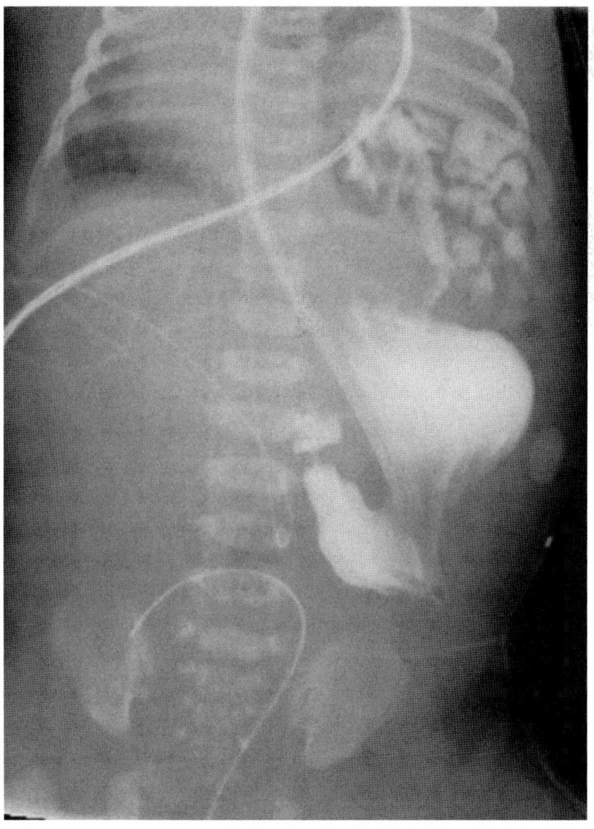

Figure 1–46 This radiograph of a newborn's lower chest and abdomen was obtained following injection of low-osmolar contrast through the orogastric tube. The stomach is normally positioned, but the proximal small bowel is in the left hemothorax in this patient with a congenital diaphragmatic hernia.

synovitis. Another example of a primarily inflammatory disorder is the various forms of vasculitis that can cause lesions in any organ system of the body. Many of these disorders, including both rheumatoid arthritis and vasculitides such as systemic lupus erythematosus, are immunologic in nature.

◇ Tumorous

From the Latin for "swelling," tumor simply implies an abnormal growth. From a differential point of view, two distinctions must be drawn. First, a tumor may be benign or malignant. In the case of a smooth, round lung nodule discovered on chest radiography, one would need to include in the differential diagnosis benign tumors such as a hamartoma, as well as malignant tumors such as an adenocarcinoma. The second distinction is between primary and metastatic lesions, which vary in relative frequency depending on the organ involved. In the case of the brain, primary malignancies are somewhat more common than metastases, whereas in the skeleton metastases outnumber primary malignancies by a factor of more than 50:1. In many cases, tissue biopsy is necessary to establish a definitive diagnosis. The importance of this differential diagnostic category is reflected in the fact that cancer is the leading killer of adults under the age of 85 in the United States, resulting in approximately one quarter of all deaths, or 575,000 deaths per year.

◇ Infectious

In 1900 the leading cause of death in the United States was infectious diseases, which now rank well down the list; however, it is worth recalling that the roles of infectious agents in human pathology are still being elucidated; for example, it was only in 1983 that human immunodeficiency virus (HIV) was identified as the agent underlying acquired immunodeficiency syndrome (AIDS) and *Helicobacter pylori*'s role in chronic gastritis was proved. Major categories of infectious disease include viral, bacterial, and protozoal disorders, among others. The immune status of the host is an important factor, because atypical or opportunistic infections become much more likely in the setting of impaired host response. Generally, clinical factors such as fever and an increased leukocyte count will favor an infectious etiology.

◇ Metabolic

Metabolic disorders relate to the endocrine system, nutritional disorders, and ion balance. Examples include diabetes, rickets, and osteoporosis. In many cases, laboratory test results are crucial in establishing the diagnosis.

◇ Iatrogenic

From the Greek meaning "physician-caused," iatrogenic disorders result from medical interventions. Examples include cystitis from bladder catheterization, and drug reactions such as bleomycin-induced interstitial lung disease. Certain findings in hospitalized patients such as pneumothorax (from central venous catheter placement) and small bowel obstruction (from postsurgical adhesions) are more often due to medical interventions than any other cause (**Fig. 1–47**).

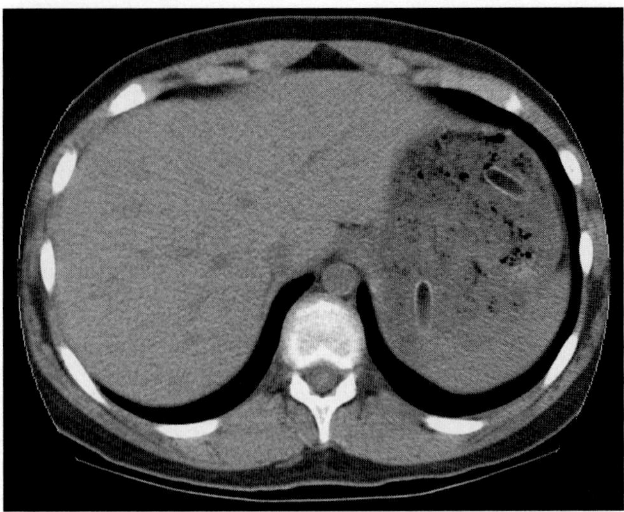

Figure 1–47 This axial CT image demonstrates two bright-rimmed central-low-density ovoid lesions in the gastric lumen, which is otherwise filled with the patient's lunch. Are they parasites? No. They are medication capsules.

◇ Traumatic

In the United States, trauma is the most common cause of death under the age of 34, acounting for over 150,000 deaths annually. The leading setting is motor vehicle accidents, although violence and falls are major contributors. Usually a history of trauma is obvious, but in some cases, such as a bone lesion that could reflect remote trauma, questioning may be required; otherwise, a healing avulsion fracture could be mistaken pathologically for an osteosarcoma. The possibility of intentional trauma should not be overlooked, particularly in the pediatric setting, because the radiologist may be the only physician who sees direct evidence of child abuse.

◇ Vascular

The vascular category includes the number 1 and number 3 causes of death in the United States, coronary artery disease and stroke, as well as pulmonary embolism. Findings as diverse as edema, hemorrhage, infarction, and shock may all be traced to vascular etiologies. The fact that inflammation is clearly a major factor in many cases of acute thrombosis of atherosclerotic plaques serves as an important reminder that these pathologic categories frequently overlap.

Radiologic Error

Error is a topic too rarely addressed in medicine, perhaps in part because both physicians and patients have vested interests in its infallibility. Generally, radiology is probably even less forgiving of error than other specialties. If an internist fails to pick up a subtle breast nodule on physical examination, the existence of the finding is unlikely to be noted anywhere in the patient's medical record. A year later, when the nodule has grown into a mass, no one can be certain that the nodule was even present or large enough to be detectable when the initial physical examination was

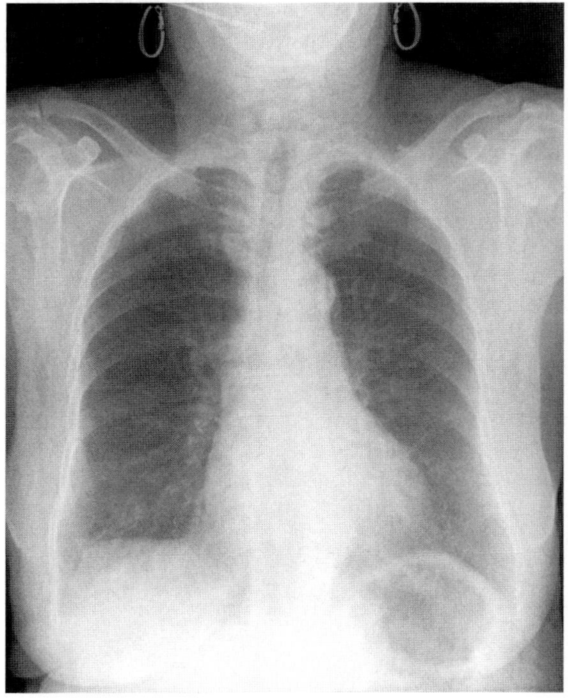

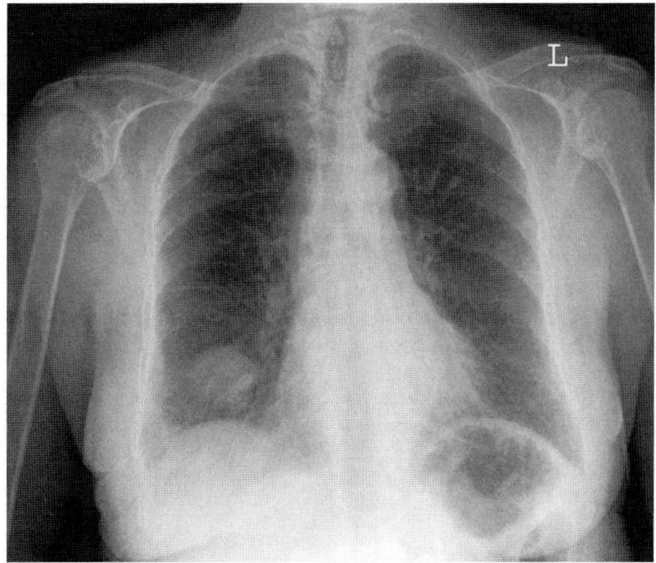

Figure 1–48 This elderly woman presented with a cough. **(A)** Her chest radiograph was interpreted as showing no pneumonia. **(B)** When she returned a year later with worsening cough, a mass was detected in the right lung base. In retrospect, a smaller nodule is visible in this location on the previous exam.

performed. By contrast, when a radiologist reading a mammogram misses subtle microcalcifications associated with a breast carcinoma, he or she has nowhere to hide. The microcalcifications will be on the image and available for detection by any physician (or malpractice attorney) by whom the study is subsequently reviewed. Failure to detect an incidental abnormality such as a cervical rib is of no clinical significance, whereas failure to detect a small primary lung carcinoma may deprive the patient of the opportunity for a curative resection (**Fig. 1–48**).

The purpose of studying radiologic error is not to assign blame, but to improve performance. The three most common types of error are search errors, recognition errors, and decision-making errors.

Search errors occur when radiologists fail to fixate their central vision on the area of the image where the abnormality lies. These errors include so-called corner signs, in which the abnormality is at the periphery of the image. To avoid search errors, it is necessary to inspect each portion of the image. This typically involves ~100 gaze fixations (each lasting a fraction of a second) for a single chest radiograph. A junior medical student will typically perform fewer fixations, centered on only a portion of the film—often the brightest areas (e.g., the heart on a chest radiograph) and regions with high-contrast borders. An experienced radiologist, on the other hand, will distribute gaze fixations more evenly and will pay attention to darker and lower-contrast regions of the image as well (**Fig. 1–49**).

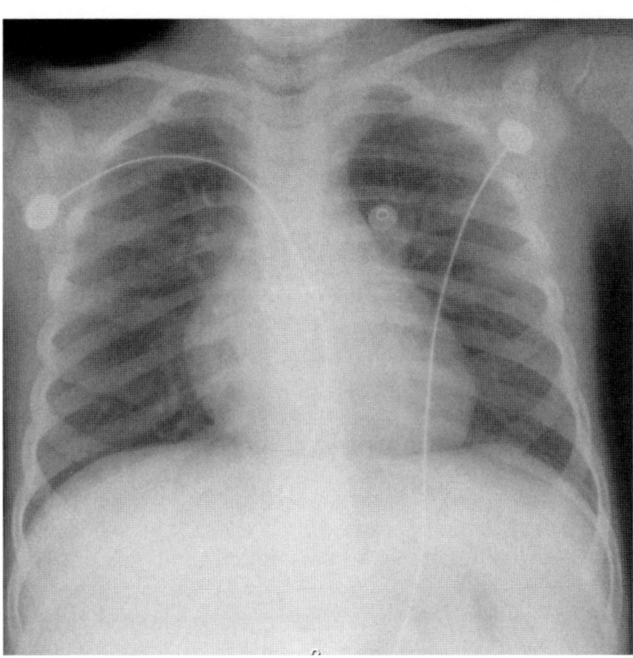

Figure 1–49 This child presented with cough and respiratory distress. The chest radiograph was interpreted as showing clear lungs. However, there is a "steeple sign" of croup at the top of the image, with the tracheal air column gradually tapering toward the glottis, rather than demonstrating an abrupt narrowing, which is normal. It is important to remember to inspect anatomy at the edges of an image.

One of the most important steps to improving radiologic performance is taking care to search each image adequately. One of the most common errors in this regard has been called "satisfaction of search." This is defined as the decreased probability of finding additional abnormalities once an abnormality has been correctly identified. Once the radiologist has found something wrong, he or she immediately launches into a discussion of that abnormality, having prematurely terminated the search through the remainder of the image. This is an especially common error among neophytes, who often have difficulty finding any abnormality, and are so pleased with themselves when they do that they stop looking further. Another potential pitfall is the simple failure to devote adequate search time to each image. Of course, most radiological examinations consist of more than one image, and many, including most cross-sectional imaging studies such as CT and MRI examinations, may contain dozens or even hundreds of images.

Recognition errors occur when an abnormality is scanned but not appreciated as an abnormality. To recognize an abnormality requires not so much visual acuity as visual memory. The radiologist is comparing this image against a mental background composed of many thousands of similar visual experiences, against which the finding either does or does not stand out. Recognition differs between different people, depending on the depth and character of their previous experience. To perform well at recognition requires an understanding of normal radiologic anatomy and the myriad ways in which various disease processes may manifest themselves.

Decision-making errors may account for slightly over one half of all errors in radiologic diagnoses. In these errors, an abnormality is both scanned and recognized, but rejected as "noise" or a normal variant. Again, an experienced visual memory and an understanding of anatomy and pathophysiology may serve as the crucial factors in avoiding such errors. In addition, clinical information may play an important role in helping the radiologist to properly evaluate the significance of such findings.

2

The Circulatory System: The Heart and Great Vessels

◆ Anatomy and Physiology

Some of the greatest figures in the history of medicine and biology, including Aristotle, Galen, and Vesalius, never knew that the blood circulates through the body. William Harvey (1578–1657), perhaps the greatest English-speaking physician in history, was the first person to prove conclusively that the blood moves away from the heart through the arteries and back to the heart through the veins, and that the heart itself is the pump responsible for the blood's motion. However, despite his great triumph, even Harvey died having left a critical piece in the circulatory puzzle unfilled, namely, how the blood moves from the arteries to the veins. It was Marcello Malphigi, using the newly developed microscope, who demonstrated the existence of capillaries (from the Latin for "hair").

The circulatory (from the Latin *circulari*, "to form a circle") system transports gases, nutrients, waste products, cells, hormones, and a variety of other substances throughout the body. It may be divided into two components, the exchange portion and the conduction portion. At any moment, only ~5% of the blood is found in the portion of the circulatory system where exchange of materials between the blood and the extracellular fluid takes place, the capillaries. Nearly all of the 75 trillion living cells in the mature human body that are not bathed in blood are located within a few cell diameters of a capillary. The capillaries allow passive diffusion of metabolites to take place simultaneously over a very short distance and a very great surface area. The capillary walls themselves are only 0.1 micron (μ) thick (an erythrocyte is 8 μ in diameter), increasing the rate at which substances may diffuse across them. It is estimated that the total surface area available for metabolite exchange in the body's 40 billion capillaries is 600 m^2. With some notable exceptions, exchange of metabolites between the blood and the extracellular fluid occurs by passive diffusion, propelled by differences in concentration.

The other component of the circulatory system, the conduction portion, functions by active bulk flow, with the heart serving as the pump and the arteries, arterioles, venules, and veins serving as conduits. The conduits are not merely passive vessels, however, as the elastic recoil of the aorta is important in sustaining forward blood flow in diastole, and the relaxation/contraction of the arterioles is critical in distributing blood flow between different organs and tissues. The right ventricle supplies the low-pressure, low-resistance pulmonary circulation, and the left ventricle supplies the high-pressure, high-resistance systemic circulation. Whereas the pulmonary circuit consists of a single pathway, the systemic circuit is actually comprised of several pathways (cerebral, coronary, mesenteric, etc.) arranged in parallel (**Fig. 2–1**). The difference in workload is manifest in the different thicknesses of the two ventricles, with the free wall of the left ventricle measuring ~1.3 cm in thickness, and that of the right 0.3 cm. The four valves permit blood to flow in only one direction through the heart (**Fig. 2–2**). Approximately 1% of cardiac muscle cells, including those in the sinoatrial (SA) and atrioventricular (AV) nodes, are autorhythmic, specialized for initiating and conducting the action potentials responsible for cardiac contraction.

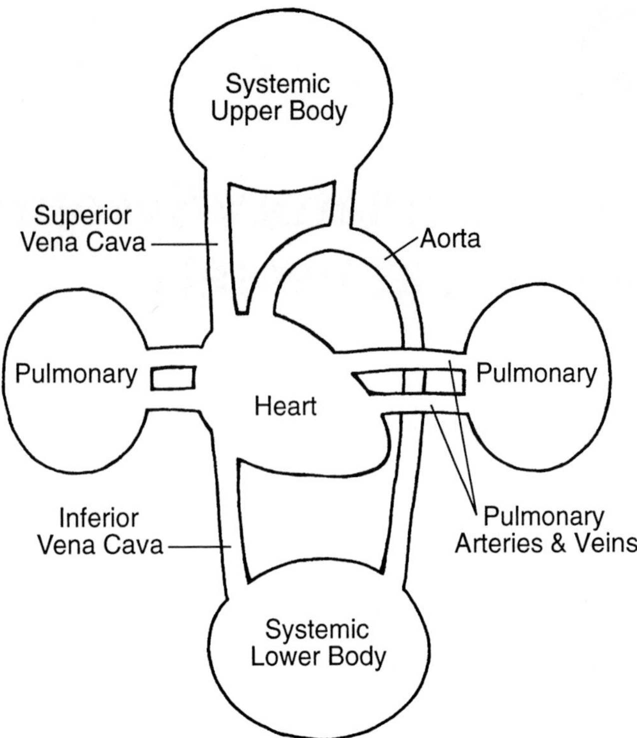

Figure 2–1 Whereas the pulmonary circulation may be conceptualized as a single circuit, the systemic circulation consists of multiple circuits arranged in parallel.

The embryonic heart begins to beat around 3 weeks after conception and over the course of a normal life span, contracts ~3 billion times, 100,000 times per day. Cardiac output is the product of stroke volume and heart rate. The normal cardiac output of 5 L/min may be increased during exercise by as much as 8 times in highly trained athletes. Stroke volume, the amount of blood ejected from the ventricle with each contraction, is determined primarily by the end-diastolic volume. The Frank-Starling law of the heart states that the heart pumps all the blood returned to it; the more blood placed in the ventricle before it contracts, the greater its stroke volume. This both balances the output of the right and left sides of the heart and allows a rapid response to increased circulatory demands. During exercise, for example, increased skeletal muscle contractions and faster and deeper breathing increase venous return to the heart. Sympathetic stimulation can further increase stroke volume by augmenting contractility, with a resultant increase in the ejection fraction (the ventricle squeezes out a greater proportion of the blood that fills it during diastole).

Heart rate is influenced primarily by autonomic input to the SA node. Parasympathetic stimulation decreases the rate of depolarization of the SA node, whereas sympathetic stimulation not only increases the SA node's rate of depolarization, but also increases the excitability of the AV and conduction pathways. In addition, sympathetic stimulation increases contractility. As the heart rate begins to exceed 220 beats per minute, the time available for ventricular filling decreases to such a degree that cardiac output actually declines.

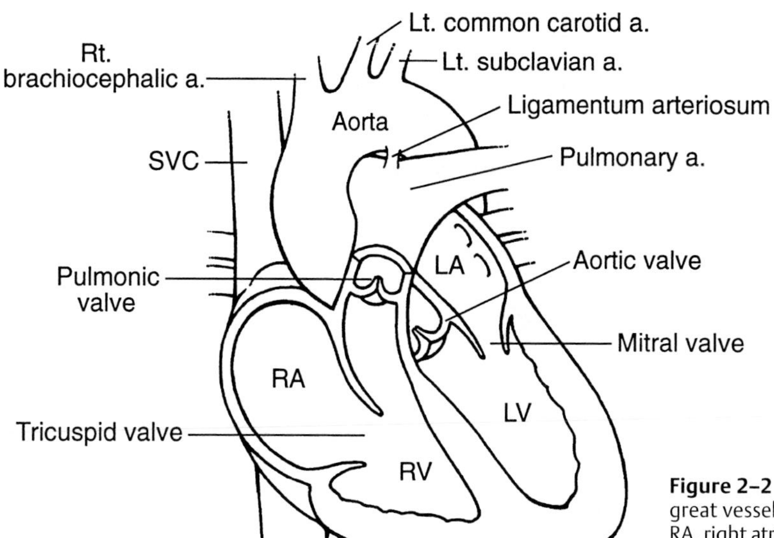

Figure 2–2 The four valves of the heart and their relationships to the great vessels. IVC, inferior vena cava; LA, left atrium; LV, left ventricle; RA, right atrium; RV, right ventricle; SVC, superior vena cava.

The heart's blood supply is the first to branch off from the aorta, with the coronary arteries (from the Latin *corona,* "crown") arising just above the aortic valve and the coronary veins returning blood to the right atrium (**Fig. 2–3**). Because of the high wall tension generated by the left ventricle during systole, ~70% of coronary blood flow occurs during diastole, propelled by the elastic recoil of the aorta (**Fig. 2–4**). This marks another reason that tachycardia ("fast heart") poses a threat to life: the percentage of time the ventricle spends in diastole decreases with increasing heart rate. Normally, increased myocardial activity produces vasodilation of the coronary arteries and increased myocardial blood flow, but the balance between myocardial consumption and coronary supply may be tipped in favor of ischemia (a term coined by

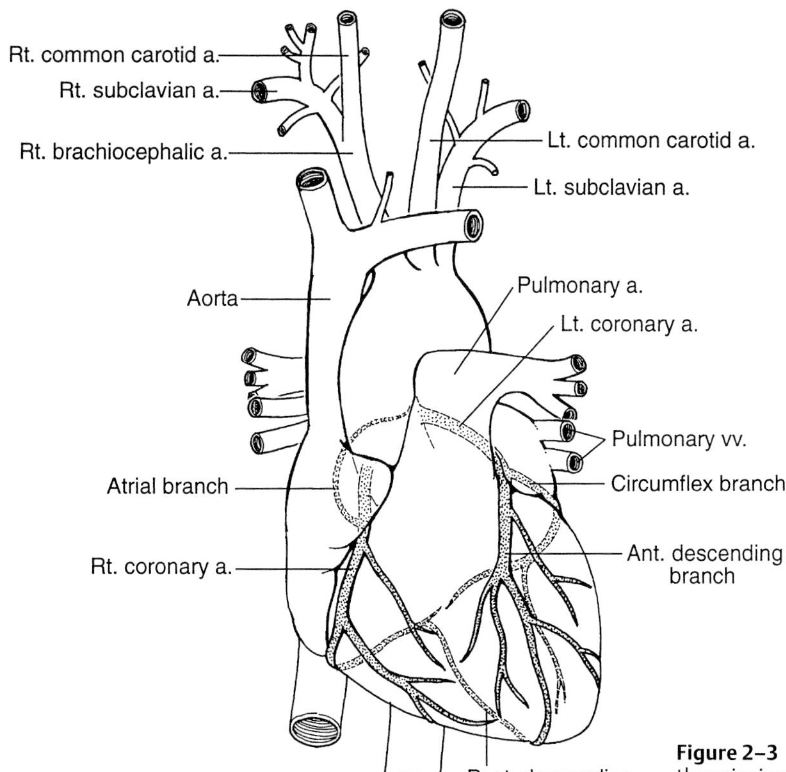

Figure 2–3 This diagram of the heart and great vessels also illustrates the principal branches of the coronary arteries arising from the aorta just above the aortic valve.

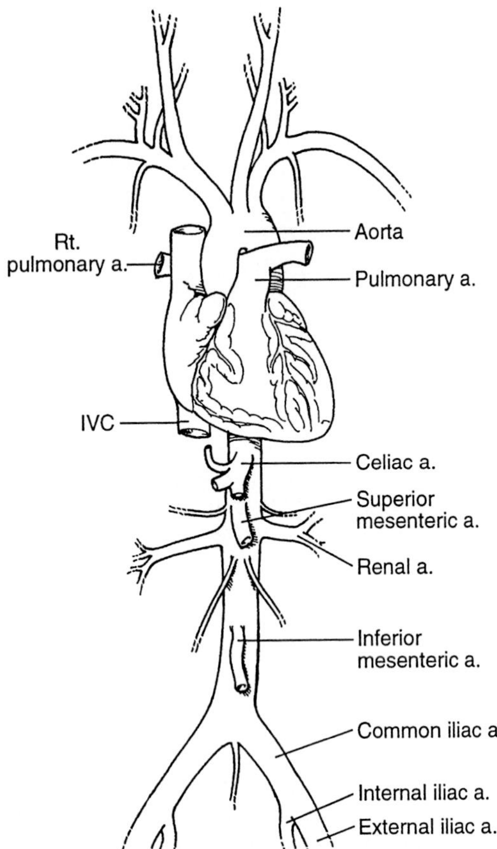

Figure 2–4 The aorta and its major branches. Note that a catheter inserted into one of the femoral arteries could be advanced upward through the aorta and into the mesenteric arteries, the brachiocephalic vessels, the coronary arteries, or the cardiac chambers themselves. This technique is employed in mesenteric angiography, cerebral angiography, coronary angiography, and cardiac angiography, respectively. IVC, inferior vena cava.

Rudolf Virchow from the Greek roots for "holding back" and "blood") by atherosclerotic disease, thrombosis, or vascular spasm.

The major resistance vessels are the arterioles, whose smooth muscle lining can be alternately tensed or relaxed to alter perfusion of a particular organ or tissue. An example of this mechanism is active hyperemia, in which increased carbon dioxide production in an area causes relaxation of arteriolar smooth muscle, with an increase in arteriolar radius, a decrease in arteriolar resistance, and increased perfusion of the area. Nonlocal modulators of blood pressure include both the nervous and endocrine systems, with the sympathetic nervous system playing a key role.

Most of the blood in the body, ~60% at rest, is found in the veins (**Fig. 2–5**). Veins serve as very low pressure conduits to return blood to the heart and contain valves that permit flow in only the cardiopetal (toward the heart) direction. Negative thoracic pressure during inspiration, the squeezing of veins during skeletal muscle contraction, and the very low or even negative intraluminal pressure of the right atrium (due to reexpansion of the right ventricle during diastole) are all forces that favor blood return.

◆ Imaging Modalities

A variety of modalities are available for cardiac imaging, each with distinctive strengths and weaknesses. Determining which study is most appropriate to a particular clinical situation requires a knowledge of these strengths and weaknesses, as well as an understanding of the particular clinical question to be answered.

Radiography

The chest radiograph, often obtained for other reasons (e.g., "rule out pneumonia"), provides a wealth of information about the heart. Although hypertrophy often produces little or no radiographic change, significant dilatation of cardiac chambers should be radiographically detectable on routine upright posteroanterior (PA; the x-ray beam enters from the patient's back and strikes the cassette in front of the patient) and lateral chest radiographs. When further information is required about specific chambers, oblique views may be helpful, although these are now only rarely obtained. On a PA view, the right heart border is made up by part of the right atrium, the upper left heart border is made up by part of the left atrium, and the mid and lower left heart borders represent the left ventricle. The right ventricle, which is located anteriorly, is not seen. On the lateral view, the right ventricle makes up the anterior border of the heart, the left atrium makes up the posterosuperior border, and the left ventricle is the posteroinferior border.

Enlargement of each chamber produces a predictable change in appearance. Right ventricular enlargement causes filling in of the retrosternal clear space on lateral views. Right atrial enlargement is the most difficult to assess but may cause bulging of the right heart border. Left ventricular enlargement causes the heart to bulge downward and to the left on the frontal view, and posteroinferiorly on the lateral view. Left atrial enlargement is manifest as a bulge below the pulmonary artery on the PA projection, as well as posterior displacement of the esophagus on the lateral view (best appreciated when the esophagus contains barium). When left atrial enlargement becomes pronounced, it may lift up the left mainstem bronchus. A guide for determining whether the heart is enlarged on an anteroposterior (AP) radiograph is the cardiothoracic ratio, the ratio of maximum width of the heart to the maximum width of the thorax. Normally, this ratio is less than 0.50. Etiologies of an increased cardiothoracic ratio other than true cardiomegaly include an expiratory radiograph and the presence of a pericardial effusion (**Fig. 2–6**).

The chest radiograph also provides information about pulmonary blood flow, with increased perfusion manifesting as increased diameter of the affected vessels. In the case of decreased flow, as in pulmonary embolism (PE), normal vasculature may be diminished or absent. Increased pulmonary vascular pressures manifest differently, depending on whether the veins or arteries are affected. Signs of pulmonary venous hypertension include enlargement of mediastinal veins such as the azygous vein; redistribution of pulmonary blood flow from the lower to the upper lung zones; perivascular edema, with associated loss of vessel

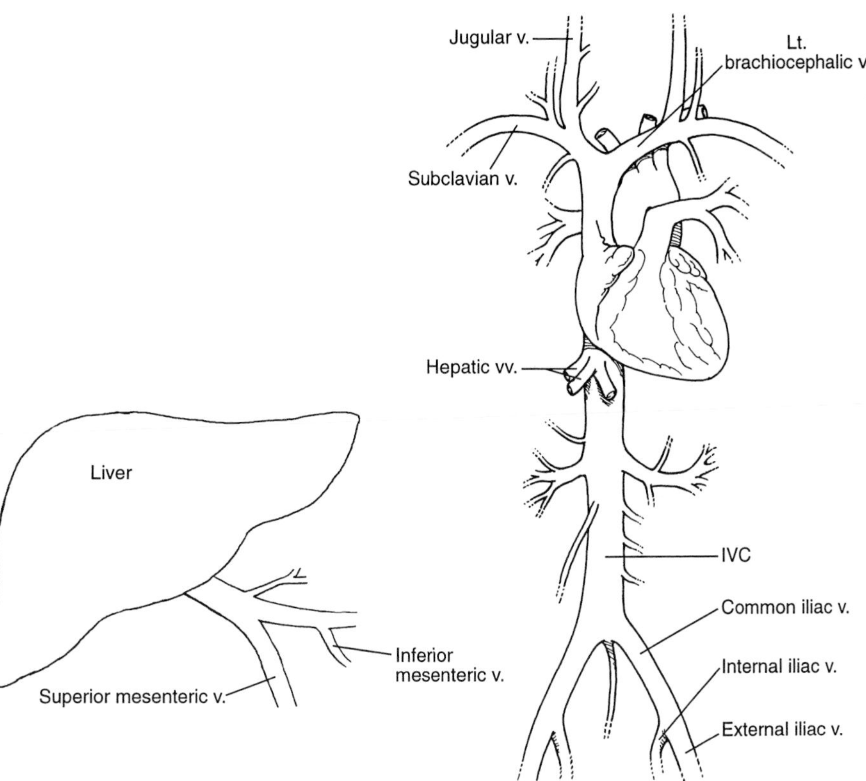

Figure 2–5 The major veins through which blood is returned to the heart. Note that a catheter inserted into the femoral vein could be advanced up through the right atrium, the right ventricle, and into the pulmonary arteries, as when a catheter pulmonary arteriogram is performed. Of course, this could also be accomplished with a catheter inserted into a neck or arm vein, as well. IVC, inferior vena cava.

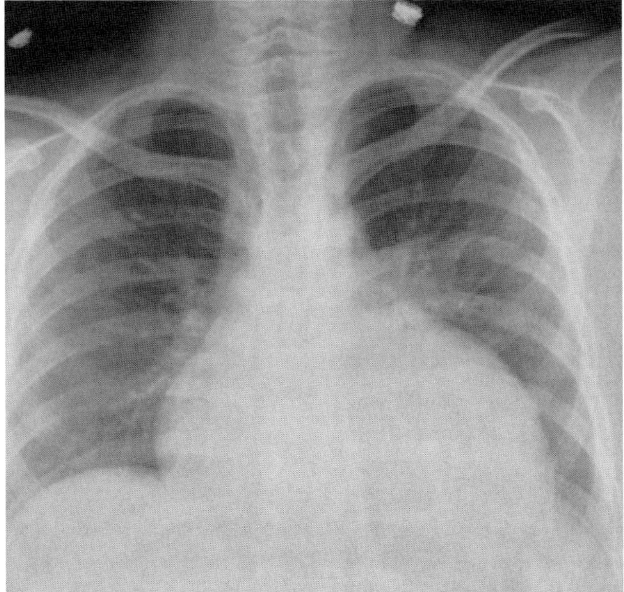

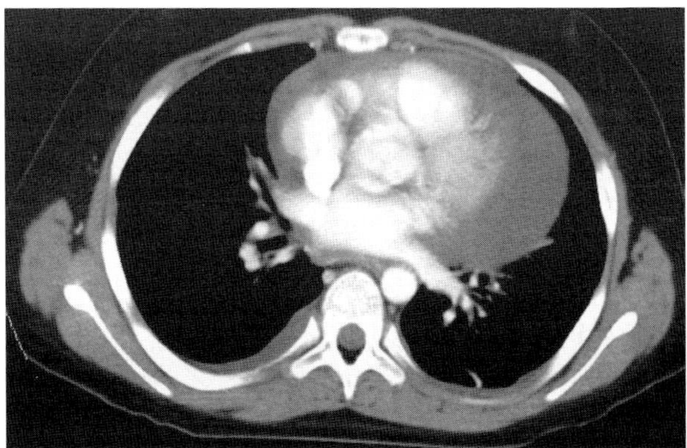

Figure 2–6 **(A)** This frontal chest radiograph demonstrates an increase in the cardiothoracic ratio, meaning that the cardiac silhouette comprises more than one half the width of the chest. Is the heart actually enlarged, or is this a mimic of cardiomegaly, such as a pericardial effusion? **(B)** This axial CT image of the chest at the level of the heart demonstrates fluid surrounding the heart, as well as a small right pleural effusion. The heart itself is actually normal in size. The effusions were due to acute histoplasmosis.

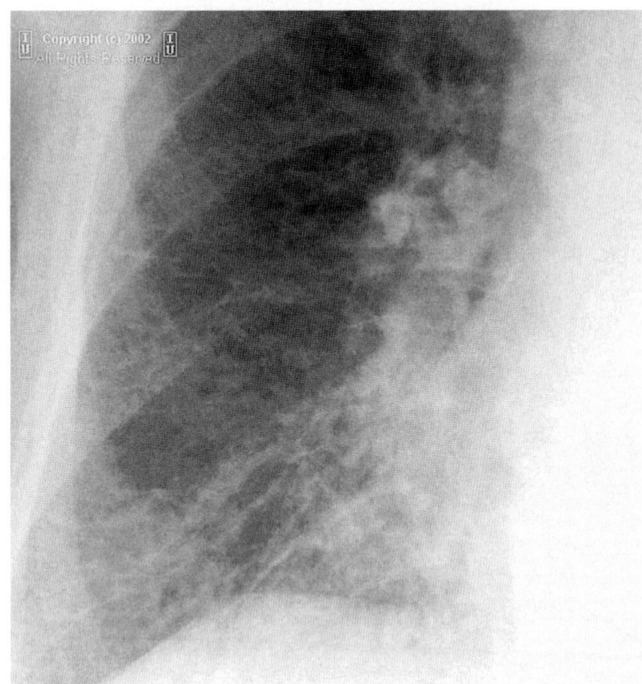

Figure 2–7 This detailed view of the right lung base of a patient in congestive heart failure demonstrates central air-space edema (fluffy, cloudlike opacities) and more peripheral interstitial edema (nodular and linear opacities). Note also several 1 to 2 cm horizontal lines at the lung periphery. These are septal lines, also known as Kerley B lines, a classic finding of pulmonary venous hypertension, most commonly due to left heart failure.

definition and subsequent development of peribronchial cuffing (fluid around the bronchi); septal lines (Kerley A lines and B lines); and frank air-space opacities, as fluid accumulates within the alveoli (**Fig. 2–7**). Pulmonary arterial hypertension produces central dilatation of the pulmonary arteries, which may be accompanied by peripheral pruning of vessels, especially when increased arteriolar resistance is the cause.

Assessment of overall cardiac size and chamber contour is less reliable on portable radiographs, which are usually obtained with the patient in varying degrees of recumbency and in the AP projection (the cassette is placed under the supine patient's back, and the x-ray beam enters from above the patient). As one would expect, the AP film tends to exaggerate the cardiac silhouette (the heart's shadow), because the greater the distance between a shadow-casting object and the screen on which its shadow is cast, the larger its shadow appears (**Fig. 2–8**). Moreover, patients who require portable films are usually sicker (which is why they cannot come to the radiology department), and hence less able to take a deep breath. The resultant underinflation is another common cause of apparent cardiomegaly, because the heart is not as stretched out along the craniocaudal axis. For these reasons, caution is warranted in assessing cardiomegaly on portable films. Furthermore, redistribution of pulmonary vascular flow from the lower lung zones to the upper lung zones cannot be diagnosed on a supine film, where it represents a normal finding (due to the loss of the gravitational gradient favoring flow to the lower lung zones).

Angiography

Coronary angiography, generally performed by cardiologists, is used to assess coronary artery disease. A catheter is usually placed into the femoral artery, advanced up through the aorta into the aortic root, and into the coronary arteries themselves. Often cannulating a particular artery requires the use of a specialized catheter, shaped to facilitate the particular maneuver being attempted. All catheter manipulation is performed under fluoroscopic monitoring, as is contrast injection. Cine films are obtained to allow the assessment of contrast flow patterns over time. Angiography visualizes only

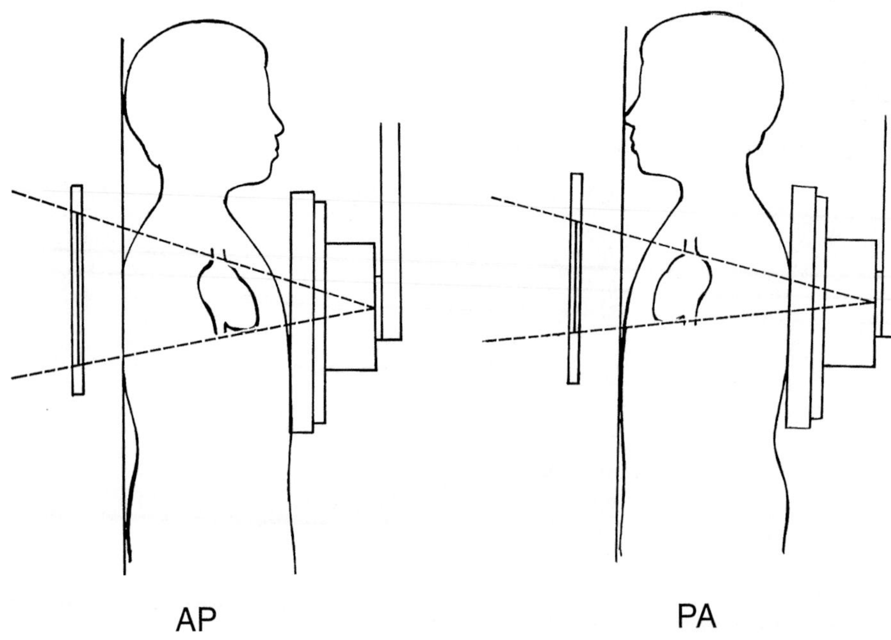

Figure 2–8 The effect of anteroposterior (AP) and posteroanterior (PA) chest radiographic technique on the size of the cardiac silhouette. The closer the heart is to the film, the less the degree of magnification, which makes the PA view the preferred technique for the assessment of cardiomegaly.

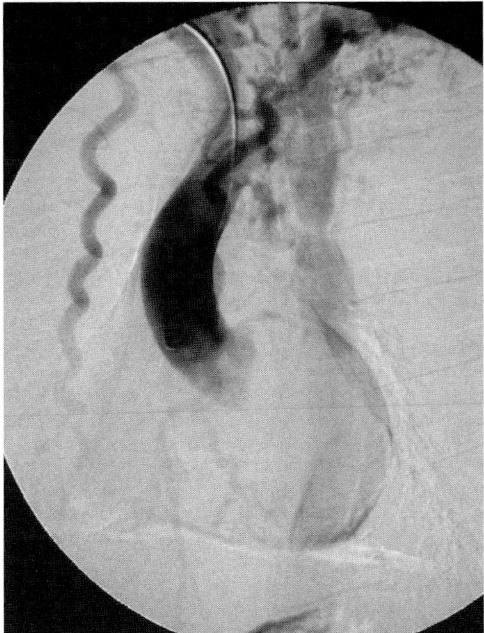

Figure 2–9 This 7-year-old boy presented with hypertension, as well as higher blood pressures in his upper extremities than his lower extremities. A digital subtraction arteriogram was performed, with catheterization of the aortic root via the right upper extremity. A frontal image demonstrates tight stenosis of the aorta just distal to the takeoff of the left subclavian artery. Note the prominent collateral vessel, the right internal mammary artery, which has enlarged in an attempt to bypass the coarctation.

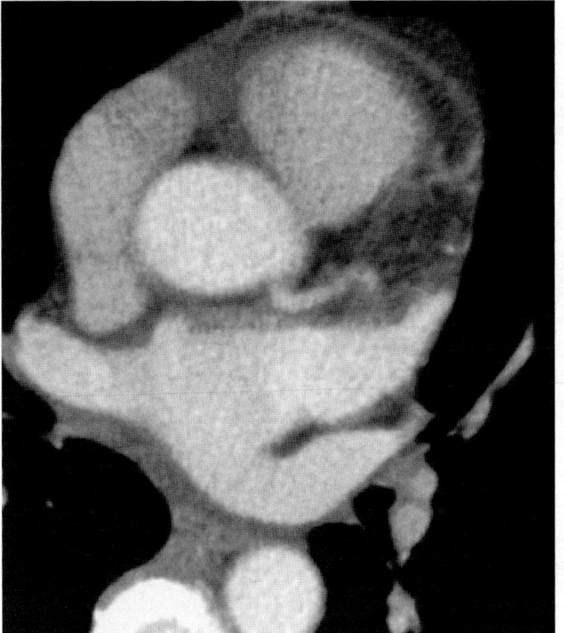

Figure 2–10 This axial image from a contrast-enhanced CT scan of the chest, with a close-up view of the heart, beautifully demonstrates the takeoff of the left main coronary artery from the left side of the aortic root.

the contrast opacified lumen of the vessel and does not provide direct visualization of the vascular wall itself (**Fig. 2–9**); however, it is often possible to infer the nature of vascular pathology based on angiographic findings, such as the presence of a focal outpouching within an area of luminal narrowing, indicating an ulcerating plaque. As CT scanners have become faster, CT arteriography is playing a growing role in evaluation of the coronary circulation (**Fig. 2–10**).

Computed Tomography

Computed tomography is playing an increasing role in cardiac imaging. Cardiomegaly, hypertrophic changes, pericardial disease, and coronary artery calcifications are frequently diagnosed on routine thoracic CT examinations obtained for other reasons (**Fig. 2–11**). Calcium scoring involves the use of CT to screen for coronary artery calcifications, a sign of coronary artery disease. Ultrafast CT, which can complete data acquisition in 0.10 or 0.20 of a second, can eliminate the problem of cardiac motion and be used in cine format to observe the changes in morphology accompanying the cardiac cycle. Examples of uses for ultrafast CT include the assessment of morphologic and functional wall abnormalities associated with myocardial infarction. These include lack of wall thickening with systole and the presence of ventricular aneurysms. Ultrafast CT may also be helpful in assessing pericardial disease, such as restrictive pericarditis, and in the determination of the patency of coronary artery bypass grafts.

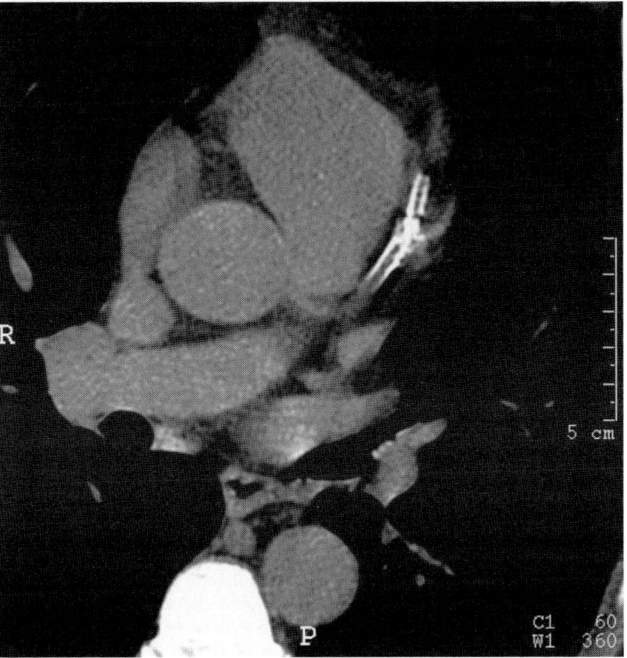

Figure 2–11 This CT image of the heart obtained without contrast infusion demonstrates severe, tram-track atherosclerotic calcification in the left coronary artery.

Echocardiography

Echocardiography, examination of the heart using ultrasound, is generally performed by cardiologists. The heart and great vessels are imaged in three different modalities. M mode, the first to be developed, produces a linear image of the changes in

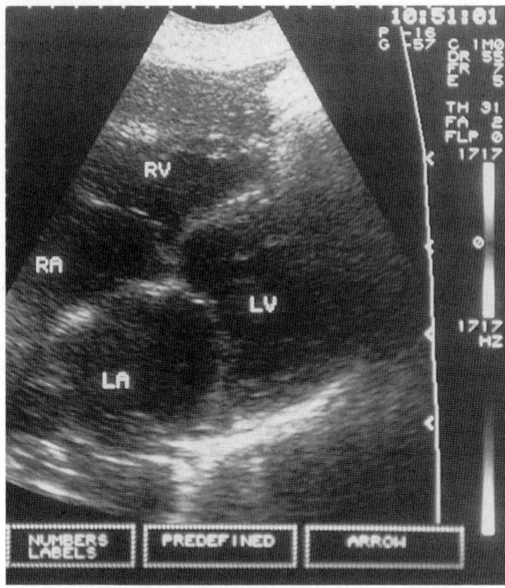

Figure 2–12 A "four-chamber" ultrasonographic view of the heart obtained via a transthoracic approach reveals the four cardiac chambers, as well as the mitral and tricuspid atrioventricular valves. LA, left atrium; LV, left ventricle; RA, right atrium; RV, right ventricle.

position of cardiac structures over time. As an example, M mode enables the assessment of changes in the position of valve cusps over milliseconds, because thousands of pulses are sent and received by the transducer each second. Using grayscale imaging, it is possible to produce two-dimensional "slice" images of the heart, which may be obtained via a transthoracic approach or from a transesophageal position, using a transducer mounted on the end of a flexible endoscope (**Fig. 2–12**). Finally, the Doppler technique enables the assessment of flow velocity and turbulence. Using the Bernoulli equation (pressure in mm Hg = $4v^2$, where v is velocity expressed in m/s), pressure changes can be estimated noninvasively.

Echocardiography is the imaging modality of choice in the evaluation of valvular heart disease, where abnormalities of valve morphology, thickness, and motion can be readily detected. Stenosis manifests as abnormally high velocity across a valve, and regurgitant flow manifests as flow in the wrong direction (e.g., blue signal when red is expected). Moreover, echocardiography permits assessment of the left ventricle, including chamber size, wall thickness, and function. It is useful in the diagnosis of the various types of cardiomyopathy (dilated, restricted, and hypertrophic). Pericardial effusions as small as 10 to 20 mL (**Fig. 2–13**) and cardiac masses, such as myxomas and rhabdomyosarcomas, are readily detected. Finally, the heart may also be stressed and visualized on echocardiography to assess exercise-related changes in wall contractility and ejection fraction.

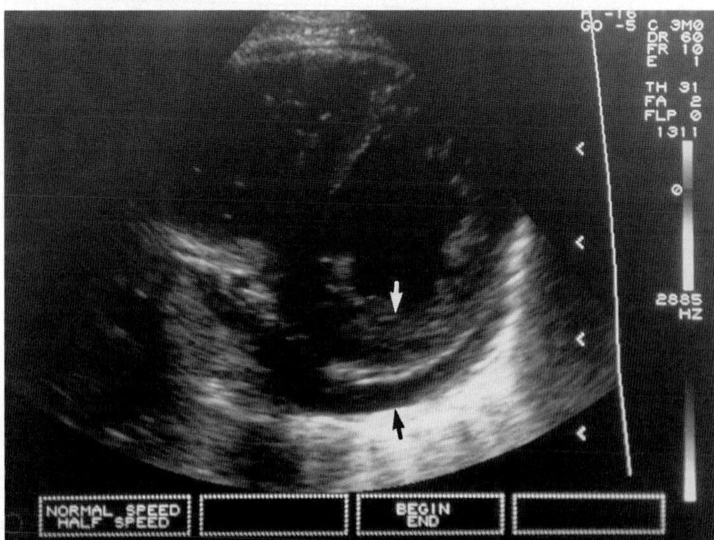

Figure 2–13 An axial sonogram of the heart reveals a rim of fluid outside the posterior wall of the left ventricle (black arrow), representing a pericardial effusion, as well as thickening of the left ventricular wall itself (white arrow).

Nuclear Cardiography

Nuclear cardiography relies on the injection of radiotracer substances whose anatomic and physiologic localization provides information about cardiac structure and function. Acute myocardial infarctions can be diagnosed using labeled pyrophosphate compounds, which bind irreversibly to molecules in damaged myocardial cells and appear as "hot spots" on scintigraphy. Myocardial perfusion imaging relies on the fact that certain molecules, such as the potassium analogue thallium 201 and newer technetium agents, are taken up by myocardial cells in proportion to regional blood flow. Ventriculography using labeled red blood cells provides assessment of cardiac size and function, with measurement of the cardiac ejection fraction. Positron emission tomography (PET) can be used to evaluate regional cardiac perfusion and metabolism.

Magnetic Resonance Imaging

Like echocardiography, MRI employs no ionizing radiation or contrast agents. Because data acquisition takes longer in MRI than in CT, cardiac and respiratory gating is essential. On conventional sequences, flowing blood appears as a signal void (black), although other "bright blood" sequences are also often employed. MRI is used to provide multiplanar imaging of cardiac anatomy and physiology, as well pathology, including aneurysms and thrombi, congenital heart disease, and aortic disease, such as dissecting aneurysms. MRI can be used to assess morphology throughout the cardiac cycle, averaging data acquisitions over hundreds of heartbeats to produce views at each phase (**Fig. 2–14**).

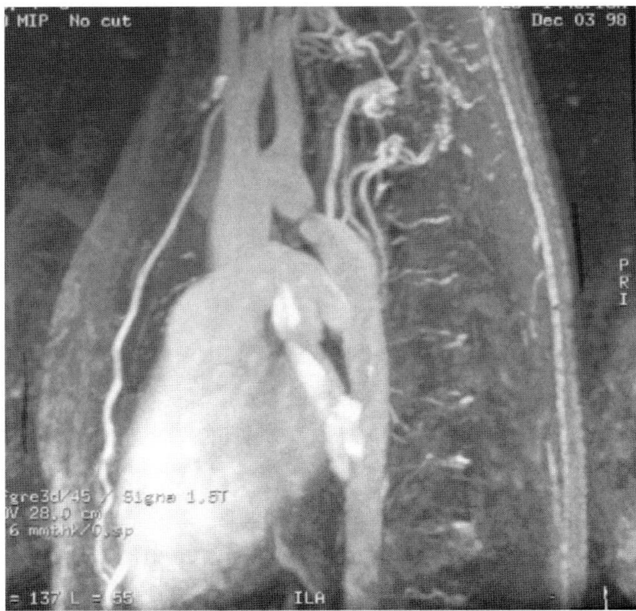

Figure 2–14 This "bright blood" oblique sagittal MR image of the aorta demonstrates a coarctation distal to the takeoff of the left subclavian artery, with prominent collateral vessels arising above the level of the stenosis. Magnetic resonance imaging can display flowing blood without the use of intravenous contrast.

◆ Heart

Pathology

Congenital

Congenital heart disease is discussed in Chapter 10.

Infectious

The pulmonary valve is rarely affected by noncongenital disease processes, leaving the mitral, tricuspid, and aortic valves as the principal sites of valvular heart disease. This discussion will focus on involvement of the mitral and aortic valves in rheumatic heart disease. The mitral valve consists of the anulus fibrosus, the valve cusps, the chordae tendineae, and the papillary muscles. In diastole, the valve opens as atrial pressure exceeds ventricular pressure, whereas in systole, when ventricular pressure exceeds atrial pressure, the valve cusps close to prevent regurgitation. The aortic valve, which has no distinct anulus fibrosus, opens when left ventricular pressure exceeds aortic pressure in systole and closes in diastole as ventricular pressure falls. Blood is then trapped in the sinuses of Valsalva, from which it enters the coronary arteries and perfuses the heart, propelled by the elastic recoil of the aorta. The surface area of the mitral valve is approximately twice that of the aortic valve, 5 versus 2.5 cm^2 (**Fig. 2–15**).

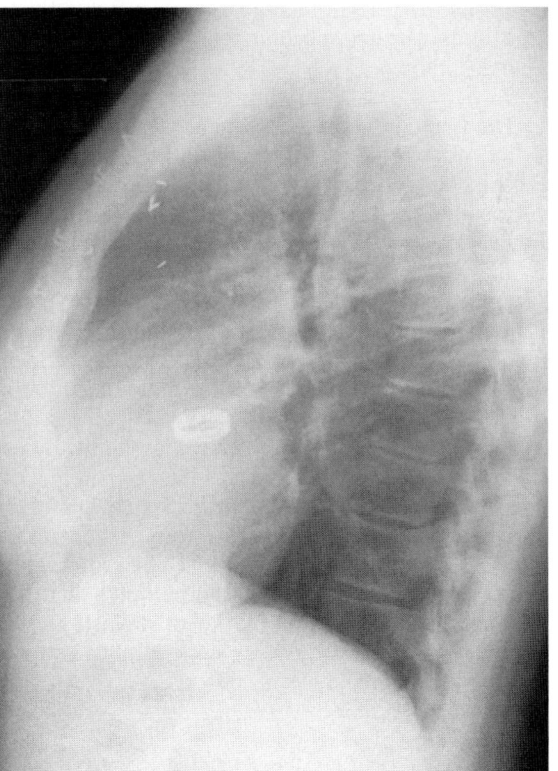

Figure 2–15 This lateral chest radiograph demonstrates multiple sternal wires and surgical clips in the anterior mediastinum. What is the ring-like metallic density overlying the heart? It represents a prosthetic aortic valve, placed to correct this patient's severe valvular aortic stenosis.

◇ Rheumatic Heart Disease

Epidemiology By far the most common cause of acquired valvular heart disease is rheumatic fever, a systemic inflammatory process associated with infection by group A β-hemolytic streptococcus and an ensuing autoimmune response. A small percentage of patients with epidemic streptococcal pharyngitis go on to develop rheumatic fever. Of patients who develop rheumatic fever, approximately one third develop the sequelae of rheumatic heart disease, with complications from valvular heart disease occurring decades later. In the United States, 99% of mitral stenosis is due to rheumatic heart disease

Pathophysiology When rheumatic fever involves the heart, all cardiac layers are affected, including the endocardium, myocardium, and pericardium. This contrasts with bacterial endocarditis, which involves the inner layer alone. The pathology of rheumatic heart disease stems primarily from fibrosis of the valve cusps and chordae, which may cause both stenosis (from fusion of the cusps) and regurgitation (from retraction of cusps and chordae). Most commonly affected is the mitral valve, which exhibits isolated involvement in two thirds of cases. Another one quarter of patients will exhibit a combination of mitral valve and aortic valve involvement. Isolated involvement of the aortic valve is uncommon.

Clinical Presentation More than 9 out of 10 patients develop rheumatic heart disease between the ages of 5 and 15 years. Following the streptococcal pharyngitis by weeks, symptoms and signs of rheumatic fever include migratory polyarthritis of the large joints, carditis, subcutaneous nodules, erythema, and Sydenham's chorea.

Imaging The hemodynamic consequences of stenosis and regurgitation, as well as their imaging findings, are all predictable, based on physiologic principles. Stenosis of a valve produces proximal pressure overload. In the case of the aortic valve, the heart responds with left ventricular hypertrophy, which manifests as thickening of the wall (detectable by cross-sectional imaging such as ultrasound) without radiographically detectable evidence of cardiomegaly. Stenotic valves are often calcific, and these calcifications may be identifiable on chest radiographs. Insufficient or regurgitant valves produce volume overload of cardiac chambers both proximal and distal to the lesion, with radiographically detectable dilation. With progressive cardiomegaly, there is often progressive distortion of the supporting framework of the valve, which further aggravates regurgitation. In contrast to stenotic valves, insufficient valves rarely exhibit radiographically detectable calcifications. It should be noted that diseased valves often exhibit a combination of stenosis and insufficiency; for example, nearly every stenotic valve will also regurgitate to some degree.

◇ Mitral Stenosis

Epidemiology Mitral stenosis, the most common form of acquired valvular heart disease, afflicts women twice as often as men and represents the most common cause of death in rheumatic heart disease.

Pathophysiology As fibrosis progresses and the mitral valve orifice is reduced by 50% (normal area is 4–6 cm^2), an increased left atrial–left ventricular pressure gradient is required to propel blood into the left ventricle. Left atrial failure and dilation may ensue. Once the valve orifice reaches 1 cm^2, a 25 mm Hg gradient is required, and the increased left atrial pressure causes increased pulmonary venous and capillary pressures and reduced pulmonary compliance. It also causes pulmonary venous hypertension, with right-sided pressure overload, right ventricular hypertrophy, and eventual right ventricular failure.

Clinical Presentation Symptoms and signs usually develop in approximately 2 decades and include exertional dyspnea, episodes of acute pulmonary edema, atrial fibrillation, and hemoptysis. On physical examination, the classic diastolic murmur includes accentuation of the first heart sound (due to snapping shut of the stenosed valve) and a middiastolic rumble (due to regurgitant flow across the valve). Once the patient becomes seriously symptomatic, death follows within 2 to 5 years unless the stenosis is relieved.

Imaging Radiographic findings include an initially normal-sized heart. The mitral valve itself is frequently calcified, and left atrial enlargement can often be detected, with elevation of the left main bronchus, a "double density" over the right atrium, and enlargement of the left atrial appendage. Another radiographic finding of left atrial enlargement is posterior displacement of the esophagus and left mainstem bronchus on barium swallow, because the left atrium forms the posterosuperior border of the heart. In advanced cases, the left atrium itself may calcify, although the high kilovoltage technique of contemporary chest radiography makes this difficult to detect. Once right ventricular failure occurs, signs of right ventricular enlargement, such as filling in of the retrosternal clear space, begin to be detected. The condition is invariably accompanied by signs of pulmonary venous hypertension.

Radiographic findings vary depending on the severity of increased pulmonary venous pressure. At pressures up to 20 mm Hg, cephalization of pulmonary blood flow is seen, with increased caliber of upper versus lower lung zone pulmonary vessels. Although the normal upper-to-lower vessel diameter ratio is ~1:3, in pulmonary venous hypertension it approaches 1:1, and may even reverse to some degree. This is thought to stem from predominantly basilar perivascular edema (see the discussion of Starling forces in the section on pulmonary edema), with reflex vasoconstriction and redistribution of blood flow to the upper lung zones. At pressures between 20 and 25 mm Hg, interstitial edema ensues, with plasma accumulating in the interstitium faster than pulmonary lymphatics can clear it. Once the pressure exceeds 25 mm Hg, alveolar edema results, with air-space infiltrates and pleural effusions.

Chronic pulmonary arterial hypertension manifests radiographically as enlargement of the arterial roots, with a paucity of peripheral lung vascular markings, the so-called pruned tree appearance.

Treatment of early mitral stenosis initially consists of penicillin prophylaxis, avoidance of physically strenuous activities, avoidance of volume overload, and treatment of atrial fibrillation. As the disease progresses and the valve orifice approaches 1 cm^2, mitral valvulotomy is generally indicated, which often results in striking symptomatic improvement and improved survival. This may be performed via cardiotomy, or percutaneously via a fluoroscopically guided balloon catheter. If valvulotomy is not sufficient, as in a patient with a significant component of regurgitation, prosthetic valve replacement may be necessary, using either a bioprosthetic or mechanical valve. Patients with mechanical valves must be maintained on anticoagulants indefinitely, due to their increased thrombogenicity.

◇ Mitral Insufficiency

Epidemiology Although rheumatic heart disease is the most common cause of mitral insufficiency, other causes include infectious endocarditis, papillary muscle rupture, and mitral valve prolapse.

Pathophysiology Regardless of the cause, valvular insufficiency results in regurgitant flow of blood into the left atrium during left ventricular systole. As expected, the left atrium and left ventricle both dilate, as both must accommodate both normal and regurgitant volumes with every cycle. Typically, the left atrium dilates more than the left ventricle, and mitral insufficiency is associated with the so-called giant left atrium. The giant left atrium is associated, in turn, with atrial fibrillation, with increased risk of thromboembolism leading to problems such as stroke. Cardiac function is generally not severely affected, because the condition develops gradually, and the left ventricle is able to accommodate the increased volume with little or no increase in end-diastolic pressure. Likewise, the left atrium simply expands, without an increase in pressure, and so the pulmonary edema and hemoptysis seen in mitral stenosis are relatively rare.

Clinical Presentation Chronic mitral regurgitation is a relatively benign condition, in which only a fraction of patients ever become symptomatic. Of all the left-sided lesions, it is the best tolerated; however, in acute mitral insufficiency, which may be seen in infective endocarditis or myocardial infarction with papillary muscle rupture, death from pulmonary edema and shock may result unless there is emergent valve replacement. The murmur of mitral regurgitation is, as expected, holosystolic.

Imaging Radiologic findings eventually include left atrial enlargement in all cases, and left ventricular enlargement in some. A chamber must double in size before enlargement is apparent on the chest radiograph. When chamber enlargement is not yet great enough to manifest on the radiograph, signs of mild to moderate pulmonary venous hypertension, such as equalization or cephalization of pulmonary blood flow, may nonetheless be apparent. In contrast to mitral valve stenosis, the valve rarely calcifies in mitral insufficiency.

In the chronic form of mitral regurgitation, clinical monitoring focuses on the evaluation of left ventricular function, with treatment of congestive heart failure (CHF) (**Fig. 2–16**). Surgery may be required in some cases.

◇ Aortic Stenosis

Epidemiology The most common causes of aortic stenosis are congenital bicuspid aortic valve and rheumatic heart disease. In advanced age, even tricuspid aortic valves may undergo degeneration. Approximately one half to three quarters of patients who develop aortic stenosis from rheumatic heart disease are males. Likewise, approximately three quarters of the 1% of persons with congenitally bicuspid aortic valves are males. By contrast, degenerative stenosis is seen with equal gender frequency and is generally less severe.

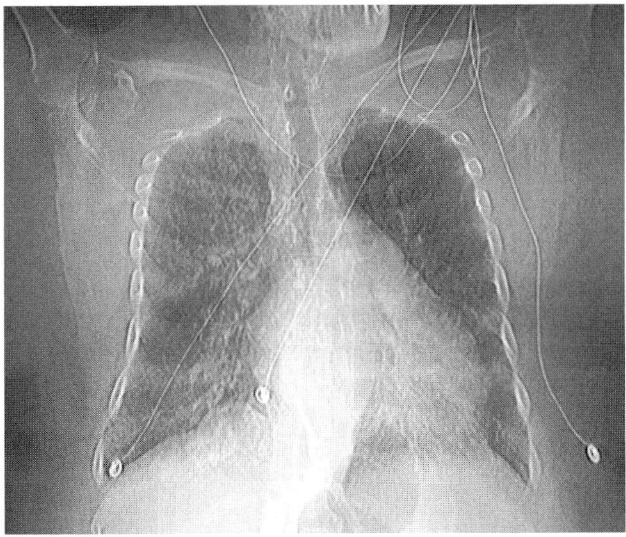
A

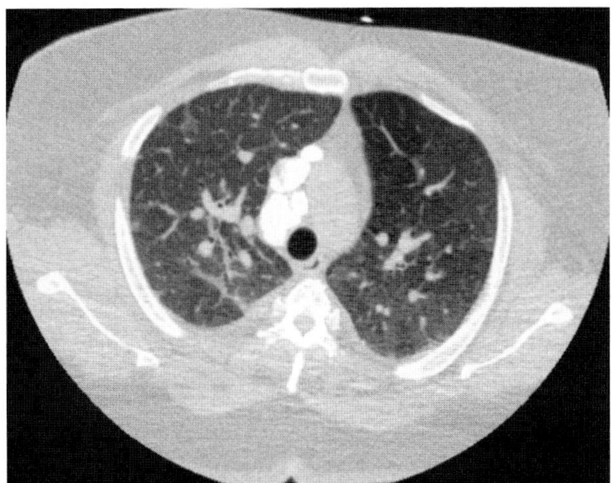
B

Figure 2–16 (A) This scout view from a thoracic CT scan demonstrates severe cardiomegaly with splaying of the main bronchi due to left atriomegaly in this patient with mitral valve insufficiency. There is pulmonary edema, most severe in the right upper lobe. There is also splaying of the carina, with the left mainstem bronchus lifted upward. **(B)** This axial CT image demonstrates bilateral hazy opacities, vascular prominence, and septal thickening, especially in the right upper lobe. In some patients with incompetent mitral valves, regurgitant flow across the value orifice is thought to be directed preferentially into the right upper lobe pulmonary view, causing findings to be more severe in that location.

Pathophysiology In the normal subject, systolic pressures in the left ventricle and aorta are equal. In the patient with aortic stenosis, a pressure gradient develops across the aortic valve. Severe stenosis is usually defined as a valve orifice that measures 0.5 cm^2 or less (normal = 2.5 cm^2). When the pressure gradient reaches 50 mm Hg, the left ventricular demand for oxygen begins to increase precipitously, the chamber hypertrophies, and end-diastolic pressure rises due to the loss of compliance. Eventually, the pressure gradient may exceed 200 mm Hg.

Clinical Presentation Patients develop angina pectoris (often without coronary artery disease), syncope (due to decreased systolic volume), and even sudden death (from ventricular fibrillation). Angina and syncope portend a survival of less than 3 to 5 years. The greater the degree of concurrent coronary artery disease, the earlier the patient presents. The murmur of aortic stenosis peaks at midsystole and is associated with a pulsus tardus et parvus (late and weak pulse). If a murmur is no longer heard, then it must be suspected that left ventricular output has declined to the point that flow across the valve is no longer sufficient to produce a murmur.

Imaging Radiologic findings include a normal heart size but a more rounded appearance to the left ventricle (**Fig. 2–17**). In adults, the aortic valve exhibits calcification. Echocardiography demonstrates a narrowed valve orifice. Doppler measurement can be used to estimate the pressure gradient across the valve. In addition, both radiography and ultrasound may demonstrate poststenotic aortic dilatation.

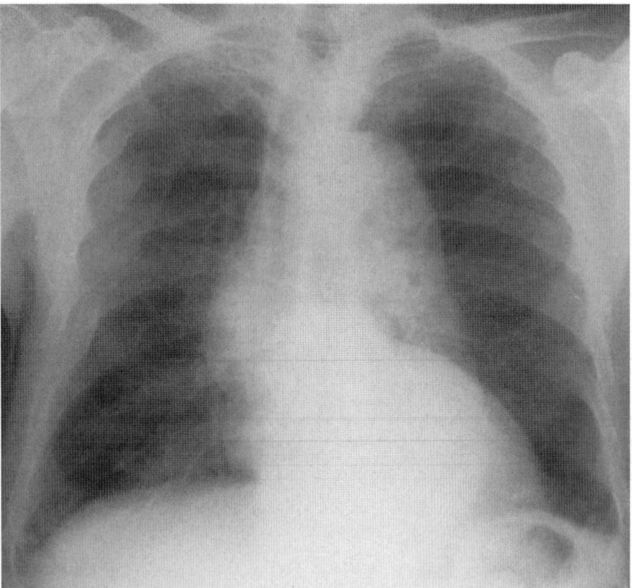

Figure 2–17 This frontal radiograph in a patient with long-standing aortic stenosis and hypertension demonstrates a left ventricular configuration of the heart, reflecting left ventriculomegaly. The ascending aorta is dilated and causes a bulge along the right side of the mediastinum. The rest of the aorta is tortuous, extending far to the left of the spine. Note also multiple right rib deformities, reflecting a remote history of trauma.

Medical management of aortic stenosis includes the use of digitalis and diuretics for CHF and the use of nitroglycerin for angina. Operative mortality is significantly reduced if valve replacement is undertaken prior to the development of heart failure, and significant improvement in long-term survival results. If the patient is a poor surgical candidate, transluminal balloon valvuloplasty may be warranted.

◇ Aortic Insufficiency

Epidemiology Causes of aortic insufficiency include rheumatic heart disease, syphilis, connective tissue diseases (such as Marfan's syndrome and ankylosing spondylitis), myxomatous degeneration, and congenitally bicuspid aortic valve. Acute aortic regurgitation, as seen in trauma with aortic dissection or in endocarditis, represents a catastrophe, due to a rapidly progressive increase in end-diastolic pressure, pulmonary edema, and loss of cardiac output. Aortic insufficiency is the earliest of the rheumatic heart disease killers, and many patients become symptomatic before the age of 20 years.

Pathophysiology Hemodynamically, chronic aortic insufficiency is associated with volume overload of the left ventricle, with resultant left ventricular dilation. In addition, there is dilation of the aortic root, which must accommodate an increased systolic volume. Left ventricular failure results from an unfavorable combination of increased cardiac output and oxygen consumption on the one hand (with every contraction, both the normal systolic volume and regurgitant volume must be pumped), and decreased coronary artery perfusion on the other (decreased aortic pressure during diastole stems from aortic dilation and aortic valvular regurgitation).

Clinical Presentation Patients manifest the consequences of a reduction in peripheral arteriolar tone, in an effort to decrease the back pressure in the systemic arteries contributing to regurgitant flow. The most reliable of these is a very wide pulse pressure, on the order of 180/50. Patients also manifest a decrescendo murmur after S_2.

Imaging Radiographically, signs include left ventriculomegaly and hypertrophy, with a boot-shaped heart and a widened ascending aorta. Left atrial enlargement may reflect both diminished left ventricular compliance and concurrent mitral valve disease. If the aorta is markedly widened, a primary aortic pathology such as syphilis or Marfan's syndrome should be suspected. Doppler echocardiography can very easily determine the presence of regurgitation. Valve replacement must be undertaken before severe left ventricular failure occurs.

Inflammatory

◇ Cardiomyopathy

The term *cardiomyopathy* (literally, "heart muscle disease") refers to heart diseases due to primary heart muscle pathology. By convention, these exclude congenital, valvular, and coronary artery processes. Several types of cardiomyopathy are recognized. Dilated cardiomyopathies account for 90% of cases in the United States, and most commonly result from toxins such as alcohol or previous infection (most commonly viral). In many patients, the cause is never clearly identified. Patients present with CHF that may be right- or left-sided, and the most common radiographic finding is global cardiomegaly. The ventricles are hypokinetic and exhibit a decreased ejection fraction—a flabby, weak heart with systolic dysfunction. Hypertrophic cardiomyopathy, by contrast, manifests as a thick, muscular heart that does not fill well during diastole. It is most commonly familial or due to pressure overload. Because portions of the heart muscle thicken but the heart itself may not dilate, nearly 50% of patients may exhibit a normal chest radiograph. Cross-sectional imaging reveals abnormal thickness of the myocardium. Restrictive cardiomyopathy, the rarest form of cardiomyopathy, causes diastolic dysfunction (inability to dilate during diastole) and exhibits physiology similar to restrictive pericarditis (**Fig. 2–18**). As in hypertrophic cardiomyopathy, diastolic dysfunction predominates. Causes include processes that infiltrate and stiffen the myocardium, such as amyloidosis and sarcoidosis. The chest radiograph often demonstrates normal cardiac size with pulmonary venous congestion.

Vascular

◇ Coronary Artery Disease

Even though the cardiac chambers are refilled with blood every second or so throughout life, the myocardium requires its own arterial supply, and the heart is in fact the first organ to receive freshly oxygenated blood from the left ventricle. The right and left coronary arteries originate in the right and left coronary sinuses of Valsalva. The right coronary artery (RCA) supplies the right ventricle and the atrioventricular node (in 90% of patients). The left coronary artery (LCA) divides into the anterior descending and circumflex arteries, the former supplying the ventricular septum and the anterior

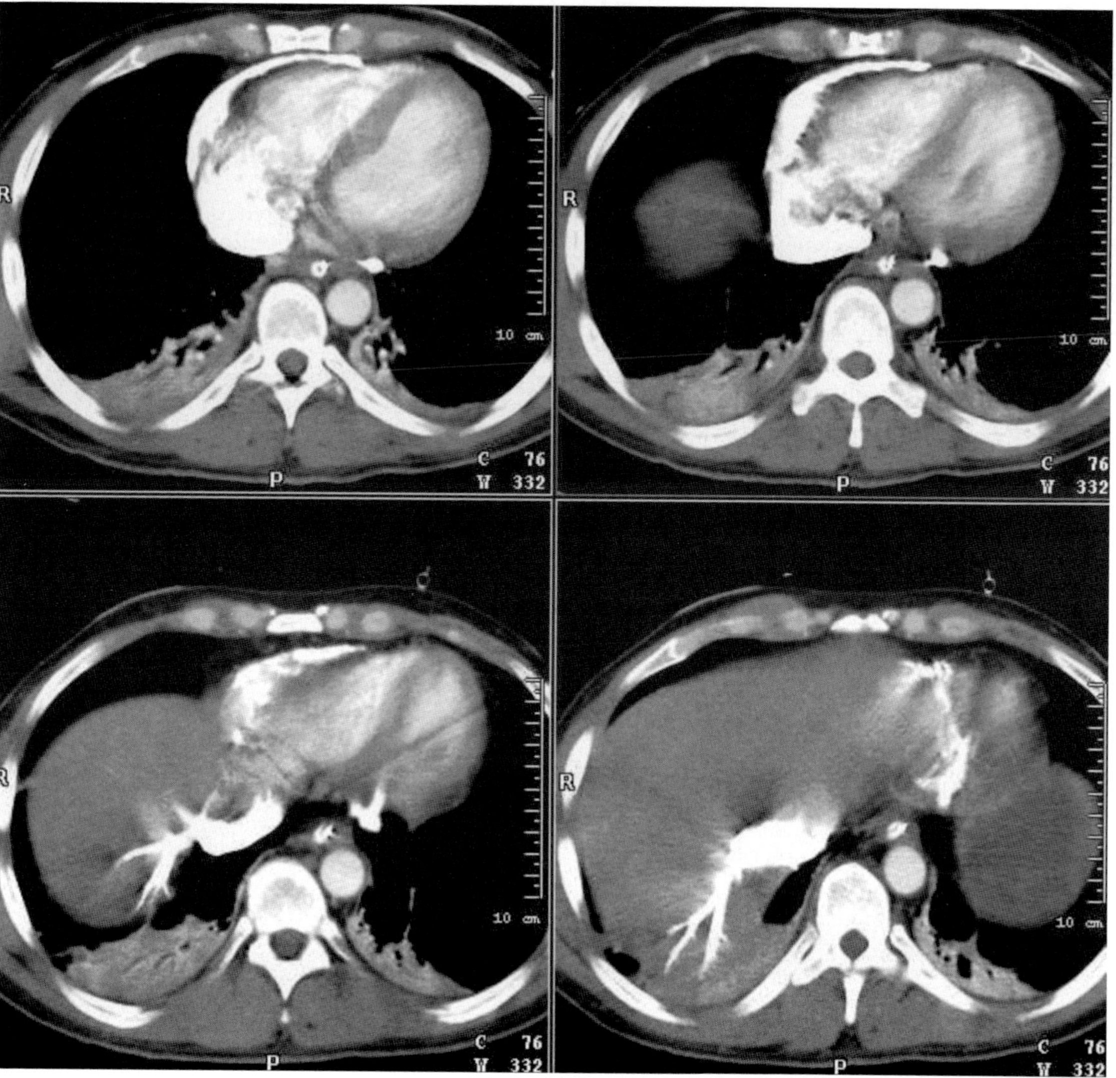

Figure 2–18 These axial CT images of the heart demonstrate thick right-sided pericardial calcification of the sort likely to cause restrictive pericarditis. This may help to explain the reflux of intravascular contrast material into this patient's hepatic veins.

wall of the left ventricle, and the latter supplying the lateral wall of the left ventricle. Patients with the more common right-dominant systems have a posterior descending coronary artery that arises from the RCA, whereas in left-dominant systems it arises from the LCA. The posterior descending artery and posterolateral branches supply the inferior and inferolateral walls of the left ventricle.

Epidemiology Ischemic heart disease is by far the most common type of heart disease in the world and constitutes the second leading cause of death in the United States. About 500,000 Americans die each year due to blockages in their coronary arteries. By far the most common cause of coronary artery disease is progressive narrowing of the coronary lumen secondary to the formation of atherosclerotic plaques, which may be complicated in the acute setting by thromboembolism. Risk factors for atherosclerosis include cigarette smoking (nearly one out of four adult Americans), hypertension (one out of four adult Americans), and diabetes (16 million afflicted in the United States).

Pathophysiology As the lumen of the coronary artery narrows, its resistance to flow increases, and the flow of blood distal to the diseased segment may be compromised. Fortunately, the coronary blood supply is relatively generous, and a severe degree of stenosis is necessary before lesions become hemodynamically significant. With distal arteriolar dilation and reduction in resistance, adequate flow can be maintained until the cross-sectional area of the lumen is reduced by more than 75%, at which point lesions become capable of causing physiologically significant ischemia; however, during exercise and increased myocardial demand, lesser degrees of attenuation may provoke ischemic symptoms and signs.

The cellular pathophysiology of myocardial ischemia helps to explain its hemodynamic effects, as well as the use of the electrocardiogram (ECG) and cardiac enzyme levels in its diagnosis. When the flow of blood to the myocardium is reduced, regions of myocardium become hypokinetic due to the lack of cellular energy supplies. If a large enough area is affected, cardiac output may decline, and signs and symptoms of CHF may appear. In addition, cellular membrane pump function and ionic permeabilities are disrupted, changes reflected on the ECG as characteristic ST-segment and T-wave abnormalities, especially ST-segment depression and T-wave inversion. When ischemia progresses to the point of infarction, changes include the appearance of Q waves, ST-segment elevation, and peaked T waves. As myocardial cells die, they release their contents, including various myocardial enzymes, into the systemic circulation. Creatinine kinase peaks within hours, and serum glutamic oxaloacetic transaminase (SGOT) and lactate dehydrogenase (LDH) peak over the first 24 hours. Dire consequences may include sudden death from dysrrhythmia (secondary to ischemia of the conducting system), massive heart failure, and papillary muscle rupture.

Clinical Presentation Classic angina pectoris is a distinct type of chest pain that patients locate in the midchest and describe as a squeezing or tightening sensation, often employing a clenched fist to embellish their description. It often radiates into the arm(s) or up to the neck, and typically lasts for a period of seconds to minutes. Generally, chest pain can be described as anginal if it is substernal, precipitated by exertion, and promptly relieved with rest or nitroglycerin. When a patient's symptoms fulfill all three criteria, the pain is typical angina; if two of the three, it is called atypical angina; if one of the three, it is probably not anginal. Although chest pain is an extremely common symptom, it indicates a significant medical problem in only a small percentage of cases. Other common sources of chest pain include anxiety with hyperventilation, esophageal pathology (reflux, spasm), chest wall problems such as costochondritis (Tietze's syndrome) and muscle strain, and pulmonary pathologies (asthma, pneumonia).

Imaging The imaging workup of myocardial ischemia is complex, and this discussion focuses on nuclear medicine imaging. The plain chest radiograph plays a limited role, due to its relatively low sensitivity. Findings on plain radiography include calcification of the myocardial wall, which indicates previous infarction, and may be accompanied by left ventricular aneurysm (**Fig. 2–19**). Calcification of the coronary arteries, when seen, is highly specific for hemodynamically significant coronary artery disease, especially in patients under the age of 55 years; however, most chest radiographs are exposed at high kilovolts peak (kVp), meaning that calcifications tend to be "burned out." CT, especially fast CT, is much more sensitive in this regard.

Radioisotope perfusion imaging relies on the availability of blood-borne tracers whose distribution corresponds to regional blood flow. Previously, thallium-201 chloride was the

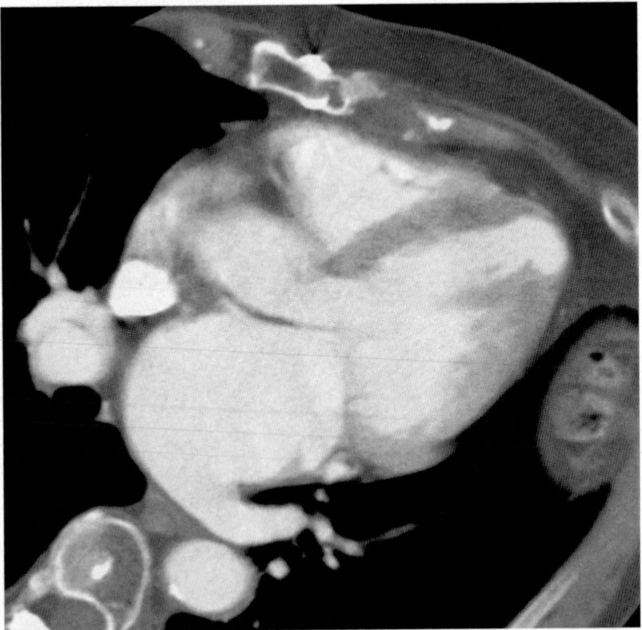

Figure 2–19 This contrast-enhanced axial CT image of the heart demonstrates an outpouching of contrast from the lumen of the left ventricular apex at a point where the heart muscle is markedly thinned. This is a left ventricular aneurysm in a patient with a history of prior myocardial infarction.

only commonly used tracer, although now technetium-99m (Tc-99m)–based agents such as sestamibi are more widely used. Each illustrates the flow of blood to each portion of the myocardium, allowing the identification of regions of relatively decreased perfusion, which appear as defects or "cold spots" adjacent to normally perfused myocardium. This is not, however, equivalent to assessing the flow of blood through each coronary artery, as the development of collaterals may produce a relatively normal-appearing examination in patients with a severely occluded coronary artery branch. Stress testing, using either exercise or pharmacologic stress, is employed to assess perfusion under conditions in which it is most likely to be abnormal. This increases the sensitivity of perfusion imaging for myocardial ischemia. The most common form of exercise testing is a treadmill test, with multiple, graded stages of increased workload. The test may be aborted if the patient cannot continue due to fatigue, dyspnea, or severe angina, hypotension, or ECG changes. A common means of determining whether the myocardial workload was adequate is to calculate the "double product," which is the product of the heart rate and blood pressure. Another means is to determine whether the patient achieved 85% of the maximum predicted heart rate (220 – age in years). One would only expect to see a perfusion deficit in a resting patient when the stenosis was greater than 85%. During exercise, however, an artery with more than 50% stenosis cannot respond adequately to the myocardial demand for increased blood supply, and a defect is seen. Hence stress testing increases sensitivity for the detection of occlusive disease at an earlier stage.

A scintigraphic image obtained soon after injection at peak exercise provides a useful "snapshot" of regional perfusion, with necrotic, fibrosed, or ischemic areas appearing as defects due to the lack of radiotracer uptake. To further determine whether the hypoperfused tissue is viable or not, a second set of images is acquired at rest. Unless the stenosis is very severe, areas of viable tissue that are cold on exercise images will "fill in" on resting images. Hence a reversible defect (**Fig. 2–20**) indicates viable tissue, whereas an irreversible or fixed defect (**Fig. 2–21**) typically indicates dead tissue, most often scar tissue from previous infarction.

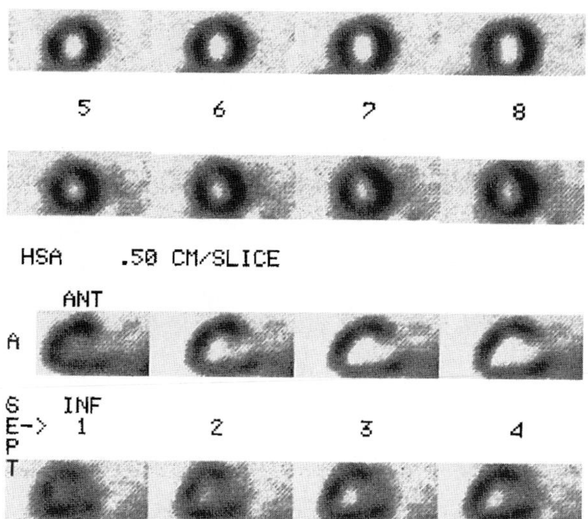

Figure 2–20 These single photon emission computed tomography (SPECT) images were obtained from a myocardial perfusion study using thallium-201 and technetium- (Tc-) 99m sestamibi as radiotracers. The top two rows of images were obtained in the short axis, with sections obtained at 5 mm intervals from the heart apex through the base (recall that the apex of the heart is caudal to its base). On these short-axis images, the left ventricular myocardium appears as a donut, with the anterior wall of the heart located superiorly, the left lateral wall of the heart on the viewer's right, the inferior wall inferiorly, and the interventricular septum on the viewer's left. The third and fourth rows represent vertical long-axis views, in which the anterior wall is located superiorly, the apex is on the viewer's left, and the inferior wall is inferiorly located. The first and third rows are stress images, which were obtained using Tc-99m sestamibi. The second and fourth rows are rest images, in which thallium 201 was used. Compare the rest and stress images, to see if there are any perfusion defects on the stress images, and then examine the rest images to determine if they are reversible or irreversible. In this case, there is a defect in the inferior wall on the stress images that fills in completely on the rest images, indicating reversible ischemia. What coronary artery is likely compromised in this patient? Because the defect is in the inferior wall, the stenotic vessel is the right coronary artery. If the lateral wall were involved, we would say that the left circumflex artery was involved, whereas an anterior defect would indicate left anterior descending artery disease. The finding of a defect on the stress images establishes that coronary ischemia is the source of a patient's chest pain. Moreover, reversible defects imply that viable myocardium is present, and that revascularization procedures such as angioplasty or coronary bypass may be of benefit. A fixed defect, on the other hand, may indicate infarcted myocardium, in which case the patient is unlikely to benefit from these procedures.

Common Clinical Problems

Congestive Heart Failure

◇ Epidemiology

CHF is a common clinical problem, which contributes to 300,000 deaths each year in the United States, and for which 2 million Americans are currently under treatment. It constitutes the leading hospital discharge diagnosis in individuals over age 65.

◇ Pathophysiology

Heart Failure Simply put, heart failure refers to the heart's inability to meet the body's demands for oxygen and nutrients and the removal of wastes. Failure of a ventricle produces increased back pressure in the vessels proximal to it, with resulting venous congestion—either systemic venous congestion from right heart failure or pulmonary venous congestion from left heart failure. Although there are myriad causes of heart failure, by far the two most common causes are ischemic damage to the myocardium and hypertensive heart disease, due to prolonged pumping against a chronically elevated systemic blood pressure.

When the heart fails, regardless of the cause, its contractility declines. As a result, it is unable to generate the same systolic pressures and stroke volumes it once did. The Frank-Starling curve describes the relationship between end-diastolic volume and stroke volume, and states that the ventricle pumps out the volume of blood with which it is filled. The greater the length to which cardiac muscle fibers are stretched during diastole, the greater the force with which

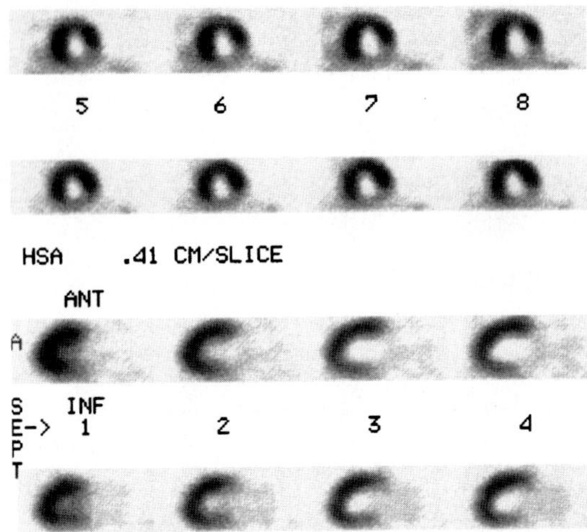

Figure 2–21 This myocardial perfusion study was performed and displayed as described in the previous figure. In this case, note the finding of an irreversible defect in the inferior wall, which most likely represents nonviable, scarred myocardium in the right coronary artery distribution.

they subsequently contract during systole. Hence filling either ventricle with more blood will cause it to contract more vigorously and eject more blood. This principle ensures that the outputs of the right and left sides of the heart are equalized, and that increased venous return (as in exercise) is accompanied by increased cardiac output. In heart failure, the Frank-Starling curve is shifted downward and to the right, meaning that the ventricle is able to eject less blood for a given end-diastolic volume (**Fig. 2–22**).

Early in heart failure, two compensatory mechanisms come into play. First, the heart's sympathetic tone is reflexively increased, with a resultant increase in contractility; however, this gambit only works in the short term, as the heart becomes progressively less responsive to the increased sympathetic input. Second, the kidneys respond to decreased cardiac output with salt and water retention, in an effort to expand circulating blood volume, and thereby increase end-diastolic volume and cardiac output. With time, the

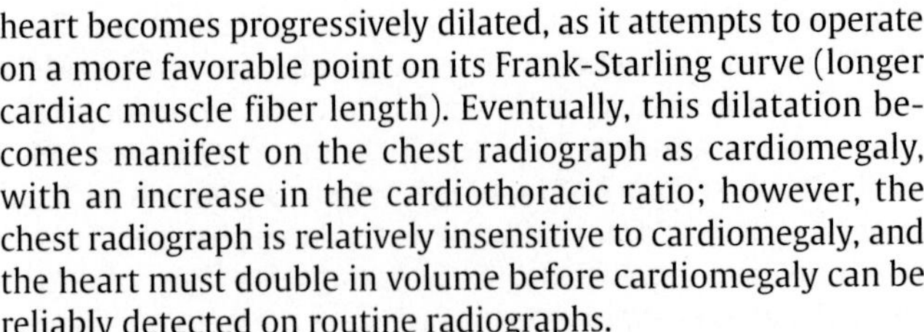

heart becomes progressively dilated, as it attempts to operate on a more favorable point on its Frank-Starling curve (longer cardiac muscle fiber length). Eventually, this dilatation becomes manifest on the chest radiograph as cardiomegaly, with an increase in the cardiothoracic ratio; however, the chest radiograph is relatively insensitive to cardiomegaly, and the heart must double in volume before cardiomegaly can be reliably detected on routine radiographs.

Two types of failure occur: forward failure and backward failure. Forward failure of the left ventricle results in inadequate systemic perfusion. Backward failure of the left ventricle results in increased pulmonary capillary pressures and an increased workload for the right ventricle. In fact, left heart failure is the most common cause of right heart failure. The pulmonary edema that accompanies left heart failure impedes gas exchange, with decreased arterial oxygenation and increased carbon dioxide.

With further progression of heart failure, the heart reaches a point at which it is no longer able to pump a normal stroke volume, despite the operation of compensatory mechanisms. For a time, the patient is precariously balanced between adequate function and failure. Often, acute exacerbations of heart failure can be traced to relatively minor inciting events, such as infections (with decreased cardiac function) and acute salt loads (a typical whole pizza contains more than a 12 g of sodium). Normally, the short-term expansion of circulating volume would exert no deleterious consequences on myocardial function, but when the heart is already stretched to its limit, it cannot compensate for any further increase in end-diastolic volume. Treatment of CHF consists of the restriction of salt intake, weight loss, and the use of drugs such as diuretics, vasodilators, and digitalis. Originally found in the foxglove plant, digitalis increases myocardial contractility.

Pulmonary Edema As discussed in Chapter 3, the pulmonary capillaries and alveoli take full advantage of Fick's law, which states that the rate of diffusion is increased as the distance across which it must take place is decreased. The alveolar walls are made up of a single layer of flattened type I pneumocytes, and the pulmonary capillaries surrounding each alveolus are also only one cell layer thick. These structural characteristics mean that the air in the

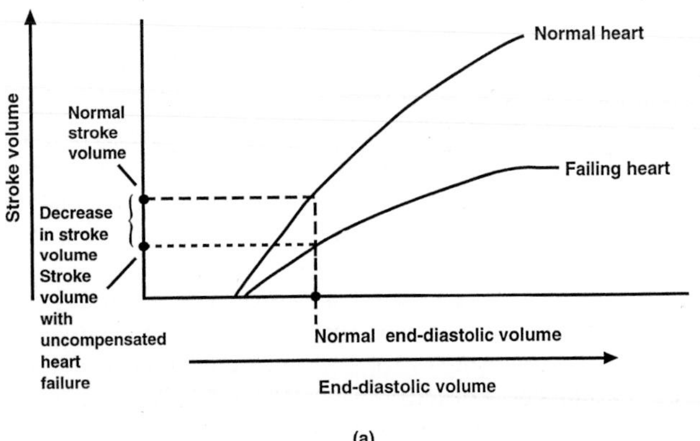

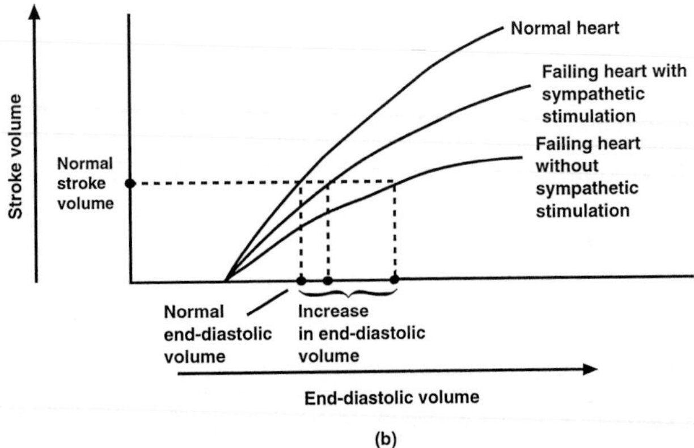

Figure 2–22 **(A)** The relationship between stroke volume and end-diastolic volume in the normal and failing heart. **(B)** The mechanisms of physiologic compensation include sympathetic stimulation (which is only temporarily effective) and further dilatation when sympathetic stimulation ceases to be effective in maintaining cardiac output. These graphs help to explain the development of cardiomegaly in congestive heart failure.

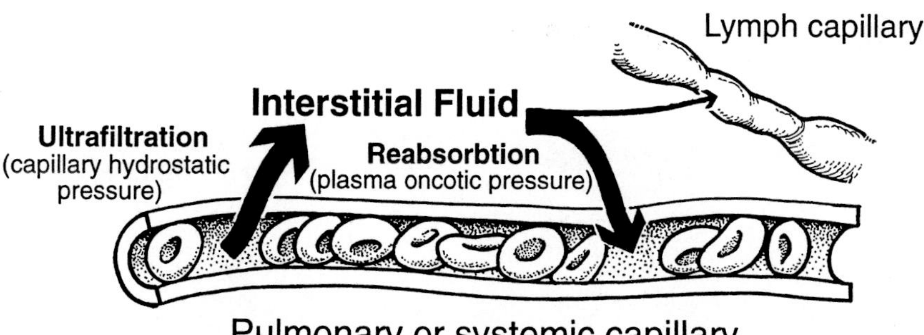

Figure 2–23 The movement of fluid between the pulmonary capillaries and the pulmonary interstitium. The most important force producing ultrafiltration of fluid from the blood into the interstitium is the pulmonary capillary hydrostatic pressure, which is higher at the arteriolar end than at the venular end of the capillary. The most important force returning fluid to the capillary is the plasma oncotic pressure, which remains constant at both ends of the capillary. The shifting balance between these two forces favors exit of fluid from the capillary at the arteriolar end and reentry of fluid at the venular end. However, the net balance is not perfect, and a small amount of fluid remains in the interstitium, to be taken up and returned to the circulation by the lymphatics.

alveolar sac is separated from the red blood cells in the capillary by only 0.5 µm.

To understand the development of pulmonary edema, it is necessary to understand the Starling forces, which determine the net flow of fluid from the pulmonary capillaries into the pulmonary interstitium and alveolar spaces (**Fig. 2–23**). Essentially, only two forces operate in each direction, the oncotic pressure (related to protein concentration) and the hydrostatic pressure (physical force exerted on the capillary walls by the blood). Like any other substance, water tends to flow from regions of higher concentration or pressure to regions of lower concentration or pressure. The concentration of water, so to speak, is highest in regions of low oncotic pressure (where the concentration of proteins is low).

The plasma hydrostatic pressure is the force exerted on the inner walls of the capillaries by the pumping action of the heart, and amounts to ~35 mm Hg at the arterial end of the capillaries and 15 mm Hg at the venous end. Hence this force tends to drive water from the capillary lumen into the interstitial tissues. The other force tending to move water into the interstitium is the interstitial oncotic pressure, which is normally close to zero, because high-molecular-weight plasma proteins cannot pass through the capillary membranes into the interstitium.

The other two Starling forces tend to move water in the opposite direction, from the interstitium into the capillary lumen. The plasma oncotic pressure is the result of the presence of high-molecular-weight plasma proteins, especially albumin, which cannot pass across the capillary membranes from the blood to the interstitial tissues. They keep the water concentration in the intravascular space lower than that in the extravascular space, thus tending to draw water from the interstitium into the blood vessels. The final force is the interstitial hydrostatic pressure, which is normally minimal.

The net Starling forces change as the blood moves from the arteriolar to the venular ends of the capillaries, due to the change in the intraluminal hydrostatic pressure. At the arteriolar end, the net filtration pressure equals the sum of the hydrostatic pressure (35 mm Hg) and the osmotic force (–25 mm Hg), which is 10mm Hg in favor of filtration, the net movement of fluid out of the capillary. By the time the blood reaches the venular end, it has lost 20 mm Hg of hydrostatic pressure, and the sum is –10 mm Hg, favoring absorption. Thus, under normal conditions, there is a nearly perfect balance between the filtration and absorption occurring along the capillary. In fact, however, a small amount of fluid is filtered into the interstitium every day, to be reabsorbed by the lymphatic vessels.

Aside from the Starling forces, two other factors are important in determining the amount of fluid that collects in the lungs. The first is the lymphatic drainage of the lung. The lymphatics remove from the pulmonary interstitium the small amount of fluid that would otherwise accumulate there every day. The flow of lymphatic fluid is useful because it facilitates the clearance of minute particulate matter, including foreign material presented to immune cells in the lymph nodes into which lymphatics drain. These lymphatics course centrally within the alveolar and interlobular septae toward the hilum. The second additional factor that may contribute to pulmonary edema is the permeability of the capillary membrane itself. If the membrane becomes more permeable to the diffusion of plasma proteins, then the interstitial oncotic pressure will rise (reducing the concentration of water outside the capillaries), and fluid will tend to accumulate within the lung.

Based on these factors, pulmonary edema may result from any one of four different mechanisms. The first, and by far the most common, is an increase in pulmonary venous hydrostatic pressure, secondary to failure of the left ventricle and "damming up" of blood in the pulmonary capillaries. The second major mechanism is a reduction in the plasma oncotic pressure, with a resultant increase in the plasma concentration of water, and an increased gradient down which fluid tends to diffuse into the interstitium. Some investigators doubt that an isolated reduction in oncotic pressure can cause pulmonary edema by itself, but there is little doubt that it acts as an important cofactor in other conditions, such as left heart failure. Common causes of a reduction in plasma oncotic pressure would include the nephrotic syndrome, with loss of proteins in the urine; hepatic failure, which decreases synthesis of plasma proteins such as albumin; and severe burns, in which proteins are lost through the damaged skin. The third common mechanism is an increase in capillary

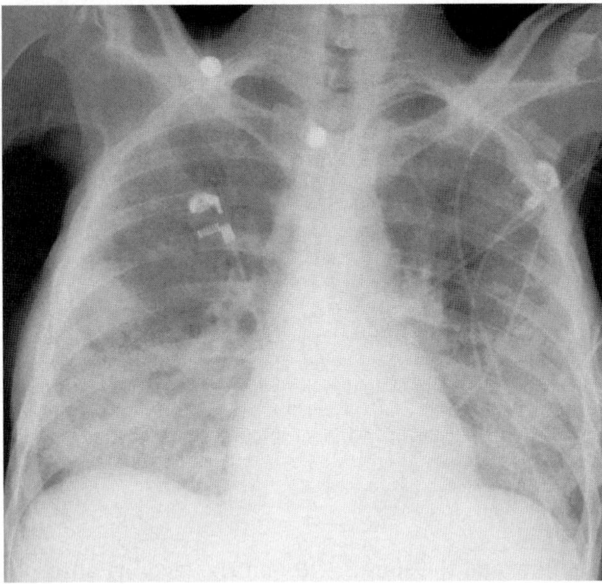

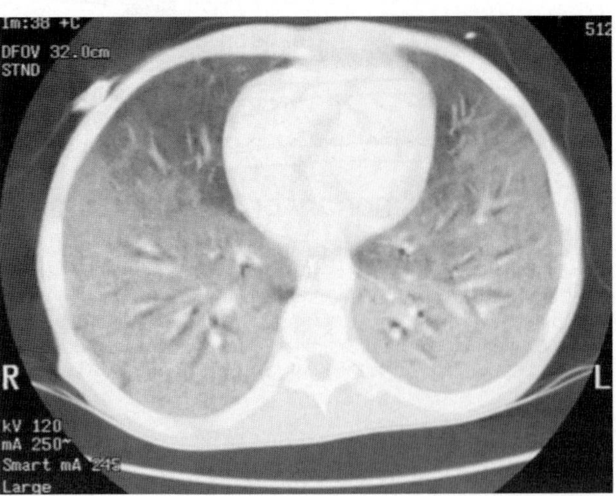

Figure 2–24 (A) This frontal chest radiograph demonstrates diffuse bilateral air-space opacities with no evidence of pleural effusions. The patient had suffered an inhalational injury in a house fire. **(B)** An axial chest CT image at lung windows also demonstrates diffuse bilateral air-space opacities but no pleural effusion. Also, the heart is not enlarged. These findings are typical of acute respiratory distress syndrome (ARDS), due to capillary leak.

permeability, with leakage of plasma proteins into the interstitium, as occurs in acute respiratory distress syndrome (ARDS). Conditions associated with ARDS include septicemia, shock, acute pancreatitis, inhalation injury, and direct chemical injury, as in aspiration or drowning (**Fig. 2–24**). The fourth mechanism is an obstruction of lymphatic drainage, for example, by a central tumor such as a bronchogenic carcinoma.

The time course over which alterations in the Starling forces occur is critical in determining whether or not pulmonary edema is likely to result. Given enough time, the pulmonary lymphatics are able to increase their drainage of interstitial fluid several-fold. This explains the fact that patients in chronic CHF may exhibit quite elevated pulmonary venous pressures, yet relatively little or no evidence of pulmonary edema. Even though an increased amount of fluid is being transudated, the lymphatics have been able to increase their capacity over time. By contrast, a previously healthy patient who suffers an acute myocardial infarction, with acutely increased left ventricular diastolic pressure and resultant increased pulmonary venous pressure, may develop radiographic evidence of pulmonary edema with only a relatively small increase in pulmonary venous pressure. In this case, the pulmonary lymphatics have not been given sufficient time to adjust to the increase in interstitial fluid.

◇ Clinical Presentation

The most common presenting symptom of CHF is dyspnea ("bad breathing"). Dyspnea refers to a subjective sensation of difficulty in breathing. It is usually accompanied by tachypnea, an increased respiratory rate, but need not be in every case. Dyspneic patients typically complain that they cannot catch their breath, or that their chest feels tight. A type of dyspnea commonly associated with CHF is orthopnea, dyspnea on assuming the supine posture, due to increased venous return to the failing left ventricle. The actual mechanisms underlying dyspnea have proven difficult to elucidate, but they probably involve abnormal activation of the neural centers of respiration in the brainstem, perhaps from stimulation of receptors in the upper and lower respiratory tracts.

The typical patient presents with a history of exertional dyspnea, which may eventually progress over years to dyspnea at rest. As we have seen, progressive failure of the left ventricle eventually produces left atrial hypertension. Left atrial hypertension causes pulmonary capillary hypertension, which in turn causes transudation of fluid into the pulmonary interstitium, reduced pulmonary compliance, increased airways resistance, and increased work of breathing. The accumulation of fluid within the interstitium and air spaces also increases the distance across which oxygen and carbon dioxide must diffuse, decreasing the efficiency of alveolar gas exchange.

Shortness of breath (SOB) can usually be attributed to one of two fundamental categories of disease, cardiac or pulmonary. This dichotomy is reflected in the legion of requisitions seen in every busy radiology practice bearing the clinical history of "SOB. Pneumonia versus CHF." When a young, previously healthy adult patient presents to the emergency department acutely short of breath, the underlying pathology is almost certainly pulmonary in nature. On the other hand, when a patient with a history of CHF and multiple previous exacerbations presents with stereotypical symptoms, an exacerbation of CHF is the working diagnosis. The distinction between cardiogenic and noncardiogenic pulmonary edema is clinically important, because the usual therapies for CHF are unlikely to be of significant benefit in noncardiogenic dyspnea. In cardiogenic pulmonary edema, the heart is usually enlarged, because cardiomegaly represents the heart's response to failure. In noncardiogenic edema, by contrast, the heart is not enlarged, because the heart itself is not diseased.

Many dyspneic patients prove less easy to categorize as cardiac or pulmonary on clinical grounds, and other clinical evidence must be sought to make this determination. One common difficulty is the fact that cardiac and pulmonary disease frequently coexist. Pulmonary function testing is often employed to determine whether the lungs are the likely culprit, and nuclear medicine and ultrasound are used to evaluate such cardiac parameters as ejection fraction. Blood gas analysis also may be helpful. However, one of the most readily available and helpful means of distinguishing between cardiac and pulmonary dyspnea is plain chest radiography, and radiology plays a crucial role in the dyspneic patient.

◇ Imaging

By far the most useful imaging study in suspected CHF is the PA and lateral chest radiograph. If CHF is the culprit, it demonstrates such characteristic findings as cardiac enlargement, pulmonary vascular redistribution (equalization or cephalization of pulmonary blood flow), unsharpness of the pulmonary vessels due to interstitial edema, pleural effusions, septal lines, and frank air-space opacities (**Fig. 2–25**).

Pulmonary edema begins within the interstitium, as the interstitial spaces immediately outside the capillaries become filled with fluid. Signs of edema at this point are subtle and include loss of definition of the vascular markings (due to accumulation of fluid around the vessel walls), peribronchial cuffing (fluid around bronchi seen on end), and tram tracking (bronchial walls that appear thickened when seen from the side). Edema within the interstitium itself produces a ground-glass type of opacity, with air spaces surrounded by a very fine network of fluid-filled interstitium. As more fluid accumulates, septal lines begin to appear, which represent the fluid-distended interlobular septae in the periphery of the lung (**Fig. 2–26**). Eventually, fluid begins to spill over into the alveoli, and fluffy air-space opacities begin to develop. These tend to be located in the mid and lower lung zones.

As noted in the discussion of valvular heart disease, the chest radiograph provides a reasonable measure of pulmonary venous pressure. At normal pressures less than 12 mm Hg, the radiograph is normal. At pressures of 12 to 18 mm Hg, redistribution of flow to the upper zones is the only finding. At pressures of 19 to 25 mm Hg, interstitial edema occurs, with loss of vascular definition, peribronchial cuffing, and septal lines. At pressures above 25 mm Hg, the alveoli begin to fill with fluid, and fluffy air-space opacities result. These findings may be associated with pleural effusion, which probably stems from the diffusion of fluid from congested visceral pleural lymphatics into the pleural space.

Noncardiogenic (nonhydrostatic) pulmonary edema will typically exhibit a quite different appearance from that seen in CHF. It is generally more peripheral, diffuse, and less gravity-dependent than cardiogenic edema. For example, ARDS, which results from the leakage of protein-rich fluid across the pulmonary capillaries, is not associated with cardiomegaly or

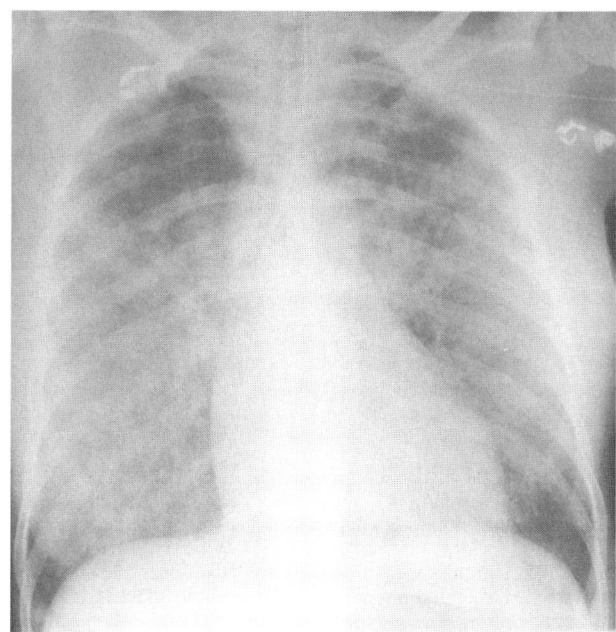

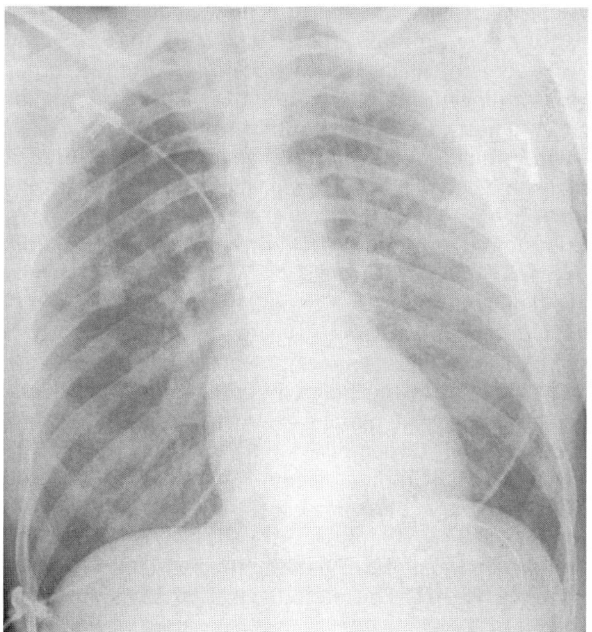

Figure 2–25 **(A)** This patient with a history of congestive heart failure presented to the emergency room with shortness of breath and soon required intubation. A frontal chest radiograph demonstrates cardiomegaly and bilateral air-space opacities in an overall pattern typical of congestive heart failure. What would you say about the endotracheal tube position? It has been inserted too far, with its tip in the right bronchus. **(B)** A second radiograph obtained 7 hours after diuretic therapy demonstrates decreased cardiomegaly and edema. Note the electrocardiogram leads and the properly positioned endotracheal tube.

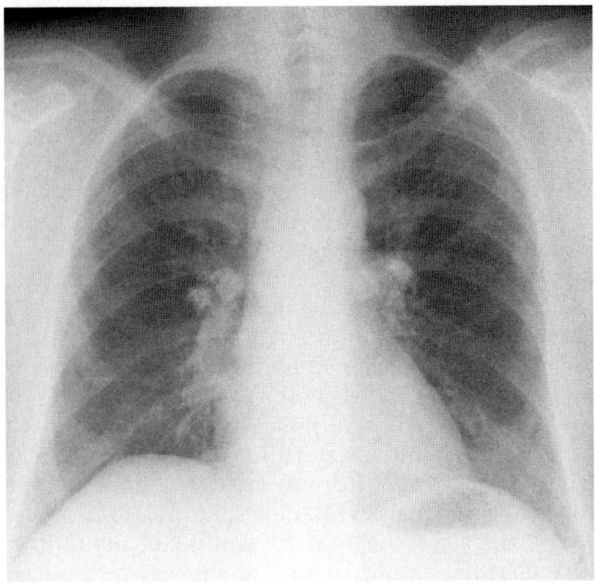
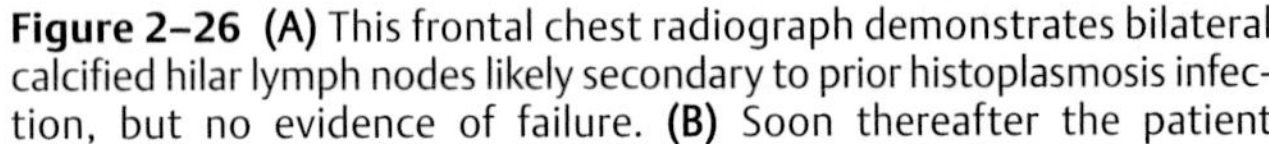
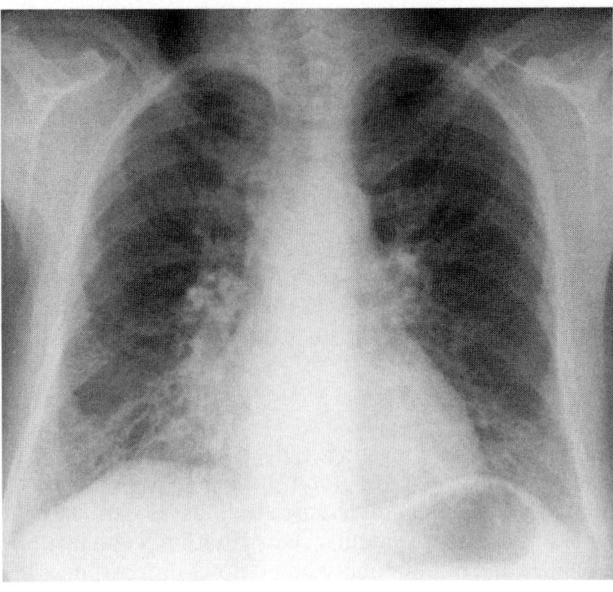

Figure 2–26 **(A)** This frontal chest radiograph demonstrates bilateral calcified hilar lymph nodes likely secondary to prior histoplasmosis infection, but no evidence of failure. **(B)** Soon thereafter the patient presented to the emergency room in congestive heart failure. Note the increase in heart size and the presence of bibasilar increased interstitial opacities, including septal lines.

pulmonary vascular redistribution. Likewise, pleural effusions are not a typical part of ARDS, and the possibility of pneumonia should be entertained in ARDS patients who develop large effusions (**Fig. 2–27**). Other examples of noncardiogenic pulmonary edema include the neurogenic and reexpansion varieties. Neurogenic edema is seen after closed head trauma, and reexpansion edema occurs after an atelectatic portion of the lung is reaerated. Aside from myocardial ischemia, other causes of cardiogenic pulmonary edema include aortic stenosis, mitral stenosis, and mitral insufficiency.

Two additional, nonradiologic maneuvers are helpful in distinguishing between cardiogenic and noncardiogenic pulmonary edema, both of which are predictable based on pathophysiologic grounds. First, the placement of a pulmonary artery catheter is extremely helpful, as the pulmonary capillary wedge pressure will be elevated only in cardiogenic pulmonary edema (due to increased left atrial pressures). The second maneuver is transbronchial sampling of edema fluid from the lungs. In cardiogenic pulmonary edema, the capillary membrane is intact, and the fluid is low in protein. In ARDS, by contrast, capillary leakage renders the fluid protein-rich. It should be noted, however, that the two types of pulmonary edema may coexist in the same patient. For example, a burn patient with ARDS is likely to be aggressively hydrated in an effort to maintain circulating volume, which may produce the distention of mediastinal veins often seen in CHF.

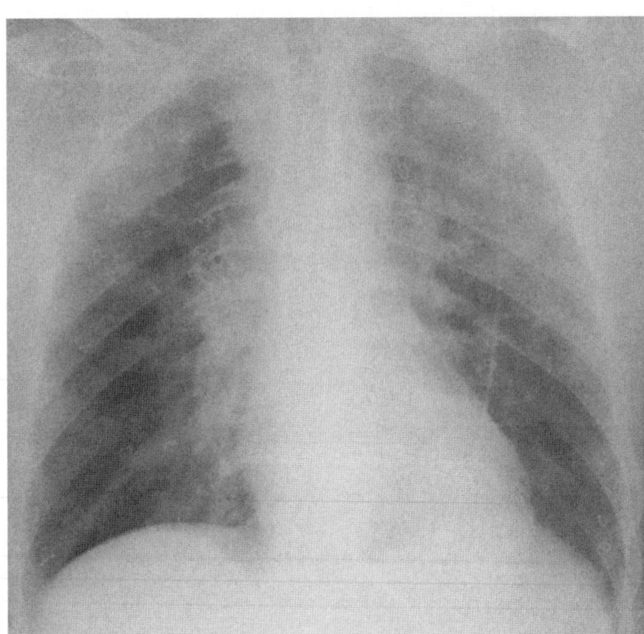

Figure 2–27 This patient's pattern of diffuse bilateral air-space pulmonary edema is not gravity dependent. If anything, the edema appears worse in the upper lobes than in the bases. What is the etiology? If you look closely, you can see many staples overlying the chest. This is a burn patient who has undergone skin grafting, and the ARDS pattern of pulmonary edema was due to a combination of smoke inhalation and sepsis.

◇ Epidemiology

Thrombosis (from the Latin for "clot") within the deep veins of the leg with embolism (from the Greek for "wedge") to the pulmonary arteries accounts for more than 100,000 deaths each year in the United States. About 10% of patients with thrombosis in the deep veins of the leg (deep venous thrombosis, DVT) develop pulmonary embolism, and ~10% of these are fatal. Pulmonary embolism is the cause of death in ~10% of hospitalized patients. It is estimated that about three quarters of PE cases go undiagnosed, with a 30% risk of recurrence. When PE is not treated, the risk of death is ~30%, whereas appropriate treatment lowers this risk to ~8%.

Most patients who develop PE suffer from an underlying condition, such as heart disease, cancer, or prolonged immobilization. Other risk factors include recent surgery, pregnancy, and history of previous DVT or PE. This explains why many high-risk patients (e.g., older patients undergoing hip or knee prosthetic joint placement) are placed in compression hose and/or given heparin prophylaxis.

◇ Pathophysiology

The pathophysiology of PE is complex. Ninety-five percent originate as DVTs, thrombi in the deep veins of the legs between the knees and hips. Once a DVT has formed, it may break free, travel up the vena cava, pass through the right heart, and lodge in the pulmonary arteries. Several outcomes are possible (**Fig. 2–28**). The first, massive embolus (with death in half of cases), results from severe impairment of right ventricular output, with cor pulmonale, distention of neck veins, and hypotension. Another outcome may be pulmonary infarction (in ~10% of cases), in which the bronchial artery component of the lung's dual blood supply is not sufficient to compensate for pulmonary artery obstruction. Most cases of PE result in neither of these outcomes, however, and although the patient may not die during the initial episode, failure to diagnose the condition and institute prophylaxis can permit recurrence.

PE typically causes some degree of mismatch between pulmonary ventilation and perfusion (V/Q mismatch), in which portions of the lung are ventilated but not perfused. This produces an immediate widening of the arterial-alveolar PO_2 gradient, and analysis of blood gases reveals an inability to achieve the expected degree of arterial oxygenation on oxygen supplementation.

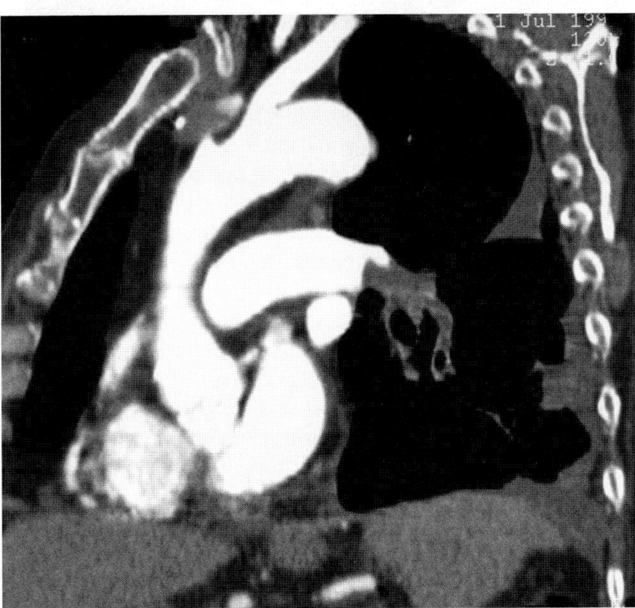

Figure 2–28 This oblique sagittal reconstruction of axially acquired CT data demonstrates a large filling defect in the lower lobe branches of the left pulmonary artery, representing acute pulmonary thromboembolism.

◇ Clinical Presentation

Leg pain and swelling (particularly if unilateral) are the typical presenting symptoms of DVT. Patients with pulmonary embolism typically present with sudden onset of dyspnea. Many patients complain of chest pain. Physical examination often reveals tachypnea and tachycardia. The ECG may demonstrate right ventricular strain or right axis deviation, although nonspecific sinus tachycardia is more common; however, the clinical diagnoses of both PE and DVT are notoriously unreliable, and the first and most crucial step is simply to suspect them.

◇ Imaging

Plain Radiography The main reason for ordering chest radiography is to rule out mimics of PE, such as pneumonia. When PE is present, the examination may be normal, although several nonspecific findings such as atelectasis are more common (due to impaired surfactant production secondary to decreased perfusion). A more specific but uncommon finding is that of the so-called Hampton's hump, a pleural-based opacity pointing toward the heart, which reflects the typically wedge-shaped pattern of infarction (**Fig. 2–29**). An even rarer but more specific sign is Westermark's sign, which consists of absent or markedly diminished pulmonary vascularity in the affected region.

Lower Extremity Ultrasound When the diagnosis is suspected and there is no other obvious etiology, such as pneumonia, one of two diagnostic courses of action should be considered. In many patients, pulmonary symptoms are mild or nonexistent, and DVT is suspected on the basis of unilateral lower extremity swelling, erythema, or a palpable venous cord. In these cases, lower extremity duplex Doppler imaging is the study of choice, focusing on the common femoral vein, superficial femoral vein (a "deep" vein despite its name), and the popliteal vein. A normal vein is thin walled and completely

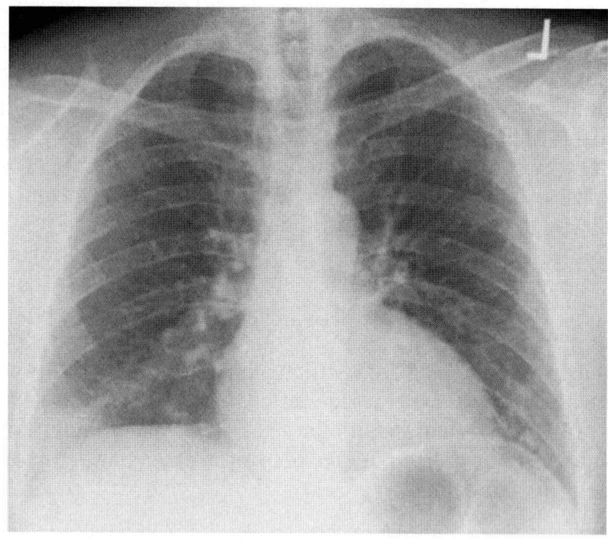

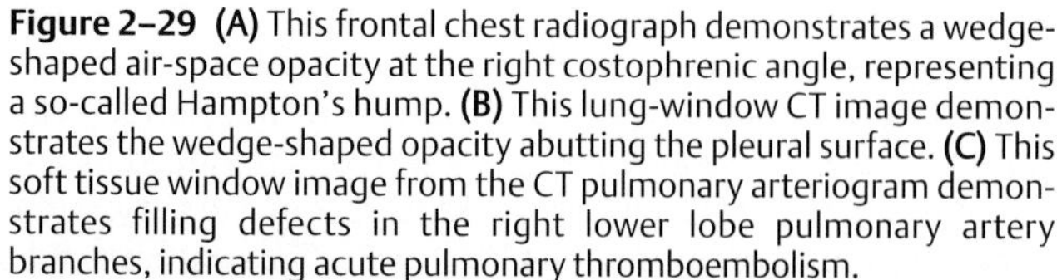

Figure 2–29 **(A)** This frontal chest radiograph demonstrates a wedge-shaped air-space opacity at the right costophrenic angle, representing a so-called Hampton's hump. **(B)** This lung-window CT image demonstrates the wedge-shaped opacity abutting the pleural surface. **(C)** This soft tissue window image from the CT pulmonary arteriogram demonstrates filling defects in the right lower lobe pulmonary artery branches, indicating acute pulmonary thromboembolism.

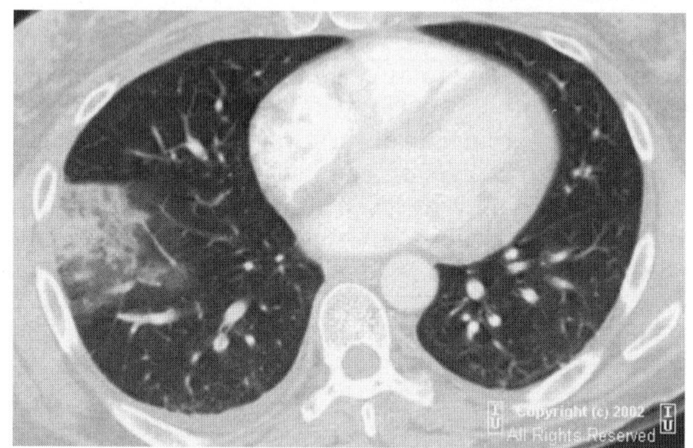

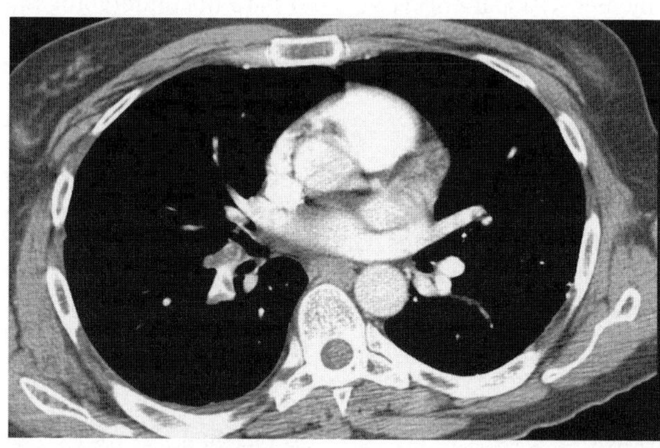

compressible (pressure applied with the transducer causes complete apposition of the far and near walls); the vessel lumen is anechoic on gray-scale images, and it fills completely with color flow; however, when a clot is present, the vessel wall may be thickened or irregular, the lumen may demonstrate internal echoes, and most importantly, the vessel is incompletely compressible and does not fill from wall to wall with color flow (because of the presence of internal thrombus) (**Fig. 2–30**). When lack of compressibility or incomplete color flow is demonstrated, therapy is warranted. Unfortunately, approximately one half of patients with lower extremity DVT have no symptoms or signs of the condition, and the diagnosis is not suspected.

Ventilation/Perfusion Scan If the patient exhibits more than minimal pulmonary symptoms and signs, the study of choice in some centers remains a nuclear medicine ventilation/perfusion lung scan (V/Q scan). The rationale behind the V/Q scan is straightforward. If there is a clinically significant PE, a segmental region of diminished or absent perfusion should be detectable. It tends to be segmental because the pulmonary parenchyma is supplied by segmental arteries, although a perfusion deficit could involve an entire lobe or even the whole lung. If there is no segmental perfusion defect, the patient does not have PE. If there is a perfusion defect, a diagnosis of PE is possible, but it must be confirmed by an assessment of the ventilation of that portion of the lung. The perfusion defect may reflect underlying lung disease, in which case the ventilation in that region will be abnormal as well. Examples of underlying lung disease include destruction of pulmonary capillaries from emphysema and filling of air spaces with pus in pneumonia. Adding ventilation scanning to perfusion scanning improves the specificity of an abnormal perfusion scan, ensuring that other causes of abnormal perfusion are not mistaken for PE. A "classic" PE, then, is an "unmatched" perfusion defect, that is, a perfusion defect without associated ventilation defect (**Fig. 2–31**). Whenever the chest radiograph shows a region of consolidation, the V/Q scan cannot be expected to provide definitive information about that region. This is why a V/Q scan should never be ordered or interpreted in the absence of a current chest radiograph.

Pulmonary perfusion is assessed by injecting Tc-99m-labeled macroaggregated albumin (MAA) into a peripheral vein. Approximately 400,000 particles are injected, and these travel through the heart, out the pulmonary outflow tract, and into the pulmonary arterioles, where they become lodged. In other words, one of the most commonly employed diagnostic test in the evaluation of PE involves the intentional production of PE. However, even this large number of

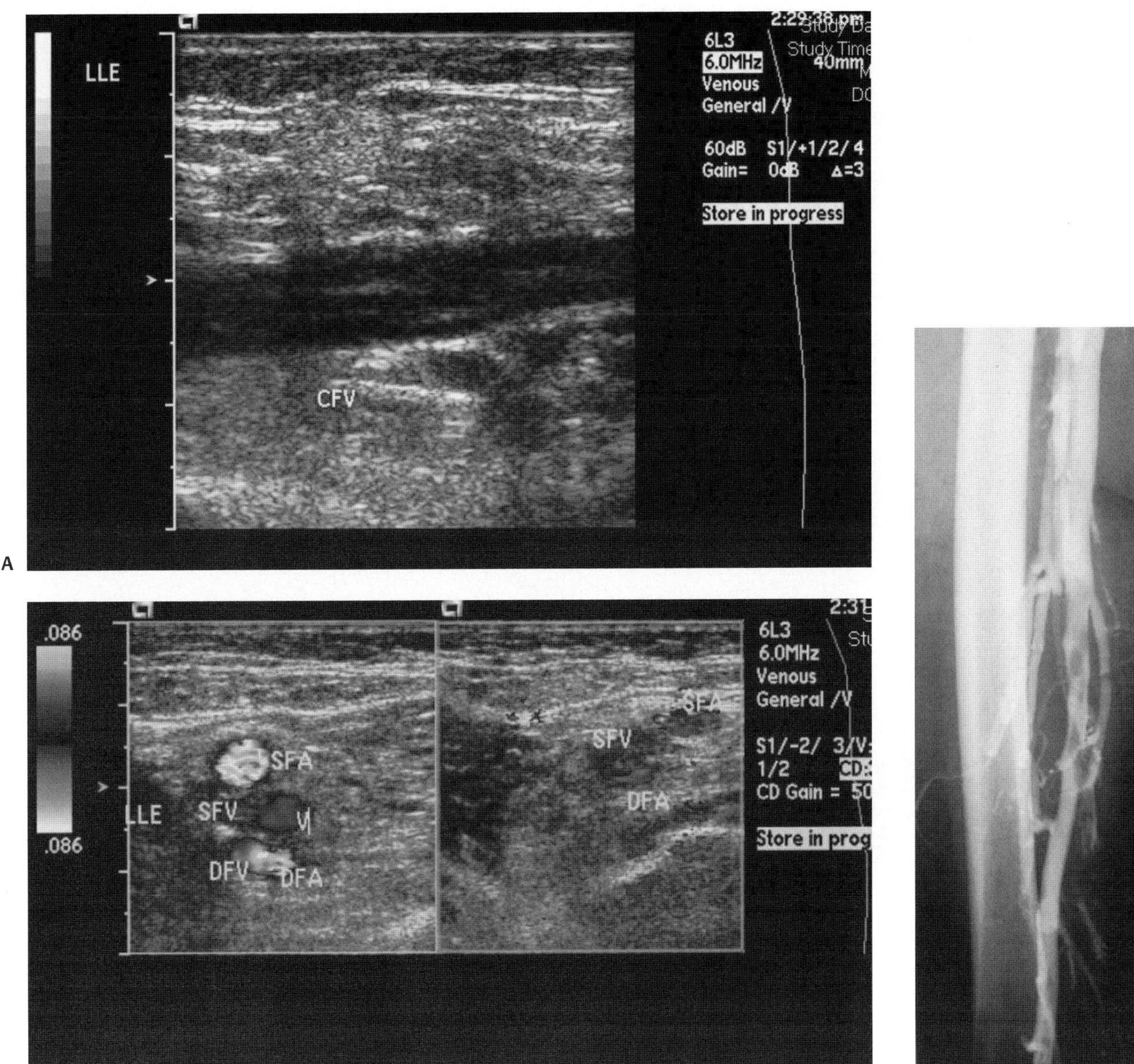

Figure 2–30 **(A)** This longitudinal sonogram of the upper thigh demonstrates echogenic material within the lumen of the common femoral vein. **(B)** These transverse images were obtained without and then with transducer-applied compression. Note that on the view with compression, the superficial femoral vein (SFV) is not compressible and contains echogenic clot. This is diagnostic of deep venous thrombosis. **(C)** This venogram in another patient was performed by starting an intravenous line on the foot and injecting iodinated contrast, then radiographing the thigh. The long filling defect visible in the SFV represents deep venous thrombosis (DVT).

particles actually embolizes only ~1 of every 1000 pulmonary capillaries, rendering the hemodynamic effect, even in the most critically ill patients, negligible. In rare cases in which a right-to-left shunt exists (raising the possibility of cerebral embolization), or when the patient suffers severe pulmonary hypertension, the number of particles may be reduced. Images are obtained in multiple projections by placing the patient in front of a scintillation detector and recording the number and location of the gamma emissions from the thorax.

Ventilation scanning is most often performed using xenon-133 gas, although Tc-99m diethylenetriamine pentaacetic acid (DTPA) aerosol is used in some centers. Imaging consists of inhalation, rebreathing, and “washout” phases obtained over several minutes, usually in a single posterior projection. Though ideally the perfusion images would be performed first to determine if there is a perfusion deficit (if not, the diagnosis of PE is already excluded), the ventilation portion is usually performed first because the higher-energy emissions

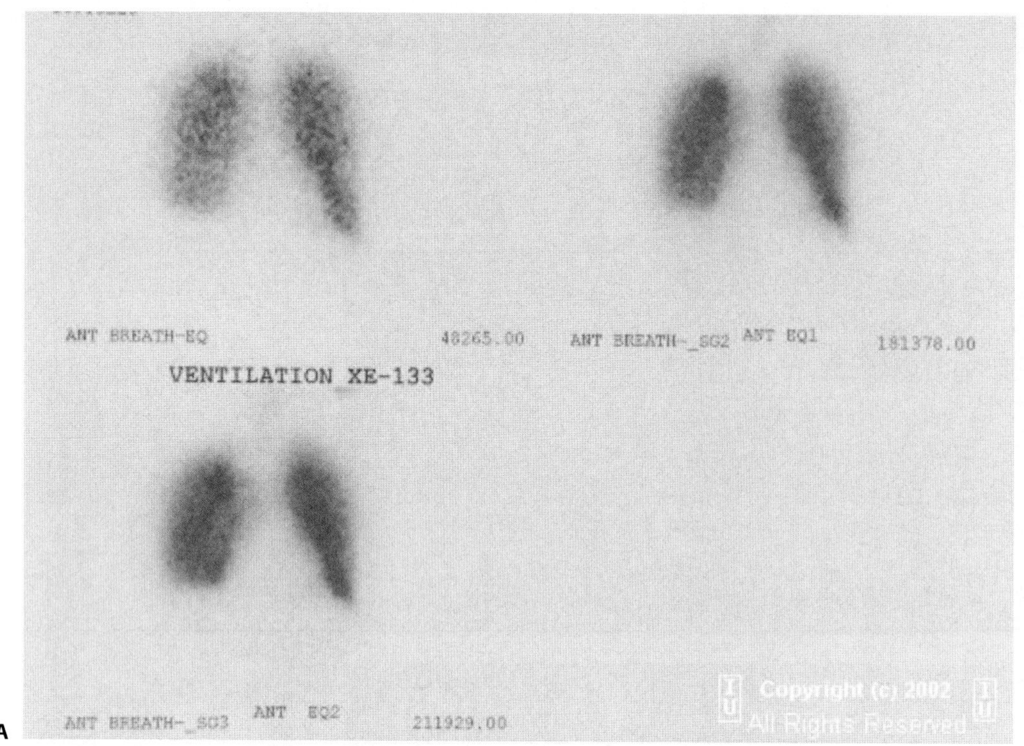

A

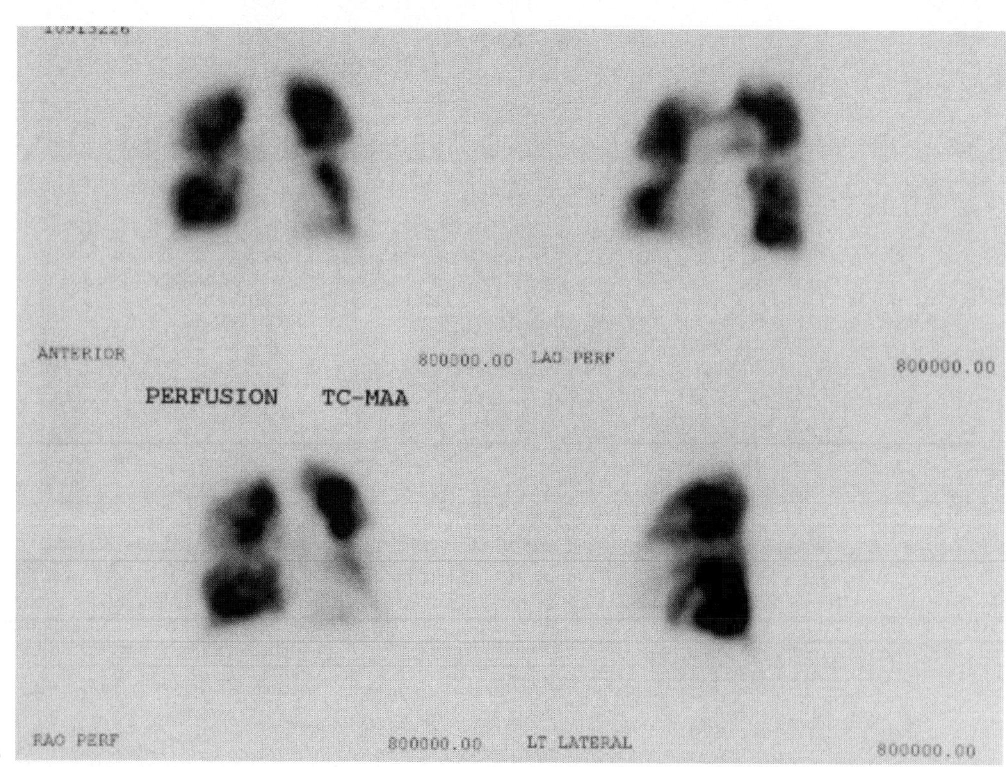

B

Figure 2–31 (A) Three images from a xenon- (Xe) 133 ventilation study demonstrate no ventilation defects. **(B)** On the Tc-99m-labeled MAA perfusion study, however, there are bilateral, peripheral, large wedge-shaped defects, diagnostic of pulmonary thromboembolism. This 40-year-old woman smoked cigarettes and was using oral contraceptives.

from the Tc 99m used in the perfusion study would interfere with detection of the xenon-133 emissions.

Broadly speaking, the results of V/Q scans are reported according to four classifications. A normal scan means that no suspicious perfusion defects were detected, and effectively rules out PE. A low-probability scan consists of perfusion defects unlikely to represent emboli, such as small defects, nonsegmental abnormalities, or larger, matched defects of the sort expected in chronic obstructive pulmonary disease (COPD) (with delayed washout of tracer on ventilation images). Low-probability scans are believed to be associated with a 10 to 15% incidence of PE. A high-probability scan consists of multiple unmatched, segmental perfusion defects, with no other likely etiology, and is associated with at least an 85% incidence of PE. Intermediate-probability scans include those in which there is extensive pulmonary consolidation or COPD, both of which compromise the specificity of the scan, as well as cases in which there is only a single defect. Unfortunately, only ~40% of patients with PE have a high-probability V/Q scan, and in up to three quarters of patients the diagnosis of PE is not definitively resolved after the study.

CT Pulmonary Arteriography In many centers, CT pulmonary arteriography has become the study of choice for the diagnosis of PE. Scanning is performed with bolus injection of intravenous iodinated contrast material timed to optimize opacification of the main pulmonary artery and its branches, and thin image "slices" are obtained to facilitate visualization of pulmonary artery branches. The increased availability of multidetector CT scanners enhances the advantages of CT angiography. Pulmonary emboli appear as filling defects ("dark" areas within the vessel lumen, which should have filled with bright contrast-opacified blood) or an abrupt cutoff of the intraluminal contrast (**Fig. 2–32**). The advantages of CT include a high sensitivity and specificity for PE, the ability to identify other disease processes that may mimic PE (pneumonia, myocardial infarction), and the ability to scan the leg veins at the same time to look for DVT (CT venography).

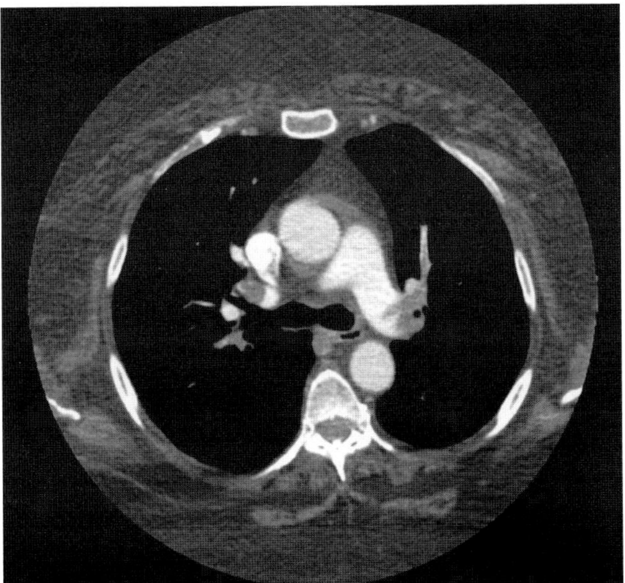

Figure 2–32 This CT pulmonary arteriogram, performed by high-flow injection of contrast into a peripheral vein, demonstrates filling defects in the right and left pulmonary arteries, diagnostic of pulmonary thromboembolism. This elderly patient had presented with dyspnea and hypoxia.

Catheter Pulmonary Angiography The gold standard for diagnosing PE is the catheter pulmonary angiogram. This study involves passing a catheter from a peripheral vein (typically the common femoral vein) through the right side of the heart and into the pulmonary outflow tract under fluoroscopic guidance, with selective catheterization of either the right or left pulmonary artery. Iodinated contrast material is then injected, and multiple rapid-sequence radiographs are obtained. Relative contraindications to pulmonary angiography include severe pulmonary hypertension, left bundle branch block (because conduction through the right branch may be temporarily disturbed as the catheter passes through the right ventricle, producing complete heart block), and a history of severe contrast reaction. The conclusive signs of PE are an intraluminal filling defect or cutoff of one of the pulmonary arteries.

◇ Treatment

Treatment of PE in most cases uses anticoagulants to prevent clot propagation and recurrence. Effective prophylaxis can be achieved in high-risk patients without symptoms or signs through low-dose subcutaneous heparin. Once DVT or PE has occurred, immediate treatment consists of higher doses of heparin. After the acute stage, patients generally receive at least 3 months of oral Coumadin therapy. These steps significantly decrease the subsequent risk of death from PE. Thrombolytic agents, such as tissue-type plasminogen activator, are playing an increasing role in DVT and PE. They activate plasminogen to plasmin, which in turn degrades fibrin to soluble peptides. Indications would include a large clot burden (multiple lobes involved) and hemodynamic instability despite adequate volume resuscitation.

Why don't we simply anticoagulate every patient with suspected PE? The answer is that anticoagulation carries a 30% risk of bleeding, with a 7% risk of major hemorrhage. Because only ~10% of patients worked up for PE actually have the condition, simply treating every patient in whom the diagnosis is suspected would carry an unfavorable risk-to-benefit ratio. In addition to the risks of bleeding with heparin, Coumadin also interacts adversely with several other drugs, which may affect its degradation (barbiturates), absorption (cholestyramine), or metabolism (disulfuram), or simply increase the risk of hemorrhage through other mechanisms of anticoagulant function (aspirin). The principal contraindications to anticoagulant therapy include a history of significant hemorrhage, as from a central nervous system (CNS) or gastrointestinal source, and recent major surgery. Inability to obtain adequate anticoagulation, as in a noncompliant patient, is another problem.

What can be done in the patient with documented DVT or PE, in whom anticoagulation is contraindicated or cannot be achieved? In these cases, percutaneous placement of an inferior vena cava (IVC) filter may be warranted, which can be performed through the same puncture site immediately after pulmonary angiography. The collapsed, netlike filter is placed into the infrarenal IVC, where it is allowed to expand and

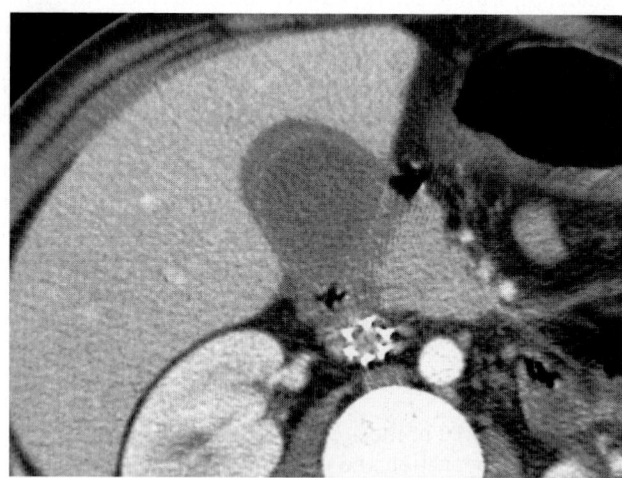

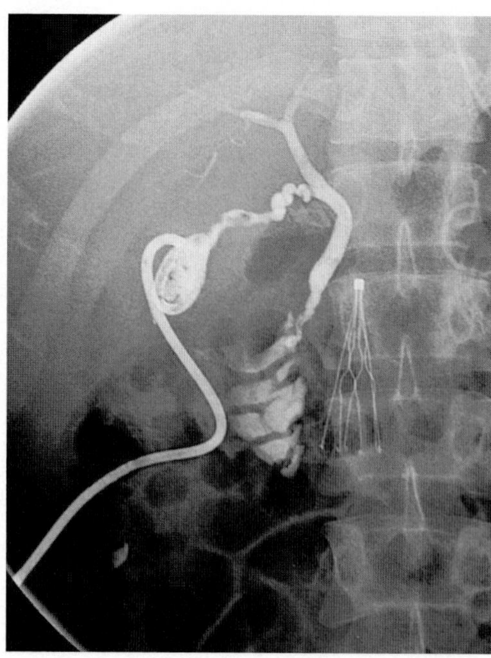

Figure 2–33 This patient with right upper quadrant pain was found to be suffering from chronic cholecystitis. **(A)** This abdominal CT scan was performed to evaluate the gallbladder. It shows abnormal gallbladder wall thickening. What are the six bright foci within the inferior vena cava (IVC), which demonstrate some streak artifact? **(B)** The answer is apparent on this spot image from a percutaneous cholecystogram/cholangiogram. There is contrast filling the gallbladder lumen and bile ducts and emptying into the duodenum. The IVC contains a filter, placed previously to prevent known DVT from becoming a pulmonary embolism.

engage the walls of the vein (**Fig. 2–33**). Thus positioned, it traps emboli originating in the legs and pelvis, preventing them from reaching the heart and lungs. Once trapped, the emboli are usually lysed by intrinsic thrombolytic mechanisms.

In centers with a multidetector CT scanner, a reasonable diagnostic algorithm for suspected PE would be to check for symptoms and signs of lower extremity DVT and, if they are present, perform a lower extremity ultrasound examination. If that is positive, the patient should be anticoagulated. If the lower extremity ultrasound is negative, a CT pulmonary arteriogram should be performed. In patients without leg findings, a CT scan should be performed.

◆ Aorta

Anatomy and Physiology

The anatomy of the thoracic aorta is divided into three portions. The most proximal is the ascending aorta, which extends from the aortic root to a point immediately proximal to the (right) brachiocephalic artery. It includes the sinuses of Valsalva and the origins of the right and left coronary arteries. The next portion is the arch, which gives rise to the brachiocephalic artery (giving rise to the right subclavian and common carotid arteries) and the left common carotid and subclavian arteries, terminating at the ligamentum arteriosum. The third portion is the descending aorta, which extends down to the diaphragm.

The thoracic aorta serves two important physiologic functions. First, it represents the conduit for the entire output of the left ventricle. Second, its elastic recoil enables it to serve as a pressure reservoir, storing the kinetic energy of systolic ejection, then releasing it during diastole. This ensures that the blood pressure never drops to zero, and maintains forward flow of blood throughout the cardiac cycle. This is especially important with respect to the heart's own blood supply, because the tension within the myocardium during systole prevents significant coronary artery blood flow. During diastole, however, when wall tension is decreased, the elastic recoil of the aorta propels blood into the myocardium.

Pathology

Although numerous disease processes may affect the aorta, three merit attention here: aneurysm, dissection, and trauma.

Aneurysm

◇ Epidemiology

An aneurysm is an abnormal dilation of a blood vessel, most commonly the aorta. The vast majority of aortic aneurysms in the United States are atherosclerotic, related to the high prevalence of tobacco use, hypertension, diabetes, and atherogenic diet. Other types of aneurysms include traumatic (penetrating trauma or deceleration injury), mycotic infection, and syphilitic aneurysms.

True aneurysm

False aneurysm

Adventitia

Figure 2–34 The morphologic distinction between a true aneurysm (left) and a false aneurysm (right). Note that the true aneurysm involves an outward bulge in all three layers of the vessel wall, whereas the false aneurysm consists of a rupture of the vessel wall, with the hemorrhage contained by the adventitia.

◇ Pathophysiology

Pathologically, there are two types of aneurysms. A true aneurysm involves all three layers of the vessel wall (intima, media, and adventitia), whereas a false aneurysm consists of a rupture of the vessel wall, with the hemorrhage contained by the adventitia (**Fig. 2–34**). Morphologically, aneurysms may be described as fusiform (circumferential dilation) or saccular (eccentric outpouching).

The treatment of thoracic aortic aneurysms consists primarily of antihypertensive medications. If the patient is symptomatic, there has been a rapid increase in size, or the aorta is greater than 6 cm in diameter, surgical resection and vascular grafting are often performed. Why are large aneurysms more worrisome? The answer hinges on the law of Laplace, which states that the tension in the wall of a vessel is proportional to the transmural pressure multiplied by the radius. Assuming the mean arterial pressure remains constant, the tension in the wall, the force promoting rupture, increases in direct relation to the radius. Hence, the larger the diameter of an aneurysm, the more likely it is to rupture. A 6 cm aneurysmal segment of ascending aorta has twice the wall tension of a healthy 3 cm segment.

◇ Clinical Presentation

Most patients with thoracic aortic aneurysms are asymptomatic, but a small minority will present with symptoms such as deep, diffuse chest pain, hoarseness, and even hemoptysis or hematemesis (secondary to communication with the tracheobronchial tree or esophagus).

◇ Imaging

Several radiologic modalities are useful in assessing for the presence of an aortic aneurysm. Patients with atherosclerotic aneurysms typically demonstrate plain radiographic signs of advanced atherosclerosis, including enlargement of the aortic silhouette, and tortuosity and calcification of the aorta and other arteries, including the coronary arteries (**Fig. 2–35**). Enlargement of the aorta or a change in its contour can be assessed by comparison to previous films. Occasionally,

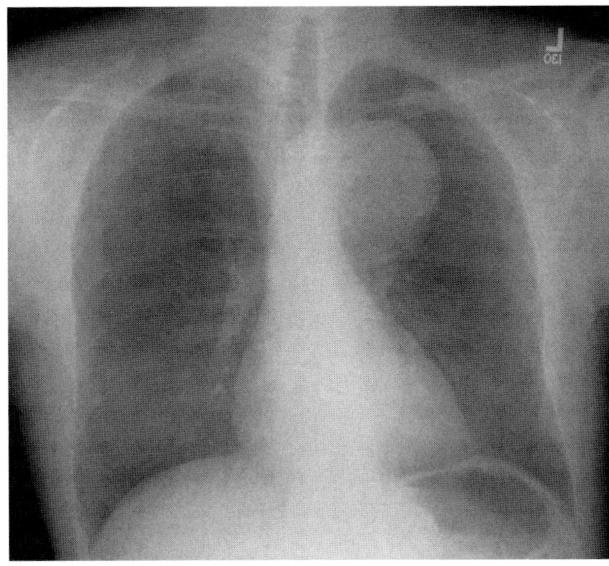

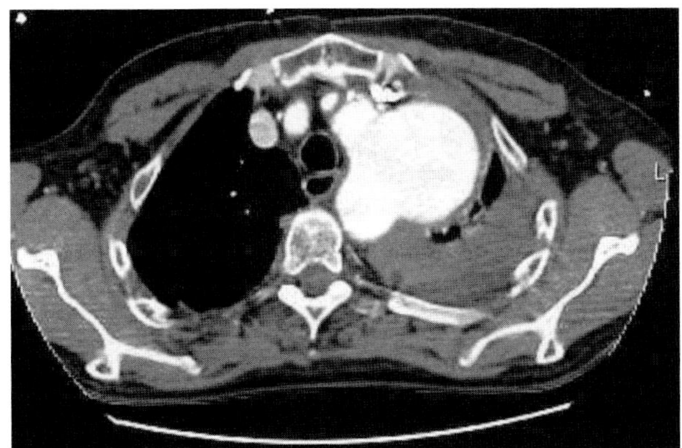

Figure 2–35 **(A)** This man with chest pain and a falling hematocrit underwent heart transplantation the previous year. His chest radiograph demonstrates a large mass originating at the level of the aortic arch. **(B)** A CT image at the level shows the large secular aneurysm extending leftward from the aortic arch, with a large left pleural effusion. The aneurysm was leaking blood into the chest.

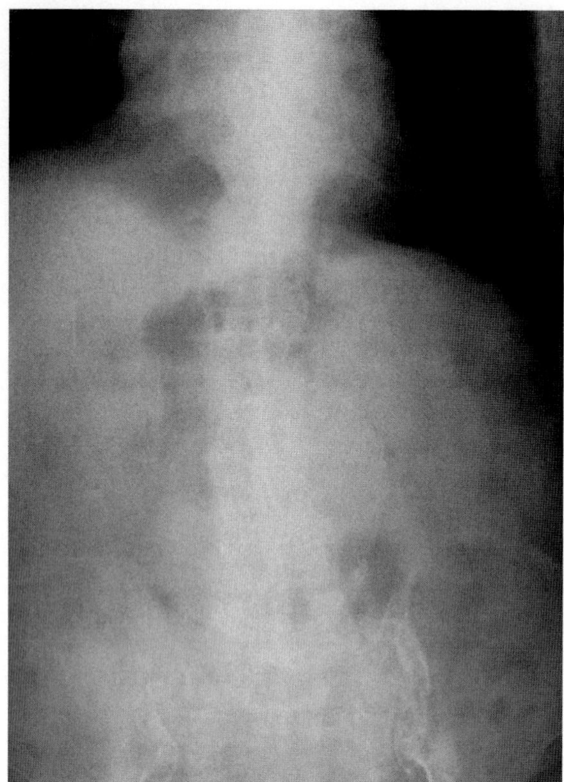

Figure 2–36 This plain radiograph of the abdomen demonstrates a faintly calcific opacity overlying the lumbar spine, creating an arclike contour on its left side. This is a large, calcific abdominal aortic aneurysm.

calcifications within the wall of an aortic aneurysm reveal its presence on plain radiography (**Fig. 2–36**). Angiography is the traditional mainstay of aneurysm assessment, although the contrast column will trace out only the patent portion of the lumen, thus underestimating the diameter of a thrombus-containing vessel. CT provides a better estimate of vessel diameter, as well as the character of any thrombus. A nontraumatic aneurysm rarely ruptures if its diameter is less than 5 cm. Signs of rupture by CT include a sudden increase in the size of the aorta, the appearance of a pleural effusion (hemothorax), and the presence of a high-attenuation hematoma around the aorta. MRI provides a similar assessment to that of CT but requires no intravascular contrast.

Dissection

◇ Epidemiology

Dissection (from the Latin for "to cut apart") denotes the splitting of the laminar planes of the arterial media, with the formation of a potentially occlusive hematoma within the vessel wall. It is most common in hypertensive men in the fifth and sixth decades of life. Other risk factors include connective tissue disorders such as Marfan's syndrome, coarctation of the aorta, and bicuspid aortic valve. Marfan's syndrome is related to an autosomal-dominant defect in connective tissue protein synthesis, resulting in an abnormal arterial media, and is associated with such physical examination findings as large height, asthenic build, scoliosis, and pectus excavatum. Untreated, patients are at very high risk of premature death from valvular insufficiency and aortic dissection, typically involving the ascending aorta.

◇ Pathophysiology

Dissection creates two "lumens": a true lumen through which blood continues to flow, and a false lumen within the vessel wall, which expands to some degree and tends to occlude flow. According to the Stanford system, aortic dissections are classified into two types: A and B. A type A dissection involves at least the ascending aorta, whereas a type B dissection does not. Type A is the most dangerous, because of three potential complications: it may extend proximally to involve the aortic root, causing acute aortic insufficiency; it may extend into the coronary arteries, compromising cardiac perfusion; and it may rupture the outer wall of the false lumen, causing hemopericardium and cardiac tamponade or even exsanguination.

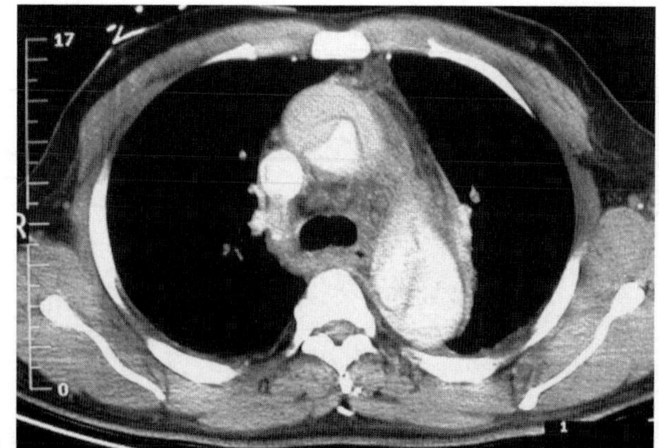

A

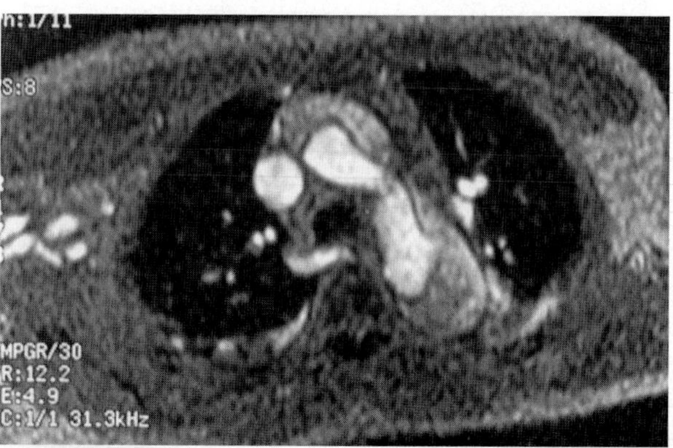

B

Figure 2–37 (A) This patient presented with ripping chest pain radiating to the back. A CT scan of the chest with intravenous contrast demonstrates a luminal flap extending through both the ascending and descending portion of the thoracic aorta. **(B)** A "bright blood" axial MR image in the same patient likewise demonstrates the luminal flap in both the ascending and descending aorta, dividing its lumen into "true" and "false" components. Both studies are diagnostic of a type A aortic dissection.

Treatment depends on the type of dissection. Type B dissections are usually treated medically, with control of hypertension to decrease the stress on the vessel. Type A dissections are typically treated surgically, which may be emergent if the patient cannot be stabilized medically. Signs of stabilization include resolution of pain and lack of radiographic evidence of dissection propagation.

◇ Clinical Presentation

Acute aortic dissection is typically heralded by the onset of severe, "tearing" chest pain, and may be accompanied by symptoms of various complications, such as myocardial infarction, stroke (if the dissection compromises the carotid or vertebral arteries), and dyspnea (from acute aortic regurgitation).

◇ Imaging

The radiologic evaluation begins with the plain radiograph, which may show aortomegaly, a disparity in the sizes of the ascending and descending portions of the aorta, a new left pleural effusion, and a change in the position of preexisting intimal calcifications due to the accumulation of blood within the vessel wall. CT with intravenous contrast material is a relatively quick and noninvasive examination that will often demonstrate the intimal flap, the extent of the tear in the vessel wall, and the presence or absence of extravasation. MRI does not necessarily require intravenous contrast (**Fig. 2–37**). Transesophageal echocardiography can be performed at the bedside by a cardiologist and constitutes the most commonly employed technique at many institutions. Angiography remains the gold standard, because the precise entry site and extent of the false lumen can be identified, the involvement of the aortic branches, including the coronary arteries, can be assessed, and the aortic valve itself can be evaluated.

Trauma

The sequelae of thoracic trauma include both aortic aneurysm and dissection, which have been discussed. Other aortic sequelae include transection and laceration, which are fatal in more than 90% of cases. Except in cases of penetrating trauma, where the mechanism of injury is obvious, it is thought that most injuries result from "pinching" of the aorta between the anterior chest wall and the vertebral column, which explains the relatively high percentage of injuries at the ligamentum arteriosum (remnant of the ductus arteriosus). Clinical findings in aortic injury include asymmetric upper extremity pulses, a disparity between upper and lower extremity blood pressures, chest pain, and dyspnea.

Radiologic findings include those previously mentioned for aneurysm and dissection. Caution is warranted in the interpretation of the chest radiograph, as even severe aortic injury may demonstrate no plain radiographic abnormalities. In addition, abnormalities such as widening of the mediastinum may reflect not traumatic rupture of the aorta, but other less serious mediastinal injuries. However, a high clinical suspicion is warranted in every case, and aortography by CT, MRI, or in the angiographic suite is generally the examination of choice. The key findings to be excluded are intimal tear, aneurysm, dissection, and extravasation.

3

The Respiratory System

- **Anatomy and Physiology**
- **Imaging**
  - The Chest X-Ray
    - *Technical Factors*
    - *Search Pattern*
    - *Pulmonary Parenchymal Patterns*
    - *Clinical History*
  - Other Imaging Modalities
- **Airway**
  - Pathology
    - *Asthma*
    - *Chronic Obstructive Pulmonary Disease*
- **Pleura**
  - Pathology
    - *Pleural Effusion*
    - *Pneumothorax*
- **Mediastinum**
  - Anatomy and Imaging
  - Pathology
    - *Mediastinal Mass*
- **Lung**
  - Pathology
    - *Congenital*
    - *Infectious*
    - *Tumorous*
    - *Inflammatory*
    - *Metabolic*
    - *Iatrogenic*
    - *Traumatic*
    - *Vascular*

◆ Anatomy and Physiology

The primary function of the respiratory system is to permit gas exchange to support cellular metabolism, including the diffusion of oxygen into the blood and the diffusion of carbon dioxide out of it. The respiratory system also performs several secondary functions, including moistening inhaled air to prevent alveolar linings from drying out, enhancing venous return to the heart during inspiration, helping to maintain acid–base balance, enabling speech, defending against inhaled foreign matter, and activating a variety of blood-borne materials that pass through it, as in the conversion of angiotensin I to angiotensin II by angiotensin converting enzyme (ACE) in the pulmonary capillaries.

The upper respiratory tract includes many of the pharyngeal structures discussed in Chapter 4, and functions primarily to conduct air to and from the sites of actual gas exchange. The trachea (from the Latin *trachia*, "windpipe") begins at the larynx in the neck and extends ~12 cm to the tracheal bifurcation in the chest (**Fig. 3–1**). It is surrounded anteriorly and laterally by U-shaped cartilages, which often calcify with age, particularly in elderly women. Lining the upper respiratory tract are ciliated cells that project into a sticky luminal layer of mucus, which constitutes the mucociliary elevator (**Fig. 3–2**). Particulate matter of a certain size is trapped in this mucous layer then propelled by ciliary motion upward toward the throat, where it can be expectorated or swallowed. The normal functioning of this apparatus is impaired in cystic fibrosis, the most common lethal genetic disease among white populations, in which the mucus is abnormally viscous and bacteria cannot be cleared. Cigarette smoking causes similar problems by paralyzing the cilia and eventually denuding the epithelium of them.

The mainstem bronchi of each lung arborize into lobar and segmental bronchi, which correspond to pulmonary divisions (**Fig. 3–3**). The right lung has upper, middle, and lower lobes, and the left lung has an upper lobe (including the lingula) and a lower lobe. Each lung is invested by a double-layered serosal membrane, the pleura (from the Greek, meaning "rib"), made up of inner visceral (from the Latin *viscus*, an

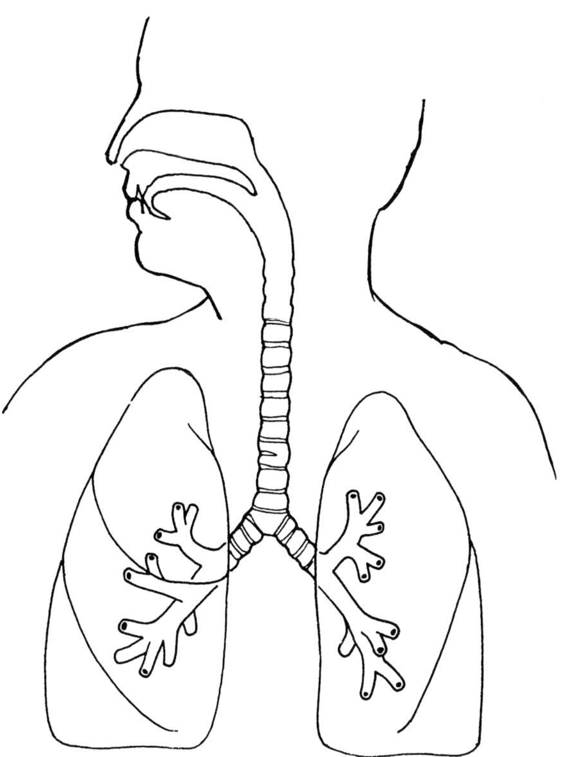

Figure 3–1 Trachea, mainstem bronchi, and segmental bronchial branches.

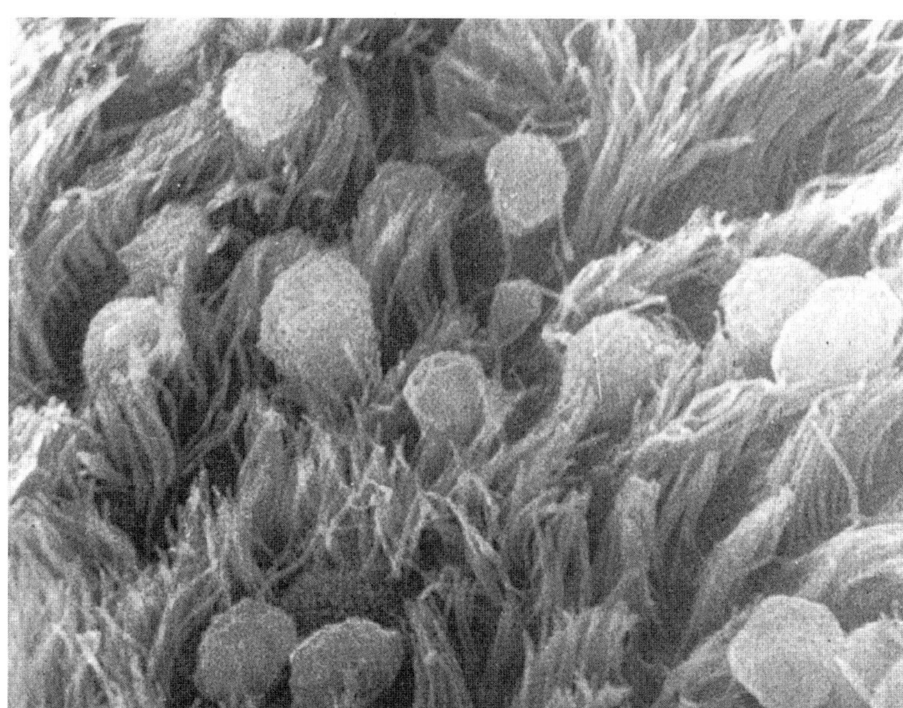

Figure 3–2 This scanning electron micrograph displays the extensively ciliated surface of the normal bronchiolar mucosa, which is integral to the function of the mucociliary elevator. (From Kuhn C. Normal anatomy and histology. In: Thurlbeck WM, Churg AM. Pathology of the Lung, 2nd ed. New York: Thieme Medical Publishers; 1995:13. Used with permission.)

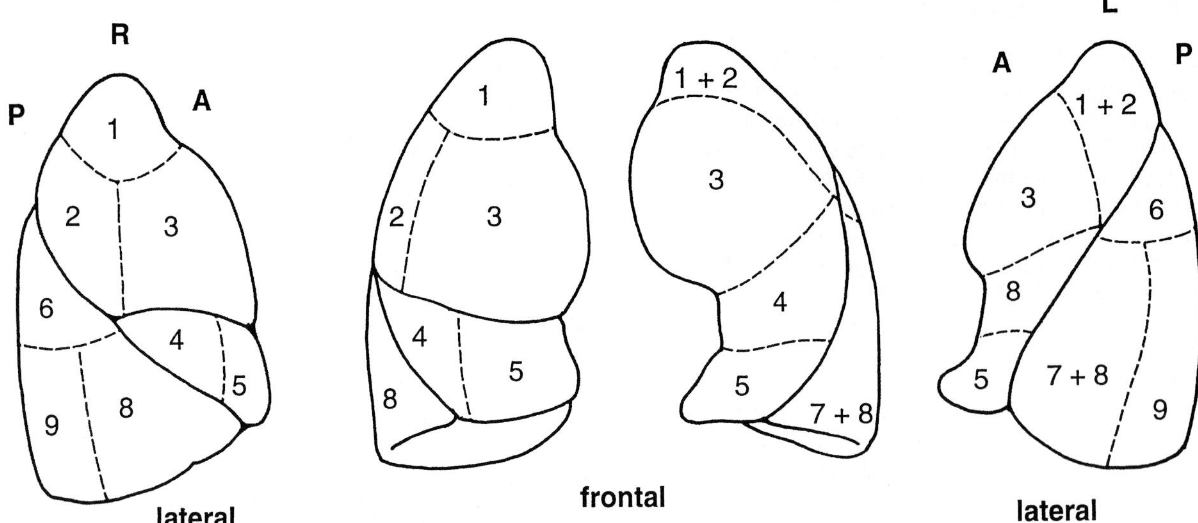

Figure 3–3 The lobar and segmental anatomy of the lung. Upper lobe: 1, apical segment; 2, posterior (P); 3, anterior (A). Middle lobe (R) or lingula (L): 4, lateral; 5, medial. Lower lobe: 6, superior; 7, medial basal; 8, anterior basal; 9, lateral basal; 10, posterior basal. Note that the left upper lobe includes the lingula, and in the left lower lobe the anterior and medial basal segments are combined. The posteromedially located posterior basal segment of the lower lobes (10) is not seen on these drawings.

inner part of the body) and outer parietal (from the Latin, meaning "wall") layers. The lobes are divided from one another by invaginations of the visceral pleura, called fissures. The right lung contains two fissures: the major fissure, which separates the upper and middle lobes anteriorly from the lower lobe posteriorly, and the minor fissure, which separates the upper lobe from the middle lobe. The left lung contains one fissure, the major fissure, which separates the upper and lower lobes. The fissures are best visualized on lateral radiographs. The lobes are then divided into segments, each of which is supplied by segmental bronchi and vessels.

Clusters of tiny alveolar air sacs are found at the end of each terminal bronchiole, the last purely air-conducting structure of the airways (**Fig. 3–4**). The acinus (from the Latin, meaning "grape") is a grape cluster–like structure distal to the terminal bronchiole. Each acinus measures ~7 mm in diameter and contains ~400 alveoli (**Fig. 3–5**). Before high-resolution computed tomography, the acini could only be seen on autopsy. With the advent of high-resolution CT, it has become possible to inspect pulmonary subsegmental anatomy during life. High-resolution CT is performed by examining very narrow slices of the lung, ~1.0 to 1.5 mm in width, and utilizing a high spatial frequency reconstruction algorithm. The secondary pulmonary lobule is the elemental pulmonary component visible by high-resolution CT and appears as a polygonal structure measuring 1.5 to 2.0 cm in diameter. Pulmonary arteries and bronchioles are centrally located within the secondary lobule, whereas the veins and

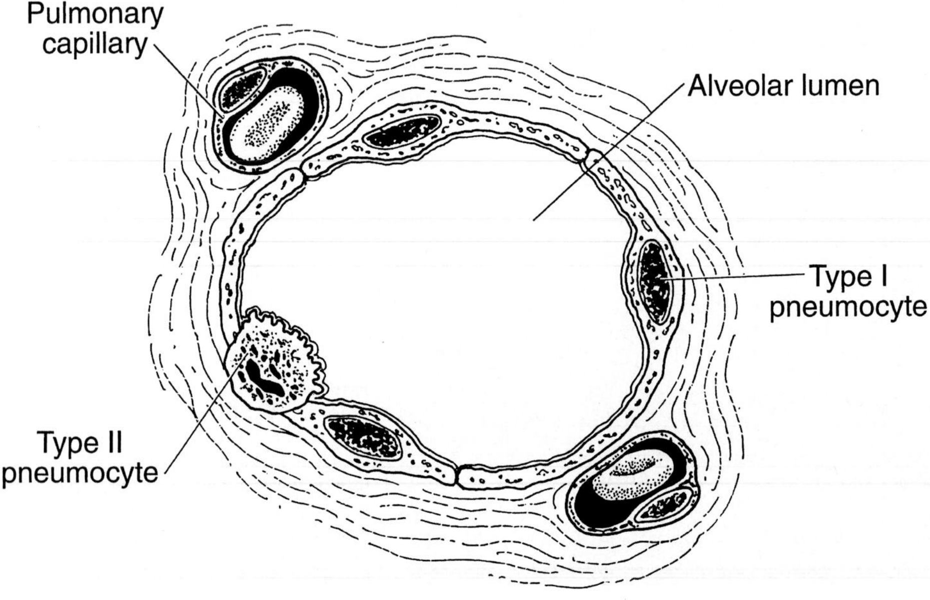

Figure 3–4 An alveolus, including type I and type II pneumocytes and the pulmonary capillaries.

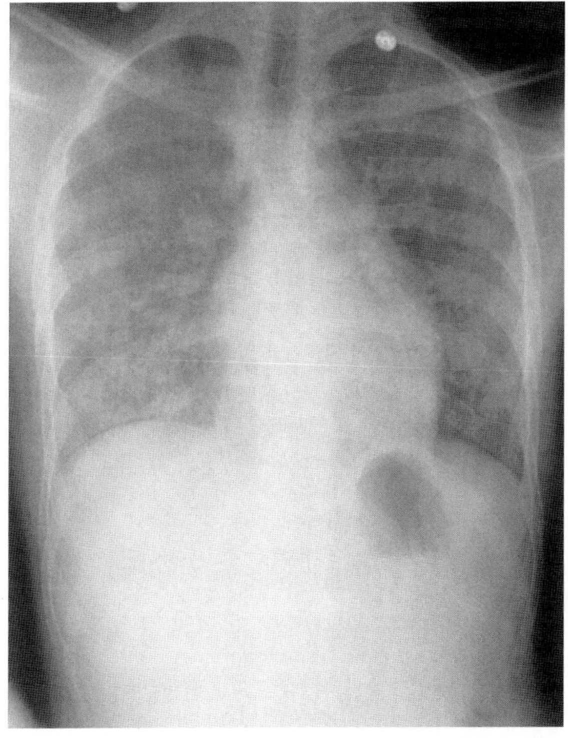

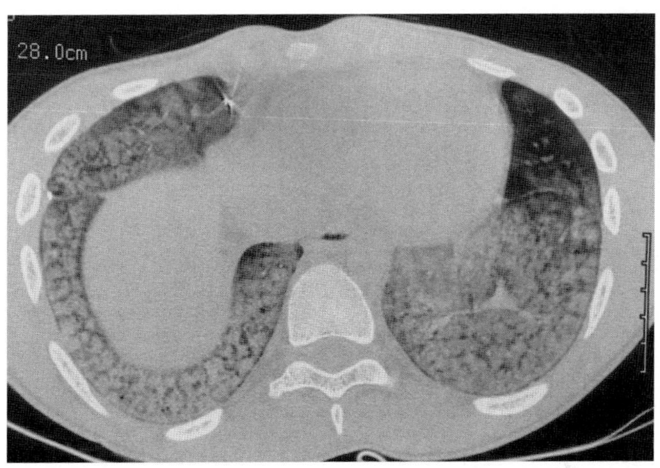

Figure 3–5 A 15-year-old male with a history of idiopathic pulmonary hemorrhage presented to the emergency room with acute hemoptysis and shortness of breath. **(A)** A portable anteroposterior chest radiograph demonstrates diffuse bilateral alveolar opacities, slightly worse on the right. **(B)** An axial image from high-resolution thoracic computed tomography beautifully demonstrates the acinar character of these opacities. Comparing the 1 cm hash marks on the right side of the image, innumerable 7 mm acinar opacities are visible, representing blood-filled acini. Each acinus contains ~400 alveoli. The relative sparing of the left upper lobe is perplexing. The two bright foci at the borders of the right middle lobe represent surgical staples from a previous open lung biopsy.

lymphatics are peripherally located. Each secondary pulmonary lobule contains three to five acini.

There are ~300 million alveoli (from the Latin for "hollow cavity") in the lungs (**Fig. 3–6**). They are adapted to two key physical parameters of diffusion: distance and surface area. Fick's law states that the shorter the distance across which diffusion must take place, the more rapidly it occurs. Atmospheric air in the alveolar lumen is separated from erythrocytes

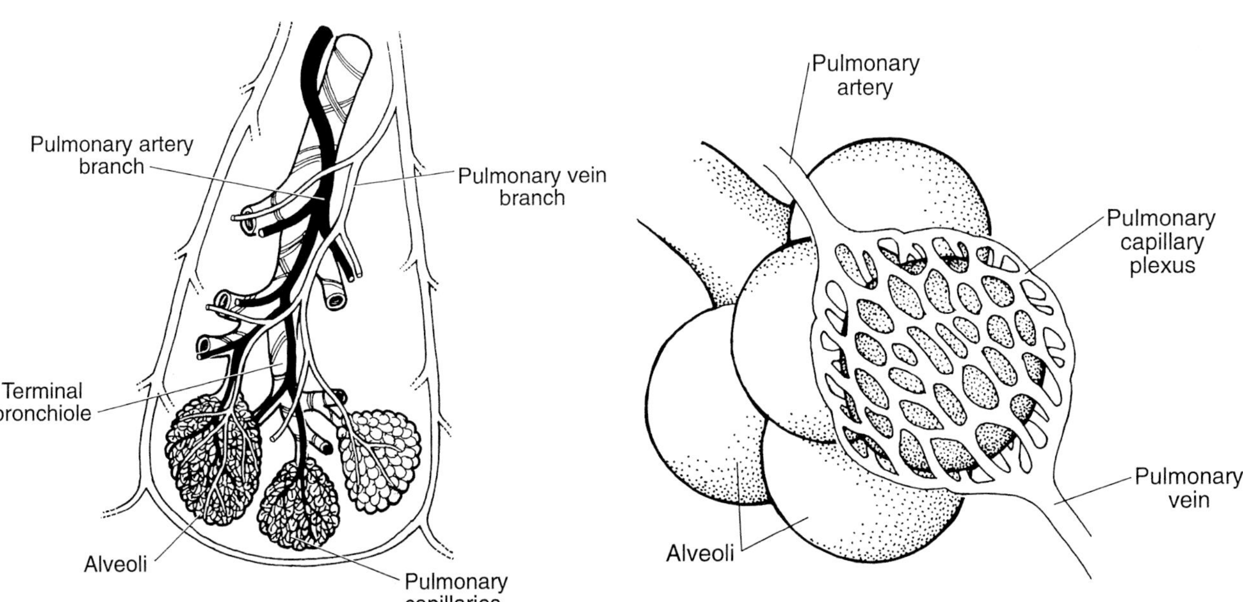

Figure 3–6 The relationship between an alveolus and its capillaries.

in the pulmonary capillaries only by the walls of the alveoli, which consist of a single layer of flattened alveolar cells, and the one cell-thick capillary endothelium, with a total width of only 0.2 μm (a red blood cell is ~7 μm in diameter). The alveoli also exploit the principle that the greater the surface area across which diffusion takes place, the more rapid its rate. The total respiratory surface area available for gas exchange in the lungs is ~75 m^2 (about the size of a doubles tennis court), but would be only ~0.1 m^2 if the lungs consisted of a single hollow chamber of the same dimensions (**Fig. 3–7**).

The epithelial cells of the alveoli are of two types, each called pneumocytes, from the Greek *pneuma-*, "to breathe," and *kytos*, "hollow," from which the combining form *-cyte*, "cell," is derived. Type I pneumocytes are the flattened squamous cells that cover ~95% of the alveolar surface area. Type II pneumocytes are cuboidal cells that secrete pulmonary surfactant, the phospholipoprotein complex that reduces the surface tension between water molecules lining the alveoli and thereby prevents alveolar collapse at low lung volumes, as well as reducing the work of breathing by increasing lung compliance. Fortunately, lung compliance is so high that only ~3% of energy expenditure is devoted to respiration during quiet breathing. Type II pneumocytes are capable of mitosis and represent the source of type I pneumocytes. Also present within the lumen of the alveoli are alveolar macrophages, which play a defensive role against microbes and particulate matter.

The air spaces are not completely isolated from one another, either functionally or anatomically. Functionally, the condition of one alveolus affects its neighbors through the

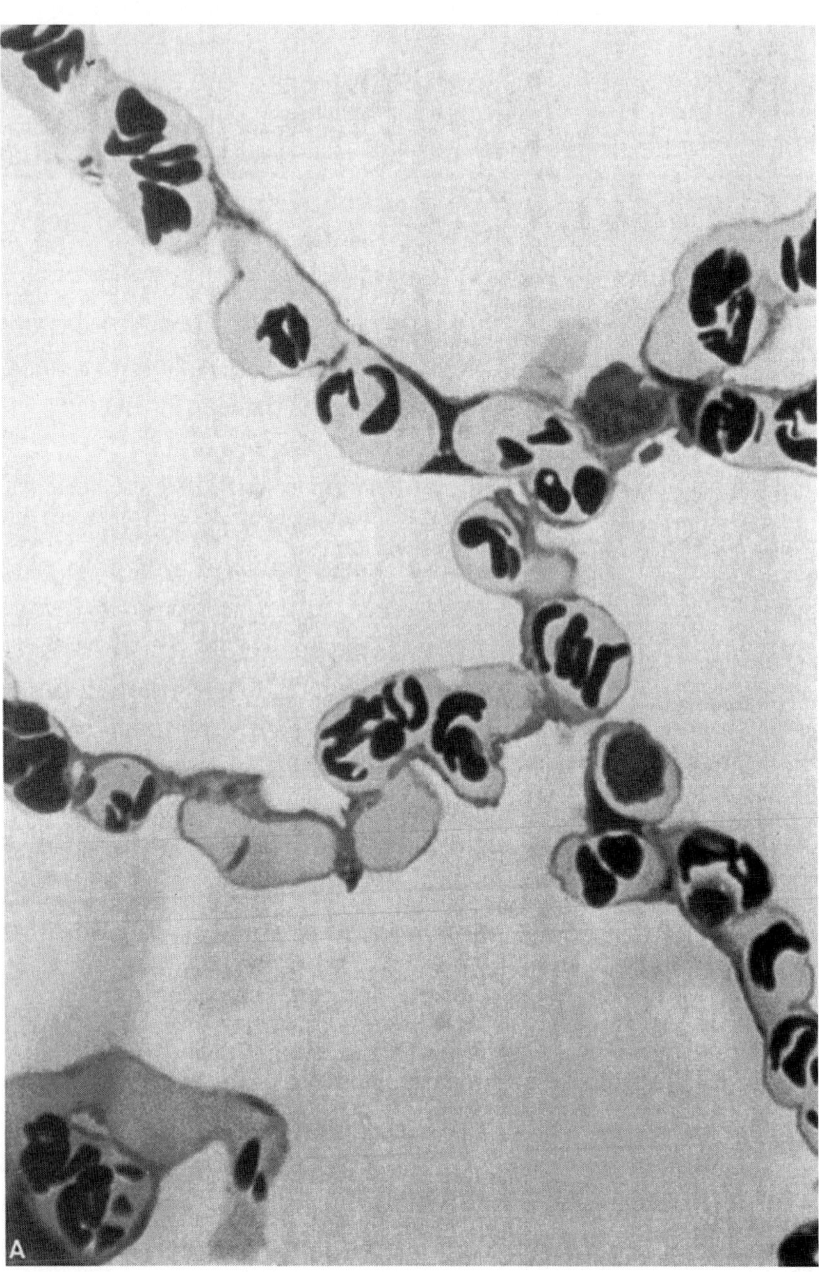

Figure 3–7 This light micrograph of the alveolar wall demonstrates the presence of numerous pulmonary capillaries and pneumocyte cell membranes across which gas exchange takes place in the alveoli. Note the erythrocytes within the capillaries. The lumen of the alveolus represents the air space, and the walls of the alveolus represent the interstitial space. (From Hogg JC. Pulmonary edema. In: Thurlbeck WM, Churg AM. Pathology of the Lung, 2nd ed. New York: Thieme Medical Publishers; 1995:376. Used with permission.)

phenomenon of interdependence. Each alveolus is surrounded by other alveoli, to which it is connected by strands of connective tissue. When any one alveolus starts to collapse, its neighbors are stretched, and their recoil in turn helps to keep the collapsing alveolus inflated. Moreover, there are anatomic channels of collateral air drift between the airways, including the pores of Kohn (interalveolar passages) and canals of Lambert (communications between preterminal bronchioles and alveoli). These communications may prove both beneficial and harmful—beneficial in that they allow collateral air drift behind an area of airway obstruction, but harmful in that they also provide a route of intersegmental dissemination in processes such as lobar pneumonia.

◆ Imaging

The Chest X-Ray

Chest radiography is the most frequently performed radiologic study in the United States, representing ~35% of examinations in many hospitals. In certain acute situations, a basic understanding of the chest radiograph may save a patient's life. In the nonacute setting, even basic radiographic findings may profoundly alter patient management. The chest radiograph's ubiquity and clinical value provide both the student and physician who understand chest radiographs well an opportunity to shine among colleagues and teachers (**Fig. 3–8**). Although the chest radiograph is routine, it also presents one of the most complex interpretive tasks faced by radiologists and nonradiologists alike. Hence a systematic approach is crucial. The following presents one reasonable algorithm for evaluating the chest radiograph. This preliminary discussion is supplemented in the remainder of the chapter with more detailed discussions of specific pathophysiologic processes and additional imaging modalities.

Technical Factors

The basic chest examination consists of two films, one taken in frontal projection and the other in lateral projection. Frontal chest radiographs come in two principal varieties, posteroanterior (PA) and anteroposterior (AP). These designations refer to the path taken by the x-ray beam through the patient, with the x-ray detector touching the front of the chest in the PA radiograph, and touching the back of the chest in the AP radiograph. The PA radiograph is exposed with the patient standing, hands on hips, with palms facing backward to rotate the scapulae out of the lung fields, and at maximal inspiration to "spread out" the pulmonary parenchyma as much as possible. If possible, PA and lateral radiographs should be obtained in essentially every patient with thoracic disease, because this combination provides optimal routine evaluation of the thorax; however, many hospitalized patients are too ill to come to the radiology department or stand for a PA film. In this case, a single frontal radiograph is generally obtained in the AP projection, because only the detector cassette and not the x-ray tube can be placed under the bed-bound patient (**Fig. 3–9**). In some hospitals, ~50% of chest radiographs are portable examinations.

Four technical factors should be evaluated on every chest radiograph: penetration, rotation, inspiration, and motion. The portable AP radiograph is generally inferior to

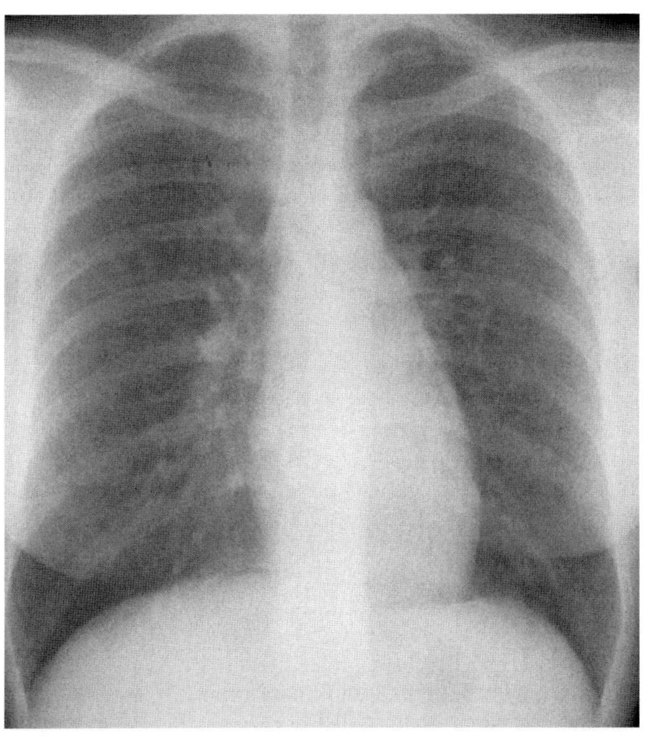

Figure 3–8 The posteroanterior (PA) chest radiograph is normal. Is the patient male or female? How can you tell? The breast shadows overlying the lower chest make it very likely that the patient is an adult female. If it turned out that the patient was male, what diagnosis would you make? The answer is gynecomastia, which means "woman's breasts."

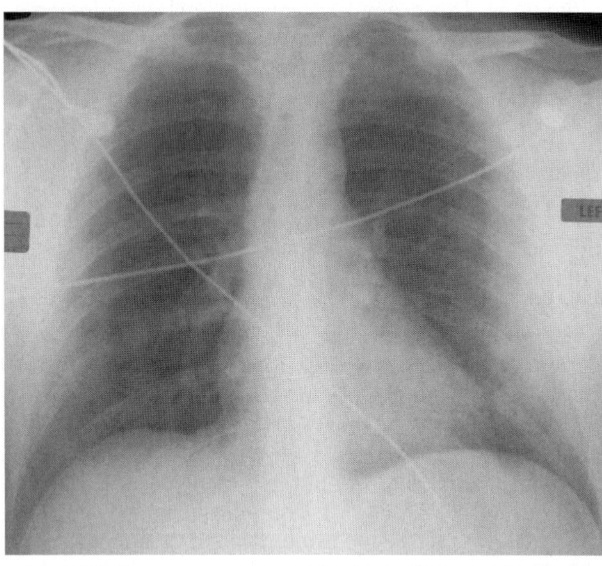

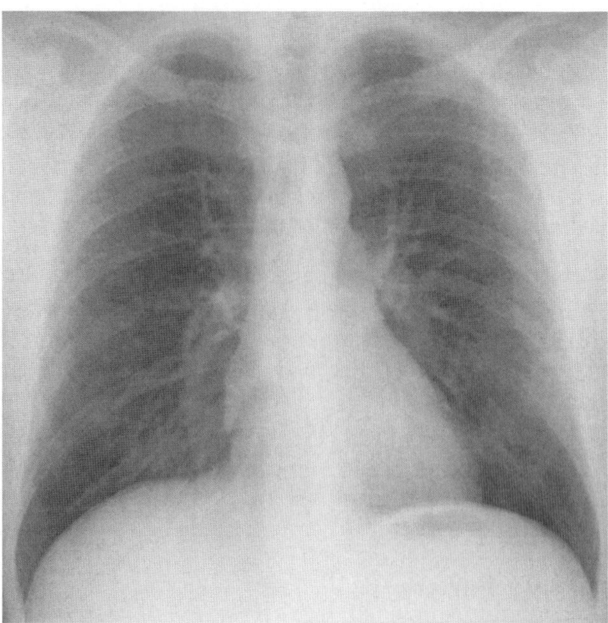

Figure 3–9 **(A)** This anteroposterior (AP) radiograph exaggerates the cardiac shadow due to magnification and underinflation of the lungs because the patient is supine. **(B)** On the PA images, made with the patient standing, the lungs are better inflated, and the heart does not appear so wide.

a standard PA radiograph in each of these respects. Penetration refers to the degree of under- or overexposure of the image. On a properly penetrated radiograph, the intervertebral disk spaces and branching pulmonary vessels should be faintly visible behind the heart. Underpenetrated radiographs make the whole chest appear too white, with inability to see the disk spaces behind the heart; if the image is overpenetrated, the disk spaces are obvious, and lung markings appear "burned out." Because the portable film is obtained under less controlled conditions, proper penetration is more difficult to achieve, although new digital techniques allow some correction for under- or overexposure.

When a patient appears rotated on a chest radiograph, it means that the patient was facing to the right or to the left instead of directly forward when the image was obtained. Rotation is detected as an asymmetry in the distance between the medial margins of the right and left clavicles and the midline spinous processes of the vertebrae. For example, if a patient is rotated to the right, the distance between the medial end of the right clavicle and the thoracic vertebral spinous process at this level is increased, while it is decreased on the left side. This would make a greater proportion of the heart appear to lie to the right of the spine.

Inspiration is assessed by counting the number of posterior ribs visible above the hemidiaphragm, which should number 10 on each side. Bed-bound patients are generally not able to inspire as deeply as ambulatory patients. Underinflation exaggerates heart size and obscures visualization of the pulmonary parenchyma, because a greater amount of lung tissue is superimposed on other lung tissue due to lower overall lung volume (**Fig. 3–10**).

Motion is assessed by noting the sharpness of the hemidiaphragms and pulmonary vessels, which appear blurred if the patient was breathing at the time the image was obtained. Because portable radiography units are generally not as powerful as fixed units, longer exposure times are necessary to obtain an adequate image, resulting in greater potential for motion artifact.

Several additional differences between PA and AP chest radiographs deserve mention. One is the magnification of the heart present on AP radiographs, which may be as great as 20%, and may be further exacerbated by underinflation. On a standard PA film, the cardiothoracic ratio should not exceed 0.5; that is, the width of the cardiac silhouette (heart shadow) should be no more than half the width of the thorax. The heart appears larger on an AP film because, being an anterior thoracic structure, it is farther away from the film, causing it to cast a larger shadow. Many patients with apparent cardiomegaly ("heart enlargement") on portable radiographs turn out to have normal-size hearts when a PA examination is obtained. Cardiac magnification may also result from anatomic anomalies such as a pectus excavatum deformity, which effectively flattens out the heart. Thus, other than AP technique, other radiographic mimics of cardiomegaly would include underinflation, pectus excavatum, and pericardial effusion (**Fig. 3–11**).

Another difference between PA and AP radiographs is the apparent pulmonary vascular redistribution present on AP films, due to the patient's supine position. On a normal upright film, the lower lung zone pulmonary vessels are approximately 3 times the diameter of the upper zone vessels, due to gravity-dependent distribution of flow. On supine films, there appears to be pulmonary vascular redistribution, with upper zone vessels equal in size to the lower zone vessels. If such redistribution were present on an upright radiograph, it would suggest pulmonary venous hypertension, as in congestive heart failure (CHF).

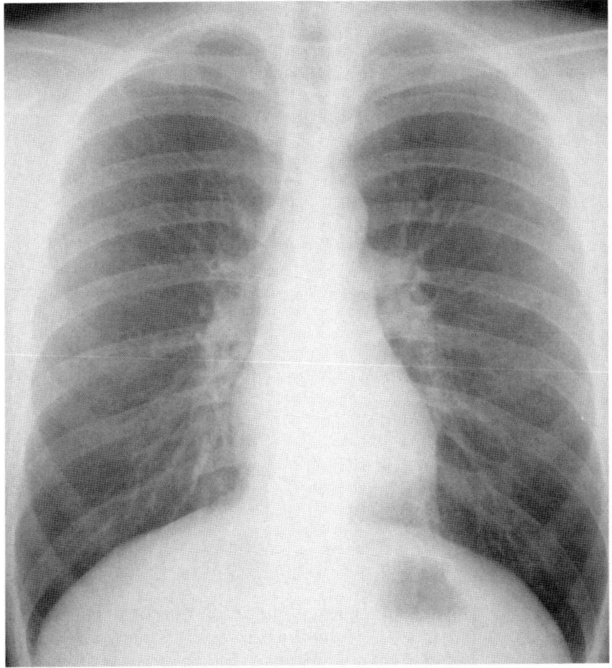

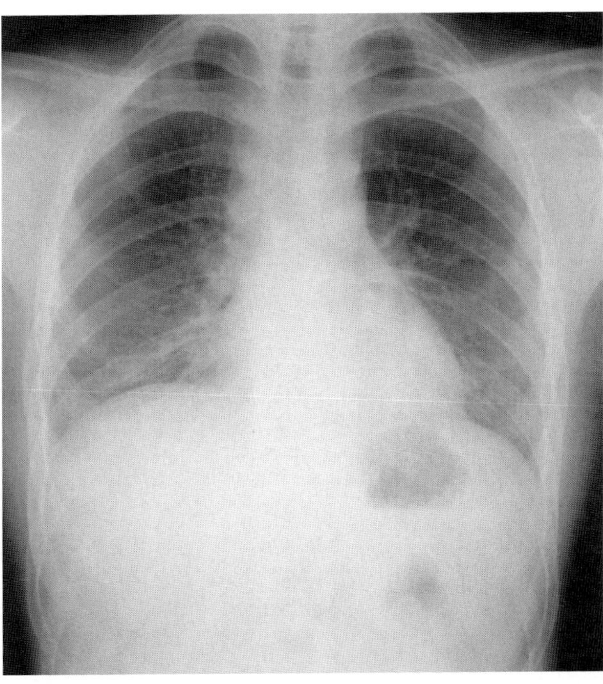

Figure 3–10 **(A)** This inspiratory image demonstrates a normal cardiothoracic ratio (the heart occupies less than 50% of the width of the thorax), and the pulmonary vessels are sharp. The lungs appear "tall." **(B)** On the expiratory view, the heart appears short and wide, the pulmonary vessels are crowded, and the lungs appear "short."

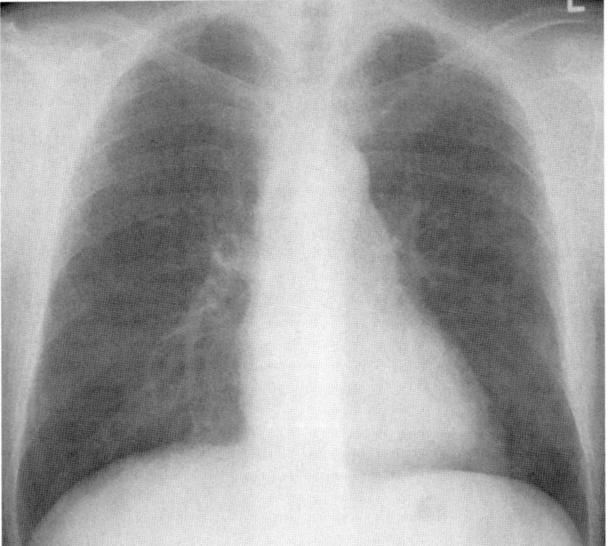

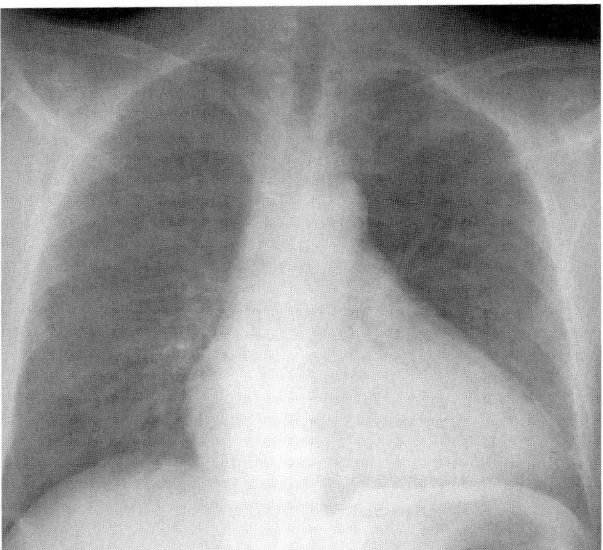

Figure 3–11 **(A)** In the first radiograph, the patient's heart appears normal in size. **(B)** Some years later, however, it appears much enlarged. This is not due to any difference in radiographic technique. In this case, the patient had developed a large pericardial effusion. The heart had not changed, but the pericardial sac had become distended over time by fluid.

Another difference between upright PA and supine AP films is the relative insensitivity of the latter to pleural effusions and pneumothoraxes. Pleural effusions can be detected in even small amounts as blunting of the costophrenic angles on upright films, but they layer out behind the lung on supine films, and thus cannot be seen in tangent. A small pneumothorax is readily detected on an upright film as air between the apex of the lung and the thoracic wall, but on supine films air within the pleural space tends to spread out along the anterior thoracic wall, and also cannot be seen in tangent (**Fig. 3–12**).

Search Pattern

A commonly employed approach to the chest radiograph utilizes an "A-B-C" (abdomen-bones-chest) approach. The value

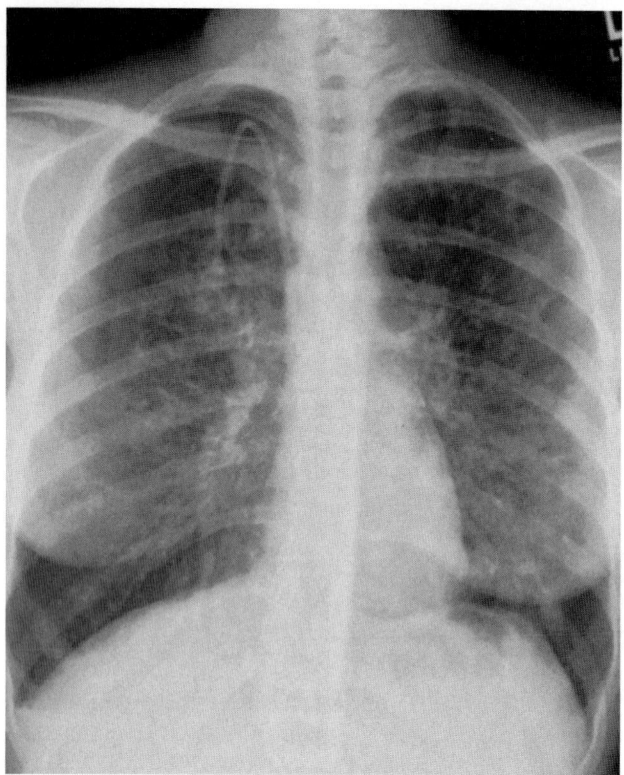

Figure 3–12 This young woman has cystic fibrosis and a right-sided central venous catheter, with its tip in the superior vena cava. Note the increased lung markings due to bronchiectasis, mycoid impactions, and increased interstitial markings. What else does she have? A large right pneumothorax. Note that the lung markings do not extend all the way to the thoracic wall on the right side.

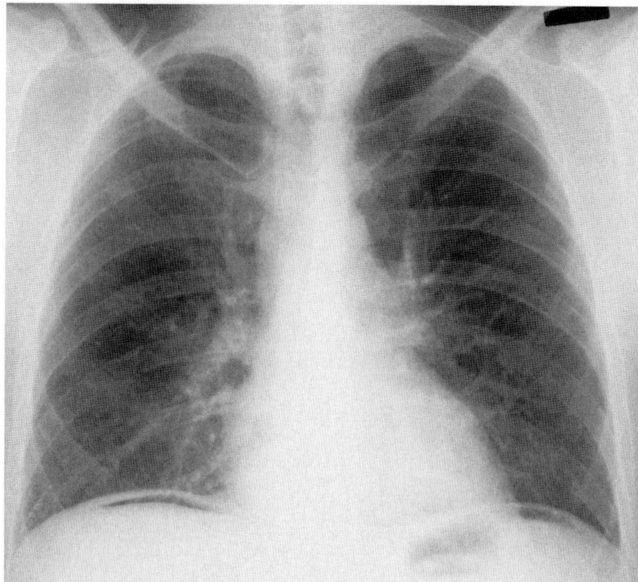

Figure 3–13 This upright chest radiograph demonstrates crescent-shaped lucencies under both hemidiaphragms. This is free intraperitoneal gas, or "free air," which rises up to the top of the peritoneal cavity when the patient is upright. Pneumoperitoneum is commonly due to recent surgery, but it may also indicate a ruptured abdominal viscus, such as a perforated duodenal ulcer.

of this approach, which puts the chest itself last, is the fact that it ensures that other easily overlooked areas outside the chest are inspected on each image. Key abdominal findings that should be sought out on chest radiographs include pneumoperitoneum, gastrointestinal (GI) dilation (possibly indicating obstruction), and masses (**Fig. 3–13**). "Bones" stands for both the osseous structures and their associated soft tissues. Examples of key osseous findings include rib fractures, vertebral compression fractures, and blastic (bone forming and hence white) or lytic (bone destroying and hence black) lesions, which might indicate infection or metastatic disease. Important findings in the soft tissues include evidence of a previous mastectomy (missing breast shadow) and calcifications in soft tissue tumors. In children, the chest radiograph should always be inspected for evidence of abuse, such as rib fractures (**Fig. 3–14**).

To ensure that easily overlooked structures within the chest are attended to, it is helpful to save the lungs for last. A good place to begin is the airway. This includes inspection of the trachea and major bronchi for evidence of foreign bodies, displacement, or compression. Next, the pleural space should be inspected, looking for processes such as pleural effusion, pleural plaque, pleural-based mass, and pneumothorax. The

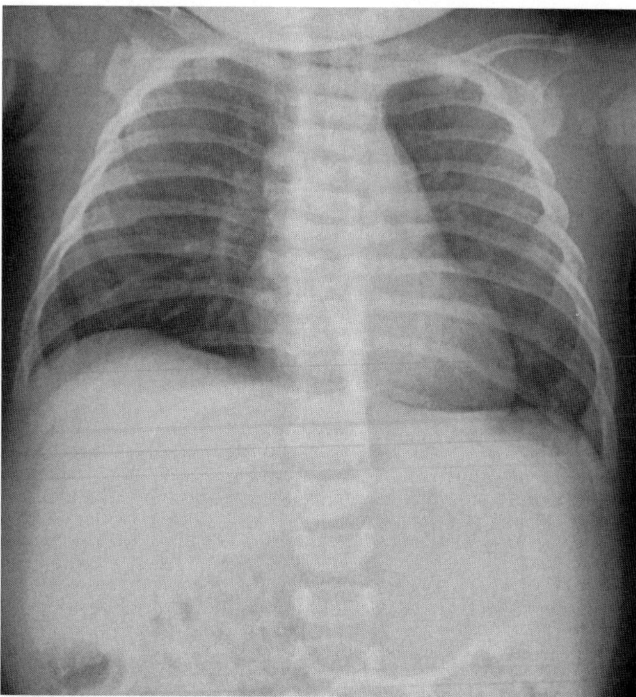

Figure 3–14 This infant's chest radiograph demonstrates healing fractures of the posterolateral aspects of the right sixth and seventh ribs, secondary to child abuse. Had this finding been missed, the child might have been returned to the setting where the abuse was taking place, and even more severe injury might have resulted.

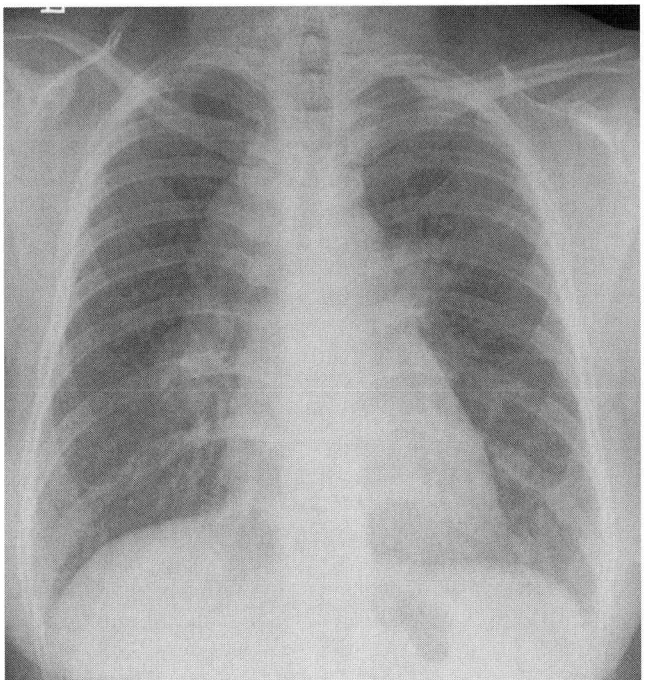

Figure 3–15 This 29-year-old woman complained of chest pain and weight loss. Her frontal chest radiograph demonstrates massive right paratracheal and bilateral hilar adenopathy, sometimes called the "1-2-3 sign" of sarcoidosis.

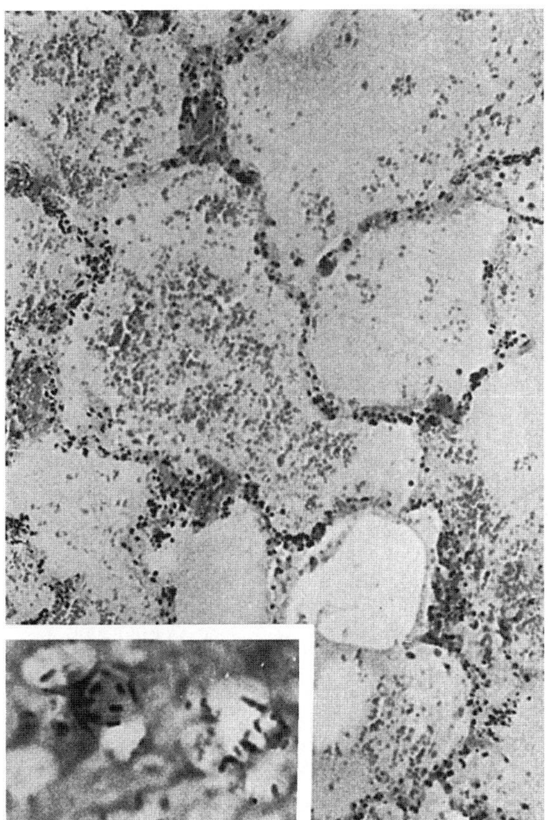

Figure 3–16 This light micrograph (×300) of the lung demonstrates filling of the airspaces with a combination of edema and hemorrhage in a patient with pneumococcal pneumonia. The inset (×2000) proves that the edema fluid teems with bacteria.

mediastinum should then be carefully evaluated, looking for widening of the paratracheal stripe (which should measure < 3–4 mm), fullness in the AP window and azygoesophageal recess, and bulging of the paraspinal lines. The hila should be inspected for evidence of fullness and for dilation of the pulmonary arteries (**Fig. 3–15**). Abnormalities in the mediastinum and hila often indicate the presence of masses or adenopathy. The general shape and size of the heart, as well as the symmetry and distribution of pulmonary perfusion, should always be evaluated (discussed at length in Chapter 2).

Finally, the lungs themselves should be examined. Key parameters include lung volumes, unilateral differences in density, and the presence of focal or diffuse opacities. Some key findings to exclude on every chest radiograph include pneumothorax, subtle nodules that may represent early lung carcinomas, and small pleural effusions that may provide the only radiographic evidence of pathology such as tuberculosis (TB). Subtle nodules that may be missed are often found in the upper lung zones, in the paramediastinal regions, and superimposed over the ribs and clavicles.

Pulmonary Parenchymal Patterns

Although numerous patterns of pulmonary parenchymal abnormality may be seen, a fundamental distinction is that between air-space and interstitial disease. Air-space disease represents filling of the pulmonary acini, the 8 mm respiratory units composed of respiratory bronchioles, alveolar ducts, and alveoli (**Fig. 3–16**). Air-space opacities appear fluffy and ill-defined, like clouds or cotton balls, and often become confluent to form larger regions of opacity. Other findings in air-space disease are air bronchograms (lucent tubular and branching structures representing aerated bronchi surrounded by opaque acini), absence of volume loss (the acini remain filled, with replacement of air by fluid or tissue), and a nonsegmental distribution (pores of Kohn and channels of Lambert allow intersegmental communication) (**Fig. 3–17**). Interstitial disease, by contrast, tends to produce opacities that can be characterized as reticular (delicate lines of opacity), nodular, reticulonodular, or "ground glass" (hazy increase in density) (**Fig. 3–18**). It represents the accumulation of fluid or tissue within the pulmonary interstitium, which includes not only the potential space between alveoli but also the lymphatics and veins. A parenchymal abnormality may be difficult to characterize as distinctly air-space or interstitial, as some combination of both is frequently present.

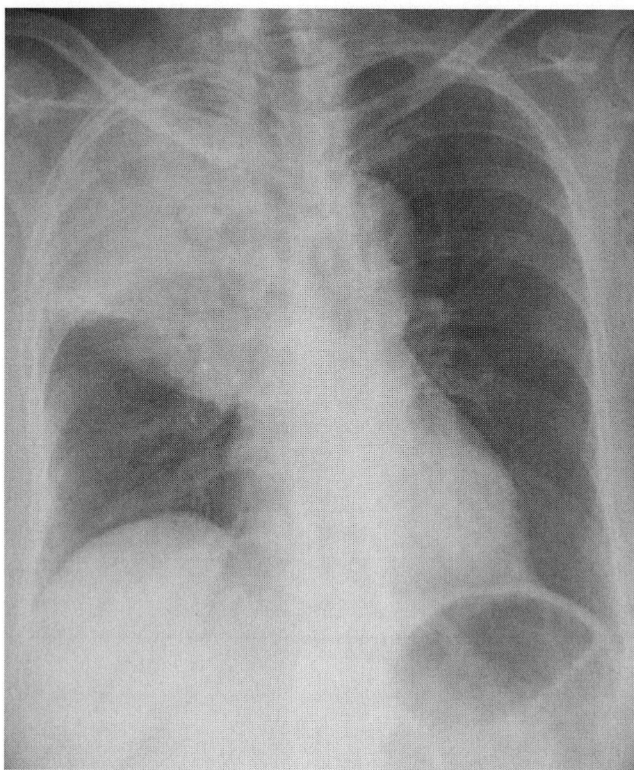

Figure 3–17 This patient's right upper lobe pneumonia demonstrates multiple air bronchograms, air-filled bronchi surrounded by fluid (pus)–filled air spaces. This finding indicates an air-space opacity.

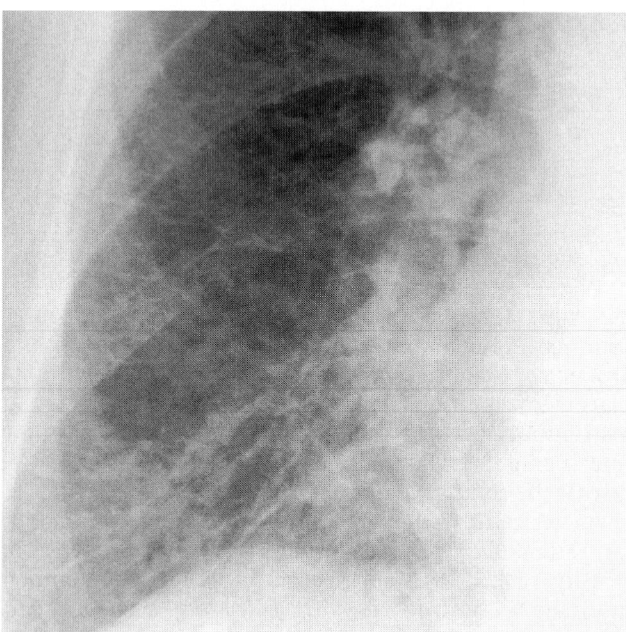

Figure 3–18 This close-up view of the right lung base demonstrates increased interstitial markings, particularly linear ones out at the lung periphery. These are sometimes called "Kerley B" lines, but they are usually referred to as septal lines. This patient has interstitial pulmonary edema from congestive heart failure.

◇ Air-Space Disease

Although the complete differential diagnosis of an air-space pattern of pulmonary opacification is quite lengthy, only five fundamental substances can be responsible for filling the air spaces. These are pus, water, blood, tumor, and protein. Pus is seen primarily in bacterial infections, such as pneumococcal pneumonia, although other infectious processes may fill the air spaces, including TB and fungal pneumonias. Water indicates pulmonary edema, including cardiogenic pulmonary edema (often accompanied by an enlarged cardiac silhouette and other signs of CHF, such as bilateral effusions and pulmonary venous hypertension) and noncardiogenic pulmonary edema, such as volume overload or renal failure. Blood may be due to trauma, bleeding diathesis, infarction, or vasculitis (as in Goodpasture's syndrome) and is a common postmortem finding, presumably due to terminal ischemia. Alveolar filling with tumor cells is seen in bronchoalveolar carcinoma and lymphoma. Proteinaceous fluid may be seen in the acute respiratory distress syndrome (ARDS), secondary to the leakage of plasma across damaged pulmonary capillary endothelium, or in alveolar proteinosis (**Fig. 3–19**).

◇ Interstitial Disease

While the differential diagnosis of interstitial disease extends to encompass over 100 distinct pathologic processes, most cases can be traced to one of several major categories of disease (**Fig. 3–20**). Infectious causes of interstitial disease include viruses, mycoplasma, TB, and *Pneumocystis carinii*. Tumor cells may fill the interstitium, as in lymphangitic spread of breast carcinoma. Inflammatory causes include collagen vascular diseases such as rheumatoid arthritis, drugs, and the pneumoconioses. Water within the interstitium generally reflects a less severe degree of pulmonary edema than that seen in air-space disease, most commonly due to CHF. Some cases of interstitial lung disease are idiopathic, as in idiopathic pulmonary fibrosis.

◇ Atelectasis

Atelectasis refers to underaerated lung tissue, which may range in extent from a subsegmental portion of parenchyma to an entire lung, in which case it is more commonly referred to as collapse. Patients with atelectasis will become dyspneic if the degree of underaeration is sufficient to compromise total pulmonary gas exchange. Reasoning pathophysiologically, it is possible to predict all of the types of atelectasis that are seen in clinical practice.

Resorptive atelectasis refers to the collapse of air spaces distal to a complete bronchial obstruction. Important causes of obstruction in adults include mucus plugs and tumors, especially bronchogenic carcinomas (**Fig. 3–21**). Mucus plugs are commonly seen in patients with obstructive airways disorders (asthma, chronic bronchitis) and patients whose ventilatory function is compromised, rendering them unable to cough (e.g., patients on mechanical ventilation). How does

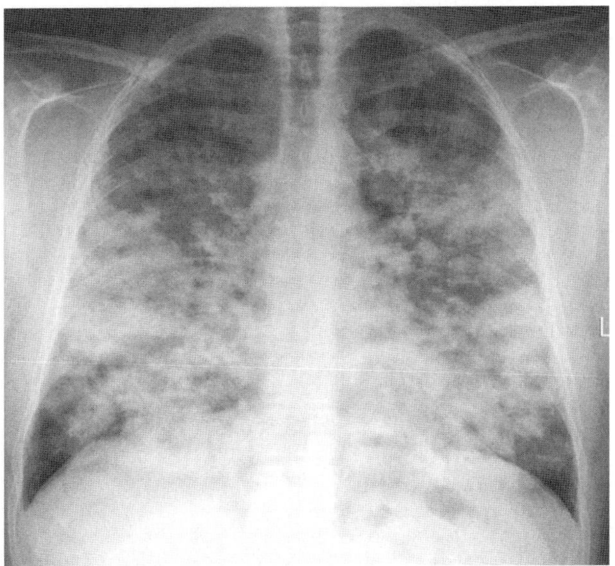

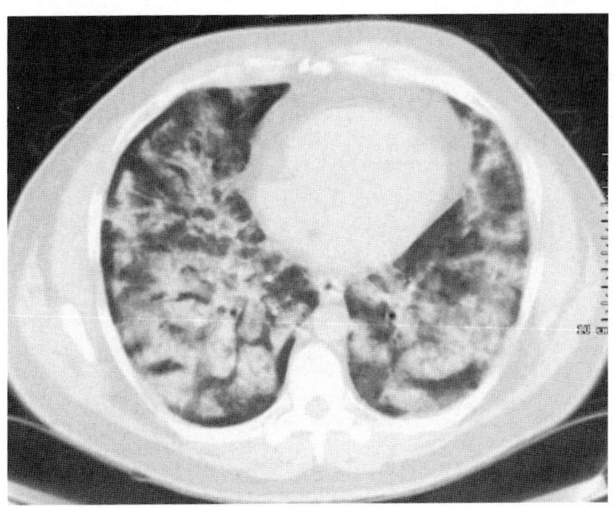

Figure 3–19 **(A)** This patient with alveolar proteinosis has patchy bilateral air-space opacities. They are cloudlike in appearance and demonstrate some air bronchograms, as in the left upper lobe. **(B)** On CT, they appear somewhat like balls of cotton scattered throughout the lungs.

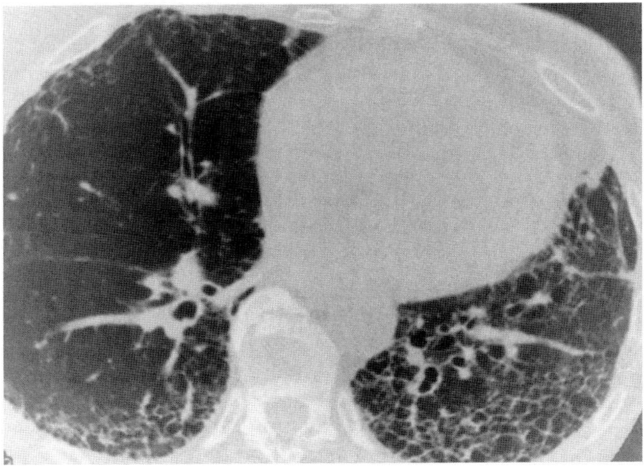

Figure 3–20 This axial image through the lung bases from high-resolution thoracic chest CT demonstrates typical changes of idiopathic pulmonary fibrosis, the result of progressive inflammation and fibrosis of the lung parenchyma of unknown etiology. Several processes, including collagen vascular diseases, drug toxicities, and inhalational lung diseases, can also produce this end-stage appearance of chronic interstitial lung disease. Once the process reaches this stage of "honeycombing" and traction bronchiectasis (from fibrosis), the prognosis tends to be poor, on the order of several years.

resorptive atelectasis occur? Regardless of the type of obstructing lesion, once an airway becomes completely occluded, the air-spaces distal to it cannot be ventilated (except perhaps by the pores of Kohn and canals of Lambert). Over a period of minutes to hours, the gas in the involved air spaces is taken up by the blood in the pulmonary capillaries. Oxygen is rapidly absorbed, due to the high oxygen affinity of hemoglobin, whereas nitrogen, which is poorly soluble in plasma, is slowly absorbed. As the gas exits the air spaces, they become progressively smaller and eventually collapse completely. Complete atelectasis of a lobe may occur within minutes in a patient breathing 100% oxygen. In intubated patients, another common cause of resorptive atelectasis is endotracheal tube malposition. For example, if the tip of the tube is located in the right mainstem bronchus, the left lung may receive no ventilation, causing it to collapse.

Passive or relaxation atelectasis occurs as a result of a space-occupying process in the (extrapulmonary) pleural space or chest wall. The two most common processes are pleural effusion and pneumothorax (**Fig. 3–22**). Another cause is tumor within the pleural space. One such tumor is malignant mesothelioma, a neoplasm related to asbestos exposure, which may completely encase the lung. In each of these conditions, inward displacement of the visceral pleura away from the chest wall results in decreased lung volume, with a resultant decrease in air-space ventilation.

The intrapulmonary counterpart of passive atelectasis is compressive atelectasis, which occurs when lung tissue is compressed by an adjacent intraparenchymal space-occupying lesion. One of the most common etiologies is a large space-occupying bulla in bullous emphysema (**Fig. 3–23**). Transthoracic bullectomy and lung reduction surgery have become important means of restoring ventilatory function to such patients. Naturally, another cause of compressive atelectasis would be a large lung tumor.

Adhesive atelectasis occurs due to loss of pulmonary surfactant, which is produced by type II pneumocytes. The water molecules lining the alveoli tend to exert an attractive effect on one another (surface tension). The effect of these attractive forces would be to increase dramatically the work of inflating the air spaces, were it not for the surfactant's ability to diminish surface tension. Respiratory distress syndrome of the newborn, also called surfactant deficiency disease, is perhaps the best-known manifestation. It occurs when the

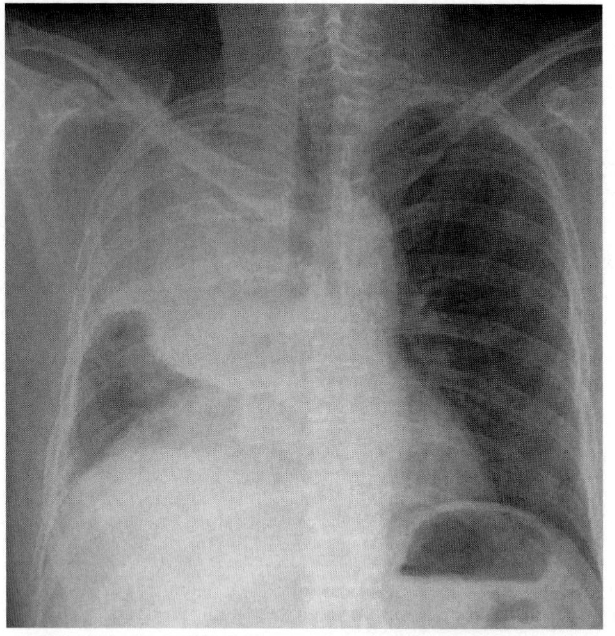

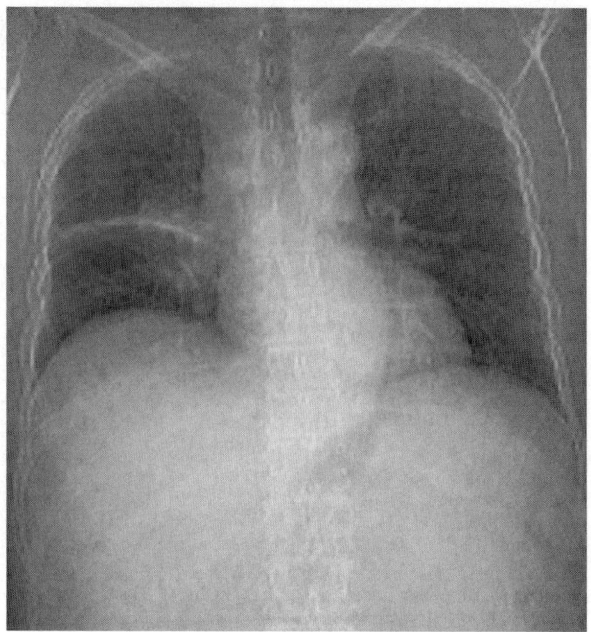

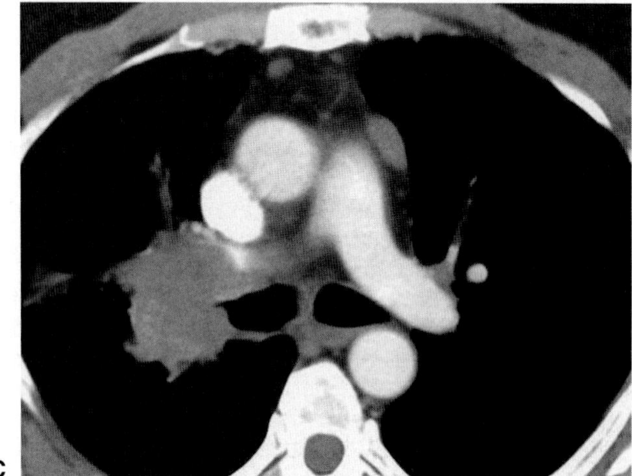

Figure 3–21 **(A)** This frontal chest radiograph demonstrates right upper lobe collapse, with rightward shift of the trachea. However, the right hilum is bulging laterally, indicating a mass. **(B)** After the atelectasis largely cleared, leaving only a residual platelike area of atelectasis, the right hilar mass is seen to better advantage. **(C)** A close-up view of the mediastinum and hila from a CT scan with intravenous (IV) contrast demonstrates the right upper hilar mass compressing the right bronchus and right pulmonary artery. This was a bronchogenic carcinoma.

immature lung, not yet producing sufficient quantities of surfactant, is forced to take on the task of respiration prematurely. Atelectasis in pulmonary embolism also results in part from a local surfactant deficiency in infarcted lung. One of the most common manifestations of adhesive atelectasis is a “platelike” linear opacity, representing underinflation or collapse of a subsegmental portion of lung (**Fig. 3–24**).

Cicatricial atelectasis is exactly what its name implies—the loss of volume in lung tissue produced by pulmonary parenchymal scarring. Cicatricial atelectasis is most commonly postinfectious, from TB or necrotizing pneumonia. Another common cause of cicatricial atelectasis is radiation therapy. High pulmonary parenchymal doses may be seen in the treatment of mediastinal Hodgkin’s lymphoma and lung carcinoma, particularly small cell carcinoma. When radiation therapy is directed at the mediastinum, a characteristic paramediastinal pattern of atelectasis and scarring, paralleling the radiation port, is often seen. In the acute phase of radiation injury, damage to type II pneumocytes causes adhesive atelectasis. Over the course of the succeeding months, pulmonary scarring and cicatricial atelectasis ensue, probably due to capillary endothelial damage.

The most reliable of the radiographic findings in atelectasis is displacement of one or more of the interlobar fissures, pulled toward the collapsed lobe. Another is displacement of pulmonary vessels, such as downward and medial displacement of the interlobar pulmonary artery in lower lobe collapse. Other signs include ipsilateral elevation of the hemidiaphragm and shift of mediastinal structures such as the heart or trachea toward the involved side. Often the collapsed portion of lung will be evident as a region of increased opacity, whereas the unaffected portion may appear more lucent, due to compensatory hyperexpansion. A common finding is the presence of linear, platelike opacities in

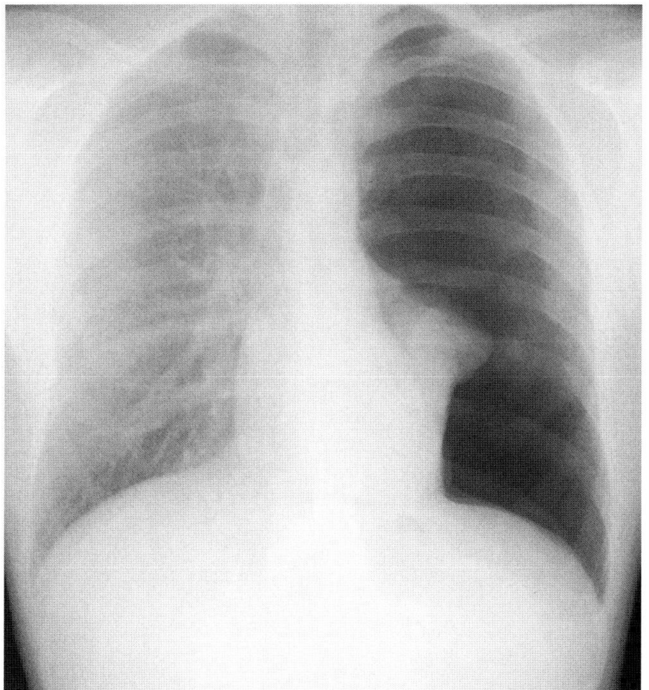

Figure 3–22 This chest radiograph demonstrates complete collapse of the left lung due to a very large left pneumothorax. Note the absence of lung markings in most of the left hemithorax. The left lung has collapsed due to the accumulation of air in the left pleural space following a failed attempt at placement of a central venous catheter in the left subclavian vein.

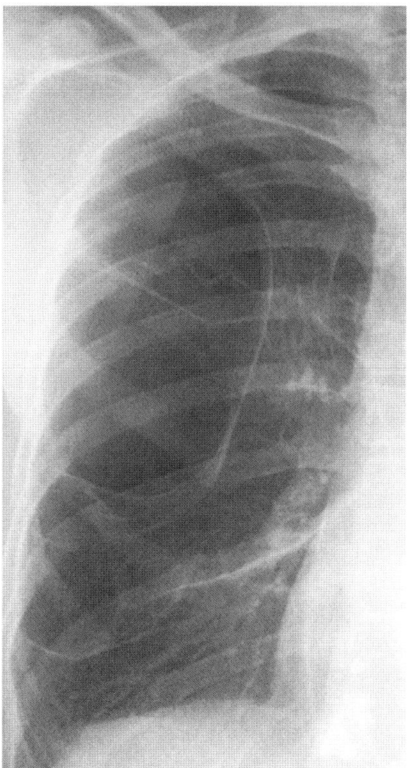

Figure 3–23 This close-up view of the right lung demonstrates compression of the lung by multiple large bullae in a patient with severe dyspnea due to bullous emphysema.

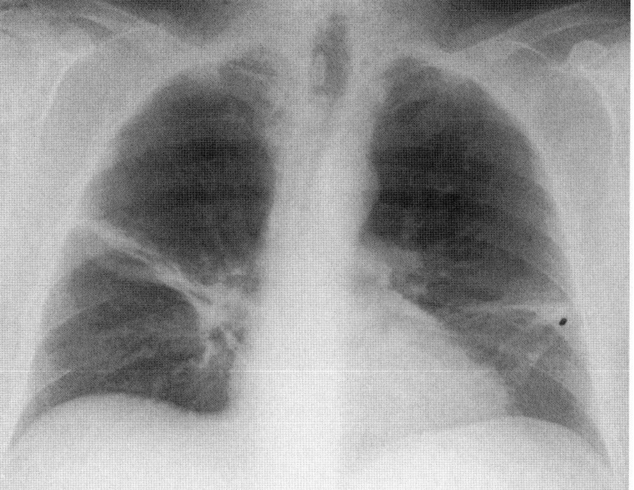

Figure 3–24 This frontal chest radiograph demonstrates "platelike" subsegmental atelectasis in both midlungs.

one or both lungs, which may represent either atelectasis or scarring. As always, comparison with previous radiographs can prove extremely helpful, as can follow-up examination. When the finding is new, or if it resolves subsequently, the diagnosis of atelectasis is quite likely; if the finding was present years before or does not change on follow-up, it likely represents scarring.

Clinical History

The importance of the clinical history in interpreting chest radiographs cannot be overemphasized. Absent such a history, the radiologist often can do little more than describe the findings and provide a long list of possible etiologies, which offers relatively little help to the clinician. Even a brief clinical history often enables the radiologist to provide a much more tightly focused differential diagnosis. Critical parameters to be included on every chest radiograph requisition include the following: age, gender, acute or chronic presentation, febrile or afebrile, significant medical and surgical history (e.g., immune compromise, collagen vascular disease, malignancy), pertinent occupational history (e.g., exposure to silica or grain silos), drug therapy (e.g., penicillin or Adriamycin), pertinent test results (e.g., TB, human immunodeficiency virus [HIV], blood coagulation profile), and, where possible, a clinical question that the study is obtained to answer (**Fig. 3–25**).

Examples of a good clinical history include "55-year-old retired shipyard worker with 80 pack-year smoking history who presents with 20 lb weight loss over 3 months and new onset of right pleuritic chest pain," and "35-year-old HIV-positive woman with acute onset of cough and chills." The former points toward a malignancy such as lung carcinoma or mesothelioma, and the latter suggests an infectious etiology, including the possibility of an opportunistic organism. An example of a suboptimal clinical history in both of these settings would be "Rule out infiltrate."

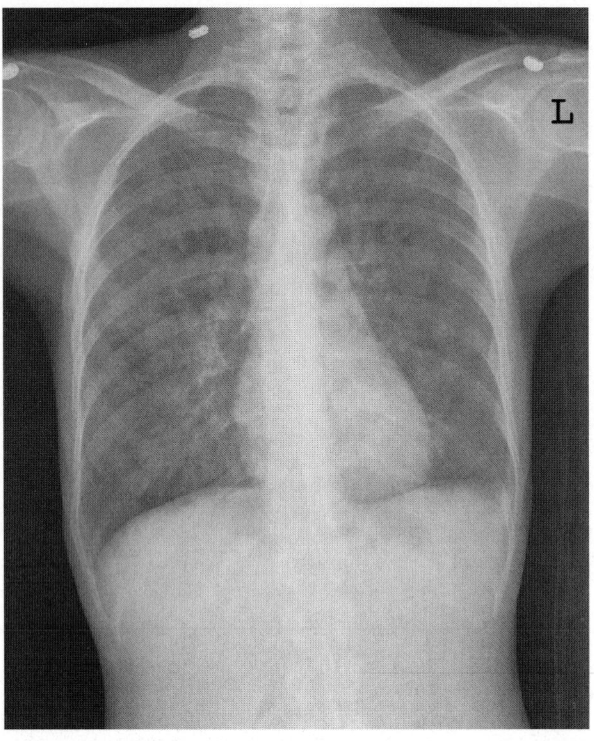

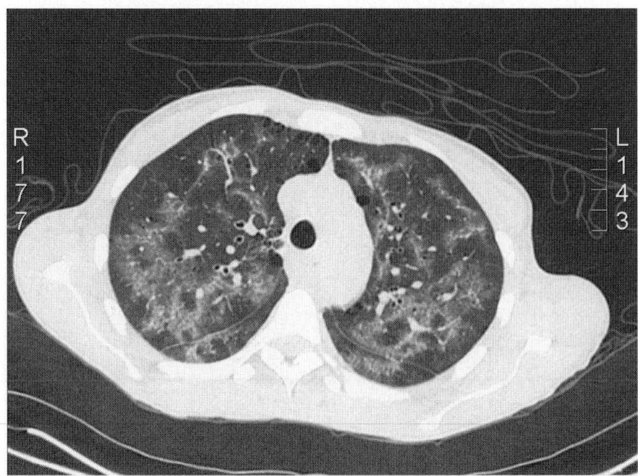

Figure 3–25 **(A)** This frontal chest radiograph demonstrates patchy bilateral, somewhat nodular air-space and interstitial opacities. The differential diagnosis, which could be long, is considerably shortened when we learn that the patient is positive for human immunodeficiency virus (HIV). The diagnosis is *Pneumocystis carinii* pneumonia. **(B)** The process has a similar appearance on chest CT.

Other Imaging Modalities

Digital radiography has provided several benefits over conventional techniques, including more consistent quality and reduced repeat rates, particularly in portable radiography. Digitization enables postprocessing of image data to provide edge enhancement, improved contrast resolution, and manipulation of window and level settings to enhance visualization of the different regions of the chest, such as the lungs and the mediastinum.

Computed tomography and high-resolution CT have dramatically enhanced thoracic imaging because of their vastly superior contrast resolution and ability to distinguish between anatomic and pathologic structures. Cross-sectional images eliminate the superimposition of structures that characterizes chest radiographs. Iodinated intravenous contrast material is used to evaluate vascular disease, to characterize the enhancement characteristics of lesions, and to distinguish hilar lymph nodes from vascular structures. CT is commonly employed to better evaluate lesions detected on plain radiography, such as pulmonary nodules and hilar or mediastinal masses, to stage lung cancers, to rule out radiographically occult thoracic metastases in malignancies with a propensity to metastasize to the lung, and to evaluate vascular pathology such as suspected aortic dissection. Three-dimensional reconstructions in the sagittal and coronal planes occasionally prove helpful, for example, in evaluating hilar lesions and suspected diaphragmatic injury. Recently, contrast-enhanced CT has emerged as a sensitive and highly specific means of evaluating suspected pulmonary embolism. High-resolution CT provides more precise characterization of calcifications within pulmonary nodules and more precisely characterizes parenchymal lung diseases and bronchiectasis. It represents the most sensitive method for the in vivo detection of emphysema.

Magnetic resonance imaging enjoys several advantages over CT, which can prove helpful in select situations. Its ability to image directly in multiple planes provides assessment of many apical, hilar, and subcarinal lesions. Its superior contrast resolution can often clearly distinguish between tumor and normal adjacent tissue such as muscle and fat. Its ability to distinguish between various tissue types and between flowing blood and stationary tissue without exogenous contrast can prove quite helpful in patients with a contraindication to iodinated contrast material (**Fig. 3–26**). MRI also permits better evaluation of possible intraspinal involvement of posterior mediastinal masses.

Disadvantages of MRI include decreased spatial resolution, insensitivity to calcification, and profound motion artifacts if good electrocardiographic and respiratory gating of image acquisition are not achieved. MRI is also more time-consuming and expensive than CT. CT is generally the preferred modality in noncardiovascular situations.

In adults, ultrasound is used primarily in the evaluation of pleural effusions and masses, anterior mediastinal masses, and chest-wall processes.

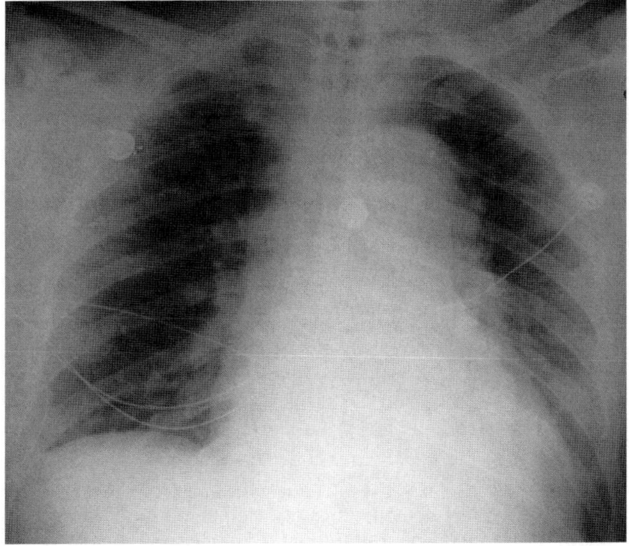

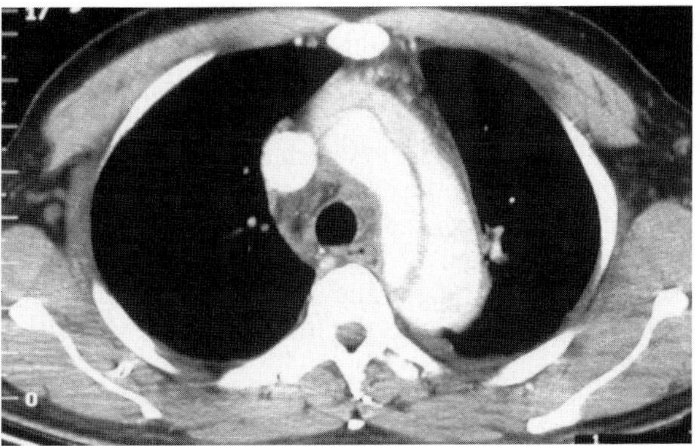

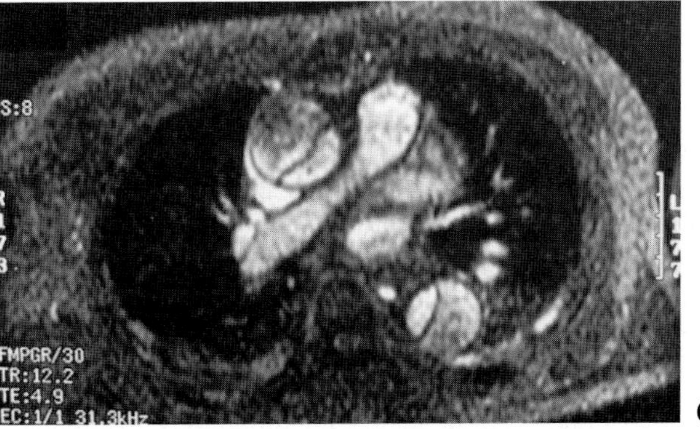

Figure 3–26 **(A)** This elderly hypertensive man presented with severe ripping chest pain that radiated to his back. His AP chest radiograph shows probably cardiomegaly and perhaps an enlarged aorta, but provides no definite explanation. **(B)** High clinical suspicion of aortic dissection leads to a chest CT with IV contrast. This axial image shows an intimal flap in both the ascending and descending aorta, indicating a type A aortic dissection. **(C)** An axial MR image also demonstrates intimal flap in both the ascending and descending aorta.

◆ Airway

Pathology

Asthma

◇ Epidemiology

Afflicting nearly 7% of the adult U.S. population, asthma is the most important cause of acute airway obstruction, one of the most common presenting complaints in U.S. emergency rooms. Precipitants of acute attacks vary from patient to patient, but include airway irritants such as dust and noxious chemicals, inflammatory mediators such as histamine, and a variety of antigens associated with allergy, such as ragweed pollen. Additional stimuli include exercise, cold, and, in some patients, nonsteroidal anti-inflammatory agents. Many patients will give a family history of the disorder or report a history of allergic symptoms.

◇ Pathophysiology

The airways obstruction has two components. The first is bronchospasm, mediated by hyperreactivity of smooth muscle surrounding both the small and large airways. The second component of obstruction is chronic inflammation, which includes excessive mucus production and thickening of airway membranes. Several different factors contribute to the clinical picture, including increased airways resistance (which increases in inverse proportion to the fourth power of the radius), decreased airflow rates and forced expiratory volumes, hyperinflation of the lungs (which may remain inflated at autopsy even when the pleural cavity is opened), increased work of breathing, and ventilation/perfusion (V/Q) mismatches.

◇ Clinical Presentation

The asthmatic suffering an acute exacerbation presents with dyspnea ("difficult breathing"), wheezing, and cough. Clinical signs of more severe airway obstruction include the recruitment of accessory muscles of respiration, such as the sternocleidomastoids, and the development of a pulsus paradoxus (a greater than 10 mm Hg drop in systolic blood pressure with inspiration). Only ~3% of metabolic energy expenditure is normally devoted to respiration in quiet breathing, but this may increase to 30% or more in patients with obstructive disease (or poorly compliant lungs), with the result that breathing itself becomes exhausting. In severe cases, blood gases typically reveal hypoxemia and hypercarbia, and a rise in the arterial carbon dioxide (partial pressure of carbon dioxide, $PaCO_2$) is an indication that the patient is decompensating and may require transfer to the intensive care unit. If the attack progresses to the point that the airways are plugged with mucus, the patient becomes refractory to bronchodilators, and status asthmaticus ensues. At this point, intubation is often required.

◇ Imaging

Radiologic evaluation consists almost exclusively of chest radiography. The radiographic signs of an acute asthma exacerbation are predictable, based on the pathophysiology. Air trapping and hyperinflation are produced by the tendency of narrowed airways to collapse under the increased positive intrathoracic pressures necessary to exhale against increased airways resistance (which explains why wheezes are most prominent in the expiratory phase of respiration). Signs of hyperinflation include flattening of the hemidiaphragms, attenuation of vascular markings, and an increase in both lung height and anteroposterior diameter, manifesting as expansion of the retrosternal clear space on the lateral view.

Atelectasis is a frequent finding and is related to the resorption of oxygen from respiratory bronchioles and alveoli distal to a plugged airway. Bronchial wall thickening may be visualized as peribronchial cuffing and tram tracking, which refer to thickened bronchi seen on end and lengthwise, respectively. In rare cases, mucus plugs with a branchlike structure may be visualized within the bronchial tree.

Chest radiography is not performed to diagnose an asthma exacerbation, which can be done on strictly clinical grounds. Instead, it is performed to rule out other possible etiologies of dyspnea, such as pneumonia, and to assess for the complications of asthma, such as pneumothorax and pneumomediastinum (**Fig. 3–27**). Excluding asthma mimics is important because the therapy for pneumonia or extrinsic tracheobronchial obstruction is usually quite different from the standard asthma regimen. Complications such as pneumothorax and pneumomediastinum result from alveolar rupture due to high expiratory pressures or positive pressure ventilation. When such complications arise, radiographs are also needed to ensure proper positioning of endotracheal tubes and chest tubes.

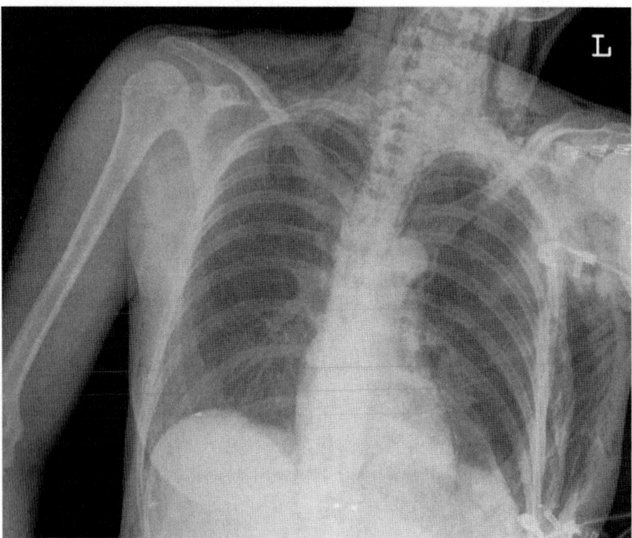

Figure 3–27 This asthmatic patient presented with severe respiratory distress. There is extensive pneumomediastinum, with air tracking along the heart and aorta up the mediastinum into the neck and supraclavicular fossae and along the thoracic wall. On physical exam, pressure on the skin of the neck elicited "crackling" sounds, sometimes called tactile crepitus.

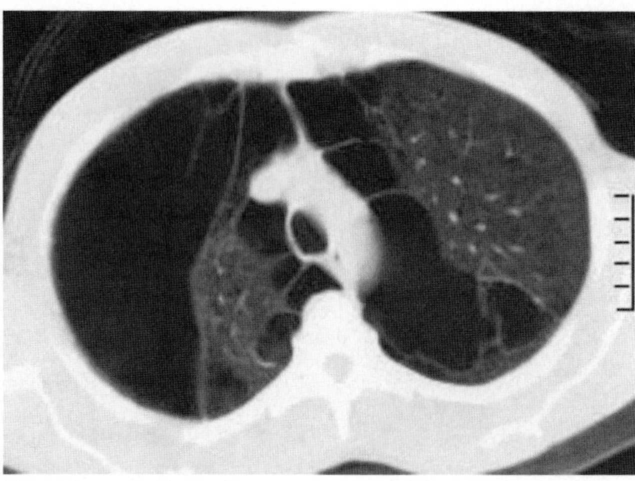

Figure 3–28 This axial chest CT image from a patient with severe bulbous emphysema demonstrates replacement of much of both upper lobes with large bullae. The amount of lung tissue available for gas exchange is markedly reduced.

Chronic Obstructive Pulmonary Disease

◇ Epidemiology

Chronic obstructive pulmonary disease (COPD) is the fourth leading cause of mortality in the United States and a major contributor to health care costs. Common causes of chronic and unremitting airway obstruction include chronic bronchitis and emphysema, which usually coexist in varying proportions in affected patients. Most cases are related to cigarette smoking. Chronic bronchitis is a clinical diagnosis, defined as cough and sputum production during at least 3 months in 2 consecutive years, and produces obstruction through inflammation, inspissated mucus, and bronchospasm. Emphysema is a pathologic diagnosis, defined as destruction of gas-exchanging lung tissue with enlargement of air spaces (**Fig. 3–28**). Emphysema is considered an obstructive disease because the loss of lung elasticity promotes airway collapse during expiration.

◇ Pathophysiology

Both diseases are characterized by chronic alveolar hypoventilation, which results in a tendency to hypercarbia and hypoxemia. In chronic bronchitis, blood is shunted past unventilated alveoli, whereas in emphysema, the alveoli themselves are destroyed. Early in the course of the disease, the V/Q mismatch is less severe in emphysema than in chronic bronchitis, because both air spaces and capillaries are destroyed. An intriguing cause of emphysema is α-1-antitrypsin deficiency, in which patients with a homozygous genetic defect exhibit a marked propensity to develop emphysema, aggravated by cigarette smoking (**Fig. 3–29**). Alpha-1-antitrypsin is an endogenous protease inhibitor that, in effect, prevents pulmonary autodigestion by endogenous proteases.

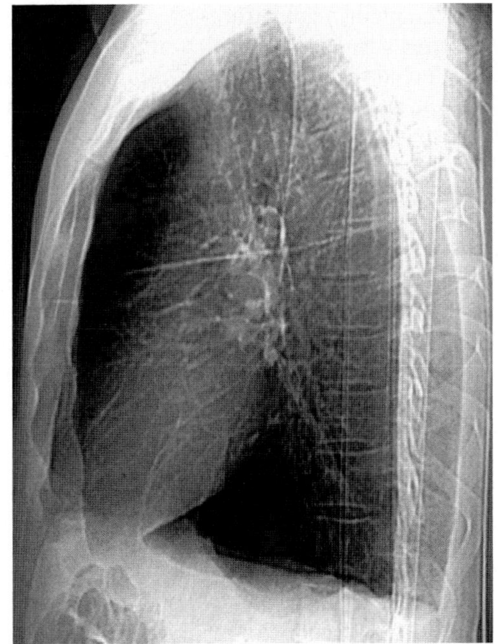

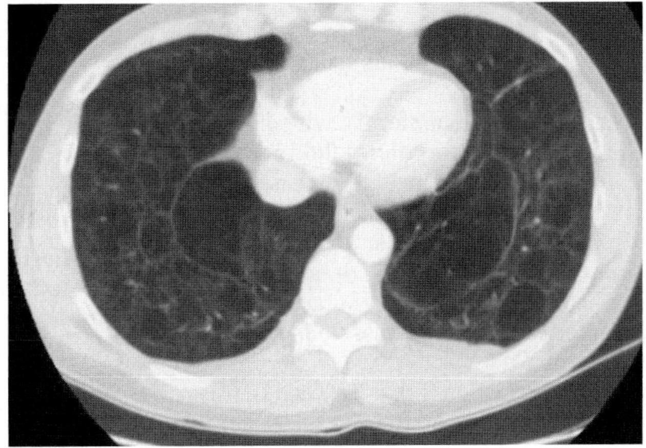

Figure 3–29 This middle-aged man presented with progressively increasing dyspnea. The patient had smoked cigarettes for many years. **(A)** A lateral view of the chest shows marked hyperexpansion, with flattening of the hemidiaphragms and widening of the retrosternal clear space (the space between the sternum and the heart/great vessels). **(B)** On CT there is severe diffuse destruction of lung tissue with bulla formation. The patient had α-1-antitrypsin deficiency.

◇ Clinical Presentation

Although both disorders are chronic and unremitting, patients tend to present during exacerbations, generally precipitated by upper respiratory infections (with increased sputum production and bronchospasm), episodes of CHF, or even pulmonary embolism. Patients with chronic bronchitis are especially likely to be chronically colonized by bacteria, probably due to a combination of defective mucociliary clearance and impaired immune response. Pulmonary function testing in chronic bronchitis reveals a prominent deficit in forced expiratory volume, and in emphysema a loss of diffusing capacity (measured with carbon monoxide).

◇ Imaging

The chest radiograph is insensitive in the diagnosis of chronic bronchitis and emphysema, and many patients with clinically diagnosed COPD will have normal chest radiographs. Radiography is employed primarily to assess complications of these disorders, such as pneumonia, pneumothorax (thin-walled bullae may rupture into the pleural space), and lung cancer (both emphysema and bronchogenic carcinoma are tobacco-related); however, the chest radiograph can suggest the diagnosis.

Radiographic signs suggestive of chronic bronchitis include bronchial thickening, such as peribronchial cuffing and tram tracking, and there is often a diffuse but nonspecific increase in lung markings. Plain radiographic findings in emphysema include hyperinflation with flattening of the diaphragms and expansion of the retrosternal air space, diffuse lucency from destruction of lung tissue, and bullae (thin-walled cysts left in the wake of lung destruction).

Because pulmonary artery hypertension is often a feature of COPD, prominent central pulmonary arteries may be noted in both chronic bronchitis and emphysema. High-resolution CT is the most sensitive in vivo technique available in detecting and characterizing the morphologic changes of emphysema.

◆ Pleura

Pathology

Pleural Effusion

◇ Epidemiology

Pleural effusion is the abnormal accumulation of fluid between the visceral and parietal layers of the pleura. Strictly speaking, a pleural effusion is not a disease, but a sign of disease that usually requires further diagnostic evaluation. Statistically, the most common causes of pleural effusions are, in descending order of frequency, congestive heart failure (CHF), bacterial pneumonia, malignancy (especially lung and breast cancer), pulmonary embolism, viral pneumonia, and cirrhosis of the liver.

◇ Pathophysiology

The normal amount of fluid in the pleural space of each lung should not exceed 15 mL. Its accumulation is governed by the Starling forces (discussed in Chapter 2), with flow of fluid from the parietal pleura and resorption of fluid at the visceral pleura. Causes of pleural effusion include increased hydrostatic pressure (as in CHF), decreased oncotic pressure (as in nephrotic syndrome), increased capillary permeability (as in pneumonia), and decreased lymphatic drainage (as in lymphatic spread of carcinoma). When thoracentesis is performed, the aspirated fluid may be classified as bloody, chylous, purulent, or serous.

Another important distinction is that between transudative and exudative effusions. Transudates are characterized by low protein (effusion/serum protein < 0.5) and are most commonly produced by elevated pulmonary venous pressures in CHF. Another means of determining if an effusion is transudative is by measuring its lactate dehydrogenase (LDH), which should be less than two thirds the upper limit of normal for blood. Exudates are produced by inflammatory or infiltrative processes, and have a higher protein concentration due to increased capillary permeability. When an exudative effusion is found in an adult, bacterial pneumonia (*Klebsiella, Staphylococcus aureus,* and anaerobes), tuberculosis, and cancer are common etiologies (**Fig. 3–30**). The finding of malignant cells within the fluid generally signifies diffuse tumor involvement. Infections within the pleural space may result in calcified pleural plaques.

◇ Clinical Presentation

Large effusions often present with dyspnea, because the fluid beneath or around the lung prevents its normal inspiratory expansion and tends to produce passive atelectasis of adjacent lung. Other common presenting complaints in patients with pleural effusions include cough and chest discomfort or pain, which is often pleuritic in nature (aggravated by inspiration). Signs raising suspicion for pleural effusion on physical examination include diminished breath sounds and dullness to percussion, with adjacent increased breath sounds due to overlying atelectatic lung.

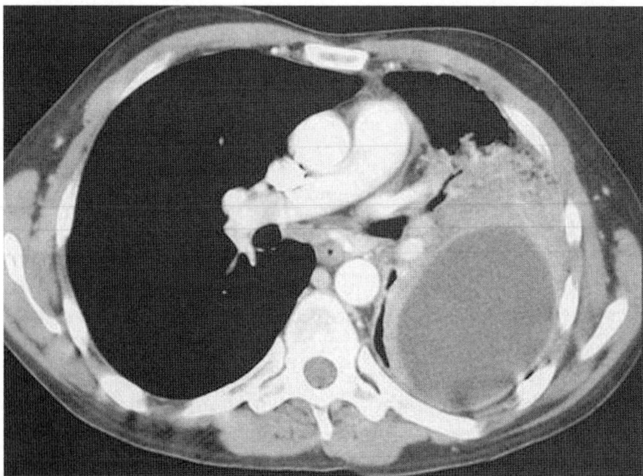

Figure 3–30 This axial CT image of the chest (soft tissue windows) after IV contrast demonstrates a large pleural fluid collection on the left surrounded by a thick enhancing rind. This proved to be an empyema. Empyema is characterized by fibrinopurulent exudates and generally requires surgical management.

◇ Imaging

Radiography is useful in the detection and quantitation of pleural effusions. Upright positioning is superior to supine, because it will cause fluid to collect at the lower end of the lung. The lateral radiograph is more sensitive than the frontal, because the posterior aspect of the costophrenic sulcus, the most dependent portion of the pleural space in the upright position, is much better visualized. A small amount of pleural fluid, less than 75 cc, will tend to collect in a subpulmonic location, between the lung and the diaphragm, and may be undetectable, although its presence is suggested when the hemidiaphragm appears to be elevated, especially laterally, or when the gastric bubble appears unusually distant from the base of the left lung; however, as the amount of fluid approaches 100 cc, it tends to spill into the costophrenic sulcus, and becomes visible as a blunting of the usually sharp posterior angles on the lateral radiograph, with a meniscus-like appearance. As more fluid accumulates (> 200 cc), the costophrenic angles will become blunted on the frontal projection as well.

If an effusion is suspected but cannot be demonstrated on routine upright views, a decubitus ("down on the elbow") film, with the patient lying on the side, may show a small amount of fluid layering out along the lateral chest wall (**Fig. 3–31**). This technique is sensitive for effusions as small as 10 cc, making it the most sensitive plain radiographic test for pleural effusion. In large effusions, fluid may be seen tracking into the fissures, especially on the lateral view.

On portable radiography, with the patient in a supine position, sensitivity for the detection of pleural effusion is markedly decreased. If clinical concern is high, decubitus or upright radiographs should be obtained, if at all possible. If not, ultrasound may warrant consideration. Plain radiographic findings in the supine position include diffuse opacification of the hemithorax, because the effusion layers out behind the lung, and blunting of the costophrenic angle. On occasion, the fluid will accumulate at the lung apex, in which case it produces a white "apical cap."

A common clinical problem is an effusion that has become loculated due to adhesions between the visceral and parietal pleura, which is commonly seen in infectious and neoplastic effusions. Loculated fluid may simulate a pleural mass. The presence of loculations can make diagnostic thoracentesis more difficult and may also render therapeutic thoracentesis (aimed to relieve dyspnea by withdrawing a large amount of fluid) unsuccessful, due to the presence of multiple noncommunicating loculations. In this case, a decubitus film will demonstrate whether the fluid is loculated, because trapped fluid will not layer out along the lateral chest wall.

Ultrasound and CT may prove helpful in guiding thoracentesis in cases of loculation, because they can help to select out the largest pocket. They may also be necessary to determine whether an area of presumed pleural fluid may in fact

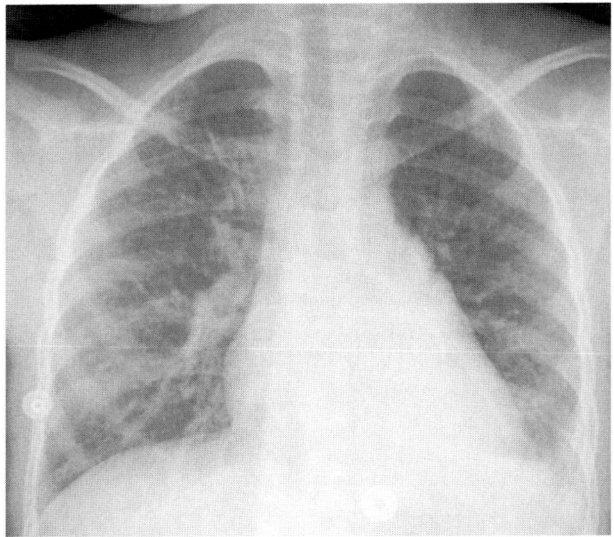

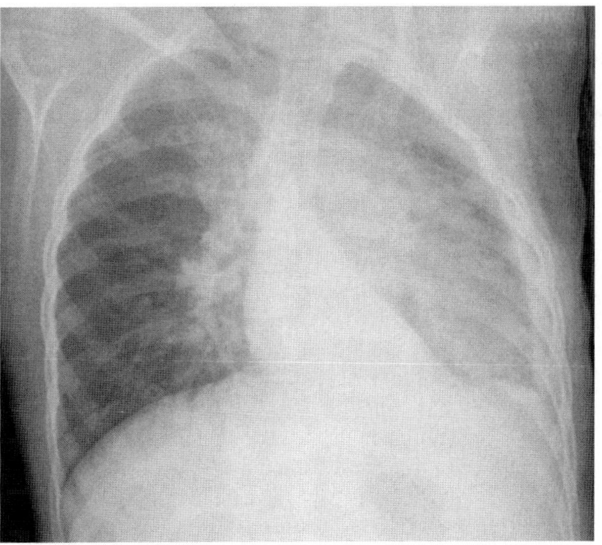

Figure 3–31 **(A)** On the frontal chest radiograph there is blunting of the left costophrenic angle, as compared with the right. **(B)** On the left lateral decubitus view, the effusion "layers out" along the left lateral chest wall, indicating that it is free flowing. The effusion appears as a white stripe along the left lung just inside the ribs.

consist, at least in part, of collapsed lung or a soft tissue mass. Imaging guidance increases the probability of obtaining fluid and decreases the rate of complications, such as hepatic or splenic laceration, pulmonary hemorrhage, and pneumothorax. In the case of a diagnostic tap, what should be done with the fluid? Because the range of possible etiologies for effusions is fairly broad, pleural fluid should be routinely sent for chemistry, cell count and differential, culture and sensitivity, Gram's stain, acid-fast bacilli, and cytology.

Pneumothorax

◇ Epidemiology

Pneumothorax, the presence of air within the pleural space, may occur spontaneously, or it may result from trauma. A high percentage of pneumothoraces in hospitalized patients are iatrogenic, occurring in such situations as central venous catheter placement (**Fig. 3–32**).

◇ Pathophysiology

In the setting of penetrating trauma, pneumothorax may result from the introduction of air through the chest wall. If the wound does not seal itself, there is a leakage of air through the chest wall and into the pleural space, creating a so-called sucking chest wound. In this situation, the negative intrathoracic pressure created with each inspiration causes additional air to enter the pleural space, which may rapidly produce a tension pneumothorax. The continued accumulation of air in the pleural space causes complete collapse of the affected lung, with a shift of the mediastinum toward the contralateral side (**Fig. 3–33**). Death may rapidly ensue, largely due to the compromise of venous return to the heart from distortion of normal mediastinal anatomy, as well as V/Q mismatching and hypoxemia. Blunt trauma may cause pneumothorax when a rib punctures the pleura or when tracheobronchial rupture results. The latter condition is associated with pneumomediastinum and persistence of pneumothorax even after chest tube placement.

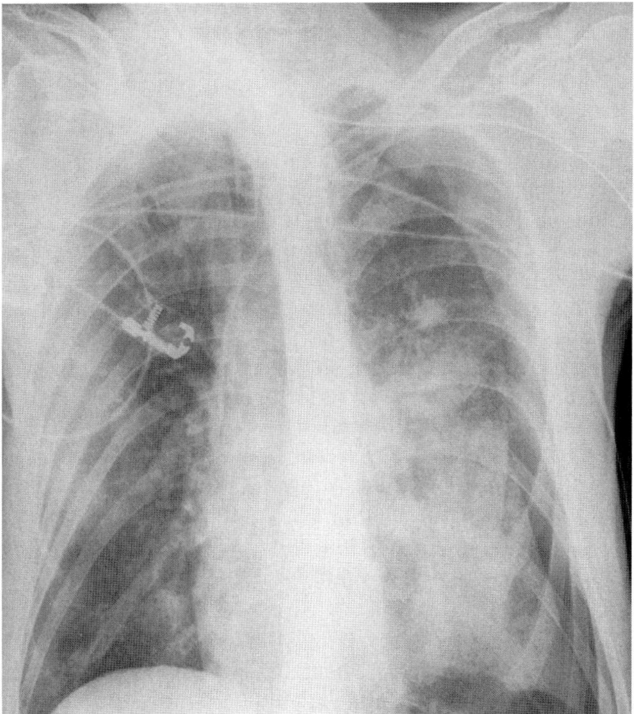

Figure 3–32 This frontal chest radiograph is typical of acutely ill or injured patients, in that there are many wires crossing the patient (electrocardiogram leads), and positioning is poor. A left subclavian central line was just placed, the tip of which is at the level of the lower superior vena cava. There is a left pneumothorax, with the edge of the opacified left lung paralleling the left chest wall.

Spontaneous pneumothorax may be idiopathic or related to preexisting lung disease. Idiopathic pneumothorax typically occurs in men in the third or fourth decades, especially in tall

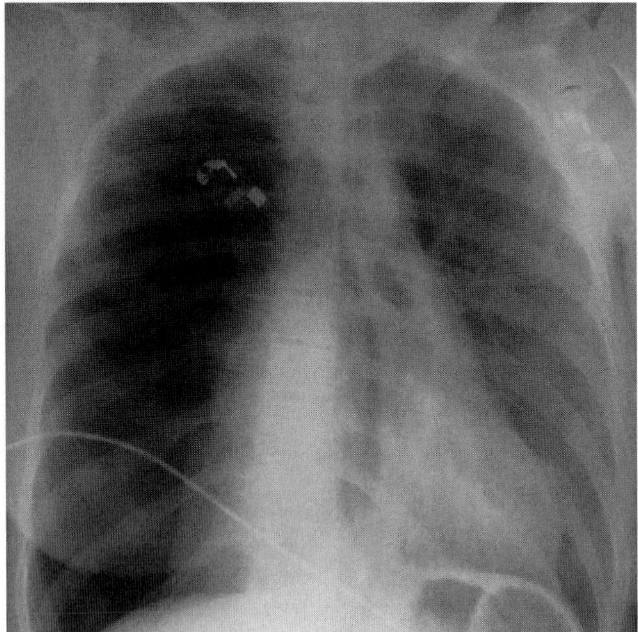

Figure 3–33 This frontal chest radiograph reveals complete collapse of the right lung due to a massive right pneumothorax, which is also shifting the heart and other mediastinal structures to the left, a tension pneumothorax.

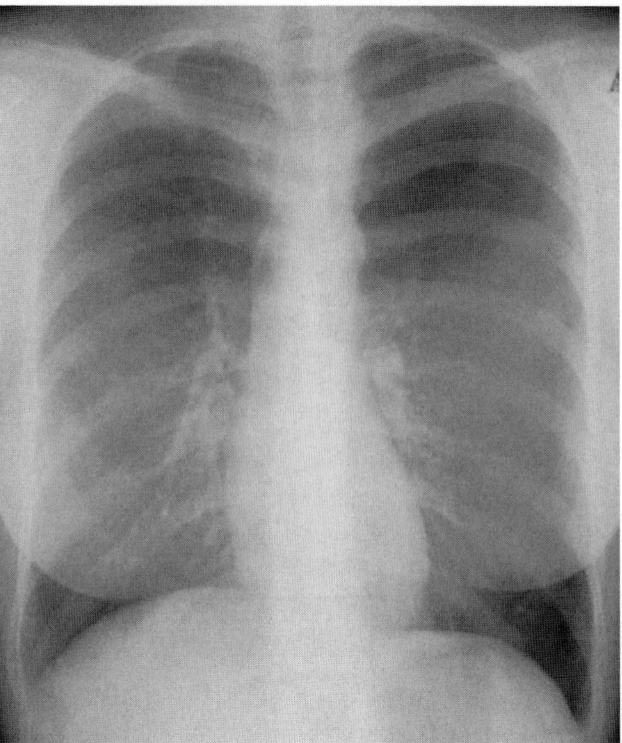

Figure 3–34 This frontal chest radiograph reveals that the left hemithorax is more lucent (darker) than the right. The left costophrenic sulcus at the inferiolateral corner of the left hemithorax is also deeper and wider than the right. On closer inspection, the lateral edge of the left lung is medially displaced by a pneumothorax.

and asthenic individuals. Such patients are sometimes found to have bullae or blebs in the lung apices. A bulla is defined as a thin-walled gas collection that is greater than 1 cm in diameter, and a bleb is a collection of gas less than 1 cm wide within the layers of the visceral pleura. COPD is the most common predisposing condition in spontaneous pneumothorax, and there is an association with Marfan's syndrome.

Regardless of the patient's underlying condition, positive pressure ventilation is a risk factor, and intubation should generally be avoided in patients with pneumothorax if a chest tube is not in place. Because so many pneumothoraces in hospitalized patients are iatrogenic, an upright chest radiograph should be obtained in every patient who has undergone placement of a central line. This not only rules out pneumothorax, but also confirms appropriate line position.

◇ Clinical Presentation

The usual presentation of pneumothorax is the sudden onset of dyspnea and chest pain. Patients with more serious tension pneumothorax are tachypneic, tachycardic, hypotensive, and cyanotic.

◇ Imaging

Whenever possible, upright radiographs should be obtained in suspected pneumothorax, because up to one third of pneumothoraces may be inapparent on supine films. An upright chest radiograph demonstrates a small pneumothorax as an apical visceral pleural line displaced away from the chest wall, with an absence of lung markings peripheral to it. Larger pneumothoraces are also suggested by asymmetrical lucency of the involved hemithorax (**Fig. 3–34**). Potential mimics include skin folds, which often extend peripherally beyond the chest wall, and bullae. If a patient cannot sit or stand upright, a lateral decubitus film should be obtained with the affected side up, which will cause intrapleural air to collect just below the lateral chest wall. CT is more sensitive than plain radiography, but also more costly.

◆ Mediastinum

Anatomy and Imaging

The mediastinum is the narrow, vertically oriented, "white" midportion of the chest located between the two lungs on a frontal chest radiograph. Its contents include the heart and great vessels, the trachea and main bronchi, the esophagus, and numerous lymph nodes. Understanding the anatomy of the mediastinum on the frontal and lateral chest radiographs is critical to detecting and evaluating abnormalities. The mediastinum is usually divided into anterior, middle, and posterior compartments (**Fig. 3–35**). The middle mediastinum contains the pericardium and its contents, as well as the great vessels and trachea and mainstem bronchi. Structures anterior to it are in the anterior mediastinum, and posteriorly located structures are in the posterior mediastinum.

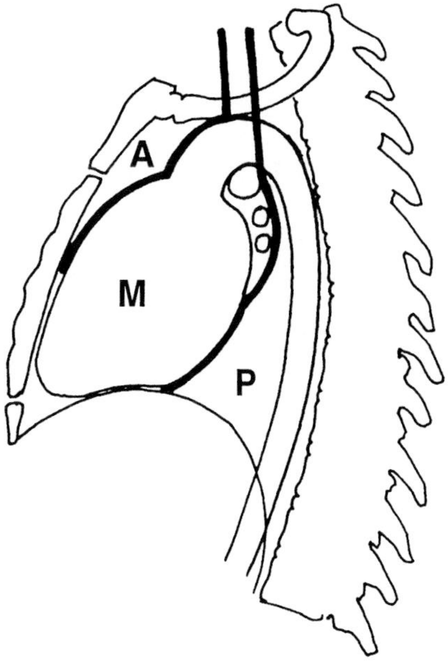

A = anterior to heart & great vessels

M = heart, aorta & branches, pulmonary arteries, trachea

P = behind heart

Figure 3–35 The three compartments of the mediastinum, as revealed on the lateral chest radiograph. Although these divisions do not correspond to any intrinsic anatomic divisions, they are extremely useful in formulating appropriate differential diagnoses for masses in the different compartments. A, anterior; M, middle; P, posterior.

The compartmental location of a mass is often suggested on the frontal radiograph; for example, a left-sided anterior mediastinal mass will not efface the border of the descending aorta, whereas a posterior mediastinal mass often will. This stems from the fact that, because the descending aorta is located in the posterior mediastinum, only a posterior mediastinal mass will be contiguous with it. However, the key radiographic projection for determining the location of a mediastinal mass is the lateral, which eliminates the superimposition of the mediastinal compartments characteristic of the frontal view.

Examples of relatively common mediastinal abnormalities include mass, infection, and hemorrhage, any one of which may manifest as diffuse mediastinal widening or a more focal contour abnormality. CT is generally the examination of choice in further evaluating an abnormality seen on chest radiography. MRI may be superior in the evaluation of suspected vascular pathology, such as aortic dissection, as well as in the evaluation of masses in the posterior mediastinum, and in patients for whom iodinated contrast poses special risk. This discussion focuses on the differential diagnosis of mediastinal masses, based on the compartments of the mediastinum—a classic radiologic differential diagnosis.

Pathology

Mediastinal Mass

◇ Anterior Mediastinum

The anterior mediastinum, often referred to as the prevascular compartment, is bounded by the sternum anteriorly and the heart and great vessels posteriorly. The normal anterior mediastinum is a relatively "empty" compartment, containing only the internal mammary vessels and lymph nodes and the thymus. Aside from the lymph nodes and thymus, two additional types of tissue may be present within the anterior mediastinum and give rise to masses: thyroid tissue and germ cells. Thyroid tissue may be present due to the extension of a goiter or carcinoma from the relatively confined space of the neck through the thoracic inlet into the relatively capacious anterior mediastinum (**Fig. 3–36**). Germ cells may be found in the anterior mediastinum due to a failure of complete descent of gonadal tissue during embryogenesis.

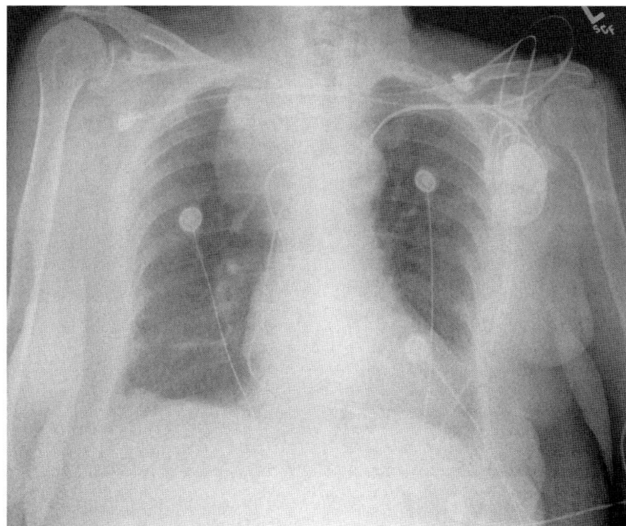

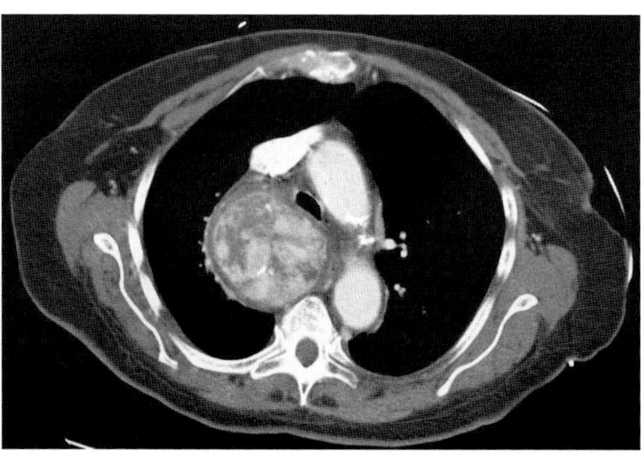

Figure 3–36 **(A)** This elderly patient has a cardiac pacemaker with leads in the right atrium and right ventricle. There is a large superior mediastinal mass displacing the trachea to the left. This proved to be a substernal goiter. **(B)** Axial CT demonstrates the large goiter displacing the trachea anteriorly.

Lymphoma is the most common primary mediastinal malignancy in adults. Although both Hodgkin's and non-Hodgkin's lymphoma (NHL) may involve the mediastinum, Hodgkin's lymphoma does so in a much higher percentage of cases (~75%), and mediastinal nodes are involved in NHL in only 20% of cases. A critical distinction between the two is that Hodgkin's disease tends to spread to contiguous nodal groups in an orderly fashion, whereas NHL often behaves as a multifocal process, skipping nodal groups. Although the finding of characteristic giant, bilobed Reed-Sternberg cells on lymph node biopsy once carried a death sentence, Hodgkin's disease now represents a highly curable condition. Local Hodgkin's disease is treated with radiation therapy or surgical resection, with a 90% response rate. NHL carries a less favorable prognosis.

Though relatively large in infants and often mistaken by neophytes for cardiomegaly in the pediatric setting, the thymus atrophies by adulthood and is usually not visible, having been replaced by fat. Thymoma is the second most common primary mediastinal neoplasm in adults, and typically presents around the ages of 40 to 50 years. Thymomas may be benign or malignant, with ~70% falling into the former category. There is a strong association between thymoma and myasthenia gravis (MG): ~15% of patients with MG have a thymoma, and ~40% of those with thymoma have MG. The tumors are typically found at the junction of the heart and great vessels and are calcified in 25% of cases. By contrast, calcification in untreated lymphoma is rare (**Fig. 3–37**).

The vast majority of anterior mediastinal thyroid masses are substernal goiters located at the thoracic inlet, which typically displace the trachea and often contain some calcification. Some patients may present with dyspnea or dysphagia, although most patients are asymptomatic, and the masses are detected incidentally on chest radiography performed for some other reason. One key imaging characteristic is continuity of the goiter with the cervical thyroid. When the diagnosis is in doubt, radionuclide thyroid scanning is definitive; however, performing a contrast-enhanced thoracic CT prior to the thyroid scintigraphy is likely to create difficulties, because the avid uptake of iodine in the CT contrast may severely compromise the usual uptake of radiotracer for many weeks. Contrast-enhanced CT scanning often demonstrates pronounced and prolonged thyroid enhancement, due to a combination of rich vascularity and iodine uptake by the gland. The thyroid gland also appears relatively bright on precontrast images, due to its normally high iodine content.

Teratomas and other germ cell neoplasms such as seminomas and choriocarcinomas are typically found in patients under the age of 40 years. Malignant germ cell tumors are seen almost exclusively in men. Teratomas contain ectodermal, mesodermal, and endodermal tissues, and often demonstrate calcifications, fat, and even teeth. Choriocarcinoma is usually associated with elevated levels of human chorionic gonadotropin, which may produce gynecomastia.

◇ Middle Mediastinum

The middle or vascular compartment of the mediastinum contains the heart and pericardium, the aorta and its great branches, the central pulmonary artery and veins, the trachea and mainstem bronchi, and numerous lymph nodes. Due to the presence of the aorta and its great branches, the differential diagnosis of middle mediastinal masses includes vascular lesions. Among the most common vascular lesions is generalized aortomegaly, often seen in very old or hypertensive

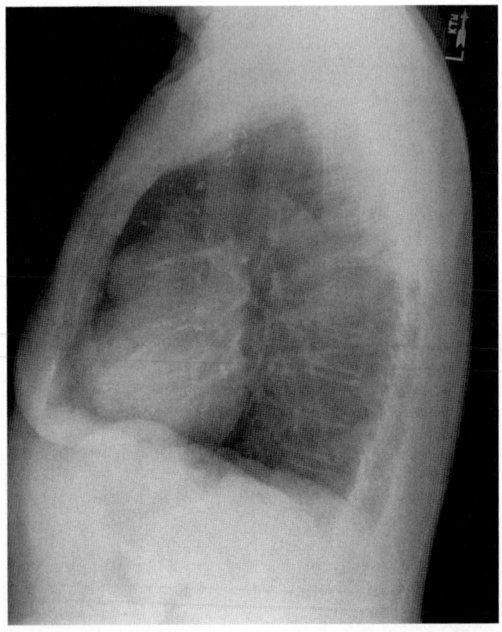

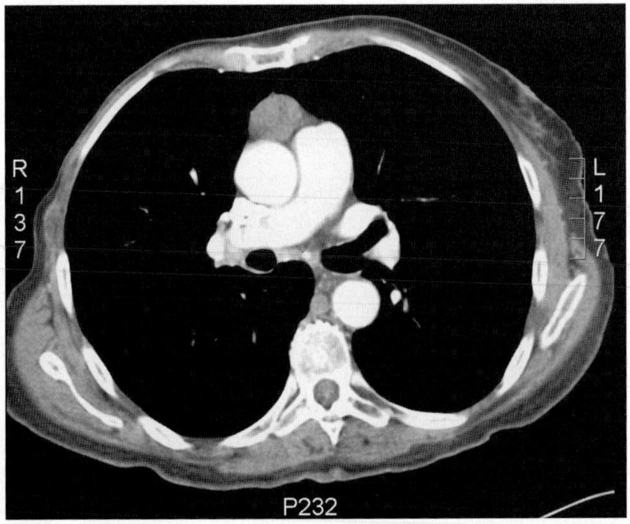

Figure 3–37 **(A)** The lateral chest radiograph demonstrates a soft tissue bulge anterior to the great vessels, extending anteriorly toward the sternum. This would be a characteristic location for a thymoma. Note the surgical clips, the result of a previous mastectomy and axillary lymph node dissection for breast cancer. **(B)** An axial image from a chest CT after administration of IV contrast material shows the mass just anterior to the ascending aorta and main pulmonary artery. This was a benign thymoma.

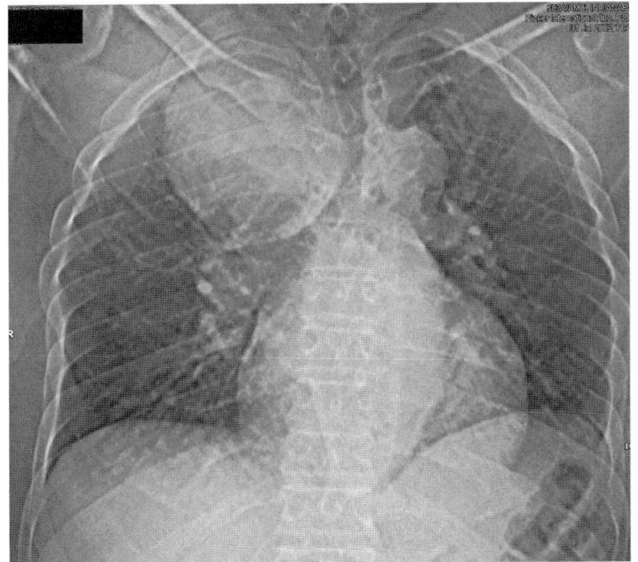

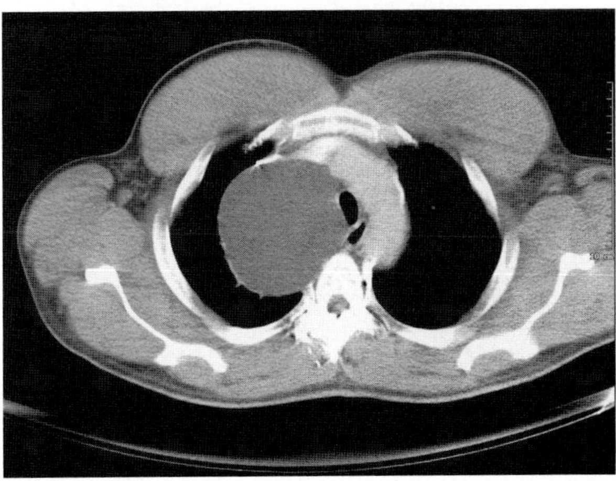

Figure 3–38 **(A)** Frontal view of the chest obtained as a "scanogram" for CT following blunt trauma demonstrates a large, round, smooth-walled mass in the right lung apex, displacing the trachea to the left. **(B)** Axial CT image after IV contrast administration demonstrates that the mass is water density (less than muscle). This was an incidentally discovered bronchogenic cyst.

patients. As the aorta enlarges, it often becomes tortuous, swinging out farther laterally than normal on the frontal projection and farther posteriorly on the lateral view. Such tortuosity is particularly worthy of comment in patients less than 50 years of age, where such changes cannot be ascribed to normal aging, and likely stem from hypertension, increased cardiac output (as in chronic anemia), or accelerated atherosclerosis. The presence of a focal aneurysm merits concern largely due to the danger of rupture, which increases in proportion to the size of the aneurysm. Aortic aneurysms are further discussed Chapter 2.

Congenital malformations of the foregut may also produce middle mediastinal masses. Bronchogenic cysts result from aberrant budding of the tracheobronchial tree, producing a cystic structure lined by respiratory epithelium (with a pseudostratified columnar epithelium containing mucous glands) and containing cartilage within its walls. They do not communicate with the tracheobronchial tree unless infected. The lesions are usually subcarinal in location, contain water-density fluid, and do not enhance with contrast administration (**Fig. 3–38**). Neurenteric cysts are lined by enteric epithelium, usually do not communicate with the GI tract, and are associated with vertebral body abnormalities such as anterior spina bifida or hemivertebrae.

Adenopathy is by far the most common middle mediastinal mass, the differential for which includes bronchogenic carcinoma, lymphoma and leukemia, metastases, sarcoidosis, and infection. The primary tumor is usually readily apparent in patients with middle mediastinal adenopathy due to lung carcinoma; however, in some cases of small cell carcinoma, the adenopathy may be much more conspicuous than the primary lesion. Bilateral involvement is associated with a poorer prognosis than unilateral involvement, which is generally on the same side as the tumor. Nodes tend to calcify in patients with treated malignancies, granulomatous diseases, and the pneumoconiosis silicosis.

Sarcoidosis is a granulomatous disease of unknown etiology that is more common in blacks than whites (10:1) and is commonly seen in the age range of 20 to 40 years. It is a multisystem disease that may involve not only the lymph nodes and lung, but also the spleen, the skeleton, and the skin. TB may exhibit an appearance similar to that of sarcoidosis, although the granulomas in sarcoidosis are noncaseous ("not cheeselike," that is, hard). Patients commonly present with malaise, fever, and erythema nodosum, although many patients with early disease are asymptomatic. Approximately one quarter of patients will also have pulmonary symptoms such as dyspnea and cough. In 80% of patients, radiographic findings include enlargement of the mediastinal and hilar nodes, the so-called 1-2-3 sign of right paratracheal and right and left hilar adenopathy (**Fig. 3–39**). Involvement of the lung is less frequently seen, manifesting as an interstitial abnormality that tends to spare the lower lung zones, and progresses to fibrosis in 20% of cases of long-standing involvement. The staging of sarcoidosis correlates with the probability of resolution. Stage I disease, with bilateral hilar nodal enlargement, resolves in 75% of cases. Stage II disease, with both hilar and pulmonary parenchymal disease, resolves in 30%. In stage III, when strictly parenchymal disease is seen, only 10% of patients resolve.

Among the infectious causes of middle mediastinal adenopathy are TB, histoplasmosis, and coccidiodomycosis. Primary TB manifests as homogenous lobar opacification with ipsilateral mediastinal or hilar adenopathy, both of which may eventuate in calcified granulomata, producing the so-called Ranke complex. Reactivation TB is seen most commonly in the upper lung zones and often cavitates. Histoplasmosis is endemic in the Ohio, Mississippi, and

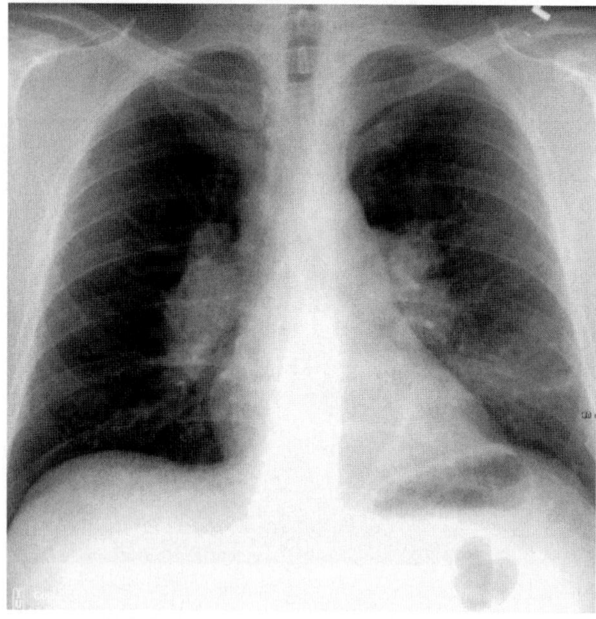
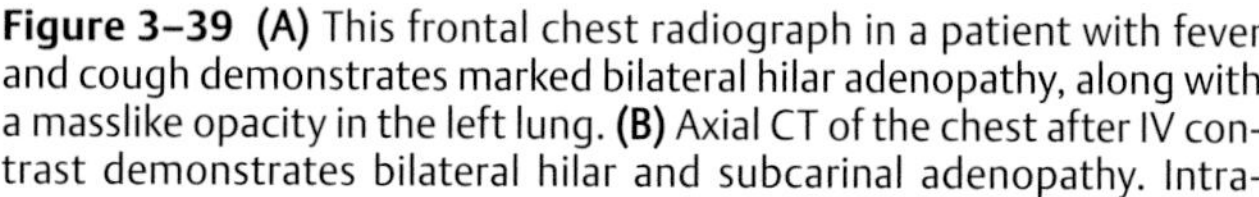
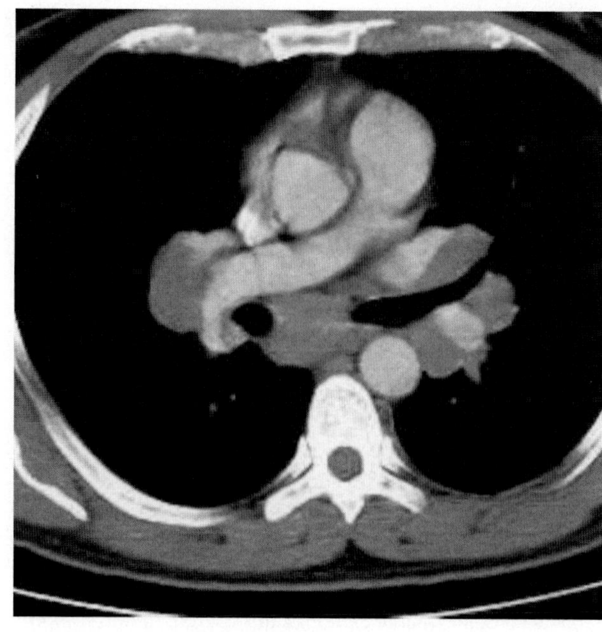

Figure 3–39 **(A)** This frontal chest radiograph in a patient with fever and cough demonstrates marked bilateral hilar adenopathy, along with a masslike opacity in the left lung. **(B)** Axial CT of the chest after IV contrast demonstrates bilateral hilar and subcarinal adenopathy. Intravenous contrast can be helpful in identifying adenopathy, because lymph nodes do not enhance to the same degree as the blood vessels. This patient suffered from sarcoidosis.

St. Lawrence river valleys in the United States, and typically produces a flu-like syndrome that resolves with no sequelae save for the presence of calcified granulomata within the lungs, mediastinal lymph nodes, and/or spleen and liver. Coccidioidomycosis is endemic to the southwestern United States, and may produce "valley fever" when associated with arthralgias and erythema nodosum. Adenopathy is seen in ~20% of infected individuals.

◇ Posterior Mediastinum

The posterior mediastinum lies behind the heart and great vessels, and includes the esophagus, descending aorta, azygous and hemiazygous veins, and the intercostal and paraspinal nerves.

The most common posterior mediastinal masses are neurogenic tumors. Tumors arising from peripheral nerves are neurofibromas or schwannomas, whereas those arising from the sympathetic ganglia are usually neuroblastomas (in children) and gangliomas (**Fig. 3–40**). The former are usually seen in the 20 to 40 year age range, and the latter are usually seen before age 20 years. Both neurofibromas and schwannomas are more common in patients with type I neurofibromatosis (NF-I), the most common of the phakomatoses. The phakomatoses include NF-I, an autosomal dominant disorder including café au lait spots, neurofibromas, optic gliomas, and spinal lesions; NF-II, the so-called central NF, which includes bilateral eighth cranial nerve masses; tuberous sclerosis, which manifests with seizures, mental retardation, and adenoma sebaceum; Sturge-Weber syndrome, which consists of a facial angioma and ipsilateral cerebral atrophy and calcification; and von Hippel-Lindau disease, which is associated with central nervous system (CNS) and retinal hemangioblastomas and renal cell carcinoma. Both neurofibromas and schwannomas appear as round paraspinal soft tissue masses. Biopsy of these lesions may prove quite painful, secondary to their neural origin.

Other paravertebral abnormalities include infection, enlargement of the azygous vein, and extramedullary hematopoiesis. Paravertebral abscesses are often related to spinal infection, with *Staphylococcus* the most common organism. *Salmonella* is often seen in sickle-cell disease. Both present with rapid onset of fever and leukocytosis. TB presents more indolently, with Pott's disease manifesting as slow collapse of one or more vertebral bodies, often with acute kyphosis or "gibbus" deformity, and a paraspinal mass. Enlargement of the azygous vein may reflect increased venous pressure or flow (e.g., volume overload in a renal failure patient who has missed a dialysis appointment), as well as either inferior or superior vena caval obstruction. In inferior vena cava (IVC) obstruction, the azygous vein provides venous drainage into the superior vena cava (SVC) for structures below the level of the obstruction. The azygous vein may also drain supradiaphragmatic structures, when the SVC is obstructed between its junction with the azygous vein and the heart. Extramedullary hematopoiesis is seen with ineffective production or excessive destruction of erythrocytes, such as thalassemia and sickle-cell disease. In these situations, the paraspinal mass represents hyperplastic marrow that has extruded from the vertebrae or ribs.

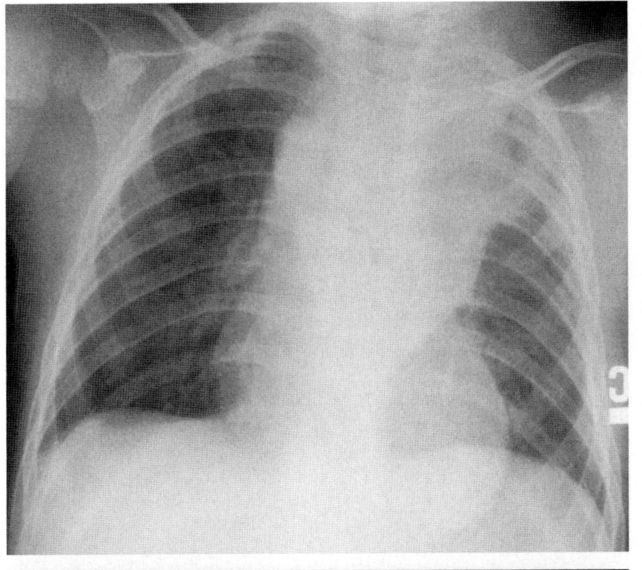

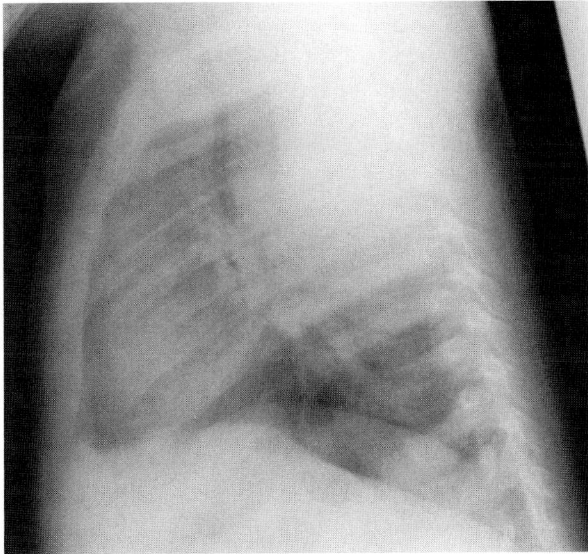

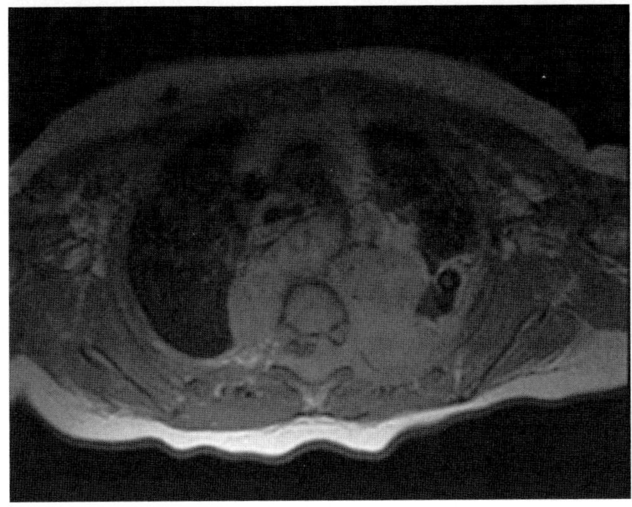

Figure 3–40 This 10-month-old presented with decreased movement in the extremities. **(A)** The frontal chest radiograph reveals a large posterior mediastinal mass, located predominantly on the left, which effaces the normally visible lateral margin of the aorta and erodes the posterior aspects of the fourth and fifth ribs on the left (compare with the contralateral ribs). **(B)** The lateral view confirms that the mass arises from the posterior compartment of the mediastinum. **(C)** An axial MR image reveals a large bilateral paraspinal mass that invades the neural foramina and compresses the spinal cord.

◆ Lung

Pathology

Congenital

Congenital diseases of the lung are discussed in Chapter 10.

Infectious

◇ Infectious Pneumonia

Epidemiology It has been estimated that the typical city dweller inhales at least 10,000 microorganisms per day, including bacteria, viruses, and fungi that represent potential causes of disease. Perhaps it is not surprising, then, that 2.5 million cases of pneumonia are diagnosed each year in the United States, and pneumonia represents the sixth most common proximate cause of death.

Pathophysiology The respiratory tract may be divided into upper and lower divisions, separated at the level of the tracheal bifurcation. Generally, the lower respiratory tract is sterile, and pneumonia may be defined as clinical infection of the lower respiratory tract. Pneumonias can be divided into community-acquired and nosocomial ("next to disease," that is, hospital- or institution-acquired infections). Most pneumonias result from inoculation with inhaled or aspirated microorganisms. Although pneumonia may occur in otherwise perfectly healthy patients of any age, certain factors predispose to its development, including impairment of specific immune responses of the sort seen in HIV disease or organ transplantation with immunosuppression, disruption of nonspecific airway defenses such as mucociliary clearance by cigarette smoke or tracheal intubation, and chronic lung diseases such as chronic bronchitis and cystic fibrosis, which interfere with local pulmonary defense mechanisms and render the lung a more microbially hospitable environment. The very young and very old are at particular risk, as are patients suffering from chronic debilitating diseases. Another important risk factor for pneumonia is impaired oropharyngeal function, as seen, for example, in alcohol intoxication, stroke, and head and neck

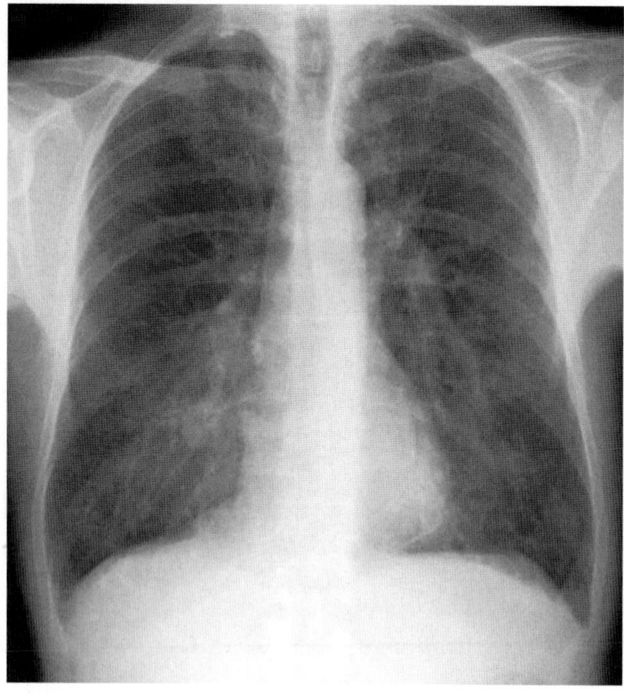

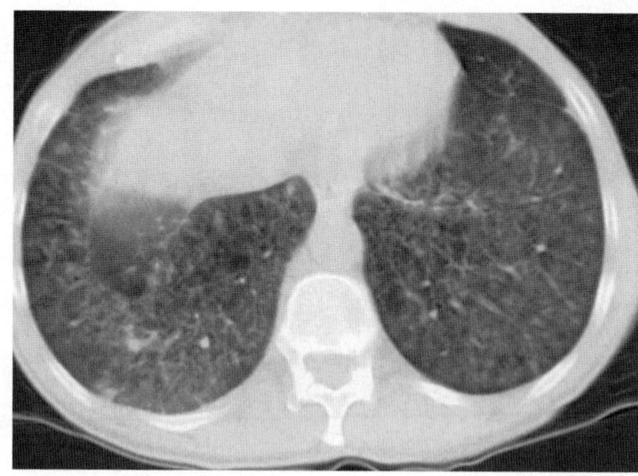

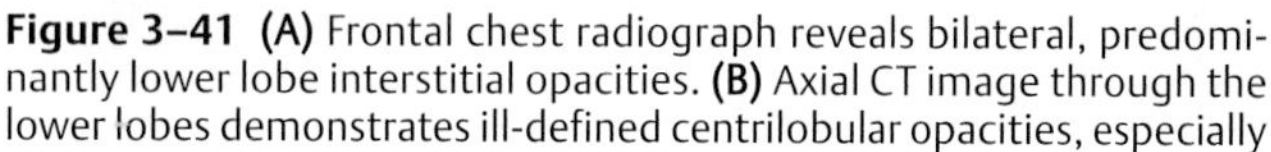

Figure 3–41 **(A)** Frontal chest radiograph reveals bilateral, predominantly lower lobe interstitial opacities. **(B)** Axial CT image through the lower lobes demonstrates ill-defined centrilobular opacities, especially on the right, associated with "ground glass" opacity. This patient had a history of head and neck cancer and was aspirating oropharyngeal contents when he drank liquids.

cancer, all of which predispose to aspiration of pharyngeal contents into the airway (**Fig. 3–41**). An important risk factor for pneumococcal pneumonia is splenectomy, which may be post-traumatic or occur spontaneously as part of the natural history of sickle-cell disease.

Clinical Presentation The patient who contracts bacterial pneumonia usually presents with sudden onset and rapid progression of symptoms, with little or no prodrome. A patient who feels well in the morning may appear toxic by evening, with high fever and complete prostration. Pneumococcal pneumonia in particular often manifests initially by one or several bouts of rigors (shaking chills), presumably reflecting bacteremia. The *Pneumococcus* represents the most common cause of community-acquired pneumonia in virtually all age groups. Staphylococcal and gram-negative pneumonias are common in hospitalized or debilitated patients, and *Klebsiella* is often seen in alcoholics. Anaerobic bacterial pneumonias usually arise from aspiration, and patients with poor dental hygiene are at increased risk. The so-called atypical pneumonias include viral and mycoplasmal infections, which present with a more insidious onset, usually over several days.

Imaging From a diagnostic point of view, pneumonia may be defined as respiratory infection with chest radiographic evidence of pulmonary involvement. If the chest radiograph is negative, the patient will be treated for an upper respiratory infection. A chest radiograph is frequently obtained in suspected upper respiratory infection, such as acute bronchitis, only to rule out the presence of a coexisting pneumonia.

Prior to the discovery of the x-ray, lower respiratory tract infections were diagnosed based on history and physical examination findings, including constitutional symptoms such as malaise and fever, respiratory symptoms such as productive cough and pleuritic chest pain, and auscultatory findings such as tubular breath sounds. An old radiologic adage, "One look is worth a thousand listens," conveys the central role now played by the chest radiograph in the diagnosis of pneumonia.

The chest radiograph not only determines whether a patient has a pneumonia, but also suggests what pathogens are likely to be involved, based on the radiographic pattern. Two classic patterns of pulmonary opacification are recognized: air-space pneumonia and interstitial pneumonia. While in difficult cases other tests such as blood and sputum cultures may play an important role in guiding therapy (although both are often nondiagnostic), the chest radiograph alone often proves adequate to select an effective antibiotic regimen.

◇ Air-Space Pneumonia

Air-space pneumonia, which often occupies a whole lobe and is known as lobar pneumonia, begins within the distal air spaces and spreads via the pores of Kohn and the canals of Lambert to produce nonsegmental lobar opacification. With time, the infection may spread to involve the entire lobe, producing a classic lobar pattern that is strongly associated with pneumococcal pneumonia (**Fig. 3–42**). Fortunately, rapid deployment of antibiotics arrests most cases before they have time to involve an entire lobe, rendering such

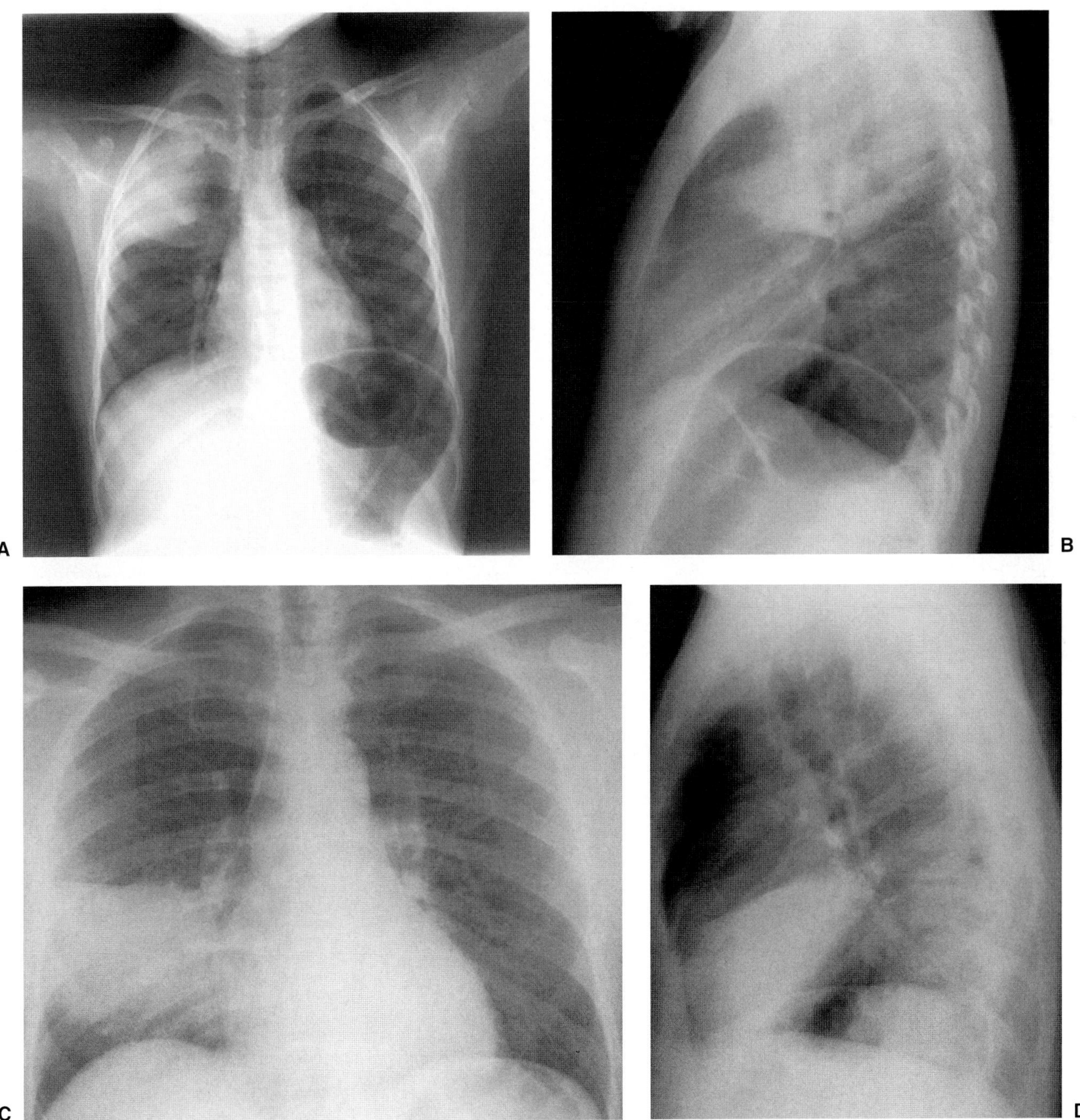

Figure 3–42 **(A)** This frontal radiograph demonstrates air-space opacity in the cranial half of the right lung, marginated inferiorly by the minor fissure. **(B)** The lateral view shows the opacity above the minor (anterior) and major (posterior) fissures. Therefore, this is a right upper lobe pneumonia. **(C)** This frontal radiograph demonstrates air-space opacity in the caudal half of the right lung, bordered superiorly by the minor fissure, with effacement of the right heart border but preservation of the sharp border of the right hemidiaphragm. **(D)** The lateral view shows the triangular opacity overlying the heart in the front half of the lung base, and bordered superiorly by the minor fissure and inferiorly by the major fissure. This is a middle lobe pneumonia.

(Continued)

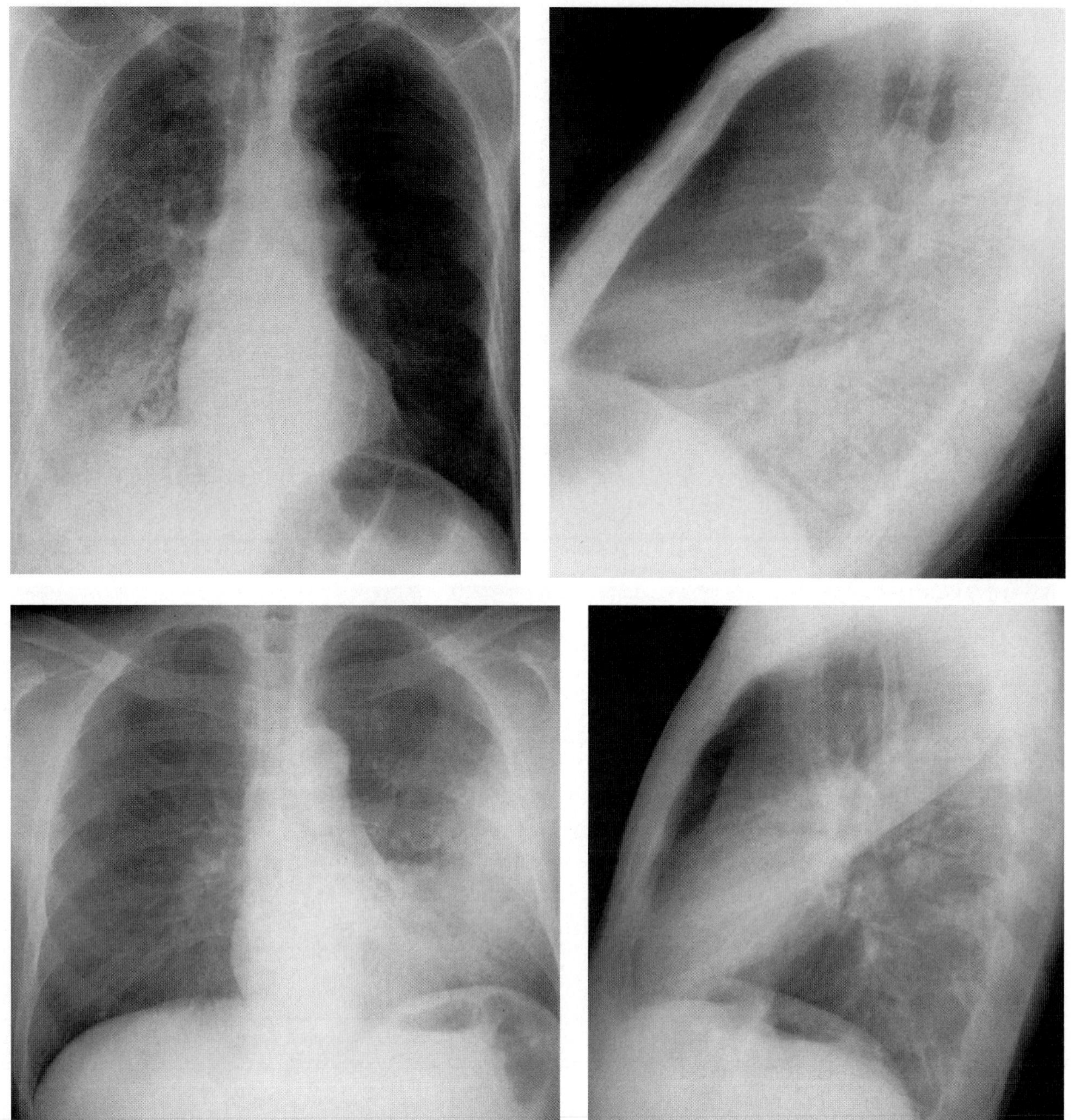

(E) This frontal radiograph demonstrates air-space opacity concentrated in the right lower lung, preserving the right border of the heart but effacing the margin of the right hemidiaphragms. **(F)** On the lateral view, there is no opacity overlying the heart, and most of the opacity is located posterior to the major fissure. This is a lower lobe pneumonia. Note that there is some upper lobe disease as well. Pneumonias tend to obscure the borders of structure they touch. Hence a right middle lobe pneumonia obscures the heart border, and a lower lobe pneumonia obscures the hemidiaphragm. **(G)** This frontal radiograph shows air-space opacity in the left midlung. Is it in the upper or lower lobe? On the left, the lingula is part of the upper lobe and touches the heart. Because the opacity obscures the heart border but not the hemidiaphragm, we can be confident that it is in the upper lobe. **(H)** The lateral view confirms this, showing the opacity overlying the upper part of the heart and extending anterior to the major fissure.

(*Continued*)

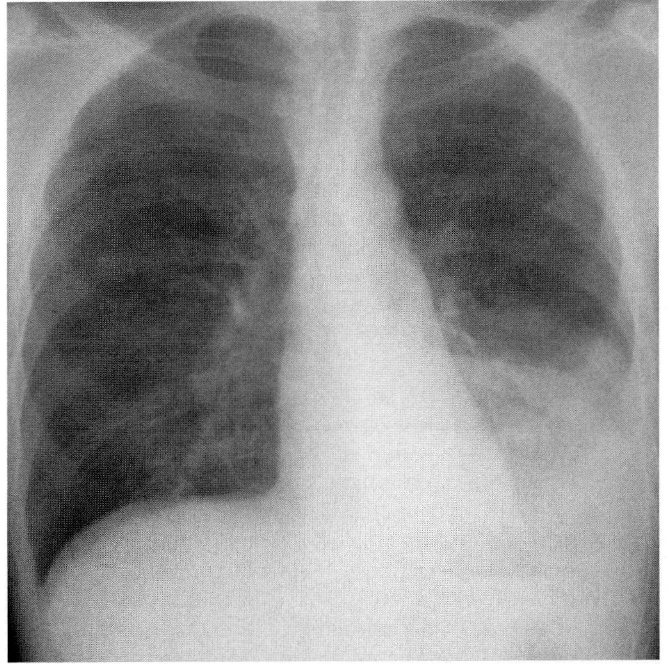

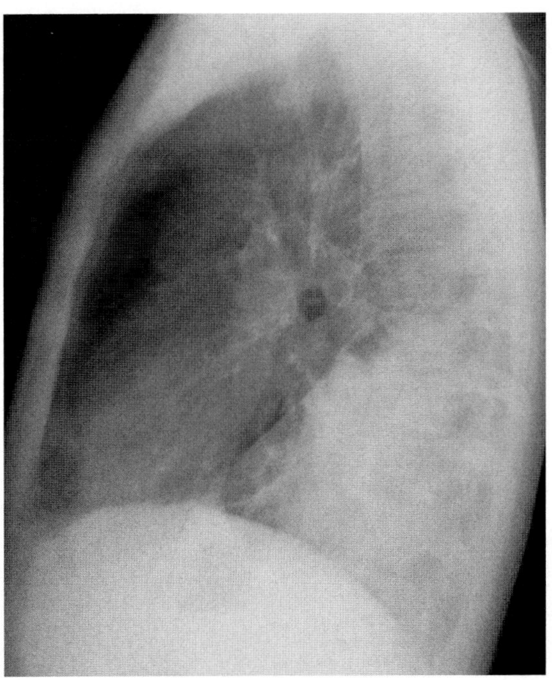

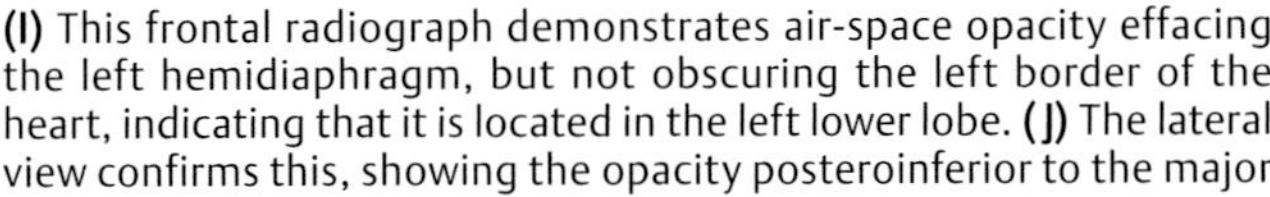

(I) This frontal radiograph demonstrates air-space opacity effacing the left hemidiaphragm, but not obscuring the left border of the heart, indicating that it is located in the left lower lobe. **(J)** The lateral view confirms this, showing the opacity posteroinferior to the major fissure. Normally, on a lateral radiograph, the chest should appear progressively more lucent (dark) as the eye travels down the spine. In lower lobe pneumonia, the reverse is true.

classic presentations relatively less common. Because only the terminal air spaces are usually involved, with sparing of the bronchi, so-called air bronchograms are often seen, which represent air-filled bronchi surrounded by pus-filled air spaces. Air bronchograms appear as tubular and branching lucencies within the consolidation (**Fig. 3–43**). Likewise, the lack of airway involvement renders postobstructive atelectasis uncommon, and lung volumes are usually preserved. Pneumococcal pneumonia generally manifests a dramatic clinical response to antibiotics within 1 or 2 days. The chest radiographic abnormality may lag behind the clinical response, and residual radiographic abnormality may be seen for weeks, particularly in older patients.

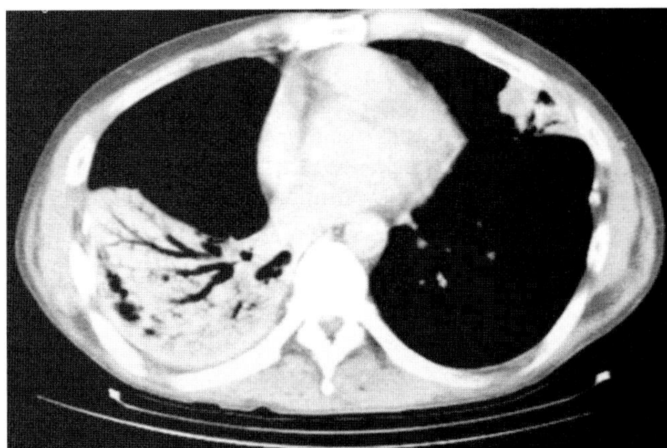

Figure 3–43 An axial chest CT image after IV contrast administration viewed at soft tissue settings demonstrates air-filled bronchi surrounded by pus-filled lung, producing the air bronchograms typical of air-space opacities.

◇ Interstitial Pneumonia

Interstitial pneumonia involves not only the alveoli or airways, but also the pulmonary interstitium along the bronchi and bronchoalveolar walls. The opacities of an interstitial process are not fluffy and ill-defined, but reticular (linear) and nodular in appearance, like a white chicken-wire fence superimposed on a black background. Air bronchograms are not seen because the alveoli remain aerated, although atelectasis may be seen secondary to thickening and eventual obstruction of small airways. The most common pathogens are mycoplasma and viruses. Mycoplasma is commonly seen in young adults and decreases dramatically in incidence during the fourth decade. Most viral pneumonias are due to influenza, and hence tend to occur in epidemics, as distinct from the community-acquired bacterial pneumonias (**Fig. 3–44**). The 1918 influenza epidemic killed 20 million people worldwide.

◇ Tuberculosis

Epidemiology Resulting in three million deaths per year worldwide, tuberculosis is considered the world's most important cause of death due to infectious disease. At the turn of the 20th century, TB was one of the most common causes of death in the United States, often striking children and young adults. Fortunately, until the mid-1980s, the incidence of TB in the United States decreased at a rate of ~3% per year,

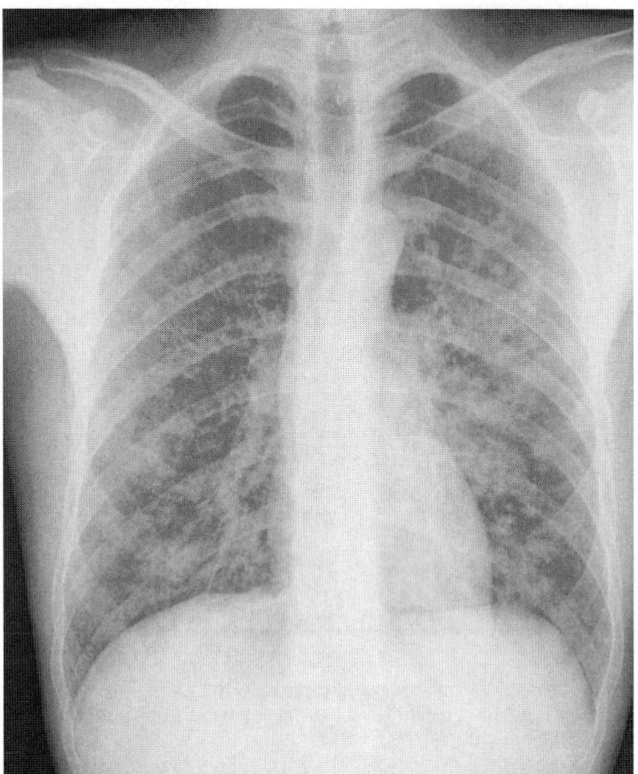

Figure 3–44 This frontal radiograph in a patient with varicella pneumonia demonstrates a patchy bilateral distribution of nodular interstitial opacities. Bilateral and patchy involvement is much more typical of atypical pneumonias due to viruses than so-called typical pneumonias due to bacteria.

most likely due to a combination of improved nutrition, less overcrowding, and increasingly effective antimicrobial therapy; however, with the advent of HIV disease and the rising number of immunosuppressed patients, the incidence of TB has increased. Individuals at increased risk include not only immunocompromised patients, but also alcoholics, intravenous drug abusers, and immigrants from areas with a high incidence of tuberculous infection. Recently, strains of multidrug-resistant TB have begun to appear. If present trends continue, TB will constitute one of the most important public health problems in the United States in the first few decades of the 21st century.

Pathophysiology Approximately 10 to 20% of cases of active disease in the United States are primary TB, which occurs by person-to-person pulmonary transmission. Infected droplets measuring ~5 µm in diameter (slightly smaller than an erythrocyte) are inhaled into the midlung and lower lung zones (where aeration is greatest). The host response leads to macrophage and lymphocyte infiltration, with the release of lysosomal enzymes and subsequent caseation necrosis and calcification. A vigorous immune response by a healthy host often terminates the infection within several months. The only sequelae may be parenchymal and nodal calcifications and an enhanced response to tuberculous antigens, manifested as greater than 10 mm of induration after purified protein derivative skin testing. Reactivation TB results when the initial infection is merely walled off but not completely irradicated. Months or even decades later, immune impairment associated with aging, disease, or immunosuppression may allow reactivation of the infection.

Clinical Presentation Primary TB, which classically afflicts children, is often asymptomatic or produces relatively slight clinical symptoms. Some patients may present with an acute pneumonic process. The patient with postprimary TB usually presents with chronic cough, weight loss, night sweats, and fever.

Imaging In primary TB, the radiographic presentation may include focal air-space opacity or an isolated pleural effusion. The parenchymal lesion is often located in the (better aerated) lower lobes. Lymphatic spread to regional lymph nodes may produce adenopathy. The combination of a calcified parenchymal opacity (the Ghon lesion) and ipsilateral hilar adenopathy is referred to as the Ranke complex.

The reactivation phase of the infection is associated with upper lobe consolidation, a distribution that is usually attributed to the higher oxygen tensions found in the higher lung zones. The upper lobe pneumonia is often necrotizing, producing cavities that range in size up to 10 cm (**Fig. 3–45**). These may exhibit thin or thick walls and may contain air–fluid levels. From a clinical point of view, cavitation—particularly with air–fluid levels—indicates that the infection is likely to be at a highly infectious stage, when coughing can spread infected particles throughout both the patient's own airways (transbronchial spread) and room air, infecting others. Diffuse hematogenous dissemination may produce a "miliary" pattern on chest radiograph, consisting of innumerable tiny opacities throughout the lung fields (**Fig. 3–46**). The term *miliary* derives from the fact that the innumerable tiny nodules were thought to resemble a host of millet seeds. Cavitary lesions may become secondarily superinfected by aspergillus, producing a "fungus ball" or mycetoma. In a small percentage of cases, the infection may erode into pulmonary arteries, producing massive hemoptysis.

Multidrug therapy is the mainstay of treatment. Although the metabolically active extracellular populations in cavitary lesions often can be sterilized within several weeks, more slowly dividing extracellular populations within caseous lesions and intracellular populations within macrophages (where the mycobacterium's coat protects it from phagolysis) often require a year of sustained therapy for complete eradication. From a radiographic point of view, the disease cannot be called inactive until the appearance of the chest has remained stable for 6 months. Pulmonary parenchymal healing is associated with volume loss, fibrosis, and bronchiectasis, especially in the upper lobes

◇ HIV Disease

Unknown as a distinct disease entity prior to 1980, it is now estimated that ~1 million Americans are infected by the human immundeficiency virus, and 700,000 cases of acquired immunodeficiency syndrome (AIDS) have been diagnosed. Worldwide, more than 40 million people are HIV-positive,

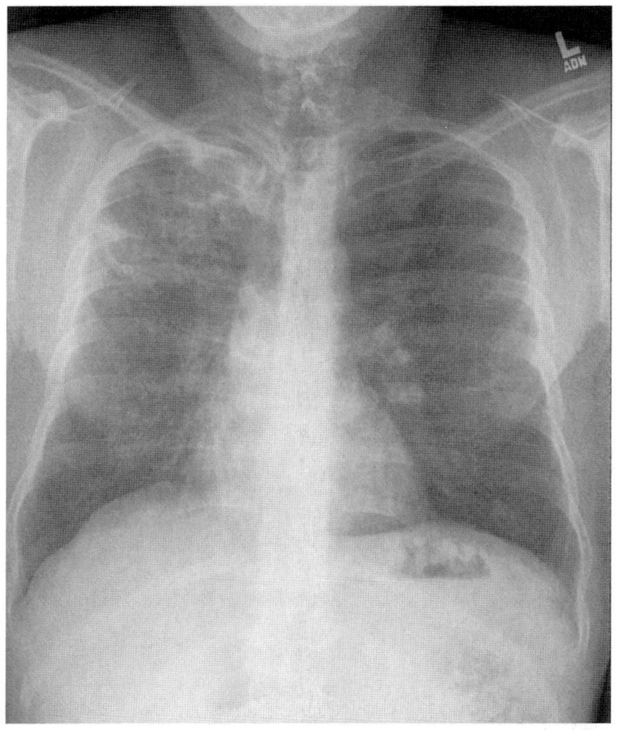

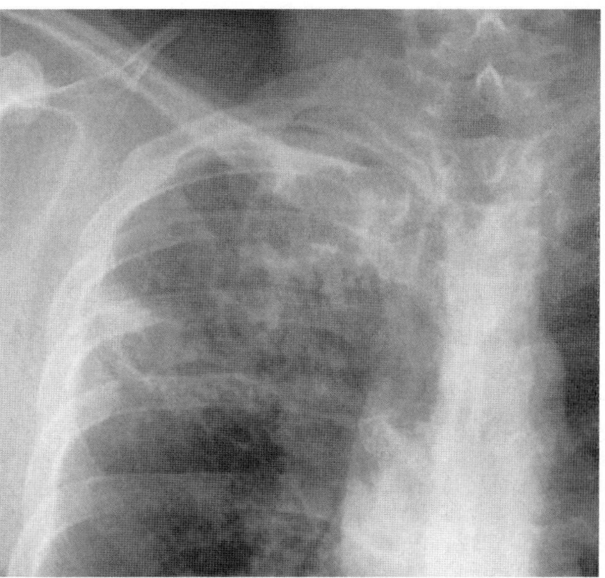

A B

Figure 3–45 **(A)** This frontal chest radiograph demonstrates bronchiectasis and multiple cavitary nodules in the right upper lobe. **(B)** This close-up view demonstrates the cavities to better advantage. The patient suffered from reactivation tuberculosis.

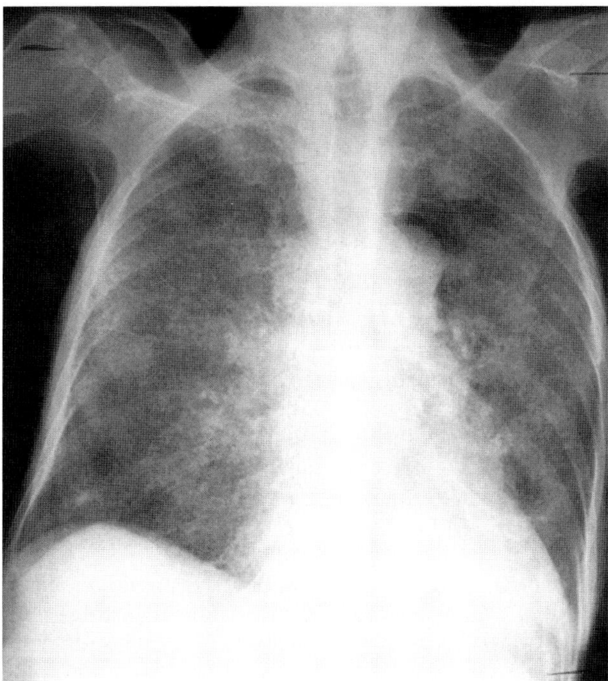

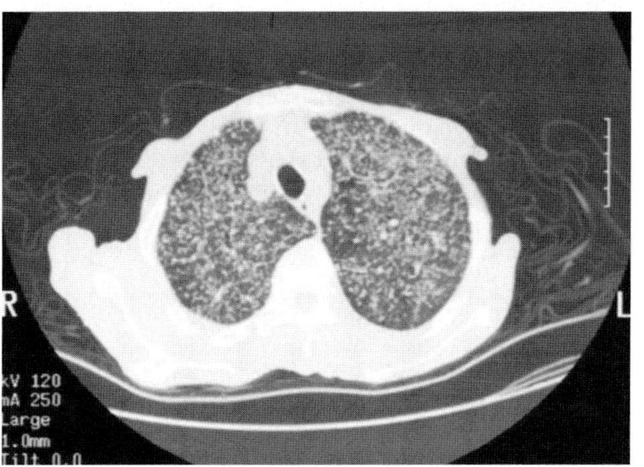

A B

Figure 3–46 **(A)** This 69-year-old woman with cough and fever has innumerable tiny opacities throughout both lungs, secondary to miliary tuberculosis. **(B)** This axial lung-window CT image demonstrates the innumerable nodular opacities.

more than 10 million cases of AIDS have been diagnosed, and ~8 million deaths have occurred. Major risk groups in the United States are men who have had sex with men, and intravenous drug users; although transmission may also occur through contaminated blood products or a mother–fetus/infant route. Worldwide, ~70% of cases are thought to involve a heterosexual route.

AIDS, which represents a late stage in the natural history of HIV infection, is seen at any one time in only a small percentage of the HIV-infected population. HIV especially targets the CD4-positive helper T cells of the immune system, whose numbers are progressively depleted over the natural history of the infection. Because the helper T cell acts as a kind of field marshal of both the humoral and cellular immune responses, this depletion results in increased susceptibility to a host of opportunistic infections and malignancies. AIDS-defining conditions include a CD4 count below 200/mm^3 and opportunistic infections such as *P. carinii* pneumonia (PCP).

Pneumocystis Carinii Pneumonia The most typical pulmonary disease seen in HIV-positive patients is PCP, which represents the initial manifestation of AIDS in up to 60% of patients, generally those with a CD4 count below 300/mm^3. It is estimated that 80% of AIDS patients develop at least one episode of PCP, which proves fatal in between 10 and 20% of patients. Pneumocystis is classified as a protozoan, and clinical infection represents reactivation of latent disease. Patients present with dyspnea, fever, and a nonproductive cough. Radiographic findings include a normal chest radiograph in 10%, but up to 80% of patients demonstrate a diffuse, bilateral pattern of reticular interstitial infiltrates, which may progress to diffuse air-space consolidation over a period of days (**Fig. 3–47**). On plain chest films, pleural effusions are rare, and their presence should prompt suspicion of another process. High-resolution CT is more sensitive and specific than plain radiography, and typically demonstrates diffuse ground-glass opacities, with thin-walled cysts in some cases. Subpleural cysts can result in spontaneous pneumothorax.

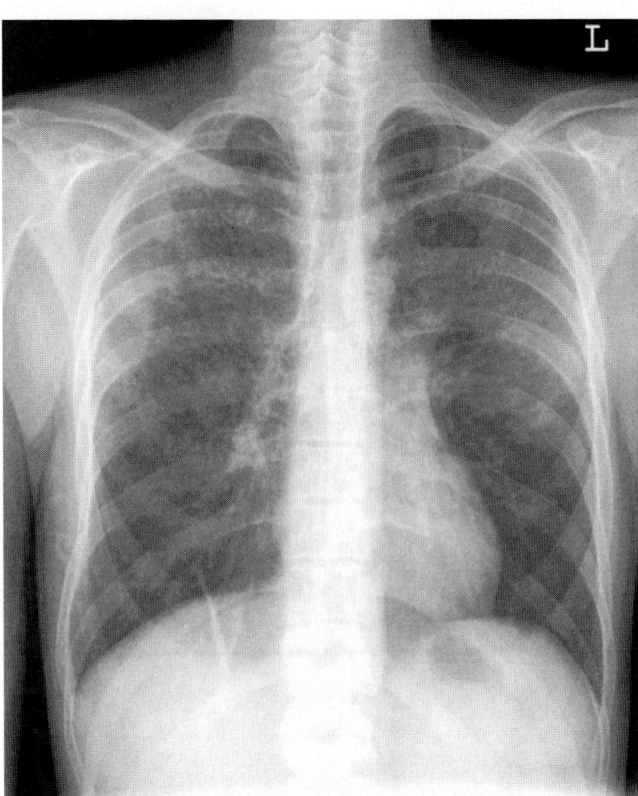

Figure 3–47 This frontal chest radiograph demonstrates patchy bilateral interstitial opacities, which, in this HIV patient, are strongly suspicious for *Pneumocystis carinii* pneumonia. Note the platelike subsegmental atelectasis in the right lower lobe.

Other Fungal Infections Other fungal infections also occur by reactivation of latent infection. *Cryptococcus* is the second most common fungal pneumonia seen in AIDS and often presents with an interstitial abnormality or isolated pleural effusion. The vast majority of patients have disseminated disease at the time of presentation, with severe headache and other signs of meningitis in most patients. Histoplasmosis most often exhibits a nodular pattern. Coccidioidomycosis most often exhibits a diffuse interstitial pattern with thin-walled cavities.

Mycobacteria Reactivation TB can occur at any point in HIV disease. In a majority of patients who eventually develop TB, TB will be the initial manifestation of HIV infection. Early in the course of HIV infection, pulmonary TB is radiographically indistinguishable from reactivation TB in the non-HIV-infected patient, with a tendency to upper lobe predominance, cavitation in up to one half of cases, and pleural effusions in one quarter. Late in HIV infection, with CD4 counts below 50/mm^3 and a virtual absence of cellular immunity, the usual host response to the organism is lacking, and atypical findings predominate. These include adenopathy and pleural effusions in over one half of patients, with no cavitation and a miliary pattern of pulmonary opacities. *Mycobacterium avium* complex rarely presents as a pulmonary disease.

Bacteria Run-of-the-mill bacterial pneumonias are common in HIV disease, with an incidence approximately 6 times that in the general population. Bacterial pneumonia is most commonly seen early in the course of HIV infection. In fact, the occurrence of more than one bacterial pneumonia in a year in a previously healthy patient may be an indication for HIV testing, and multiple bacterial pneumonias constitute an AIDS-defining illness. The most common organisms are the usual organisms seen in non-HIV-infected patients, including *Staphylococcus pneumoniae* and *Haemophilus influenzae.*

Lymphoma AIDS-related lymphoma is an aggressive non-Hodgkin's B-cell disorder with extranodal involvement in nearly all patients. Approximately 10% of patients demonstrate thoracic involvement, including single or multiple masses, interstitial or alveolar opacities, and effusions, with adenopathy in 20%. On nuclear medicine testing, lymphoma is both thallium- and gallium-avid, which distinguishes it from Kaposi's sarcoma. The prognosis is poor, with a median survival of ~6 months.

Lymphocytic Interstitial Pneumonitis Lymphocytic interstitial pneumonitis (LIP) is an AIDS-defining illness in children, in whom it is most common. Pathologically, it consists of a mixed infiltrate of lymphocytes, plasma cells, and histiocytes in the pulmonary interstitium. The disorder is also seen in non-AIDS conditions such as Sjögren's syndrome (immune-mediated destruction of exocrine glands resulting in mucosal and conjunctival dryness), in which it can be associated with malignant transformation. This is not the case in AIDS-associated LIP. LIP is an indolent process that persists for months, without response to antibiotics. Radiographic findings consist of nonspecific persistent reticulonodular opacities. The diagnosis is established by biopsy.

Tumorous

◇ Metastatic Disease

Pulmonary malignancy arising from another primary tumor is more common than primary lung carcinoma. In fact, the lung is the single most frequent site of metastatic disease in the human body. Why? The lung constitutes the first capillary bed distal to the circulation of most organs and tissues. The most important exception to this statement is the liver, which, because of the hepatic portal system, represents the first capillary bed distal to most of the GI tract, including the stomach, pancreas, and colon. Because the liver "sees" the venous blood from the pancreas first, it would be unusual to find pulmonary metastases in a pancreatic carcinoma patient whose liver was free of disease. Neoplasms that commonly metastasize to lung include GI tract malignancies, melanoma, sarcomas, and carcinomas of the breast, kidney, and lung. Plain chest radiography, and in many cases CT, is mandatory in any patient diagnosed with such a tumor, because the presence of pulmonary metastases dramatically alters prognosis and therapy.

Hematogenous dissemination is the most common route of metastatic spread to the lung. Additional paths of metastasis include direct extension, pleural spread (typically producing a malignant pleural effusion), transbronchial spread (a frequent route for bronchoalveolar carcinoma), and lymphogenous dissemination. At least three quarters of patients with lung metastases will have implants elsewhere in the body as well. Hematogenous spread occurs when a tumor invades venules or lymphatics, and cells break off and travel in the blood, become trapped in a distal capillary bed, take root, and spread beyond the capillary into surrounding tissue. It is estimated that only 1 in 100,000 malignant cells released into the bloodstream is able to complete this course.

Where are metastases most frequently found in the lungs? Predictably, in the regions that enjoy the greatest perfusion: the bases. Most metastases will be multiple and bilateral as well, although up to 10% of metastases may be solitary (**Fig. 3–48**). Cavitation is a common feature of squamous cell carcinomas, whereas calcification may be seen in osteogenic sarcoma and mucin-producing tumors such as certain gastric, colorectal, and ovarian carcinomas.

◇ Primary Lung Cancer

Epidemiology Often called bronchogenic carcinoma because these malignant neoplasms can be traced to exposure to inhaled carcinogens, lung cancers have dramatically risen in incidence. Although only several hundred cases were reported annually in the United States at the turn of the 20th

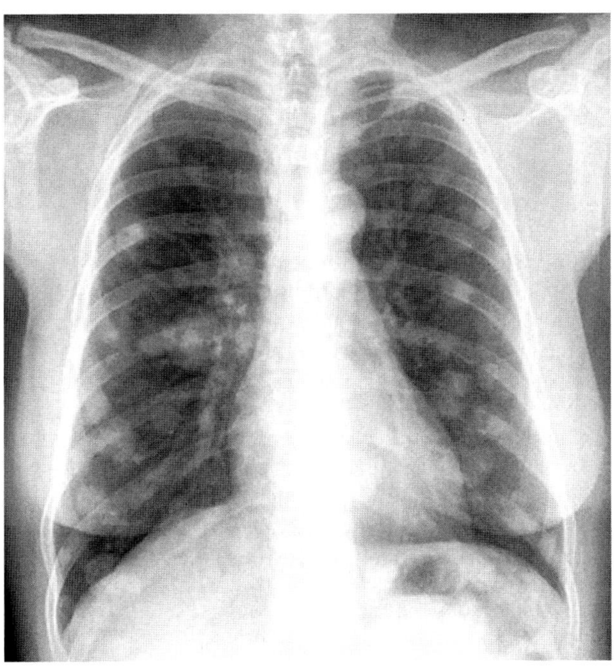

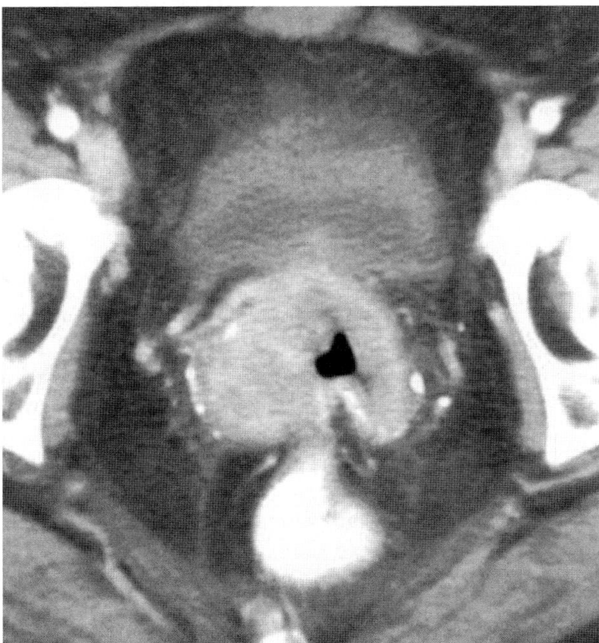

Figure 3–48 **(A)** This frontal chest radiograph in a woman with cervical carcinoma demonstrates multiple bilateral pulmonary nodules, indicating hematogenous metastases. Note that some of the nodules are visible behind the hemidiaphragms. **(B)** This axial CT with oral and IV contrast demonstrates the irregular, hyperemic cervical mass between the bladder and rectum.

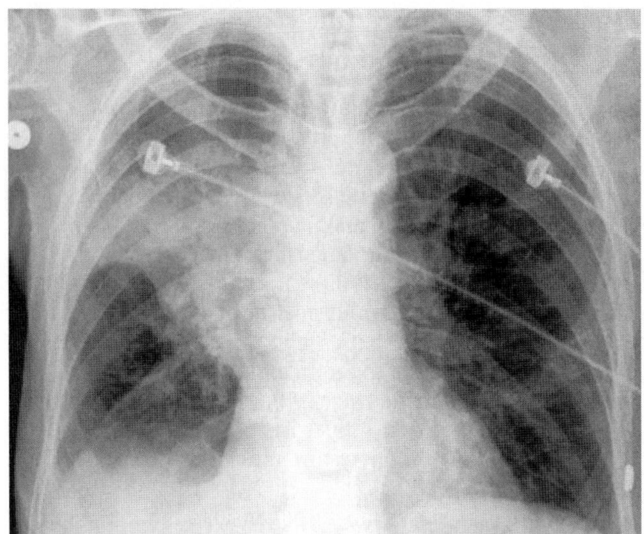

Figure 3–49 This 79-year-old woman presented with weight loss and increasing shortness of breath. A frontal chest radiograph demonstrates a large right hilar mass with air-space opacification and obstructive atelectasis of the right upper lobe.

century, ~180,000 lung cancers are now diagnosed each year, and lung cancer is the leading cause of cancer mortality. It results in 95,000 deaths per year among men and 60,000 deaths per year among women. In the 1980s, it surpassed breast cancer as the number one cancer killer of American women, a distinction it has held for decades in men (**Fig. 3–49**).

Pathophysiology The trends in lung cancer incidence are traceable to cigarette smoking. Approximately 90% of lung cancer deaths are directly attributable to tobacco, with a strong correlation between the level of risk and the number of pack-years smoked, and a decline in risk with smoking cessation (although it takes 10 years for risk to return to normal). Tobacco use in American men and women has dramatically declined since 1965, when more than 60% of men and 30% of women smoked, but cigarette use has dramatically risen in other nations, such as the Philippines, Korea, and Poland, which must brace their health care systems for epidemics of lung cancer.

Other risk factors for the development of lung cancer include exposure to environmental agents such as radon, various occupational exposures including asbestos and uranium, and several preexisting diseases, such as pulmonary fibrosis and scleroderma. In many situations, the risks are additive. For example, while the average smoker has a relative risk of contracting lung cancer 10 times that of a nonsmoker, that risk rises to 50 times normal when the smoker has a history of occupational asbestos exposure.

Despite recent developments in medical and surgical therapies, the outlook remains bleak. The only hope for cure lies in complete resection of all tumor cells, yet three quarters of tumors are deemed inoperable at preoperative staging, to which another 10% are added based on operative findings. Five-year survival is ~10%.

Clinical Presentation Lung cancer presents with a variety of symptoms. Tumors involving central bronchi present with respiratory symptoms, such as cough, hemoptysis, and postobstructive pneumonia. Pleural involvement may produce pleuritic chest pain or local chest-wall pain, as well as dyspnea from effusions. Well-known syndromes associated with lung cancer include paraneoplastic syndromes (such as Cushing's syndrome in a patient with corticotropin-producing oat cell carcinoma), Pancoast's syndrome (pain, hand weakness, and Horner's syndrome secondary to a superior sulcus tumor impinging on the brachial plexus and sympathetic ganglia), and SVC syndrome (distention of head, neck, and upper limb veins due to compression or invasion of the SVC).

Imaging It is often said that all pneumonias in patients over 35 years of age should be followed to the point of radiographic resolution. Why? Because the pneumonia may be trying to tell us something; namely, that one of the patient's bronchi harbors an obstructing lesion. Hence, recurrent pneumonias in the same site should prompt a search for an endobronchial lesion, which will likely be either a squamous cell carcinoma, a carcinoid tumor, or a foreign body.

There are four histologic types of bronchogenic carcinoma, each with its own characteristic biologic behavior and imaging characteristics.

Histologic Types The most common primary pulmonary malignancy, adenocarcinoma, is increasing most rapidly in incidence, and now accounts for nearly 50% of lung cancers. On light microscopy, this tumor forms glandular or papillary structures. It is the most common type in women and has the weakest association with cigarette smoking. Although the primary lesion exhibits relatively slow growth, it tends to metastasize early. Radiologically, three quarters of these lesions present peripherally in the lung, most often as a solitary nodule or mass, and often in the upper lobes (**Fig. 3–50**). A variant of adenocarcinoma, bronchoalveolar carcinoma, disseminates along the tracheobronchial tree. It characteristically presents as a small peripheral nodule or as persistent air-space opacities (a "pneumonia" that fails to respond radiographically to antibiotics). It has a much better prognosis if removed before it reaches 3 cm in size.

The second most frequent form, accounting for approximately one third of cases, is squamous cell carcinoma, so named because it exhibits the keratinization and intercellular bridges one expects in squamous epithelium. Squamous cell carcinoma typically arises centrally within a bronchus, spreading by endobronchial growth. On radiographs, it often appears as a hilar or perihilar mass, and produces segmental or lobar atelectasis and/or consolidation secondary to bronchial obstruction (**Fig. 3–51**); however, up to one third of lesions may present peripherally. It is the most common type to cavitate and also constitutes the most common etiology of Pancoast's syndrome. It has the best overall prognosis, with significant potential for cure if tumors are removed prior to metastatic spread.

The third most common cell type is small cell carcinoma, including the so-called oat cell variety, so named because its cells are small, round, and possess hyperchromatic nuclei. It is the most strongly associated with

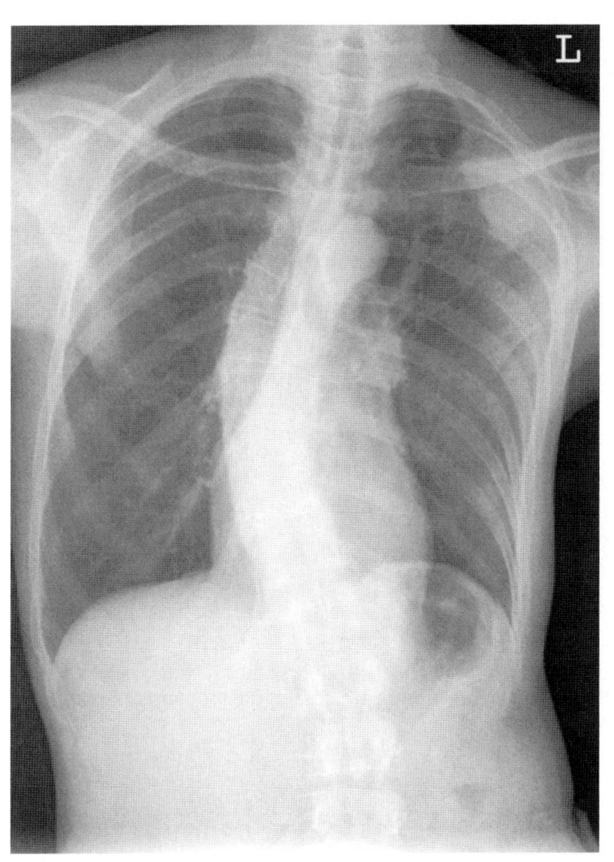

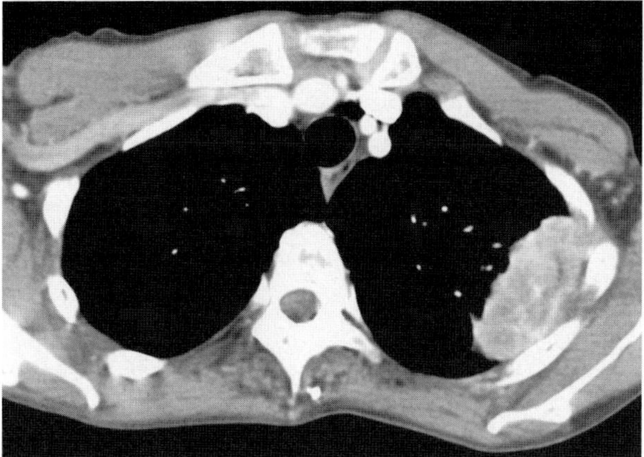

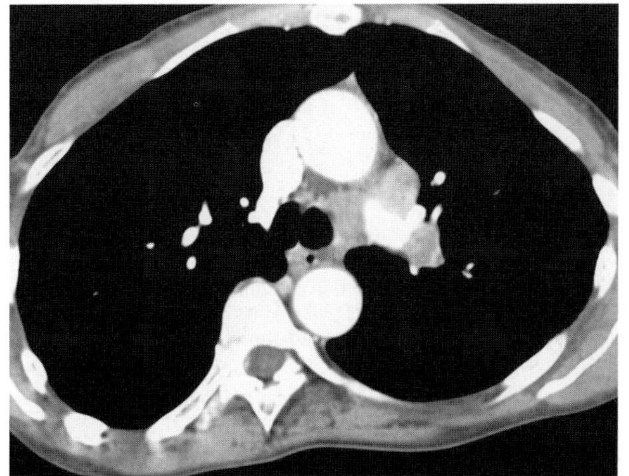

A B C

Figure 3–50 This 57-year-old woman presented with left scapular pain. **(A)** Her chest radiograph demonstrates a mass in the left upper lobe with associated pleural thickening. Note that she also has scoliosis, or curvature of the spine, an incidental finding. **(B)** Axial CT image after IV contrast shows the mass abutting the chest wall. **(C)** Axial CT image at the level of the aorticopulmonary window reveals metastatic adenopathy around the left pulmonary artery. This was an adenocarcinoma.

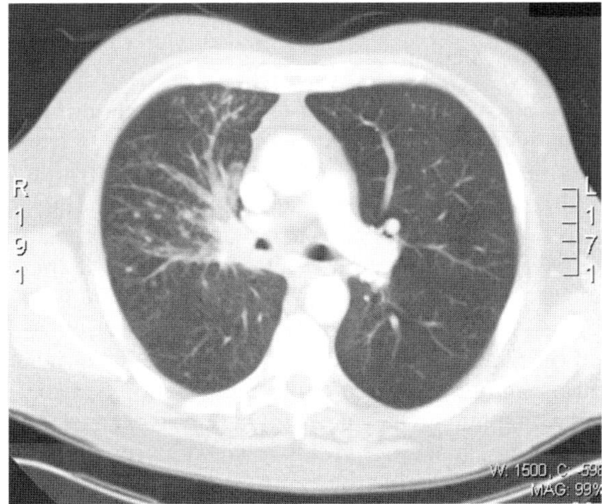

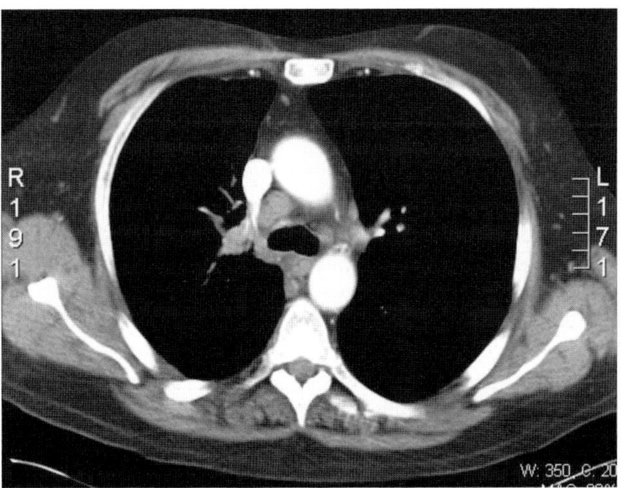

A B

Figure 3–51 This middle-aged man presented with cough and weight loss. **(A)** A lung-window axial CT image after IV contrast demonstrates a right hilar mass with endobronchial tumor spread into the lung. **(B)** A soft tissue window image shows a portion of the mass in the right hilum, as well as metastatic disease anterior to the carina. This was a squamous cell carcinoma.

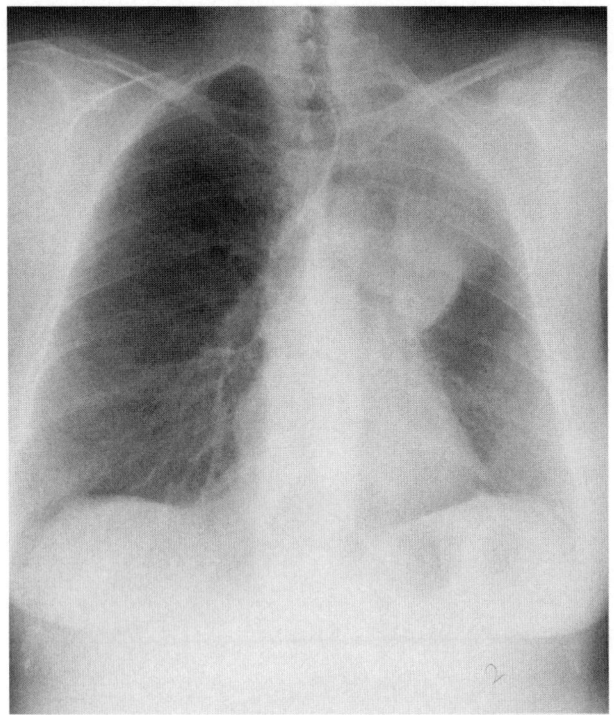

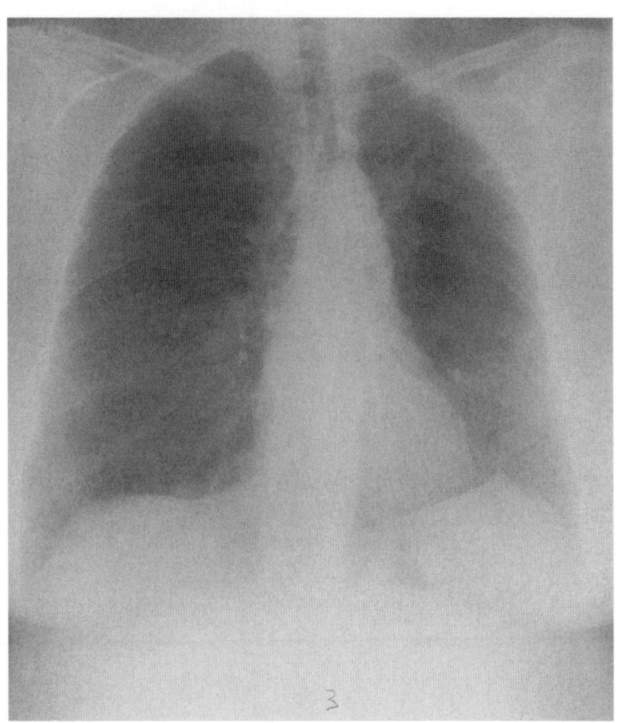

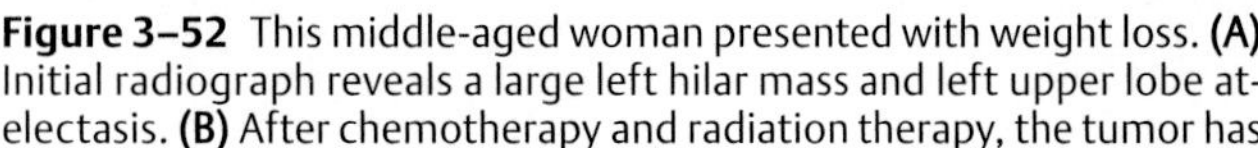

Figure 3–52 This middle-aged woman presented with weight loss. **(A)** Initial radiograph reveals a large left hilar mass and left upper lobe atelectasis. **(B)** After chemotherapy and radiation therapy, the tumor has shrunk dramatically, and the left upper lobe is largely reinflated. Despite this gratifying response to treatment, the prognosis in small cell carcinoma is very poor.

cigarette smoking. Small cell carcinoma most often presents as a large, central mass and is very likely to be metastatic at the time of detection, with 80% of patients demonstrating extrathoracic metastatic disease. It is associated with significant degrees of mediastinal and hilar adenopathy in most cases (**Fig. 3–52**). Paradoxically, while small cell carcinoma exhibits the best response to radiation and chemotherapy, it also has the shortest median survival, ~1 to 2 years.

Large cell lung carcinoma most often presents as a large, peripheral mass. Unfortunately, it exhibits the worst combination of biological behaviors, growing rapidly and metastasizing early. However, its prognosis remains more favorable than that of small cell carcinoma.

Solitary Pulmonary Nodule One of the classic differential diagnoses in radiology is that of the solitary pulmonary nodule (SPN). SPNs are defined as single pulmonary lesions measuring less than 3 cm in diameter, and at least 150,000 of these lesions are biopsied or excised each year. In descending order of frequency, the most likely etiologies for a solitary nodule are granuloma (TB, histoplasmosis, etc.), bronchogenic carcinoma, carcinoid tumor, and metastasis. The best morphologic predictor of benignity is central calcification. Other radiologic characteristics that favor benignity include small size (although every 6 cm lung cancer was once a 1 cm tumor, and this criterion should not influence diagnostic workup), well-defined borders (although many lung cancers are well-defined), and patterns of calcification, such as complete, laminated, or "popcorn" calcification (the latter indicating a hamartoma) (**Fig. 3–53**). The fact that carcinomas may arise in preexisting granulomas means that this criterion must be applied with caution. An additional criterion is the patient's age. Nodules in patients younger than 35 years of age rarely represent carcinomas. On the other hand, a nodule in a 60-year-old heavy smoker is much more likely to represent a lung cancer.

Where possible, the single most important determination to be made in the evaluation of an SPN is whether the nodule is a new or changing finding. If it has been stable for more than 2 years, it is almost certainly benign. The key to determining change is the review of previous chest radiographs. A time-consuming, worrisome, and expensive diagnostic workup can often be completely avoided if a nodule is found to have been present for years. Generally, a lesion that has been stable in size for 2 years can be diagnosed as benign, because the typical doubling time of a primary lung malignancy is ~120 days; however, changes in size may be subtle; a lesion that doubles in volume increases in diameter by only ~25%, indicating that accurate measurements are critical in assessing for change (**Fig. 3–54**).

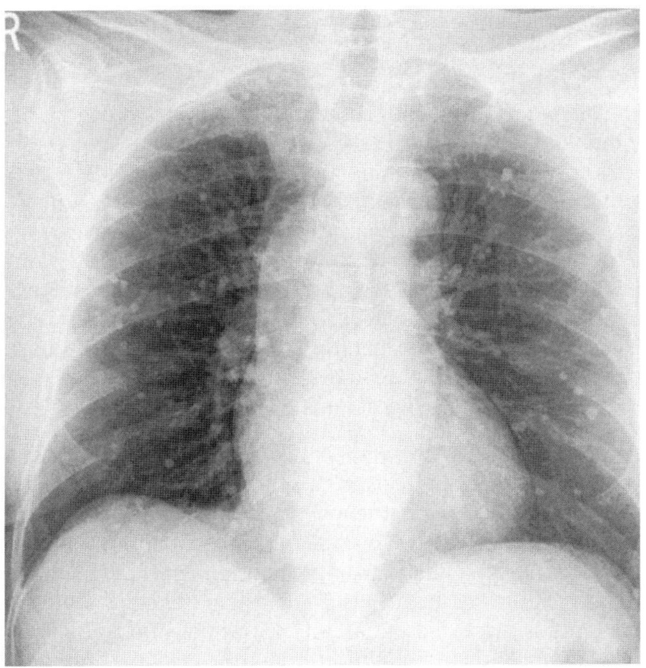

Figure 3–53 This frontal chest radiograph demonstrates multiple nodules that, though smaller in diameter than ribs, appear even more opaque. This indicates that they are very likely to be calcified granulomas, probably from remote histoplasmosis.

Tissue Diagnosis The radiologist's role in the diagnosis of lung cancer extends beyond the radiographic detection of tumors to include the acquisition of tissue for diagnosis. Using fluoroscopic or CT guidance, it is possible to obtain both fine-needle aspirates and core-needle biopsies of nodules, masses, and adenopathy, as well as suspected metastatic lesions. Such procedures enable tissue typing of most lesions, with a better than 90% rate of success, at lower cost, and with a lower rate of complication than surgical procedures such as thoracotomy. The principal complication of transthoracic needle biopsy is pneumothorax, which occurs in ~20% of cases; however, in 90% of pneumothoraces, the degree of respiratory compromise is clinically insignificant, and the placement of a pleural vent is not required. Additional complications of transthoracic needle biopsy include bleeding and hemoptysis. Other means of obtaining tissue include bronchoscopy for central endobronchial lesions, and thoracoscopy and even thoracotomy in patients for whom the risk of pneumothorax is unacceptable (as in a patient with severe bullous emphysema).

Staging Whether lung cancer is primary or metastatic, staging is another routine function of the radiologist. It is important for several reasons. First, in the case of metastatic disease, a small percentage of patients may benefit from resection of their pulmonary metastases, such as patients with melanoma or osteogenic sarcoma. In

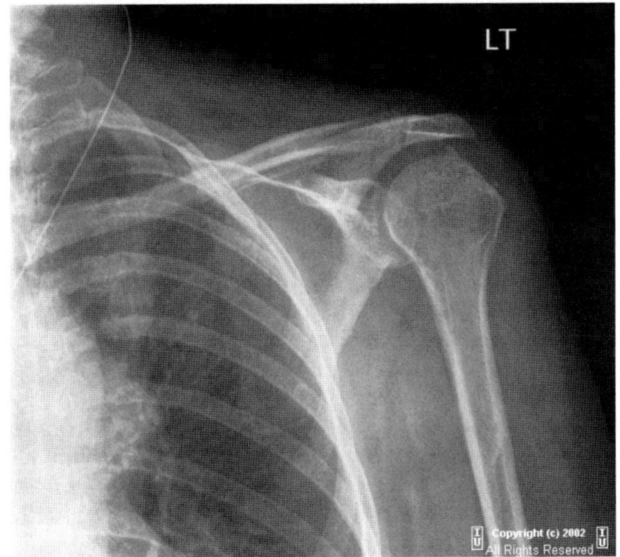

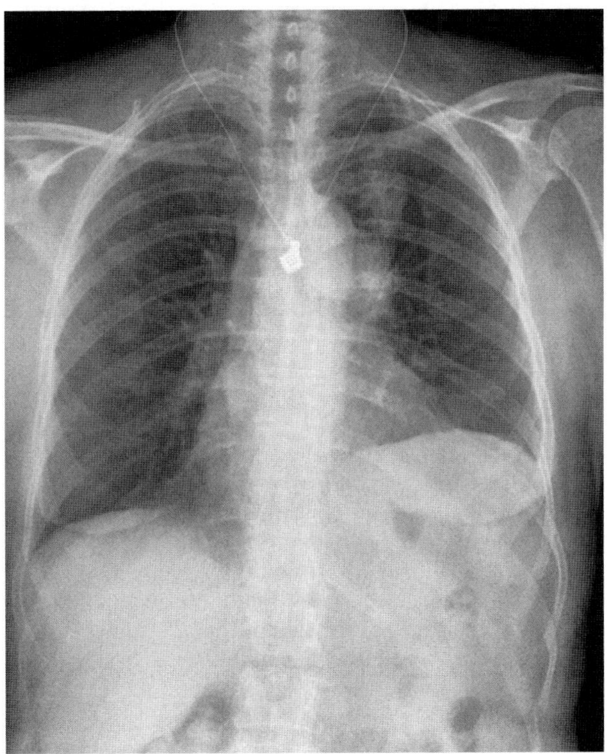

Figure 3–54 This man with a long history of smoking presented with shoulder pain. **(A)** Frontal view of the left shoulder demonstrates osteoarthritic changes in the humerus. The nodule projecting just inferior to the anterior portion of the first rib was missed. **(B)** When the patient returned with cough 1 year later, the nodule had grown. On biopsy, it was an adenocarcinoma. Note also the left hilar mass and elevation of the left hemidiaphragm.

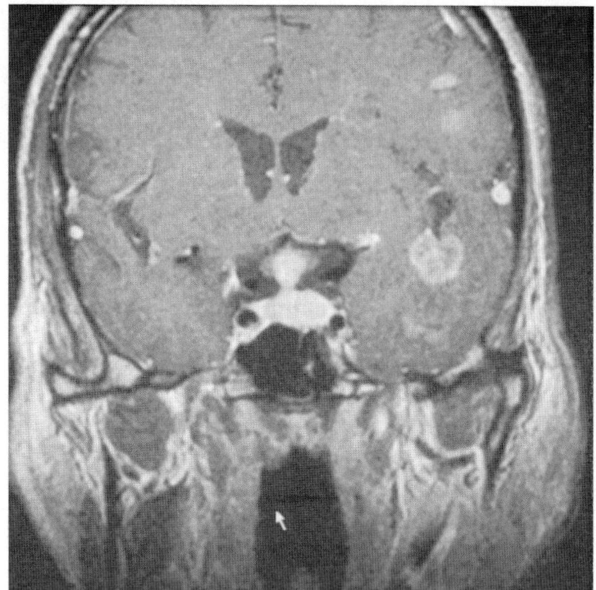

Figure 3–55 This patient with newly diagnosed lung cancer underwent brain MRI for staging. This contrast-enhanced coronal MR image demonstrates, among other findings, a large, enhancing metastasis in the left temporal lobe, making the patient's disease stage IV.

addition, patients with metastatic disease elsewhere in the body, such as the liver or CNS, generally should be spared thoracotomy. Similar reasoning applies in the staging of primary lung carcinoma, where surgery with curative intent should be undertaken only in the small minority of patients in whom cure is possible, that is, patients whose tumors have not already spread to other organs. Staging is also important in the evaluation of treatment protocols.

The staging of lung cancer employs the familiar TNM (*t*umor-*n*ode-*m*etastasis) system. *T* refers to the size, location, and extent of the primary tumor; *N* to local nodal involvement; and *M* to the presence or absence of distant metastatic disease, including lymphatic involvement (**Fig. 3–55**). Among the most common examinations used in staging are CT scans of the chest and upper abdomen, and radionuclide bone scans to assess skeletal involvement.

Unfortunately, none of the cross-sectional imaging techniques (CT, MRI, or ultrasound) can demonstrate abnormal internal nodal architecture, and the criteria for metastatic nodal involvement are based on size, which has limitations. For example, if the radiologist reports every node larger than 1 cm in short axis as probably involved, which is standard practice for most nodal groups, nearly one third of the nodes called abnormal will be free of metastatic disease, while nearly one tenth of smaller nodes will show evidence of micrometastasis. Nuclear medicine studies using tumor-specific radiopharmaceuticals may provide a more sensitive and specific means of tumor staging in the future. PET/CT is already playing an important role, permitting an assessment of metabolic activity (increased in carcinomas) within lung nodules, and assisting in the detection of metastatic disease.

Inflammatory

◇ Aspiration

Epidemiology Clinical risk factors for aspiration can be divided into two principal categories: CNS disorders and swallowing disorders. Common CNS conditions include recent general anesthesia, alcoholism, and seizure disorders. Important predisposing conditions in children are mental retardation and cerebral palsy. Common swallowing disorders include head and neck cancers, previous head and neck surgery or irradiation, and esophageal motility disorders, including gastroesophageal reflux. In hospitalized patients, the presence of endotracheal tubes and nasogastric tubes, which interfere with normal oropharyngeal function, are also risk factors.

Pathophysiology Aspiration of oropharyngeal contents into the tracheobronchial tree and air spaces poses a threat for two principal reasons. First, the normal oropharyngeal flora consists of dozens of species of bacteria, both aerobic and anaerobic, that are capable of causing pneumonia if they reach the lungs in sufficient quantities. The virulence of oropharyngeal contents is increased in patients with poor oral hygiene, in whom mixed anaerobic infections are especially common. Halitosis serves as an indicator of bacterial overgrowth, and many of these patients will have noticeably bad breath.

The second reason that aspiration poses a threat to the lungs relates to the irritative properties of gastric contents. The low pH of gastric secretions, with a hydrogen ion concentration ~10,000 times that found in the pulmonary interstitium, means that even a small quantity of aspirate can produce a profuse chemical pneumonitis in exposed regions of lung. Moreover, aspirated food particles can both induce a foreign-body granulomatous response and serve as a culture medium for bacterial growth.

Clinical Presentation A history of coughing or choking when eating or repeated unexplained pneumonias is the most important clinical indicator that an ambulatory patient may have aspirated. Patients with aspiration pneumonitis often exhibit a low-grade fever and productive cough.

Imaging Lung zones affected by aspiration will vary depending on the amount of aspirate and the patient's position at the time the episode occurred. Generally, the aspirated material will travel to the most gravity-dependent portions of the lung. In the upright position, this most commonly includes the posterior basal segments of the lower lobes. In supine patients, upper lobes are most commonly involved. The usual radiographic pattern of acute aspiration consists of air-space opacities in the affected portions of lung. Atelectasis may also be seen, presumably secondary to pneumonitic damage to type II pneumocytes or obstruction of airways by food particles. The picture usually begins to improve within several days, unless complicated by infection or ARDS. Repeated bouts may lead to a chronic aspiration pattern, characterized by interstitial opacities and scarring (**Fig. 3–56**).

Inhalational Lung Disease A variety of inhaled inorganic dust particles may overwhelm the lung's intrinsic clearance mechanisms and produce a pneumoconiosis. The pneumoconioses include silicosis, coal worker's pneumoconiosis, and asbestos-

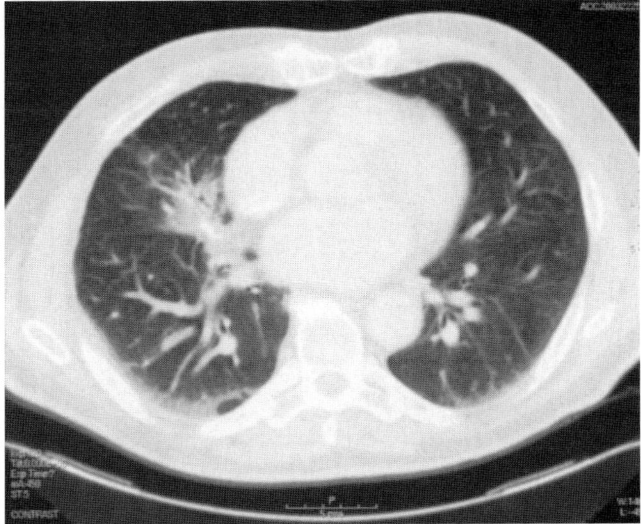

Figure 3–56 This elderly man had a right hilar mass on chest radiography. This axial CT image shows calcified adenopathy and low-density in both the right middle lobe and lung bases. Density measurements were consistent with lipid. The patient was inadvertently aspirating mineral oil and had developed lipoid pneumonia. Some lipid material is also seen in the lower lobes.

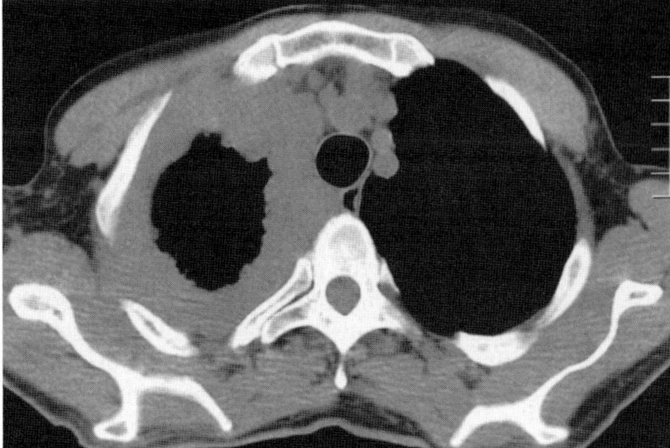

Figure 3–57 This patient had a remote history of asbestos exposure and had developed right-sided chest pain. An axial CT image of the upper chest shows lumpy soft tissue completely encasing the right lung. This proved to be malignant mesothelioma.

related disease. All produce tiny nodules that may progress through inflammation to fibrosis to end-stage lung disease. Macrophages ingest the dust particles but are unable to digest them, with the release of phagolysosomal enzymes and the formation of granulomas.

Asbestos exposure may cause not only interstitial lung disease, but also pleural diseases. These include pleural plaques (which may calcify), pleural effusions, and malignancies. The most common malignancy in asbestos exposure is lung cancer, although malignant mesothelioma has a more specific correlation with asbestos exposure, with a 5000 to 10,000 times increased incidence (**Fig. 3–57**). The risk of bronchogenic carcinoma and carcinomas of the GI tract is also increased. Radiographically, mesothelioma manifests as pleural thickening and/or effusion, diffuse encasement of the lung with volume loss, or pulmonary metastases.

Metabolic

Cystic fibrosis is often called the most common fatal genetic disease in Caucasians, with an incidence of 1 in 2000 live births in the United States. It is caused by a defect in a membrane ion transport protein of mucus-secreting cells, which results in the production of thick, tenacious mucus by exocrine glands and resultant impaired mucociliary transport. Pulmonary manifestations are universal and include mucus plugging, recurrent infections, especially with *Pseudomonas,* and progressive respiratory failure. Other clinical manifestations include pancreatic insufficiency, sinusitis, and infertility in males. Radiographic findings include bronchiectasis, disordered aeration (secondary to mucus plugging), pneumonia, and predominantly upper lobe involvement (**Fig. 3–58**). Complications include pneumothorax,

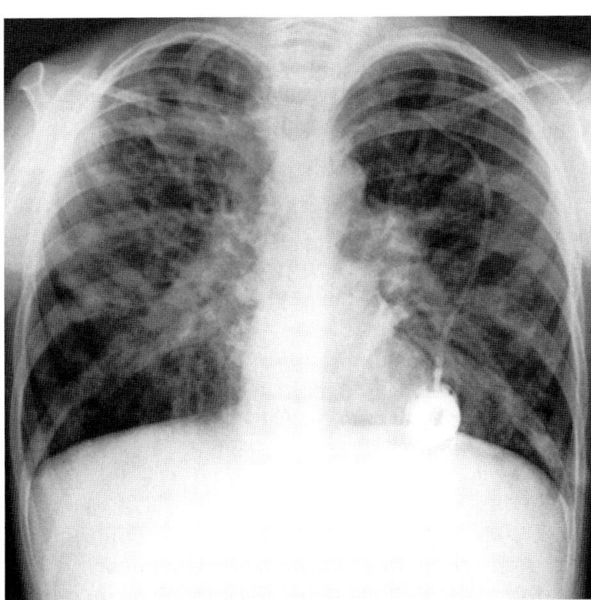

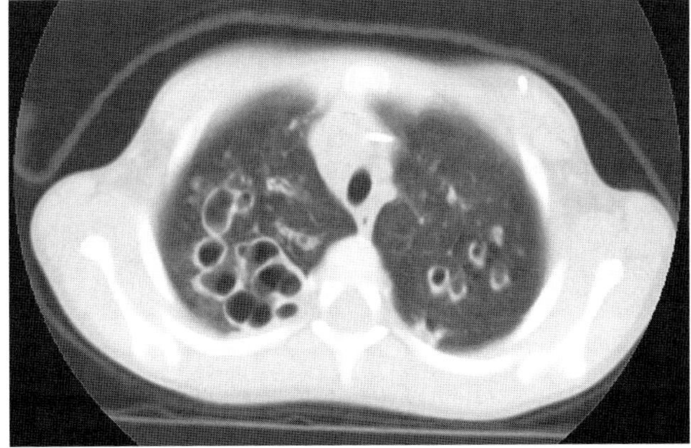

Figure 3–58 **(A)** This frontal radiograph reveals severe cystic bronchiectasis, worse in the upper lobes, particularly on the right. Note the left subclavian central venous port with its tip at the level of the superior vena cava. **(B)** An axial CT image confirms severe cystic bronchiectasis.

hemoptysis, *Aspergillus* superinfection, and pulmonary hypertension and cor pulmonale.

Iatrogenic

◇ Medical Devices

One of the most common reasons for obtaining a chest radiograph in hospitalized patients is to assess the results of medical interventions, such as the placement of central venous catheters and intravascular monitoring devices. The first order of business in reading the chest radiograph of any intensive care unit patient is to verify the correct position of medical devices and ensure the absence of placement complications.

Central Venous Catheters The most frequent use of central venous catheters is the administration of medications, such as antibiotics and cytotoxic chemotherapeutic agents, although other uses such as parenteral feeding and central venous pressure monitoring are also common. Both intravenous medications and feeding solutions are often too irritating to smaller peripheral vessels and must be administered centrally, where they are immediately diluted in larger volumes of blood. By far the most common routes of catheter insertion are the jugular and subclavian venous approaches (**Fig. 3–59**). The latter is generally more comfortable for the patient, who may have a catheter in place for weeks or months, although jugular catheters are less likely to cause thrombosis. The use of smaller-caliber peripherally inserted central catheters (PICCs), which might be inserted near the elbow but extend to the SVC, has become popular.

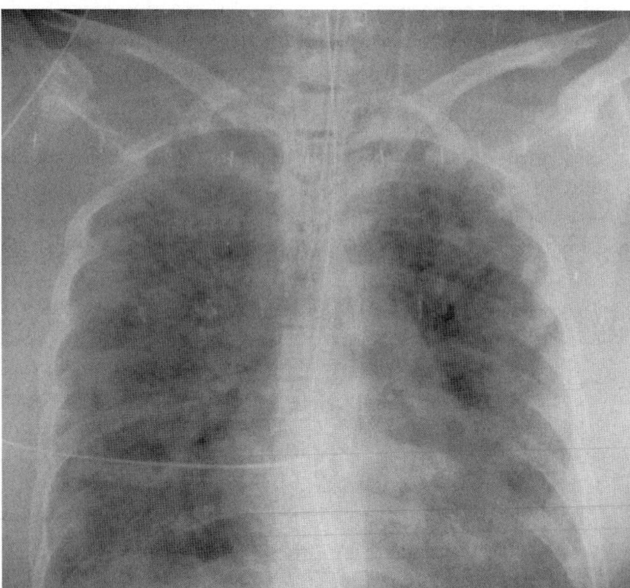

Figure 3–59 Where is this patient in the hospital? Note the endotracheal tube tip several centimeters above the tracheal bifurcation, as well as multiple staples overlying the upper chest. This patient also has an acute respiratory distress syndrome–like pattern of bilateral pulmonary opacities. The patient is in the burn intensive care unit, having undergone skin grafting (staples). There is a left jugular central line with its tip in the left brachiocephalic vein. The right jugular line, however, crosses the midline and runs cardially along the expected course of the descending aorta. This results from the fact that it was inadvertently placed in the right carotid artery. The patient also has a nasogastric tube. A well-positioned central venous line should usually terminate in the superior vena cava.

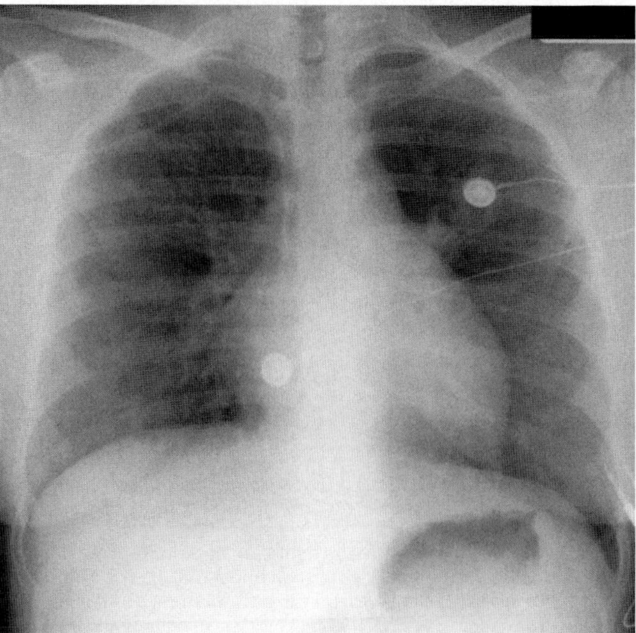

Figure 3–60 This patient's right subclavian central catheter is as caudal in position as should be tolerated, at or just below the junction of the superior vena cava and right atrium. Advanced any farther, it might provoke dysrhythmias.

Regardless of the route of insertion of a central venous catheter (assuming it is above the heart), the optimal position of its tip is the SVC, between the brachiocephalic veins and the right atrium (**Fig. 3–60**). The normal SVC extends craniocaudally along the right side of the mediastinum, and the distal portion of the catheter should follow this route. Types of malposition include location outside the SVC, such as in smaller vessels or in the heart (which can precipitate dysrhythmias), or outside the vascular space altogether, in which case hematoma formation is likely. An extravascular location is often associated with poor blood return following catheter insertion. Another important complication of central venous catheter insertion is pneumothorax, produced by puncture of the pleura. This risk is reduced with PICC-type lines.

Pulmonary Artery Catheters Pulmonary artery catheters are routinely employed in critically ill patients to monitor pulmonary hemodynamics and cardiac output. The catheter is usually placed into the right subclavian or jugular vein and allowed to follow the flow of blood through the right heart and into the pulmonary outflow tract. The key consideration in placement of a pulmonary artery catheter is to ensure that the tip is not located more peripherally in the lung than the proximal pulmonary arteries. If it is located more peripherally, inflation of the balloon to obtain pulmonary artery "wedge" pressures may rupture the vessel, causing pulmonary hemorrhage (**Fig. 3–61**). Moreover, the tip itself may occlude a smaller vessel and cause thrombosis or even infarction. The finding of a wedge-shaped opacity distal to the catheter tip is highly suggestive of such an infarction.

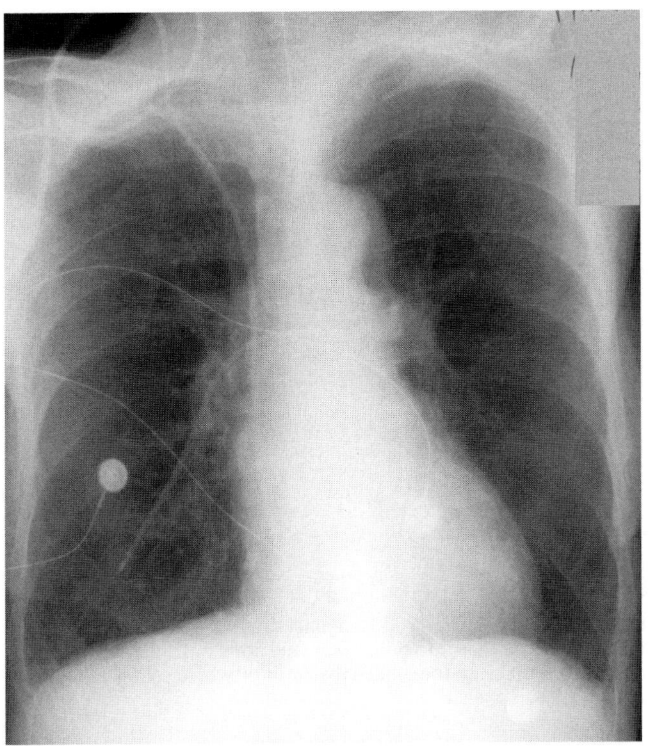

Figure 3–61 This patient's pulmonary artery catheter travels down the right jugular vein into the superior vena cava, right atrium, right ventricle, pulmonary artery, right pulmonary artery, and a branch of the right upper lobe pulmonary artery. It should be retracted to the level of the right pulmonary artery.

Balloon Pumps In patients with cardiogenic shock, an intra-aortic counterpulsation balloon pump may be inserted to augment cardiac output. The balloon is pneumatically inflated during diastole, which increases intra-aortic pressure and augments coronary perfusion. During systole, it deflates, thereby reducing afterload and left ventricular work. The catheter is generally placed from a femoral approach and should be positioned so that its radiopaque tip is distal to the left subclavian artery, the last of the great vessels branching off from the aortic arch. If the tip is placed proximal to the left subclavian artery, it may cause dissection or occlusion of the carotid and subclavian arteries.

Pacemakers Cardiac pacemakers are commonly employed to treat arrhythmias, and are generally implanted under the skin of the chest or abdomen, with leads tunneled subcutaneously up to the subclavian vein site where they enter the central veins and descend to the heart. A similar device is the implantable automatic defibrillation device, which can cardiovert the patient automatically in the field. Pacemakers may be unipolar or bipolar. Unipolar pacer lead tips should be located near the apex of the right ventricle, whereas bipolar leads are generally located in the right atrial appendage and the right ventricular apex. Aside from the usual complications of central line placement, complications with the placement of pacer wires include puncture of the myocardium and the development of hemopericardium, which manifests radiographically as an abrupt increase in the size of the cardiac silhouette. In addition, the pacemaker device and leads should be inspected to ensure that there is no disruption in the wiring that could render the device nonfunctional.

Endotracheal Tubes Patients on mechanically assisted ventilation generally require endotracheal intubation to ensure that only the respiratory tract, and not the digestive tract, is ventilated. The radiopaque walls of the endotracheal tube are generally visible on portable chest radiographs descending through the pharynx into the trachea. The tip of the tube should be located ~5 cm above the carina in most adult patients. The tip of the tube will change in position with changes in head position. With the chin tilted down toward the chest, the tip will move closer to the carina, whereas elevating the chin will cause the tip to move away from the carina. A tip located too high may allow the balloon cuff to impinge on the vocal cords (**Fig. 3–62**). A tip located too low may move into one of the mainstem bronchi, almost always the right, causing underventilation of the contralateral lung (**Fig. 3–63**). Another concern is the degree of inflation of the cuff. An overinflated cuff can press on the tracheal mucosa with sufficient force that it overcomes capillary perfusion pressure and causes necrosis, with resultant tracheomalacia. At a minimum, the cuff should not cause the walls of the trachea to bow laterally.

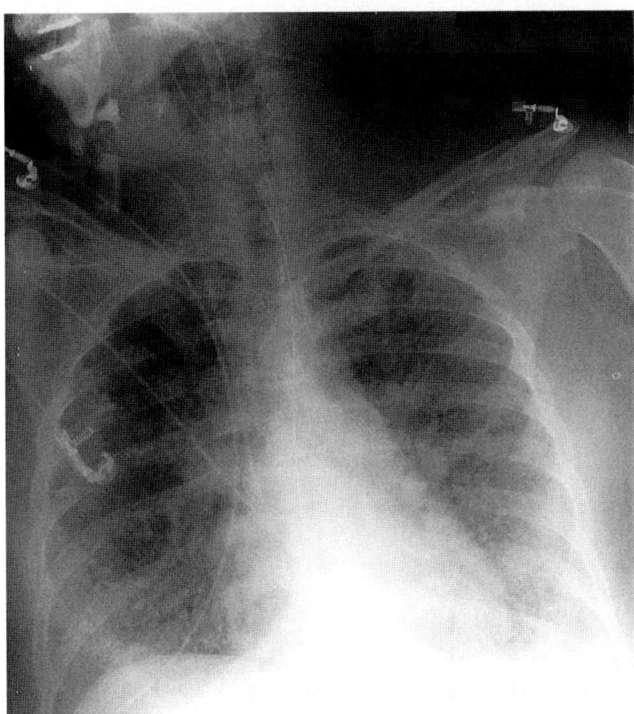

Figure 3–62 This patient's endotracheal tube is positioned too high, in the hypopharynx, which probably explains the bibasilar atelectasis. Note also a right jugular line with the tip at the lower superior vena cava, a left subclavian line in the brachiocephalic vein, and a nasogastric tube headed for the stomach.

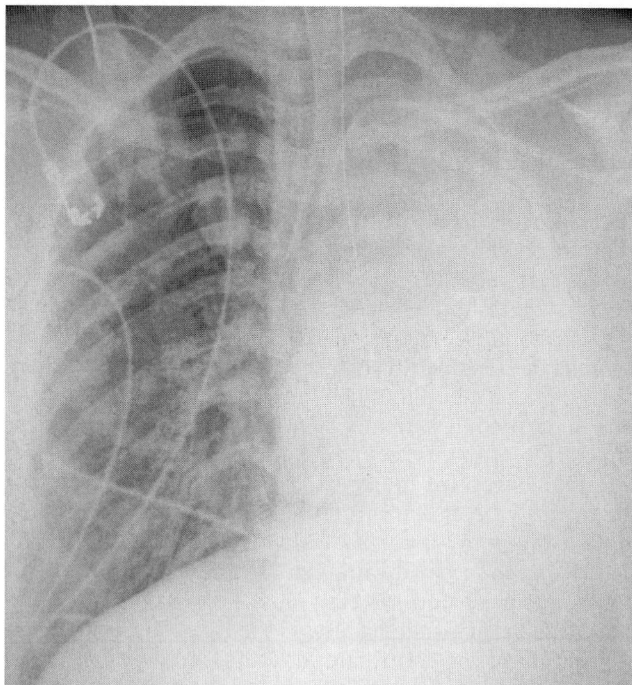

Figure 3–63 There is collapse of the patient's left lung, with leftward shift of the mediastinum. Why? The endotracheal tube is positioned in the bronchus intermedius on the right, depriving the left lung of ventilation. Note that a left subclavian central venous catheter is in the brachiocephalic vein.

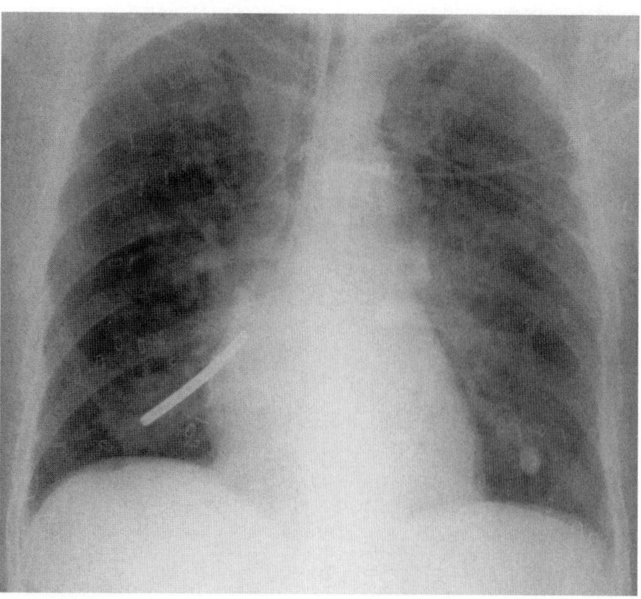

Figure 3–65 This patient's nasojejunal tube was inadvertently placed through the trachea into a right lower lobe bronchus. Infusing an enteral feeding solution with the tube in this position would cause "aspiration" pneumonitis.

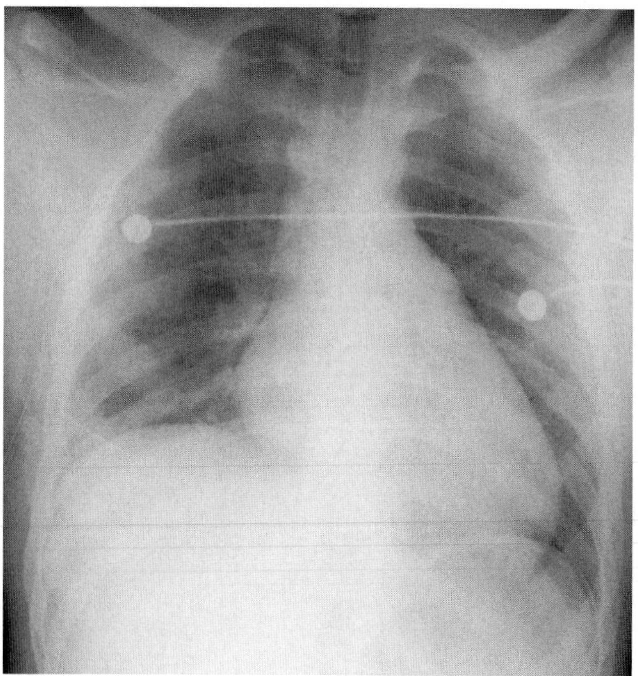

Figure 3–64 This patient's right chest tube is positioned outside the rib cage and therefore cannot assist in draining pleural air or fluid.

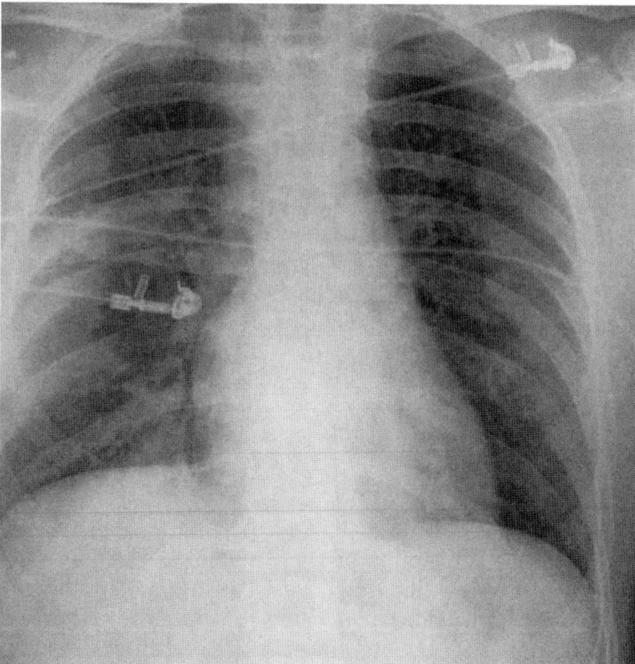

Figure 3–66 The patchy right-sided air-space opacities in this patient who suffered blunt chest trauma represent pulmonary contusion. They resolved completely over several days.

Chest Tubes Chest tubes are inserted primarily to drain gas or fluid from the pleural space. Thus, the tube can only perform its intended function if it is located in the pleural space, in communication with the collection it is intended to drain (**Fig. 3–64**). One sign that the tube is improperly positioned is persistence of the pneumothorax or hydrothorax. An even more worrisome sign is an increase in pleural gas, which may indicate more serious complications, such as an air leak from the tracheobronchial tree.

Nasogastric Tubes Nasogastric tubes are commonly inserted to decompress the stomach, as in bowel obstruction, or for aspiration or lavage of gastric contents, as in upper GI bleeding. The tip of the tube is routinely visualized on portable chest radiographs and should be located in the gastric body or antrum. If the tip is located within or below the pyloric channel, the tube may not achieve its intended purpose. Similarly, a tube located too high, within the esophagus, may not communicate with the gastric lumen at all. Strictly speaking, the tip of the tube is less important in this regard than its side port, which is generally located 5 to 7 cm above the tip. It is the side port, and not the tip, that is used for injection or aspiration. Enteric feeding tubes, such as Dobhoff tubes, are positioned in the distal duodenum or, ideally, the proximal jejunum (**Fig. 3–65**).

Traumatic

Trauma may injure the lung by a variety of mechanisms, including direct impact by a penetrating object and shear injuries due to torsion at interfaces between fixed and mobile structures. Aside from skeletal fractures and pneumothorax, one of the most common manifestations of chest trauma is pulmonary contusion. Contusion occurs when vessels rupture, with filling of adjacent interstitium and alveoli with blood and associated edema. Interstitial and air-space opacities usually appear ~6 hours after the injury, and require ~1 week to resolve (**Fig. 3–66**). When abnormalities persist beyond that point, consideration should be given to the possibility of superinfection and ARDS.

Vascular

The lung is prey to injury in collagen vascular diseases and vasculitides. The most common collagen vascular disease to involve the lung is rheumatoid arthritis. Common findings include rheumatoid lung nodules and fibrosing alveolitis, in addition to pleuritis and pleural effusions. Like other collagen vascular diseases such as ankylosing spondylitis and systemic lupus erythematosus, rheumatoid arthritis tends to involve the lower lung zones, where blood flow is greatest. An important vasculitis affecting the lung is Wegener's granulomatosis, which is a systemic disease that involves the upper respiratory tract and kidneys as well. Vascular destruction manifests in the lungs as multiple cavitating nodules and interstitial lung disease.

4

The Digestive System

- **The Digestive Tract**
  - Oropharynx
    - *Anatomy and Physiology*
    - *Imaging*
  - Esophagus
    - *Anatomy and Physiology*
    - *Imaging*
  - Stomach
    - *Anatomy and Physiology*
    - *Imaging*
  - Duodenum
    - *Anatomy and Physiology*
    - *Imaging*
  - Mesenteric Small Bowel
    - *Anatomy and Physiology*
    - *Imaging*
  - Large Intestine
    - *Anatomy and Physiology*
    - *Imaging*
  - Basic Patterns of Gastrointestinal Tract Abnormalities
    - *Filling Defects*
    - *Polyps*
    - *Masses*
    - *Intrinsic Wall Abnormalities*
    - *Extraluminal Projections*
    - *Distention*
    - *Narrowing*
  - Select Pathologies
    - *Esophagus*
    - *Stomach*
    - *Small Bowel*
    - *Colon and Rectum*
- **The Solid Organs of Digestion**
  - Search Pattern
  - Select Pathologies
    - *Liver*
    - *Pancreas*
- **Abdominal Trauma**
  - Diagnosis
    - *Diagnostic Peritoneal Lavage*
    - *Computed Tomography*

The abdomen extends inferiorly from the diaphragm through the pelvis and includes tissues from most of the major organ systems. This chapter focuses on the imaging of the digestive system, including both the alimentary canal and the solid organs that participate in digestion. A mainstay of the imaging of the alimentary canal is barium, a term used colloquially to refer to barium sulfate preparations that also contain emulsifying and coating agents. The mucosa of a viscus that would normally be difficult to visualize radiographically can be imaged in exquisite anatomic detail when filled or coated with barium.

◆ The Digestive Tract

The digestive tract begins at the lips and ends at the anus. From a strict anatomic point of view, the luminal contents of the digestive tract are not inside but outside the body and do not become truly internalized until they enter into capillaries or lymphatics by passing through the mucosal cells lining the gut. The major functions of the digestive system include (1) motility of luminal contents, (2) secretion of digestive juices, (3) mechanical and chemical breakdown of foodstuffs into absorbable units (digestion), and (4) absorption. The layers of the gut include (1) the mucosa, the luminal surface that functions in secretion and absorption and protects the body from luminal contents; (2) the submucosa, which provides distensibility and elasticity; (3) the muscularis externa, comprised of an inner circular layer and outer longitudinal layer, which is responsible for motility; and (4) the serosa, which secretes a serous fluid that reduces friction between segments of the gut and surrounding viscera.

The major divisions of the digestive tract include the mouth, the oropharynx (from the Latin for "mouth" and "throat"), the esophagus (from the Greek *oisophagos,* "passage for food"), the stomach (from the Greek *stoma,* "mouth"), the duodenum (from the Latin *duo,* "two" + *den,* "ten," because it is 12 fingerbreadths long), the jejunum (from the Latin *jejunus,* "empty," because it was thought to be empty at death), the ileum (from the Latin *ileus,* "flank"), the colon, the rectum (from the Latin for "straight," as in rectitude), and the anus (from the Latin for "ring," as in annular) (**Fig. 4–1**).

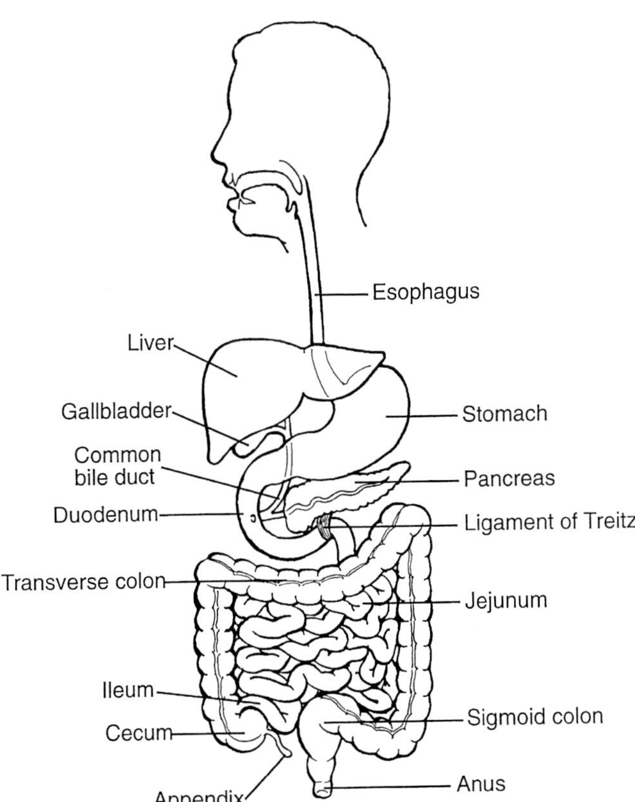

Figure 4–1 Parts of the gastrointestinal (GI) tract.

Oropharynx

Anatomy and Physiology

The pharynx is usually divided by anatomists into three segments, the nasopharynx (from the skull base to the soft palate), the oropharynx (from the soft palate to the hyoid bone), and the hypopharynx (from the hyoid bone to the cricopharyngeus muscle). The oropharynx functions in the mechanical breakdown of food through chewing, in the chemical breakdown of food by salivary amylase, in speech, and in swallowing. Because the digestive and respiratory systems share a common pathway in the oropharynx, normal swallowing is critical, because it keeps ingested material out of the airway. Aspiration refers to the passage of liquids or solids into the trachea.

Imaging

Though not a standard part of a barium swallow examination, double-contrast pharyngography is performed in cases where symptoms are suspicious for a pharyngeal abnormality. Such symptoms include difficulty initiating swallowing, hoarseness, and coughing or choking. Pharyngography involves double-contrast views of the oropharynx and hypopharynx in both anteroposterior (AP) and lateral projections, with and without phonation and the Valsalva maneuver (**Fig. 4–2**). Structures to be evaluated include the valleculae (the symmetric pouches in the recess between the base of the tongue and the epiglottis) and the pyriform sinuses (the lateral pouches between the larynx and hypopharynx). Asymmetry or displacement of these structures suggests neuromuscular impairment or a space-occupying lesion such as a carcinoma (**Fig. 4–3**).

An important type of imaging in this area is the oropharyngeal motility (OPM) study, which is frequently employed to evaluate patients with swallowing difficulties due to disorders such as head and neck cancer and stroke. The patient is monitored fluoroscopically in the lateral projection while boluses of barium or food mixed with barium are transferred from the lips to the upper esophagus. The OPM study can be used to determine whether patients can be fed orally and to counsel patients regarding appropriate types of food to eat, as well as compensatory chewing and swallowing maneuvers. For example, a patient who aspirates with

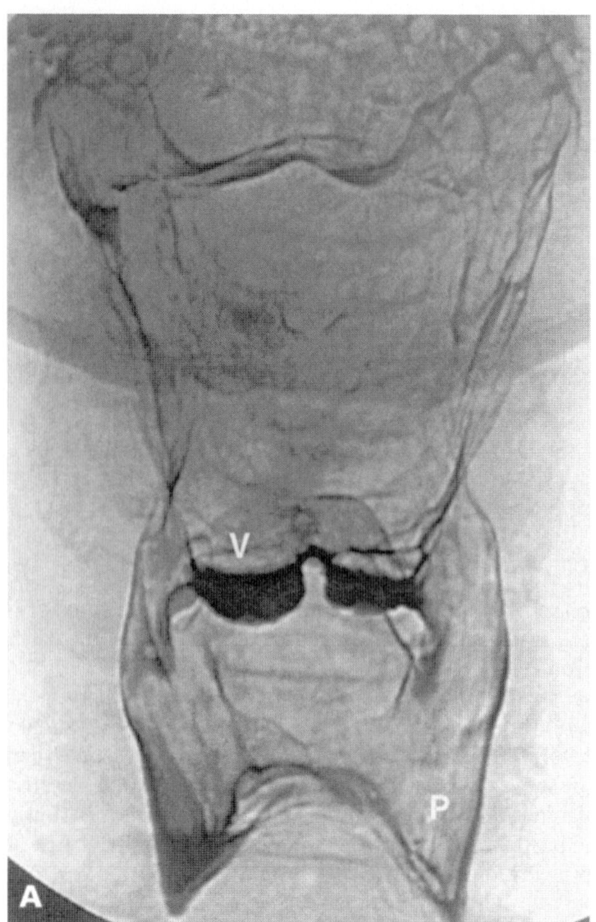

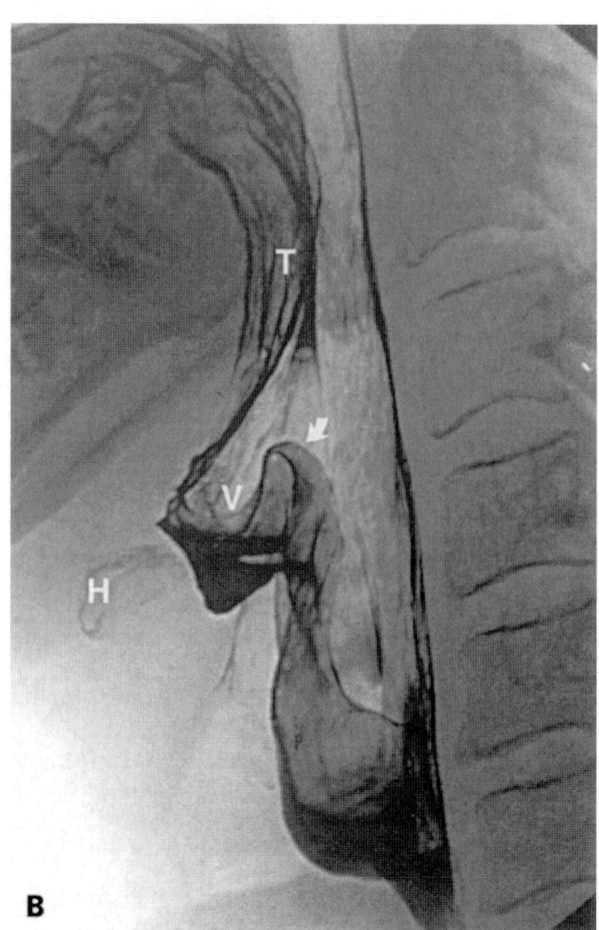

Figure 4–2 These **(A)** frontal and **(B)** lateral projection digital radiographs from a double-contrast pharyngogram exquisitely demonstrate the normal structures of the pharynx. The epiglottis is designated by the white arrow. The hyoid bone (H) separates the oropharynx from the hypopharynx. P, pyriform sinus; T, base of tongue; V, vallecula.

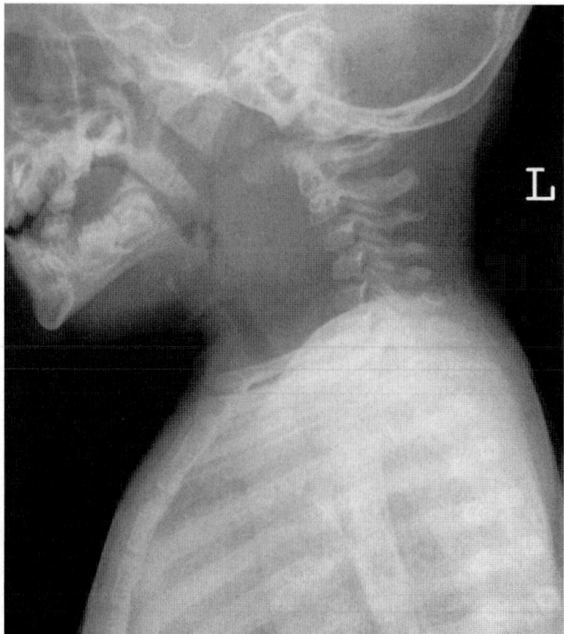

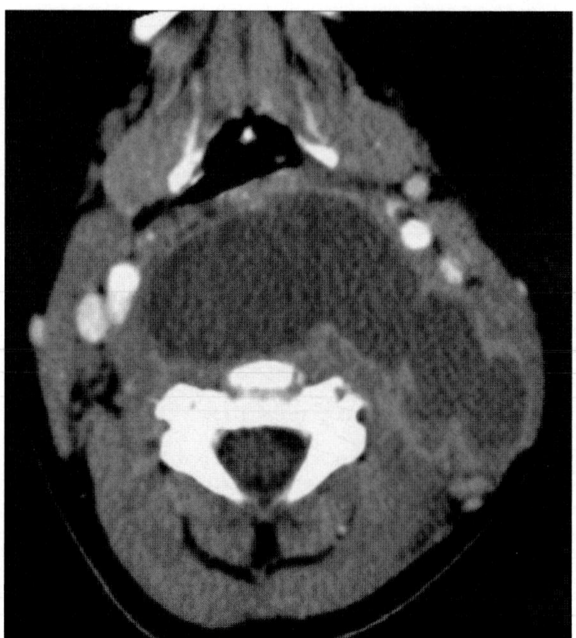

Figure 4–3 This toddler presented with fever and difficulty swallowing. **(A)** This lateral radiograph of the soft tissues of the neck demonstrates marked anterior displacement of the air-containing pharynx and trachea by a prevertebral soft tissue mass. **(B)** This postcontrast axial CT image of the neck shows a large low-density mass with a thin enhancing wall, consistent with a retropharyngeal abscess, which extends into the left side of the neck.

thin-consistency liquids may be able to swallow thickened liquids safely. Patients who exhibit significant aspiration with all consistencies should not be fed orally, due to the risk of aspiration pneumonitis and pneumonia.

If swallowing is to occur normally, food must be prevented from reentering the mouth, from entering the nasal passages, and, most importantly, from entering the trachea. Normal swallowing involves (1) suppression of respiration by the medullary swallowing center; (2) elevation of the uvula to prevent nasal reflux; (3) positioning of the back of the tongue to prevent oral reentry; and (4) posteroinferior reflection of the epiglottis and apposition of the vocal cords to prevent penetration into the glottis, which would result in aspiration.

Esophagus

Anatomy and Physiology

The esophagus extends from the pharyngoesophageal sphincter at the level of C5–C6 to the gastroesophageal (GE) junction. Its proximal one third contains predominantly striated muscle, and the distal two thirds contains smooth muscle. The fact that it lacks an outer serosal layer is often invoked to explain the tendency for esophageal malignancies to spread to other mediastinal structures. The most important function of the esophagus is to transport swallowed material from the pharynx to the stomach, through the coordinated muscular contractions known as peristalsis (from the Greek *peri-*, "around," and *stallein,* "to place").

In a normal individual, esophageal peristalsis is so efficient that it is possible to drink liquids while suspended upside down. The primary wave requires 5 to 9 seconds to move the bolus into the stomach. If the bolus becomes lodged for some reason, or if an esophageal motility disorder is present, a secondary wave arises, which is more forceful than the primary wave. The primary wave is initiated by the central nervous system swallowing center through the vagus nerve, while the secondary wave is initiated by the intrinsic nerve plexuses of the esophagus. Tertiary contractions are nonproductive fasciculations seen exclusively in motility disorders.

Imaging

Indications for esophagography include chest pain, heartburn, dysphagia (difficulty swallowing, such as the feeling that food boluses "get stuck" in the chest), and odynophagia (painful swallowing). Radiologic evaluation of the esophagus is routinely performed using both single- and double-contrast techniques, with the patient in both upright and prone positions. Double-contrast views are obtained with the patient upright (**Fig. 4–4**). With adequate air distention and luminal coating, double-contrast visualization of mucosal detail and subtle mucosal lesions is excellent. Single-contrast views with the patient prone are performed to assess motility and to aid in the demonstration of mass lesions and filling defects, which are often best evaluated with a greater degree of luminal distention than double-contrast views provide. In addition, the presence and degree of GE reflux, the major cause of heartburn, is best assessed at this stage. The esophagus, stomach, and duodenum are often imaged together in a

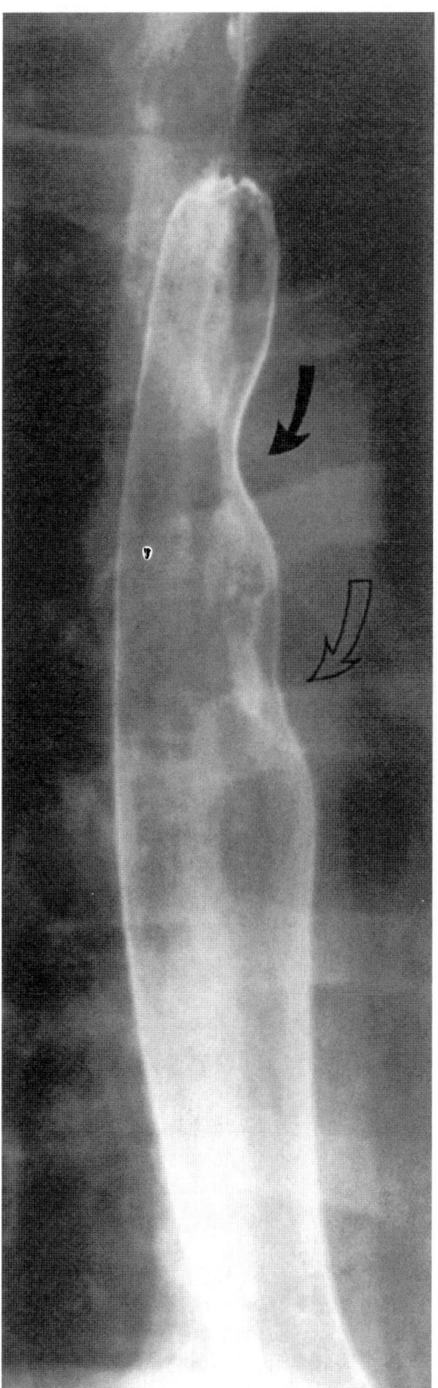

Figure 4–4 This spot film from a double-contrast esophagogram demonstrates two prominent indentations along the left side of the proximal esophagus. They are quite smooth and form obtuse angles with the esophageal lumen, suggesting that they reflect pressure from structures extrinsic to the esophagus. What is the differential diagnosis of these contour abnormalities? In this case, there is no differential, because these represent normal impressions on the esophagus by the aortic arch (solid arrow) and the left mainstem bronchus (open arrow). As this case illustrates, a thorough knowledge of normal anatomy, including so-called normal variants, is critical in interpreting imaging studies.

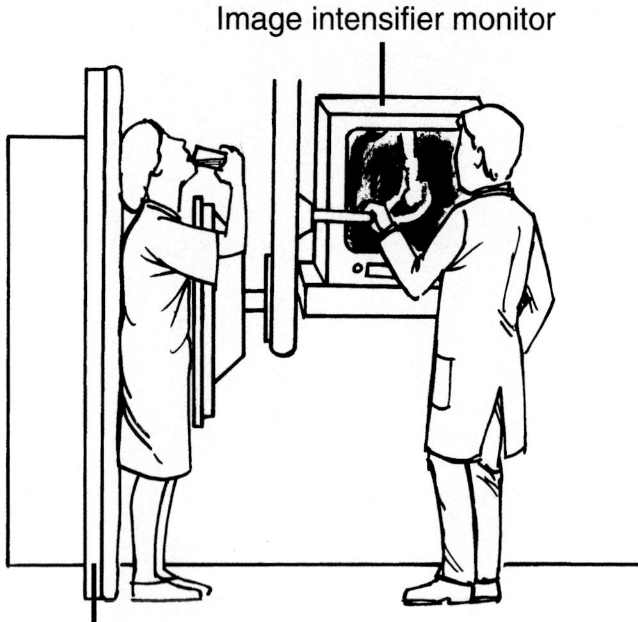

Figure 4–5 This diagram illustrates an upper gastrointestinal examination, in which a patient drinks barium, and fluoroscopic monitoring is used to obtain images of the esophagus, stomach, and duodenum.

so-called upper gastrointestinal (GI) series (**Fig. 4–5**). Computed tomography and magnetic resonance imaging are used primarily to evaluate the extent of extraesophageal disease in conditions such as esophageal carcinoma. Endoluminal ultrasonography also permits assessment of local tumor extent.

Stomach

Anatomy and Physiology

The stomach, which stores and liquefies food and initiates protein digestion, is divided arbitrarily into the cardia, fundus, body, antrum, and pylorus (**Fig. 4–6**). The cardia is the portion of the stomach adjacent to the esophagus. The fundus is that portion of the stomach that lies above the GE junction. *Fundus* means "bottom," referring to the fact that the fundus is the most posterior portion of the stomach, and the area where contrast material collects when patients are supine. The body comprises the central two thirds, extending from the fundus to the incisura angularis. The body and the fundus contain the chief cells, which secrete pepsinogen, and the parietal cells, which secrete hydrochloric acid and intrinsic factor. Normal gastric pH is ~2, with a hydrogen ion concentration ~10,000 times that of the blood. The antrum, the most thickly muscled portion, extends from the body to the pylorus and contains gastrin-secreting cells, which stimulate secretion by the parietal and chief cells. The pylorus, from the Greek for "gatekeeper," is important in regulating the rate of gastric emptying (**Fig. 4–7**).

Imaging

Indications for gastric imaging include heartburn, epigastric pain, vomiting, and hematemesis (vomiting of blood). Like the esophagus, the stomach is visualized using both single- and double-contrast techniques, the former to fill and distend the stomach to look for filling defects and areas of mural rigidity, and the latter to optimize visualization of mucosal detail. Unless a nasogastric tube is passed, gas is introduced into the gastric lumen by having the patient swallow carbon dioxide–producing crystals. When the gastroesophageal sphincter opens, gas is released into the esophageal lumen, distending the lumen and enabling double-contrast visualization.

Because different portions of gastric anatomy are best demonstrated from different points of view, multiple projections are necessary, with changes in patient positioning between each. To empty the stomach, the patient is turned right side down, because the stomach empties to the right. To move air into the duodenum for double-contrast views of the duodenal mucosa, the patient is positioned left posterior oblique, midway between left side down and supine. External compression with a radiolucent paddle is sometimes helpful to flatten out the stomach and duodenum, thereby helping to determine whether possible lesions are truly fixed or not. CT and MRI are less useful for the detection of primary gastric lesions but good for assessing disease extent. For example, CT can be helpful in determining whether a neoplastic lesion extends all the way through the wall of the stomach and whether metastatic lesions are present in the liver.

Duodenum

Anatomy and Physiology

The duodenum functions principally in digestion, the breakdown of food molecules (**Fig. 4–8**). It extends from the pyloric

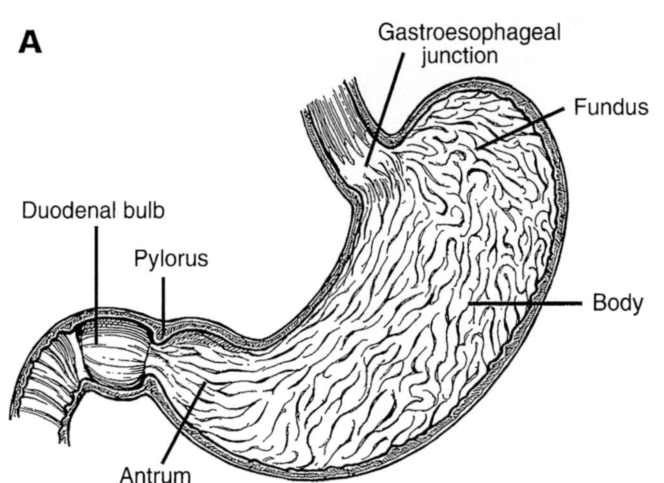

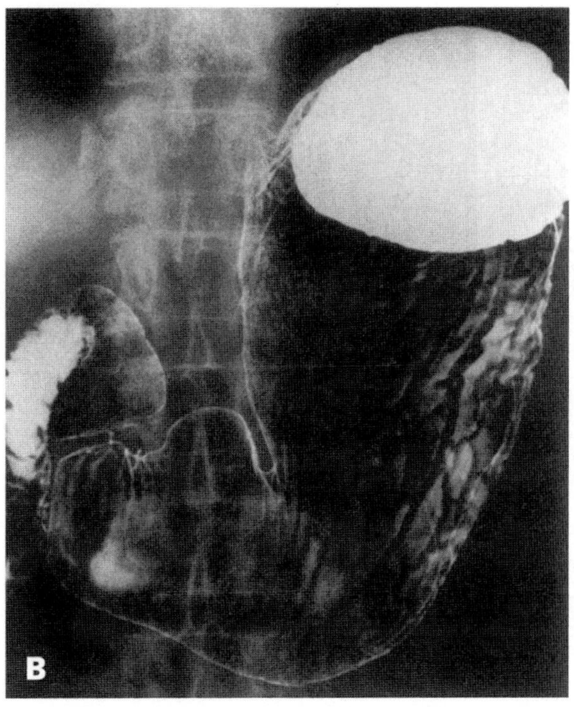

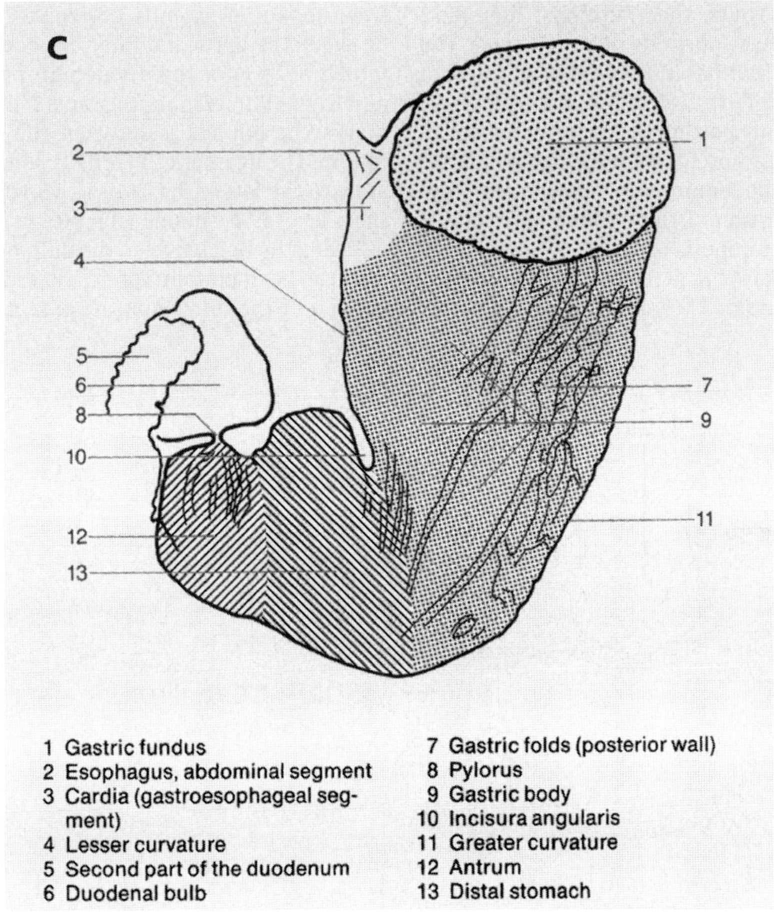

Figure 4–6 (A) Parts of the stomach. **(B,C)** Normal double-contrast view of the stomach in a supine patient.

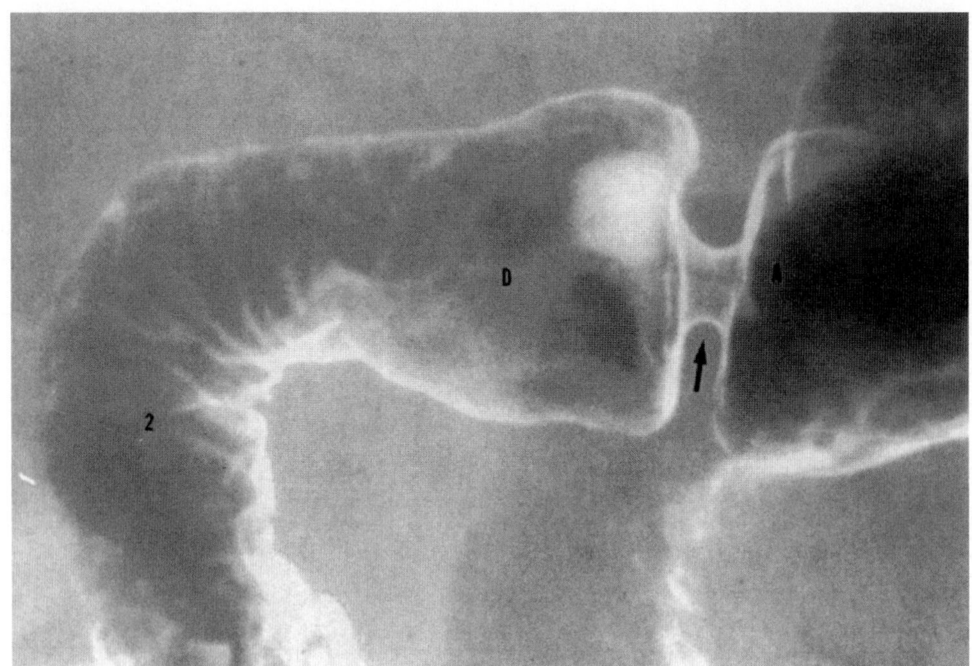

Figure 4–7 A spot film from a double-contrast upper gastrointestinal examination demonstrates the distal gastric antrum (A), pylorus (arrow), duodenal bulb (D), and upper half of the second portion of the duodenum (2). The pylorus is critical in normal digestion because it enables the small bowel to digest and absorb over a period of hours a large quantity of food that may have been consumed in only minutes, by releasing food at a slow controlled rate from the stomach into the duodenum. Patients who have undergone pyloroplasty or partial gastrectomy may experience a "dumping syndrome" due to the dumping of large quantities of gastric contents into the small bowel at once. These patients experience nausea, weakness, and palpitations, followed by reactive hypoglycemia, due to the large osmotic load and premature unregulated absorption of glucose.

canal to the ligament of Treitz, the traditional boundary between the upper and lower portions of the GI tract. The duodenum is divided into four parts. The first part, referred to as the bulb, is surrounded by visceral peritoneum on all sides, and represents the only portion that is intraperitoneal. More than 90% of peptic ulcers occur in the duodenal bulb.

The remainder of the duodenum is retroperitoneal. The second, or descending, portion of the duodenum contains along its medial aspect the ampulla of Vater, through which the biliary system and exocrine pancreas secrete their alkaline digestive juices into the small bowel. The third portion of the duodenum extends horizontally to the left to a point between the aorta and inferior vena cava. At that point, the fourth portion of the duodenum begins to ascend upward and to the left, terminating at the ligament of Treitz, which marks the boundary between the duodenum and the jejunum. The ligament of Treitz is commonly located immediately to the left of the L1 or L2 vertebral body, usually at the same level as the duodenal bulb.

The distinction between the different portions of the duodenum can be important. For example, a tumor arising in the first portion of the duodenum is quite unlikely to be malignant,

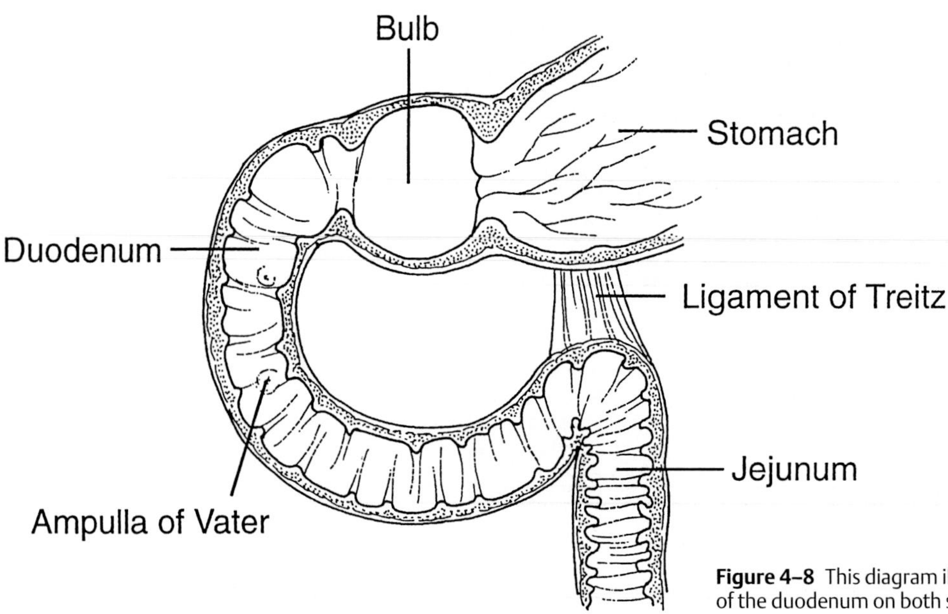

Figure 4–8 This diagram illustrates the appearance of the portions of the duodenum on both single- and double-contrast studies.

whereas a tumor in the fourth portion carries a very high risk of malignancy. Similarly, peptic ulcers in the fourth portion would suggest an unusual condition, such as Zollinger-Ellison syndrome, in which a gastrinoma causes marked hyperacidity.

Imaging

Contrast examination of the duodenum is also performed with both single- and double-contrast techniques. Mass lesions, which appear as filling defects, are well imaged on single-contrast views, as is the degree of luminal distensibility. The double-contrast technique is generally superior for the evaluation of the mucosal fold pattern and smaller mucosal lesions (**Fig. 4–9**). As in the esophagus and stomach, the primary role of CT and MRI is to assess disease extent and extrinsic processes affecting the duodenum, such as pancreatitis. To accurately characterize a primary lesion, adequate distention of the lumen is critical, because redundant folds in a collapsed viscus can easily simulate a neoplasm.

Mesenteric Small Bowel

Anatomy and Physiology

The mesenteric small bowel functions primarily in the chemical digestion and absorption of nutrients. It extends from the ligament of Treitz to the ileocecal valve. It is so named because it is suspended from the small bowel mesentery, which extends obliquely from the left upper quadrant into the right lower quadrant. Whereas the mesenteric small bowel itself measures ~7 m in length, its mesentery is only a little more than 1 ft (i.e., 30 cm) in length, indicating that the small bowel mesentery is a highly folded structure. The mesentery not only suspends the small bowel mesentery from the posterior abdominal wall, it also contains its blood vessels, lymphatics, and nerves.

The mesenteric small bowel is divided into the jejunum and the ileum, with the ileum constituting the distal 60% of its length. On intraluminal contrast studies, the jejunum has a wider lumen, a thicker wall, and more folds per centimeter than the ileum. The surface area of the small bowel is remarkably increased by the presence of mucosal folds (valvulae conniventes), villi, and microvilli. These structures increase the surface area of the small bowel ~600 times, allowing this 7 m tube to achieve a surface area equivalent to a doubles tennis court.

Imaging

Common indications for imaging the small bowel include abdominal pain, malabsorption, diarrhea, and blood in the stools. Techniques for imaging the small bowel include the so-called small bowel follow-through, a dedicated small bowel series, and enteroclysis. The small bowel follow-through represents a continuation of an upper GI series, in which the patient drinks a barium preparation under fluoroscopic monitoring, and spot images are taken of the esophagus, stomach, and duodenum. In the follow-through, the same contrast is followed beyond the duodenum into the mesenteric small bowel, with overhead images taken at 15- to 30-minute intervals until contrast is seen in the colon. Additional spot images with compression are taken of the terminal ileum and any findings of interest. The follow-through is somewhat less

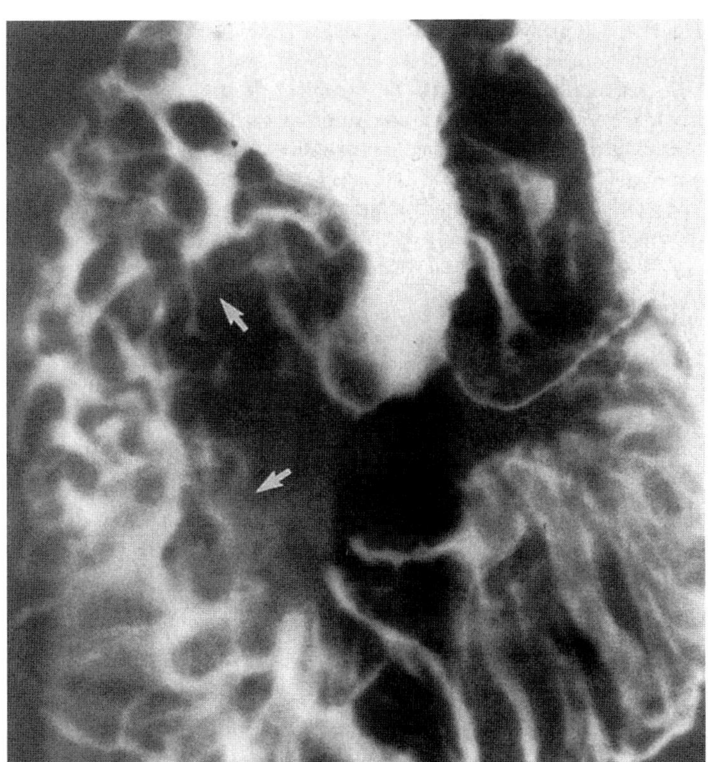

Figure 4–9 Spot film of the duodenal sweep from a double-contrast upper gastrointestinal examination reveals nodular duodenal fold thickening (arrows) in the "C" loop, indicating severe duodenitis, which in this case was secondary to peptic disease.

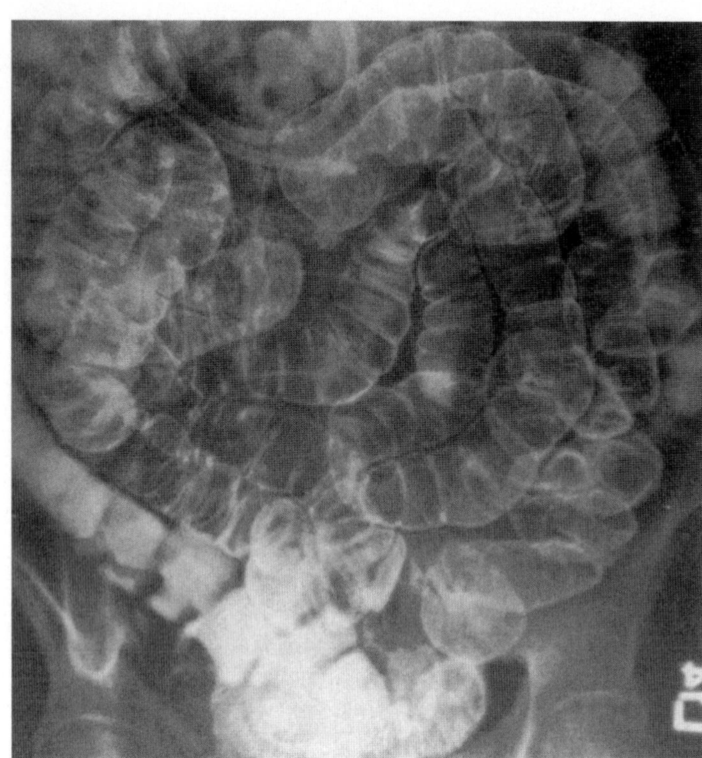

Figure 4–10 An overhead film from an enteroclysis (small bowel enema) demonstrates the exquisite small bowel mucosal detail revealed by this technique. Note that the jejunum, which contains more folds per centimeter than the ileum, is located primarily in the left upper quadrant, and the ileum, with its more rarefied fold pattern, is located primarily in the right lower quadrant.

sensitive than the dedicated small bowel series, in which a barium preparation optimized for the small bowel is employed.

The gold standard of small bowel imaging is the enteroclysis, which is performed by oral intubation of the jejunum. Barium is injected, followed by a continuous infusion of methylcellulose solution. The methylcellulose solution is used to prevent rapid absorption of water through the intestinal mucosa. As the barium shot is pushed along the lumen by the methylcellulose solution chaser, the mural surfaces are coated with barium, the lumen becomes mildly distended, and the mucosal fold pattern and areas of stenosis or dilatation are optimally visualized (**Fig. 4–10**). Disadvantages of enteroclysis include the need for more specialized equipment, patient discomfort associated with intubation, and higher cost. Enteroclysis may also be performed using CT.

Large Intestine

Anatomy and Physiology

The functions of the large intestine include absorption, storage, and elimination (**Fig. 4–11**). It measures ~1.5 m in length, and includes the cecum; appendix; ascending, transverse, and descending portions of the colon; sigmoid colon; rectum; and anal canal. From the ligament of Treitz through the splenic flexure of the colon, the intestine receives its blood supply from the superior mesenteric artery. The inferior mesenteric artery supplies the large intestine distal to the splenic flexure. Both the ascending and descending portions of the colon are extraperitoneal in location, with important implications for the spread of intraperitoneal inflammatory and neoplastic processes. Some patients have unusually long colonic segments, particularly in the sigmoid and transverse portions. They may require extra maneuvers on endoscopic or contrast examinations for optimal visualization.

Imaging

Common indications for imaging the colon include rectal bleeding, abdominal pain, anemia, and weight loss. Because a complete evaluation of the colon relies on patient mobility to direct flow of barium and/or air through the colon, some elderly and debilitated patients may be poor candidates for a barium enema. Before any contrast study is undertaken, a plain radiograph of the abdomen should be obtained to ensure that the colon is properly cleansed and that no residual contrast material from another examination is present. Fecal debris can easily masquerade as a polypoid lesion (**Fig. 4–12**). The standard preparation protocol employed for colonoscopy will interfere with a double-contrast barium enema, because the colonic mucosa is typically too wet to permit proper barium coating. The barium enema uses a barium-containing bag connected by a tube to the rectal tip. In double-contrast examinations, an insufflator is used to introduce air into the colon via the rectum (**Fig. 4–13**).

In imaging the colon, a single-contrast examination is preferred to evaluate patients with obstructing lesions and fistulas, as well as those who do not exhibit the mobility required for a double-contrast examination (**Fig. 4–14**). The double-contrast technique is especially useful for demonstrating small polypoid lesions and evaluating mucosal detail, which can be

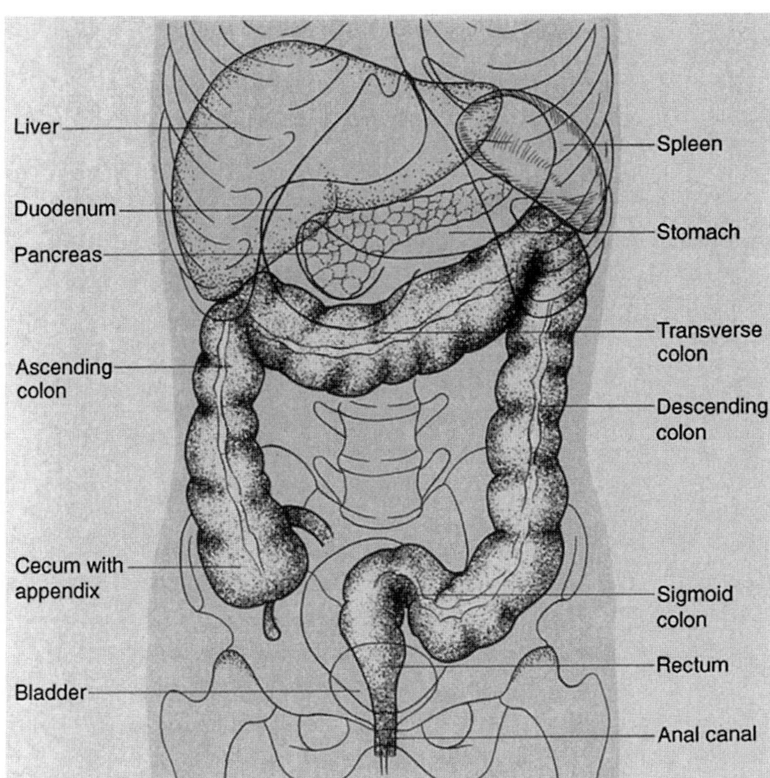

Figure 4–11 Topography of the colon in relation to other abdominal organs.

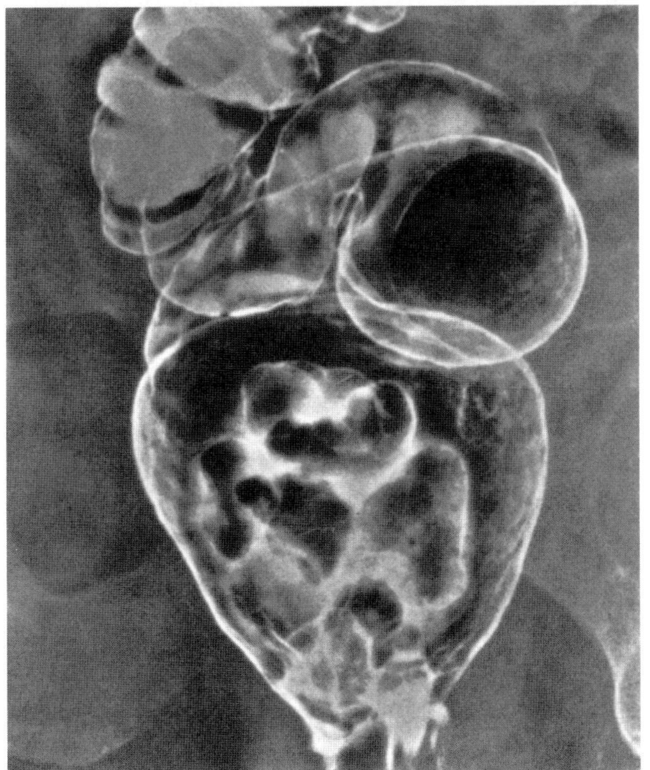

Figure 4–12 This spot film from a double-contrast barium enema seems to demonstrate a large, polypoid lesion filling much of the rectum. In fact, however, this "lesion" merely represents stool in the rectum. This image dramatizes the importance of adequate bowel preparation.

especially important in cancer surveillance and suspected inflammatory bowel disease. CT and MRI are best for evaluating the distant spread of primary colonic malignancies and determining the nature of extrinsic processes affecting the large intestine, such as pelvic malignancies. Both CT and MRI are more limited in their ability to evaluate the local extent of tumor.

Basic Patterns of Gastrointestinal Tract Abnormalities

Nearly all radiologically detectable GI tract lesions can be categorized according to a relatively small number of radiographic patterns. These patterns may be further grouped into three basic categories: lesions projecting into the gut lumen, lesions affecting the structure of the gut wall itself, and lesions projecting away from the lumen of the gut. Additional processes include distention and narrowing of the gut.

In interpreting a contrast study of the GI tract, one effective strategy for ensuring a thorough evaluation is to train the eye to follow the natural course of the contrast agent from proximal to distal. A good grasp of normal anatomic patterns is crucial. Generally, if the observer can bear in mind each of the five fundamental patterns of GI abnormalities—filling defects, intrinsic mural abnormalities, extraluminal projections, distention, and narrowing—few radiologically detectable pathologies will be missed (**Fig. 4–15**).

Filling Defects

The principle types of lesions that project into the gut lumen are polyps and masses. They are referred to as filling defects

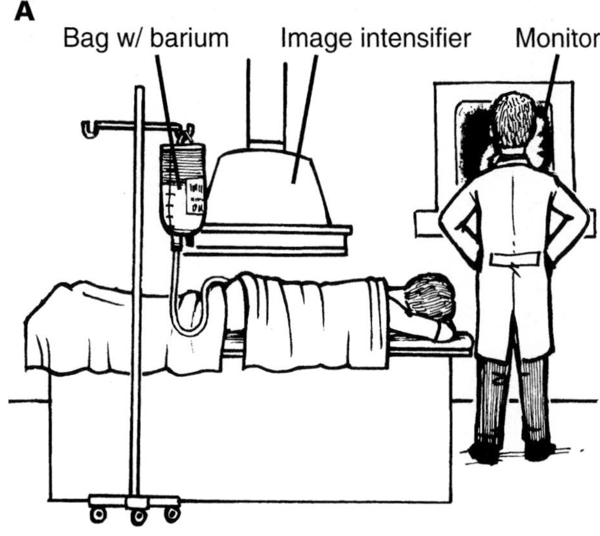

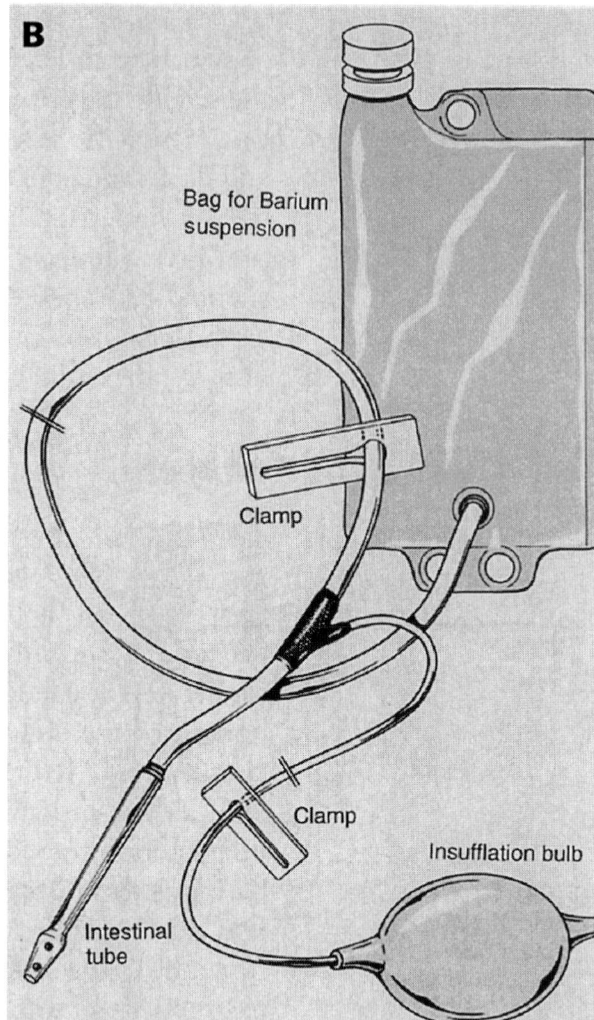

Figure 4–13 **(A)** A patient undergoing barium enema. **(B)** Intestinal tube and insufflator attached to barium reservoir.

because they represent areas that should normally fill with barium but instead are occupied by tissue and thus remain unfilled. The contour of the displaced barium provides a silhouette of the abnormal lesion.

Polyps

Polyps (from the Greek *polypous,* meaning "many-footed") are produced by excessive growth of the bowel mucosa, which may be up to several centimeters in diameter. They may be benign or malignant, and their morphology may be described as sessile or pedunculated (**Fig. 4–16**). A sessile polyp (from the Latin *sedere,* "to sit") refers to a broad-based lesion that is not attached to the mucosa by a peduncle. In contrast, a pedunculated polyp (from the Latin *pes,* meaning "foot") is attached by a stalk to the mucosa. Unless they are large, polyps are usually identified on single-contrast studies as filling defects in the contrast column, or on double-contrast studies when they are outlined by a thin layer of contrast.

Polyps come in multiple histologic types. Nonneoplastic polyps include hyperplastic polyps (overgrowth of otherwise normal cells), inflammatory polyps, and hamartomatous polyps, which represent an abnormal proliferation of tissues that are otherwise normally present.

Neoplastic polyps include adenomas and carcinomas. Adenomas are composed of benign-appearing glandular epithelium. As the polyp extends outward from the mucosal surface, its lack of attachment to deeper layers of the bowel wall enables it to be pulled farther out into the lumen. Eventually, it is pulled downstream by peristalsis, which is why so many polyps have a pedunculated appearance (**Fig. 4–17**). Histologic indicators of benignity include lack of cellular atypia, few mitotic figures (suggesting low growth rate), low nucleus/cytoplasm ratio, and lack of spread beyond the mucosa. Dysplastic polyps are those that demonstrate a greater degree of atypia. The term *carcinoma* is reserved for malignant epithelial growths. Unequivocally carcinomatous polyps will demonstrate evidence of local and/or discontinuous (metastatic) tumor spread. A carcinoma in situ is a growth of cancerous-appearing cells that appears well-contained, without evidence of local, lymphatic, or vascular invasion.

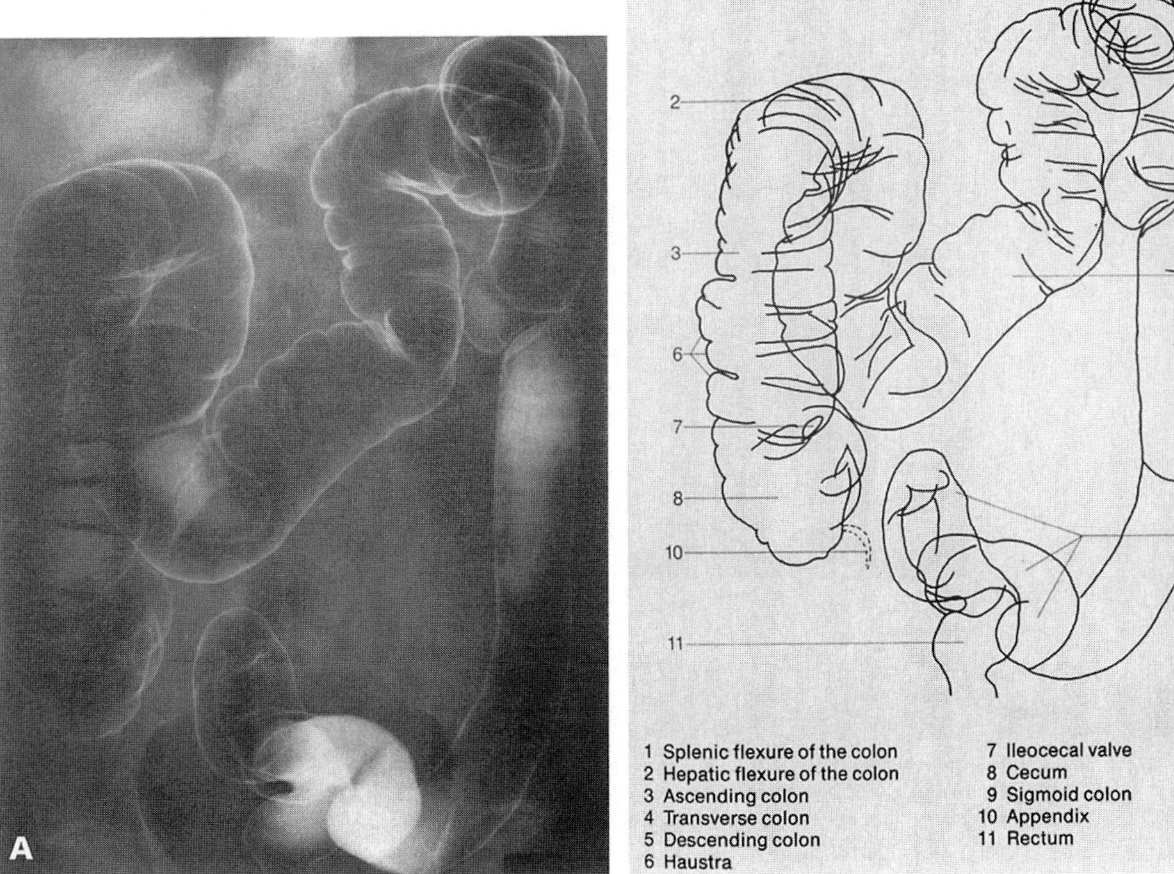

Figure 4–14 (A,B) Normal double-contrast colonic anatomy.

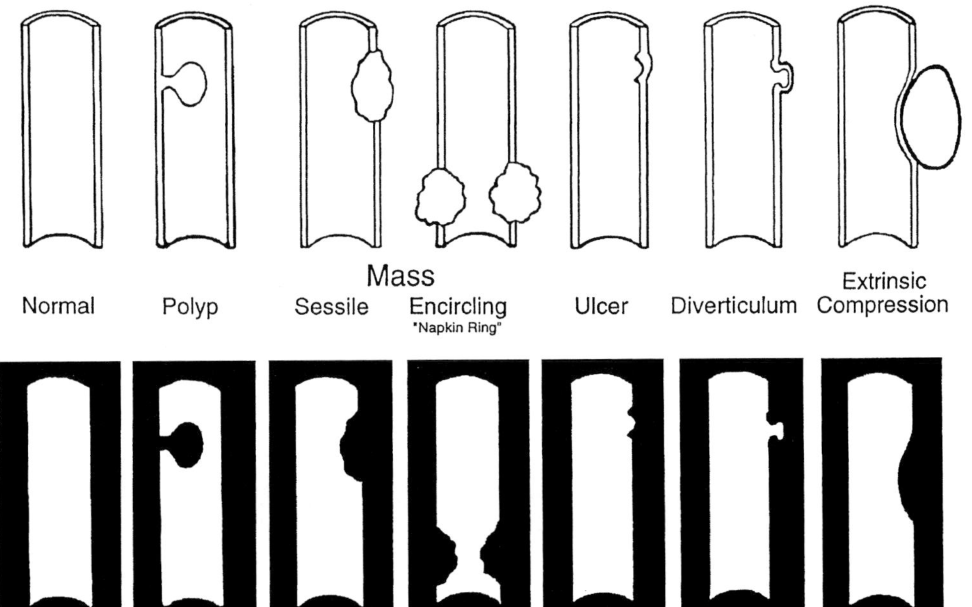

Figure 4–15 Paradigmatic abnormalities visible on barium studies: filling defects (polyps and masses) and extramural projections (ulcers, diverticula, and fistula).

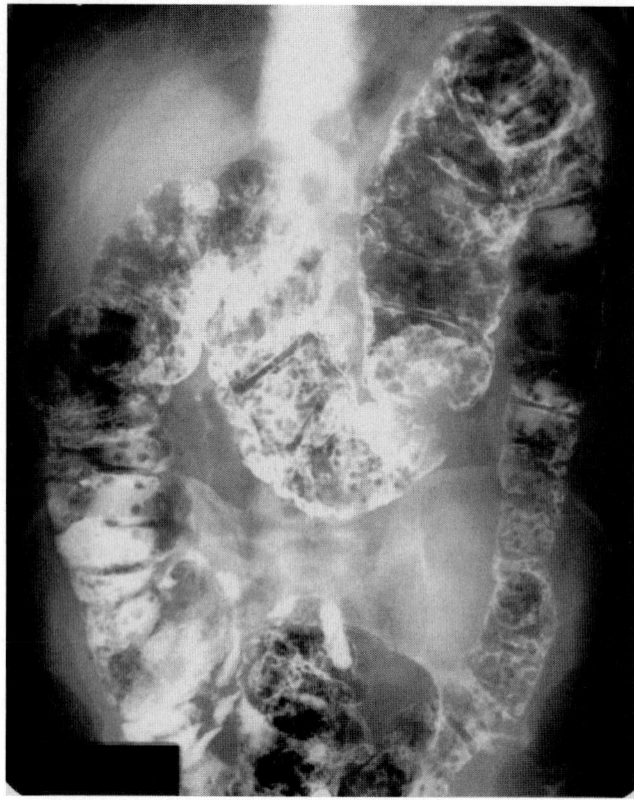

Figure 4–16 This radiograph from a double-contrast barium enema demonstrates innumerable polypoid filling defects throughout the colon in this patient with familial polyposis.

Masses

Masses are lesions measuring more than a few centimeters in size. They may spread primarily within the bowel wall or grow out into the lumen in an exophytic fashion. The term *polyp* is sometimes used as a modifier to describe masses, a polypoid mass being one with multiple excrescences or outgrowths extending from its surface.

A mass that grows exophytically into the lumen is more likely to cause early obstruction, to bleed, and to invade the wall late, if at all. Hence exophytic lesions tend to be discovered at an earlier, more resectable stage. Other tumors tend to spread intramurally, producing either an annular constricting lesion, the so-called napkin ring lesion seen in many colorectal carcinomas, or a diffusely infiltrating lesion, as in the so-called *linitis plastica*, or "leather bottle," lesion of scirrhous gastric carcinoma. (**Fig. 4–18**).

Lesions originating from below the mucosa, typically in the submucosa, have radiographic margins different from mucosal lesions. A submucosal tumor pushes a segment of the mucosa outward from beneath, tending to produce smoothly tapered, obtuse angles with the bowel wall. A mucosal tumor, by contrast, grows out from the surface of the mucosa and tends to have a more abrupt zone of transition with the luminal surface, forming acute angles.

Intrinsic Wall Abnormalities

Several processes may cause changes in the wall itself, altering the radiographic appearance of the gut. One of the most important is a change in the fold pattern, which may occur anywhere from the esophagus to the rectum. Increased

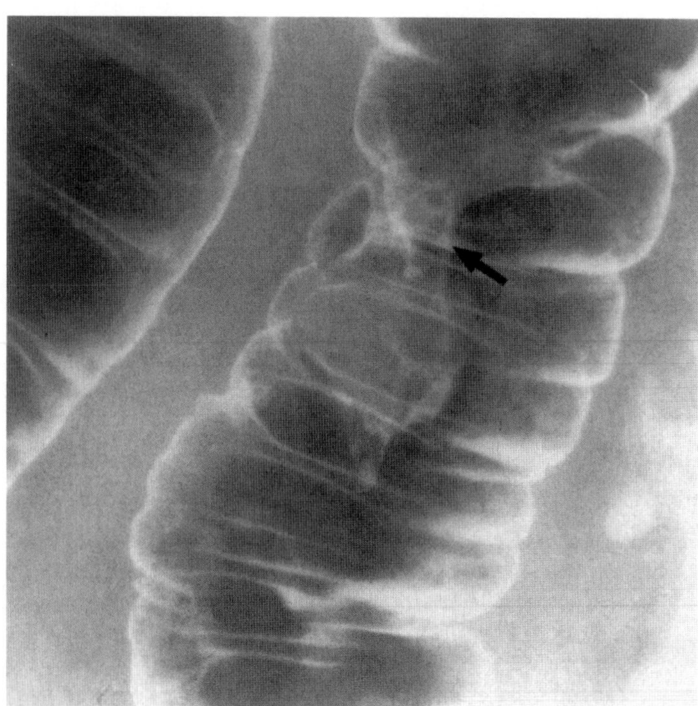

Figure 4–17 This spot film from a double-contrast barium enema reveals a classic appearance of a pedunculated adenomatous polyp, meaning that it is connected to the bowel by a stalk (arrow). When one polyp is discovered, there is a 50% chance that additional polyps will be found elsewhere in the colon. Moreover, the fact that this polyp measures more than 2 cm in diameter implies an ~40% probability of malignancy.

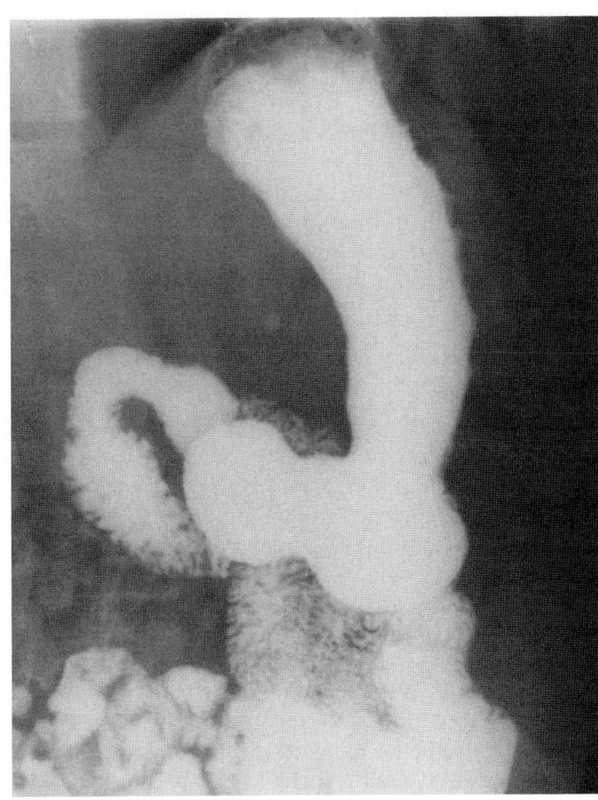

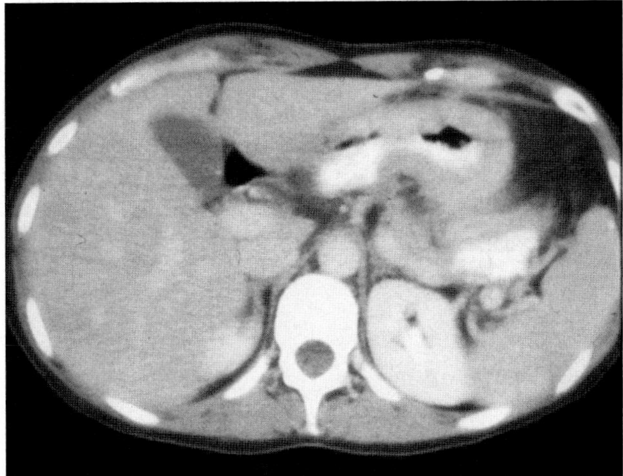

Figure 4–18 **(A)** This elderly man presented with weight loss and early satiety. A single-contrast upper GI exam demonstrates a long segment of fixed circumferential narrowing and mucosal irregularity of the entire gastric body in this patient with a "leather bottle" gastric adenocarcinoma. **(B)** This CT image from another patient with the same lesion demonstrates marked thickening of the gastric wall. Such lesions can be missed on endoscopy due to their submucosal location if deep biopsies are not taken.

prominence or thickening of the folds typically reflects either an inflammatory process (e.g., gastritis or enteritis), edema, or infiltration by cells or cellular products (**Fig. 4–19**). Edema is by far the most common cause and may result from any of the usual physiologic forces that cause interstitial fluid accumulation, including ischemia, congestive heart failure, and hypoproteinemia. Infiltration of the gut wall, manifesting as both thickening and rigidity, may result from lymphoma or amyloidosis.

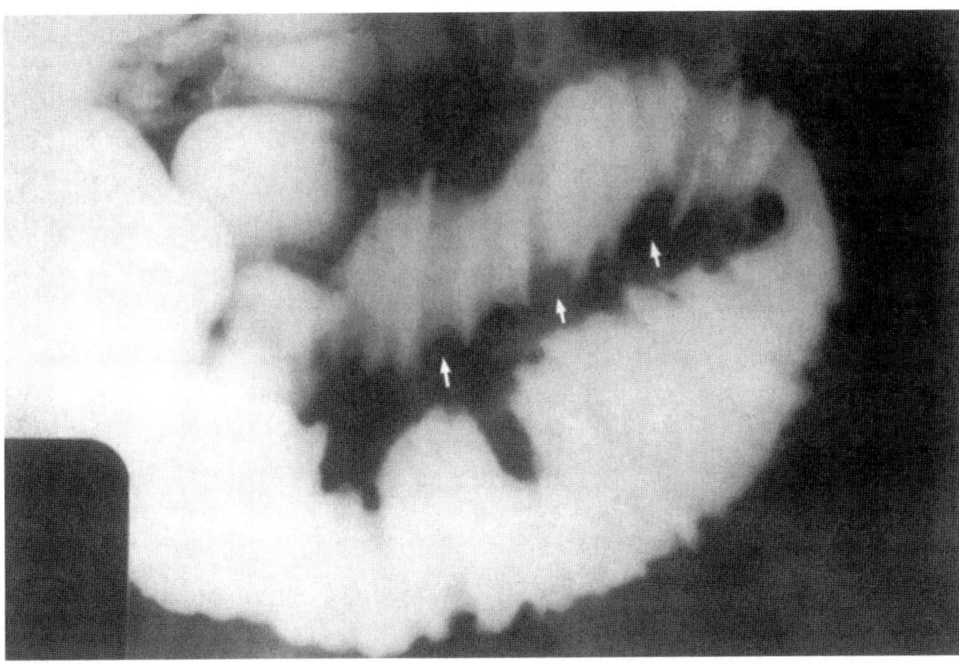

Figure 4–19 Spot film from a small bowel series demonstrates marked thickening of the folds in this segment of small bowel (arrows). The differential diagnosis of fold thickening includes causes of submucosal edema such as ischemia and enteritis, submucosal tumor such as lymphoma, and submucosal hemorrhage from such causes as coagulopathy. However, in this patient with a clinical history of malabsorption, etiologies such as Whipple disease and celiac sprue are more likely. In this case, active sprue was the culprit. Sprue reflects an intolerance to the gluten found, for example, in wheat.

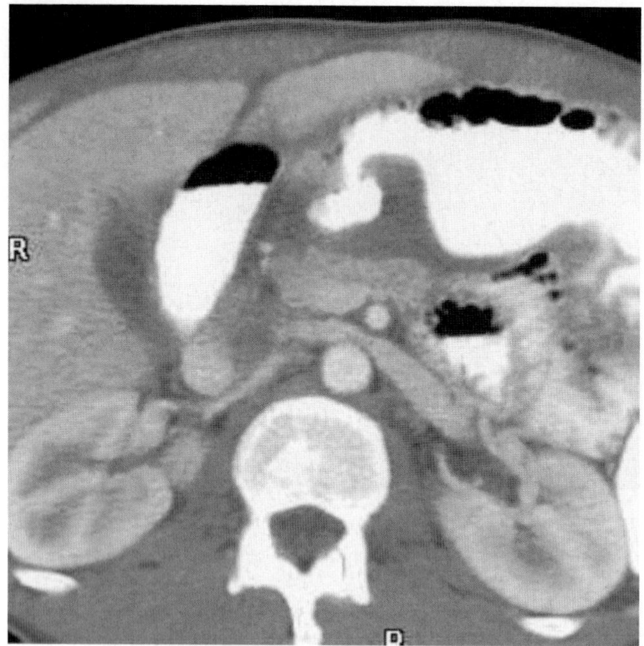

Figure 4–20 This middle-aged man presented with abdominal pain and hemoptysis. An axial CT image after oral and intravenous (IV) contrast demonstrates a large penetrating ulcer projecting posteriorly from the gastric antrum. Note the surrounding low-density edema.

Extraluminal Projections

◇ Ulcers

Common lesions extending away from the lumen of the gut are ulcers, which appear as extraluminal collections of barium. A variety of ulcer types exist, including the peptic ulcerations in peptic ulcer disease; aphthous ulcers, most commonly associated with Crohn's disease; the collar-button ulcers of ulcerative colitis; and malignant patterns of ulceration. In the case of peptic ulcers, a benign ulcer usually exhibits intact epithelium extending right up to its edge, because it is produced by the erosion of the gut wall by an intraluminal process (**Fig. 4–20**). A malignant ulcer demonstrates a heaped-up mound of irregular tissue around its edges, because it results from necrosis of the central portion of a mass. Other criteria of benignity are considered in the discussion of peptic ulcers in Chapter 6.

◇ Diverticula

Diverticula are another type of lesion that extends away from the gut lumen. The name is derived from the Latin *devertere,* meaning "to turn aside" (as in "divert"). In the presence of these lesions, the barium in the gut lumen literally turns to one side when it reaches the diverticulum, which it fills in an orientation perpendicular to the gut lumen (**Fig. 4–21**). So-called false diverticula, including the usual colonic diverticula seen in many elderly patients, do not contain all layers of the bowel wall. The most important diverticula are found in the colon. When they become obstructed by inspissated luminal material, the result may be inflammation, infection, and even perforation. Colonic diverticula are further discussed in the diverticulitis section of Chapter 6.

Distention

One of the most commonly sought findings on plain films of the abdomen in patients with obstructive symptoms such as vomiting is distention, or dilation of the bowel. Such dilation may be functional, as in a patient with an adynamic ileus

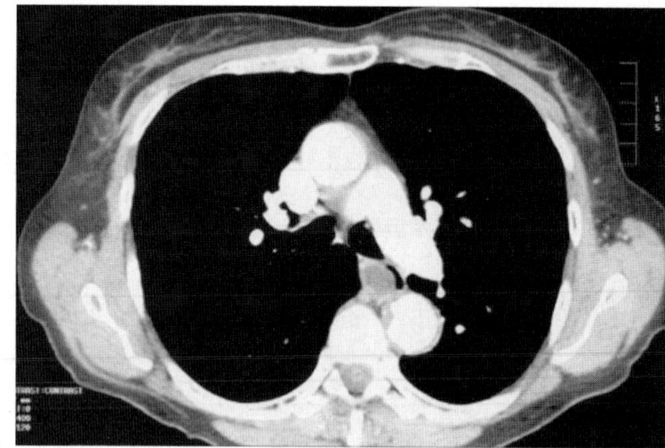

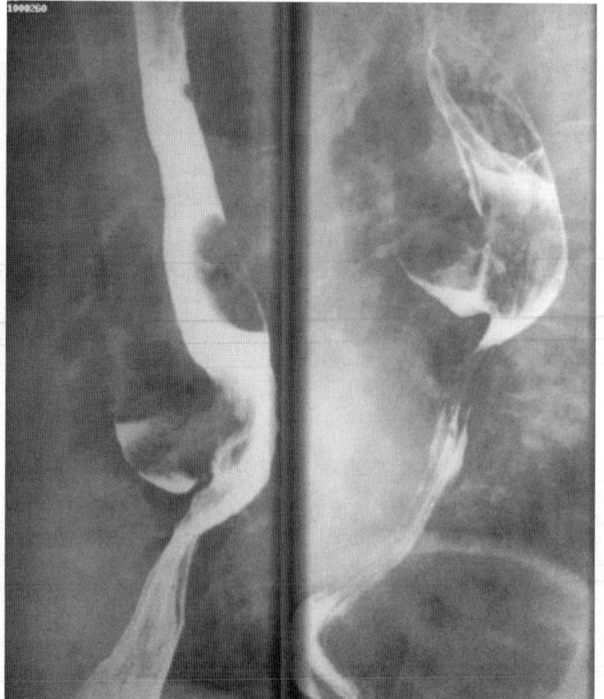

Figure 4–21 **(A)** This elderly woman presented with back pain and possible dissection of the aorta. An axial CT image of the chest demonstrates a water-density mass displacing the esophagus to the left. **(B)** Two views from a double-contrast esophagogram demonstrate a posterior right-sided diverticulum. This most likely represented a traction diverticulum in a patient with a previous history of granulomatous disease.

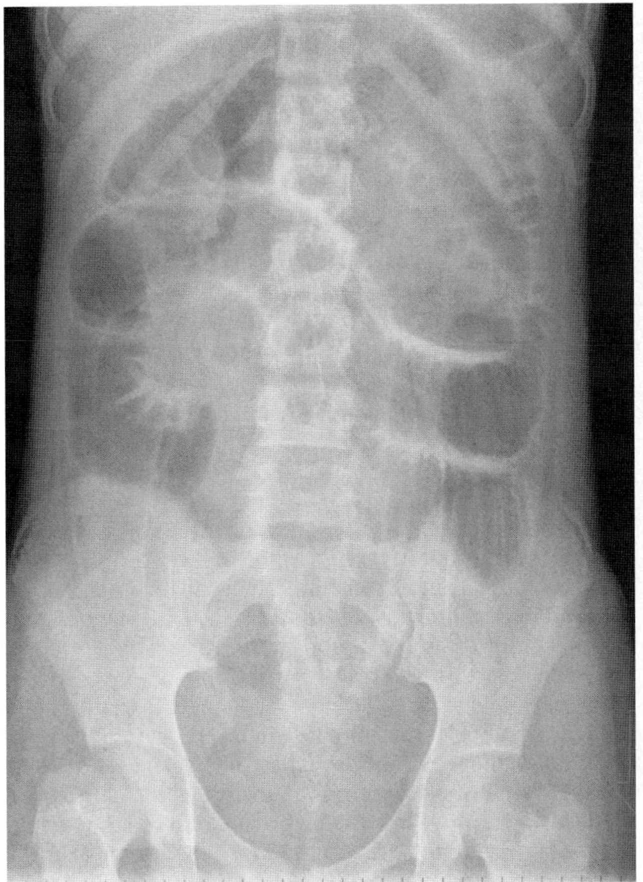

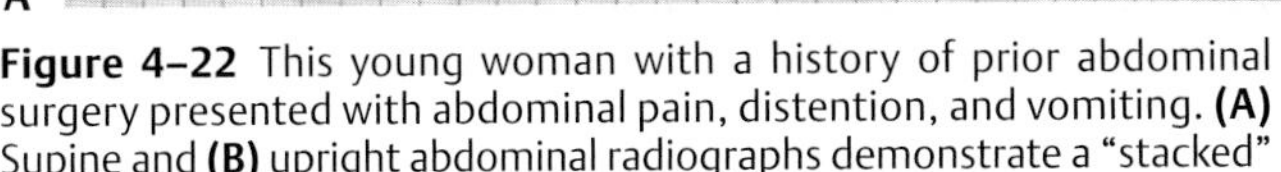

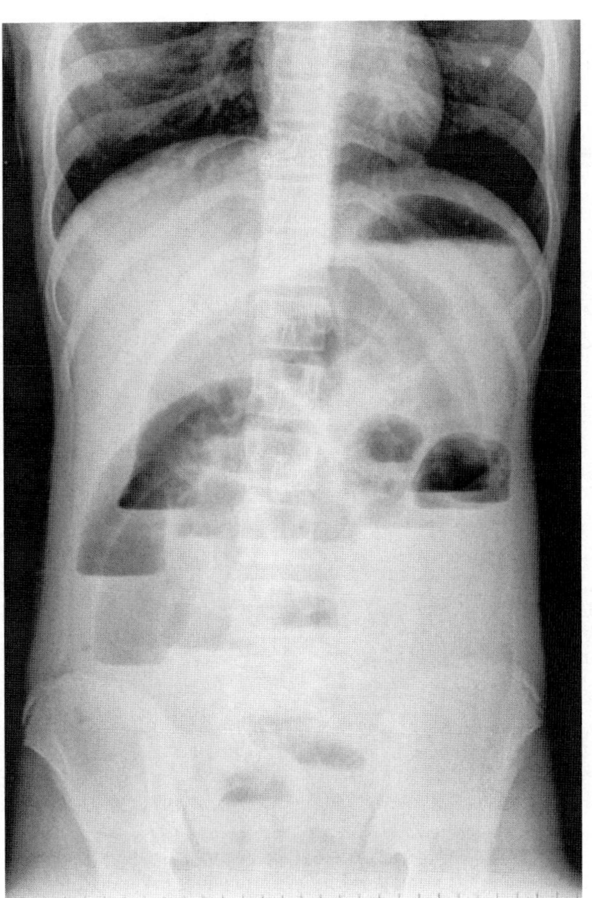

Figure 4–22 This young woman with a history of prior abdominal surgery presented with abdominal pain, distention, and vomiting. **(A)** Supine and **(B)** upright abdominal radiographs demonstrate a "stacked" appearance of multiple segments of markedly dilated small bowel with numerous air–fluid levels. The patient had developed postsurgical adhesions causing a high-grade distal small bowel obstruction.

secondary to narcotic analgesics, or anatomic, as in a small bowel obstruction secondary to postsurgical adhesions (**Fig. 4–22**). If only the stomach is dilated with gas, and the remainder of the bowel is gasless, one might suspect a gastric outlet obstruction. If the entire small and large bowel are distended down to the sigmoid region, one would expect an obstructing process in that location.

The most common causes of mechanical obstructions in adults include postsurgical adhesions, hernias, and masses. The most common cause of functional obstruction is adynamic ileus, which is often seen in the postoperative setting, or resulting from pain (e.g., an obstructive ureteral stone), inflammation (e.g., appendicitis), ischemia, and medications (e.g., narcotic analgesics). Obstruction is further discussed in Chapter 6.

Narrowing

Focal or diffuse narrowings of the bowel most often reflect either normal anatomic structures or muscular spasm. True anatomic lesions persist, whereas narrowing from spasm will typically subside over minutes. Long-segment narrowing is a common sequela of Crohn's disease, in which transmural inflammation results in fibrosis and stricture (**Fig. 4–23**). A similar appearance may occur from almost any process that results in scarring, although the narrowing is often more focal. Carcinomas may cause irregular strictures, such as the well-known "apple core" annular lesion of colorectal carcinoma.

Processes outside the bowel may also cause narrowing due to extrinsic compression. A postoperative adhesion produces dilation of bowel proximal to it, while the site of the adhesion itself appears as a tight stenosis, often with angulation and fixation of the adhesed bowel segment. Extra-intestinal tumors and fluid collections, as well as inflammatory masses, may likewise compress the bowel, producing what is often referred to as "mass effect."

Endoscopy versus Radiology

Endoscopic and radiologic methods of evaluation each have distinct advantages and disadvantages. Endoscopy, generally performed by a gastroenterologist or surgeon, offers the ability to directly visualize pathology, to obtain tissue for histologic diagnosis, and to provide certain types of therapy, such as sclerotherapy (for bleeding varices) and polypectomy. Disadvantages of endoscopy, as opposed to barium radiography, include the need for sedation, a higher (but still very low) incidence of complications such as perforation, and significantly higher cost (often 3–6 times greater). Generally speaking, endoscopy is somewhat more

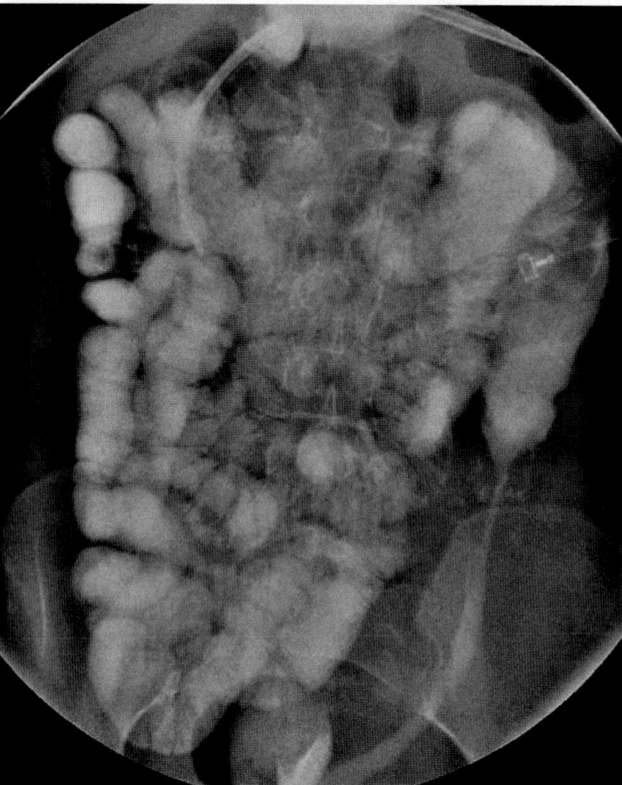

Figure 4–23 This young woman with a history of hemicolectomy for Crohn's disease presented with worsening abdominal pain. The abdominal radiograph from an enteroclysis procedure demonstrates a long segment of fixed narrowing in the descending colon, associated with multiple sinus tracts.

sensitive for several lesions, but it is unable to visualize much of the mesenteric small bowel. There are certain lesions where the sensitivity of endoscopy is much greater than barium radiography; for example, the detection of Barrett's esophagus.

Select Pathologies

Esophagus

◇ Congenital

The most important congenital abnormalities of the esophagus are esophageal atresia and tracheoesophageal fistula, which are discussed in Chapter 7.

◇ Inflammatory

The most common cause of inflammation of the esophagus is reflux esophagitis, with a prevalence of 5% in Western adult populations. It occurs when an incompetent lower esophageal sphincter allows acidic gastric contents access to the esophageal mucosa, and is often associated with symptoms of heartburn. Factors contributing to reflux esophagitis include decreased lower esophageal tone, delayed esophageal clearance, and delayed gastric emptying. Although most patients with gastroesophageal reflux do not have hiatal hernias, there is an increased incidence of reflux in this condition, in which a portion of the stomach herniates up through the diaphragm into the thorax (**Fig. 4–24**). Radiologic findings of reflux include actual visualization of retrograde flow of contrast from the stomach into the

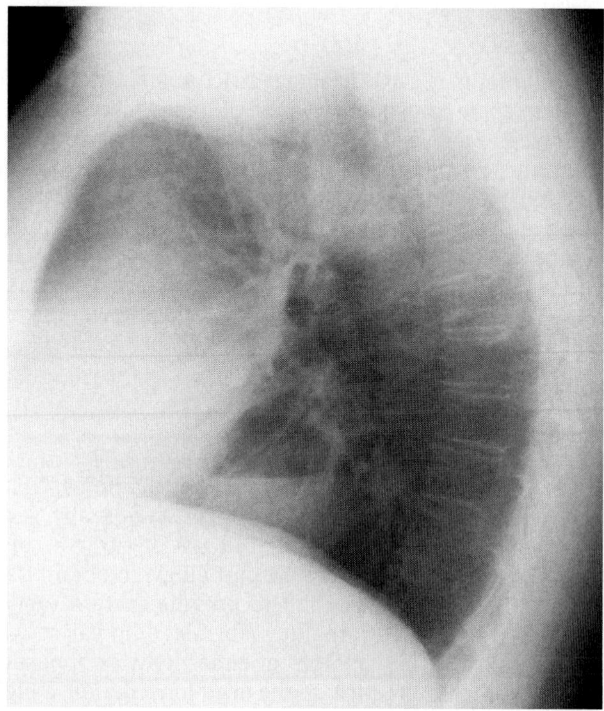

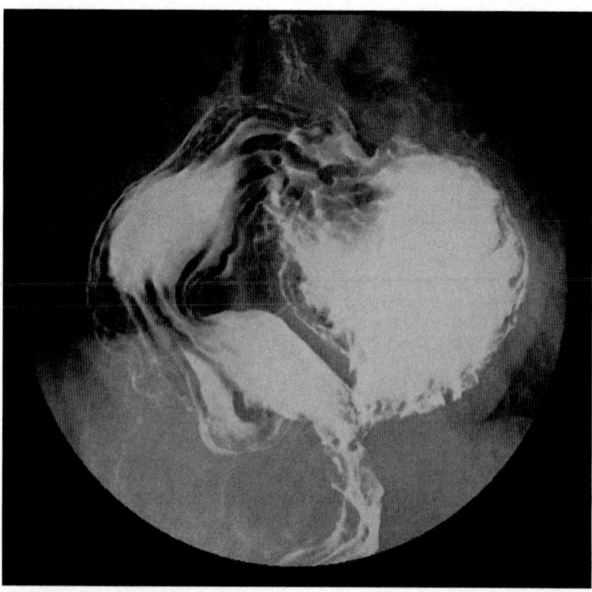

Figure 4–24 **(A)** This lateral chest radiograph demonstrates a large retrocardiac mass containing an air–fluid level. This is a classic appearance of a large sliding hiatal hernia. **(B)** This elderly patient presented with hemoptysis. A frontal image from a barium upper GI exam demonstrates the entire stomach in the lower mediastinum. The stomach has also volvulized, with the greater curvature located cephalad to the lesser curative (organoaxial volvulus).

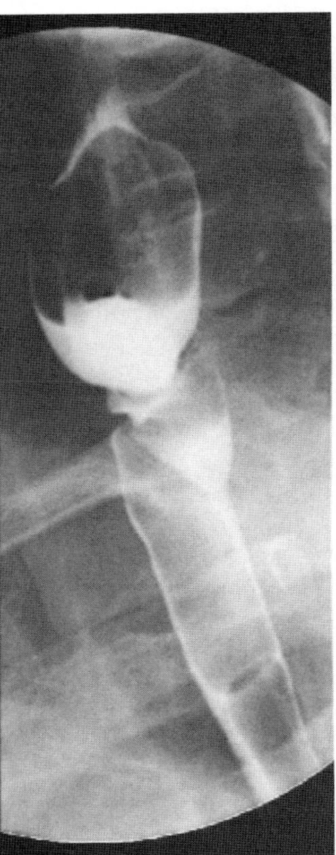

Figure 4–25 This double-contrast esophagogram in a patient with long-standing reflux esophagitis demonstrates a weblike stenosis of the lower cervical esophagus that required endoluminal dilation to relieve symptoms of dysphagia.

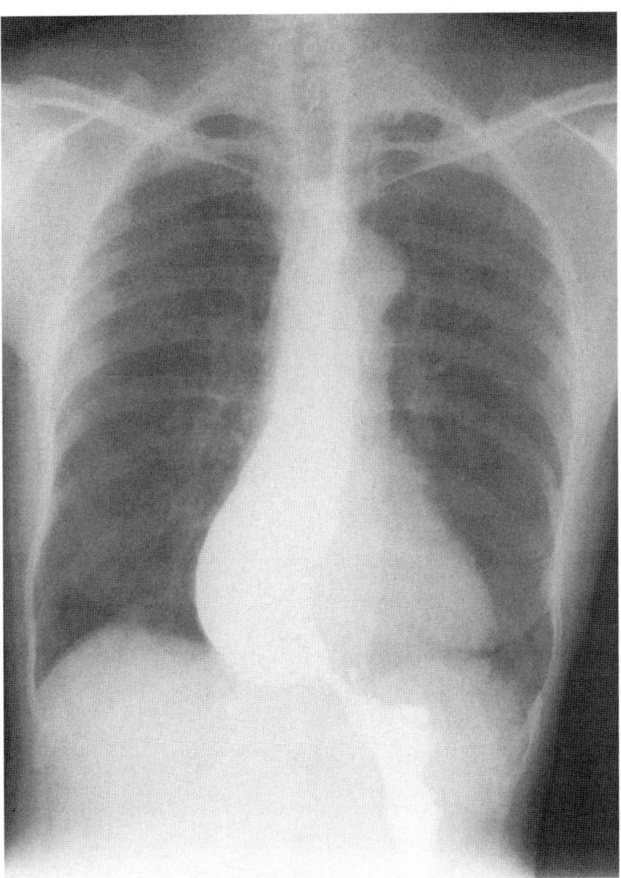

Figure 4–26 This woman complained of gradually worsening dysphagia. An upright chest radiograph obtained during a barium esophagogram demonstrates a severe, fusiform dilation of the esophagus with a "bird's beak" narrowing at the gastroesophageal junction. Note also a tiny diverticulum extending upward from the gastric cardia, as well as the scoliosis of the spine.

esophagus, thickening of esophageal folds, ulcerations, and focal strictures (**Fig. 4–25**). Another common cause of esophagitis, which is associated with postinflammatory stricture formation, is chemical ingestion, especially caustic agents such as lye. The strictures associated with lye ingestion are typically fusiform and long, often involving the whole esophagus.

Achalasia is an acquired esophageal motor disorder, characterized by failure of the lower esophageal sphincter to relax, secondary to degeneration of the myenteric plexus of the esophagus (Auerbach's plexus). Most cases manifest idiopathically in young adults, who present with dysphagia and weight loss. Secondary achalasia results from Chagas' disease, in which *Trypanosoma cruzi* destroys the myenteric plexus. Radiologic findings include absence of normal peristalsis, dilation, and a persistent beaklike tapering of the distal esophagus, often associated with an air–fluid level due to the inability of the esophagus to empty (**Fig. 4–26**). Complications include aspiration, which manifests acutely as pneumonia and chronically as interstitial lung disease, as well as squamous cell carcinoma.

◇ Tumorous

Both benign and malignant tumors are seen in the esophagus. By far the most common benign tumor is the leiomyoma, a smooth muscle tumor that is usually asymptomatic and typically presents as a smooth intramural mass.

Esophageal malignancies account for 6% of GI cancers, but they cause a greater proportion of deaths, due to their tendency to present at an advanced stage. The most common malignant tumor of the esophagus worldwide is squamous cell carcinoma, arising in the mucosal layer of stratified squamous epithelium. In the United States, squamous cell carcinomas account for about one half of esophageal malignancies, and they are more common in men (M:F = 4:1) and blacks (black:white = 4:1). Risk factors include alcohol and tobacco abuse, as well as medical conditions such as lye stricture and achalasia. The usual finding on barium swallow is a polypoid, stenotic mass in the mid- or distal esophagus that may be ulcerated. The tumor is typically advanced at diagnosis, with local spread to the trachea, aorta, or pericardium; lymphatic metastases to the mediastinal and celiac nodes; and hematogenous dissemination, especially to the liver. The primary lesion is best imaged by barium esophagography, while CT and MRI are used primarily in staging (**Fig. 4–27**).

An esophageal tumor of rapidly increasing incidence is adenocarcinoma, which now constitutes one half of primary esophageal malignancies in the United States. It is associated

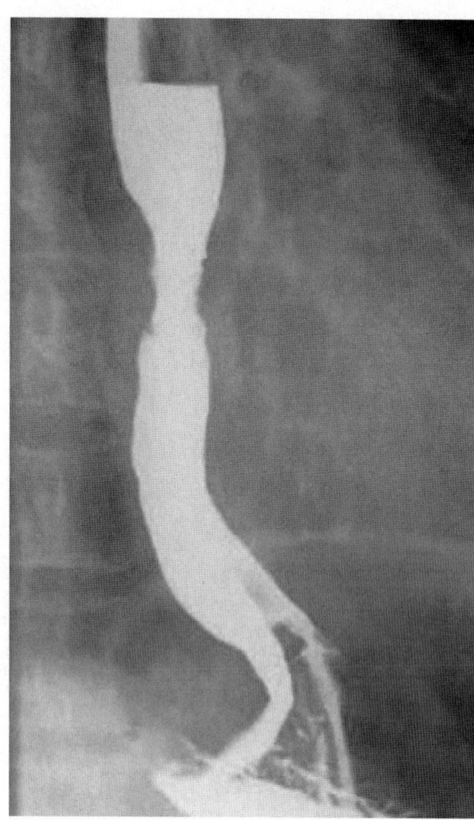

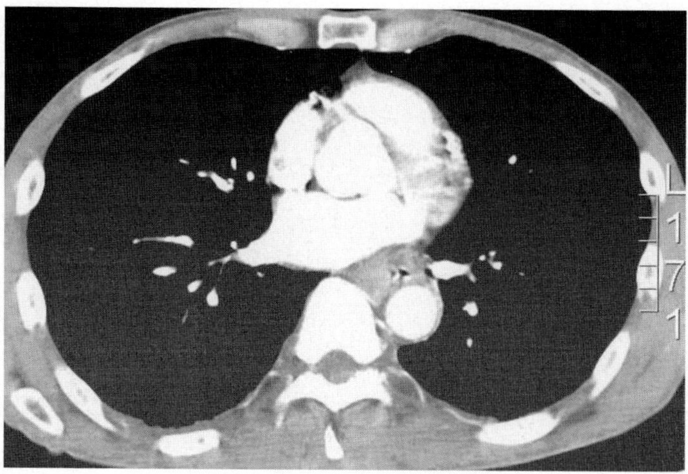

Figure 4–27 This 60-year-old man presented with weight loss and difficulty swallowing. **(A)** This single-contrast esophagogram demonstrates an annular mass of the midesophagus with multiple mucosal ulcerations. It is causing slight obstruction and dilation of the proximal esophagus. **(B)** Postcontrast axial chest CT demonstrates the circumferential thickening of the esophageal wall, as well as probable involvement of the posterior wall of the left atrium and anterior aorta. This was a squamous cell carcinoma of the esophagus.

with Barrett's esophagus, a metaplastic condition eventually occurring in ~10% of patients with symptomatic reflux disease. Barrett's esophagus consists of columnar metaplasia of the esophageal mucosa, presumably secondary to chronic reflux, and is most common among white males. The most important radiologic indicator of Barrett's esophagus in a patient with mucosal changes of reflux esophagitis is a midesophageal stricture, although diagnosis is usually by esophagoscopy. Up to 10% of patients with Barrett's esophagus eventually develop adenocarcinoma. The tumor is usually found in the distal esophagus, and typically has a polypoid or ulcerative appearance, not unlike that of squamous cell carcinoma.

◇ Infectious

Infectious lesions of the esophagus are most commonly seen in immunocompromised patients. Causative organisms include herpes simplex virus, which produces small, discrete ulcerations; *Candida,* which produces raised, plaquelike lesions; and cytomegalovirus (CMV), which often produces large ulcerations.

◇ Iatrogenic

There are several iatrogenic lesions of the esophagus. Medications such as tetracycline, aspirin, and potassium supplement tablets may produce esophagitis if they become lodged in the esophagus. For this reason, patients should be encouraged to remain upright and drink a full glass of water when taking such pills. Another important iatrogenic lesion is perforation, which is seen in a small percentage of patients who have undergone endoscopy or following dilatation for achalasia (**Fig. 4–28**). The risk of perforation is increased in patients with esophageal diverticula, such as a Zenker's diverticulum, because these luminal projections may be inadvertently intubated during insertion of a nasogastric tube or endoscope.

◇ Traumatic

There are two important traumatic lesions of the esophagus. Mallory-Weiss tear is most commonly seen in alcoholics who have experienced prolonged episodes of vomiting or retching. It involves a tear of the esophageal mucosa, which is frequently associated with hematemesis and hematochezia (blood in the stool). The radiographic finding is mucosal disruption at the tear, and the prognosis is excellent. By contrast, Boerhaave's syndrome involves a transmural rent in the esophagus, usually due to a sudden increase in intraluminal pressure from vomiting or trauma. The perforation is usually on the left side, just above the diaphragm. The patient presents with sudden onset of severe epigastric pain, which can progress rapidly to shock. Plain film findings include pneumomediastinum and a left-sided pleural effusion. Oral contrast administration demonstrates extravasation into the mediastinum and pleural space. Due to a mortality rate of 25 to 50%, emergent thoracotomy is often indicated (**Fig. 4–29**).

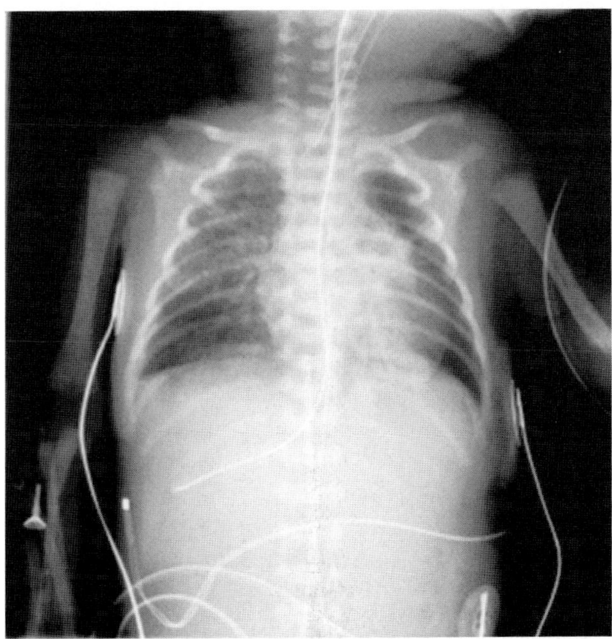

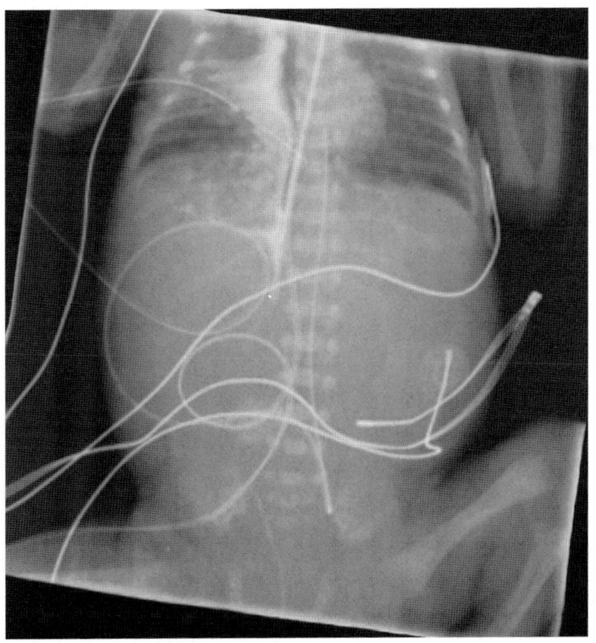

Figure 4–28 (A) What is wrong with this picture? This premature neonate underwent insertion of an endotracheal tube, umbilical artery and vein catheters, and an orogastric tube. Note that the orogastric tube is positioned in the right upper quadrant. **(B)** An abdominal radiograph obtained immediately after the injection of a few milliliters of low-osmolar contrast material demonstrates leakage of contrast into the mediastinum and pleural space, indicating an esophageal perforation.

◇ Vascular

The most important vascular lesion of the esophagus is esophageal varices (**Fig. 4–30**). It is estimated that 90% of patients with alcoholic cirrhosis eventually develop esophageal varices. Distortion of hepatic architecture in cirrhosis causes obstruction of the portal venous branches, resulting in portal hypertension. In such situations, the portal vein is usually decompressed over time by the coronary and azygous veins, which connect to the superior vena cava (SVC), producing thin-walled, dilated veins in the lower esophagus

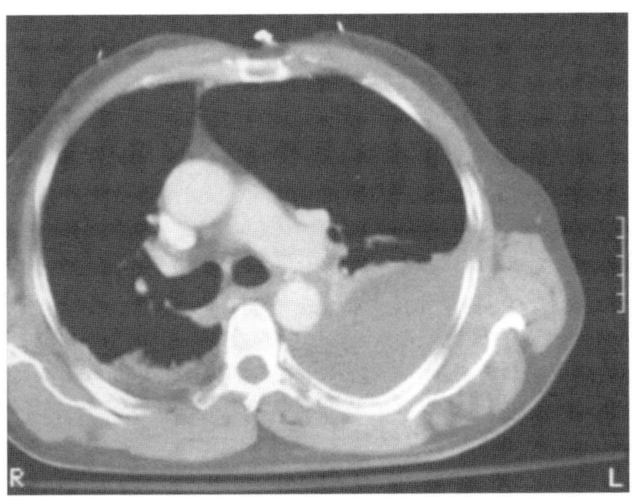

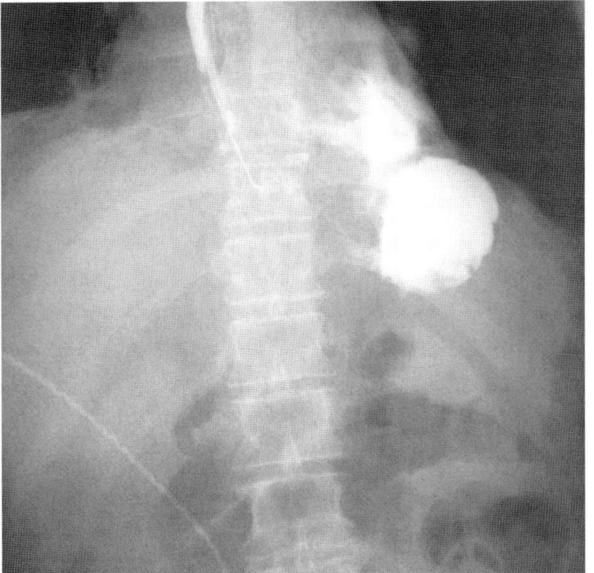

Figure 4–29 (A) This middle-aged man developed acute severe chest pain after vomiting. An axial CT image after IV contrast demonstrates bilateral pleural effusions, larger on the left. **(B)** A frontal image from an esophagogram demonstrates leakage of contrast from the distal esophagus into the mediastinum and left pleural space in this patient with Boerhaave's syndrome.

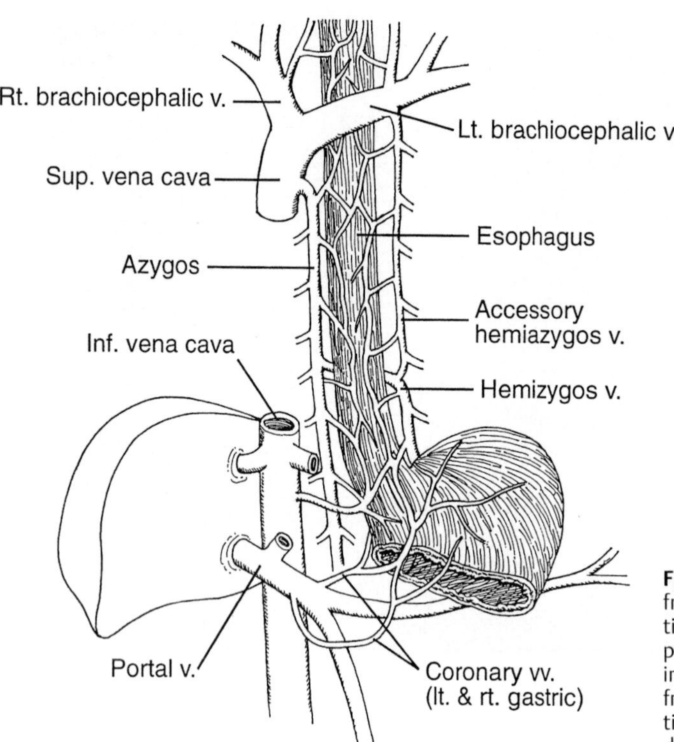

Figure 4–30 "Uphill" and "downhill" esophageal varices typically result from portal hypertension and superior vena cava obstruction, respectively. In uphill esophageal varices with portal hypertension, increased portal venous pressure is decompressed through the coronary vein and into the esophageal/azygous system, whereas downhill varices result from obstruction of the superior vena cava below the level of the insertion of the azygous vein, which allows decompression in the opposite direction.

(**Fig. 4–31**). These are called "uphill varices," because the flow of blood is from the abdomen into the thorax. "Downhill varices" occur when the SVC is obstructed caudal to its anastomosis with the azygous vein, with flow of blood from the thorax into the abdomen. One of the greatest dangers in esophageal varices is erosion of the vein walls from GE reflux, which can produce massive GI bleeding that takes the lives of about half of patients with advanced cirrhosis. An interventional radiologic treatment for varices is transjugular intrahepatic portosystemic shunt (TIPS), which decompresses the portal venous system by percutaneously creating a shunt between a relatively high-pressure portal vein and a relatively low-pressure hepatic vein. Despite the high risk of bleeding from esophageal varices, most episodes of bleeding in these patients are from other causes, such as gastritis, Mallory-Weiss tear, and peptic ulcer disease.

Stomach

◇ Inflammatory

Gastritis is a relatively common condition, with an increased incidence in patients on nonsteroidal anti-inflammatory drugs, heavy smokers and drinkers, and seriously ill patients. It consists of erosions of the gastric mucosa, which are usually rapidly reversible. Radiologic findings include small mucosal erosions and fold thickening.

A more complete discussion of peptic ulcer disease is found in Chapter 6. Peptic ulcer disease afflicts ~4 million people in the United States, with 350,000 new cases diagnosed each year. Gastric ulcers are seen radiographically as persistent collections of barium that project beyond the gastric lumen, often with a raised rim of surrounding edema. Ulcers may be benign or malignant. Signs of a benign gastric ulcer include mucosal folds extending up to the crater, penetration beyond the expected luminal margin, and normal peristaltic activity (**Fig. 4–32**). Malignant ulcers occur in the midst of a neoplasm and typically do not exhibit these signs. In patients younger than age 35, in whom the risk of malignancy is virtually nil, no imaging is indicated for suspected peptic ulcer disease, and a good response to empiric therapy is considered diagnostic. In older patients, in whom malignancy may need to be ruled out, benign-appearing ulcers can be followed up with repeat upper GI examination at 6 weeks to ensure complete healing. Malignant-appearing or indeterminate ulcers should undergo endoscopic biopsy.

Both chronic gastritis and peptic ulcer disease are associated with the presence of *Helicobacter pylori,* a urease-producing organism whose metabolic byproducts include ammonia and inflammatory toxins. The association in the case of duodenal ulcers is felt to be as high as 99%, but perhaps only as high as 90% in cases of chronic gastritis. However, the majority of people with *H. pylori* infection never develop peptic ulcer disease. Radiologic findings are nonspecific, and the diagnosis of infection can be made by endoscopic biopsy or a breath test for urease activity.

◇ Tumorous

The most common primary malignancy of the stomach is adenocarcinoma. In the first part of the 20th century, gastric carcinoma was the most common cause of cancer death in the United States, but its incidence has markedly decreased,

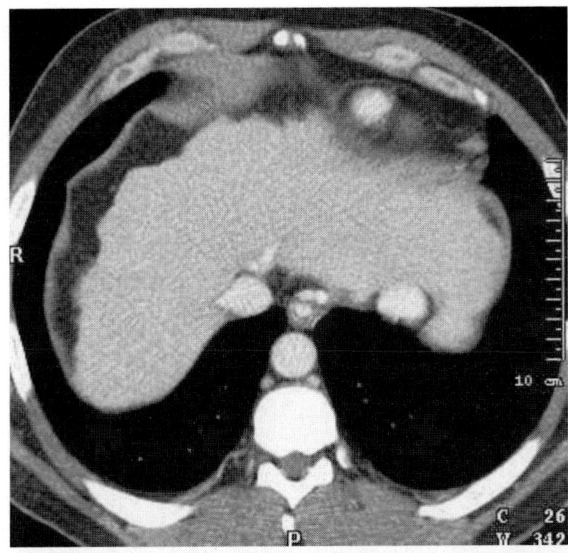

A

B

Figure 4–31 **(A)** An axial CT image through the lower chest demonstrates a small, nodular liver and dilated, contrast-opacified veins in the distal esophagus of this patient with alcoholic cirrhosis of the liver and esophageal varices. Note the nodular contour of the liver. **(B)** Four contiguous images at the level of the upper abdomen demonstrate enormous varices adjacent to the gastric fundus.

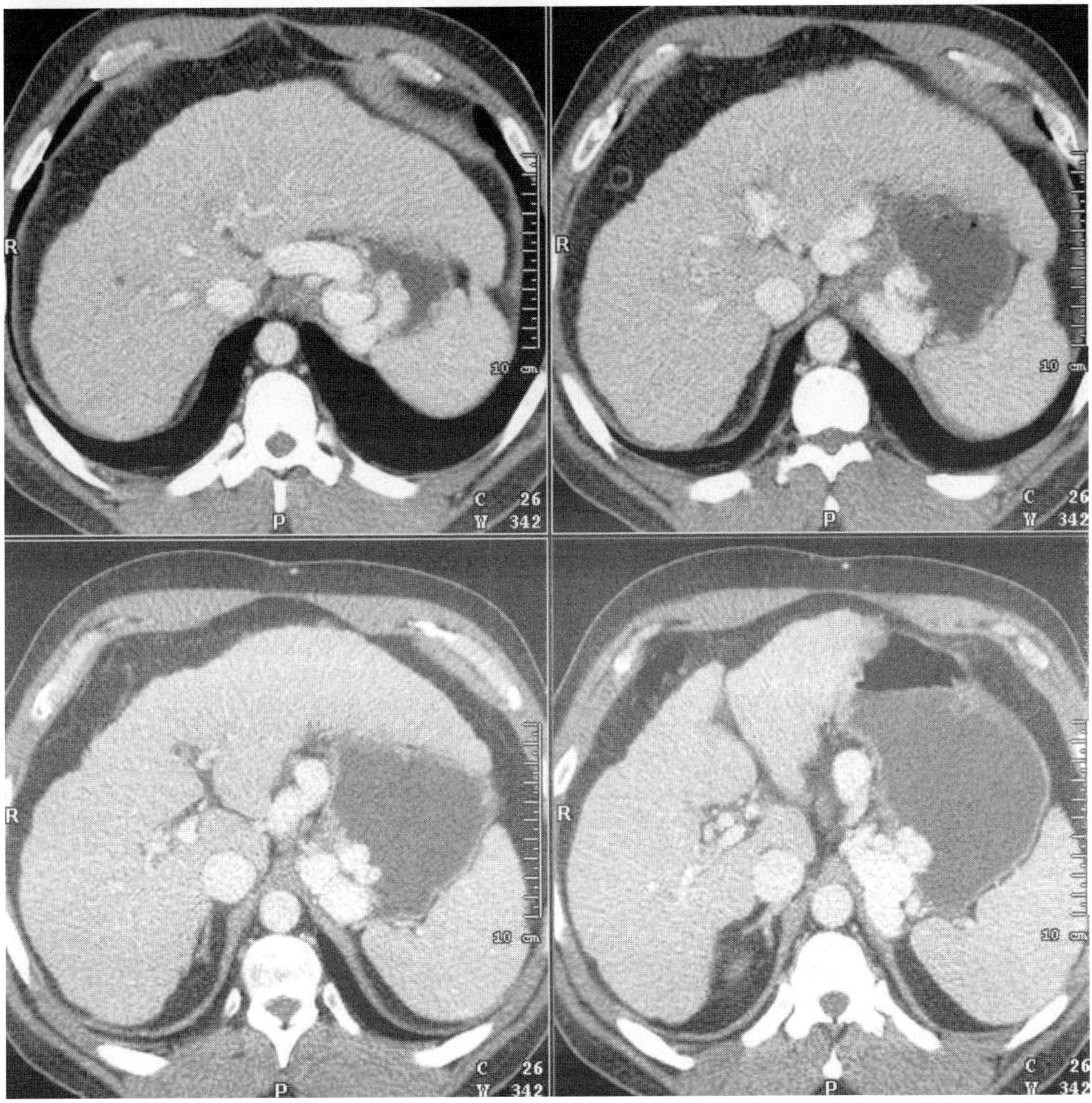

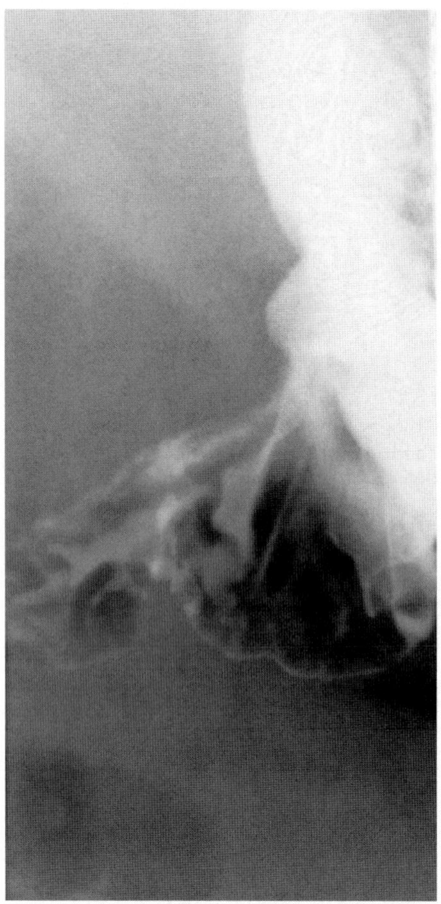

Figure 4–32 This double-contrast view of the stomach demonstrates a typical benign ulcer on the lesser curvature.

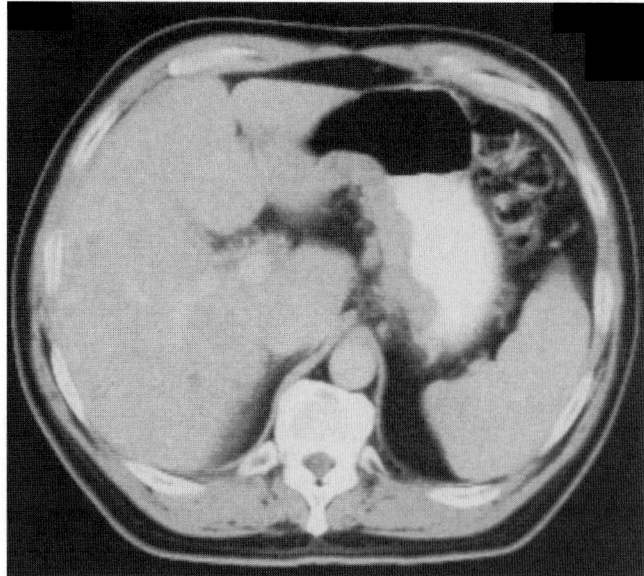

Figure 4–33 This retired man presented with left upper quadrant pain and weight loss. The axial CT image demonstrates abnormal thickening of the posterior wall of the stomach, as well as multiple hypodense lesions in the liver. This was metastatic gastric adenocarcinoma.

and now only 25,000 cases per year are diagnosed. Gastric adenocarcinoma is much more common in Japan, Chile, and China. Men are more commonly affected than women, with a peak age of incidence in the sixth decade. A key risk factor is a diet of high-nitrite smoked and salted foods, associated with lack of refrigeration. Predisposing conditions are all associated with gastritis and include achlorhydria and previous gastrojejunostomy (with reflux of alkaline bile). Two types of gastric cancer are recognized, polypoid and infiltrating (**Fig. 4–33**). Many gastric adenocarcinomas present as malignant-appearing ulcers, likely because the tumor lacks the usual mucosal defenses against gastric acid. Because the disease has usually penetrated the submucosa or spread to the lymph nodes at the time of diagnosis, 5-year survival is only ~15%.

◇ Metabolic

One "metabolic" disorder seen in the stomach is Ménétrier's disease, which involves a combination of protein-losing enteropathy, achlorhydria, and an increased incidence of adenocarcinoma. Men are more commonly affected than women, and the usual age of diagnosis is in the sixth or seventh decade of life. The loss of protein, which produces edema and an increased incidence of infection, can be traced to proliferation of the superficial layer of the gastric mucosa, which becomes "leaky." This proliferation produces characteristic giant rugal folds on barium examination. The achlorhydria is secondary to atrophy of the deeper glandular layer of the mucosa.

A second metabolic disorder of the stomach is Zollinger-Ellison syndrome, which consists of recurrent treatment-resistant peptic ulcers, diarrhea, and abdominal pain. In 90% of cases, a gastrin-secreting tumor is present, often in the pancreas or duodenum. Approximately one half of these prove to be malignant.

◇ Iatrogenic

Numerous iatrogenic conditions are seen in the postoperative stomach. Commonly performed gastric procedures include the Nissen fundoplication, in which a portion of the stomach is wrapped around the distal esophagus to prevent GE reflux; the Billroth I, in which the distal stomach is resected, and the remainder of the stomach is anastomosed to the duodenum; and the Billroth II, in which the distal stomach is resected and a gastrojejunostomy performed. Early complications for which contrast studies (not barium) are often requested include suspected anastomotic leak and obstruction (often secondary to edema). Barium is not used, because of the danger of leakage into the peritoneal cavity, where it can produce peritonitis. Later complications include gastritis (often secondary to bile reflux), recurrent ulcers, and gastric carcinoma.

Small Bowel

◇ Congenital

The most common congenital anomaly of the small bowel is a Meckel's diverticulum. Resulting from failure of closure of

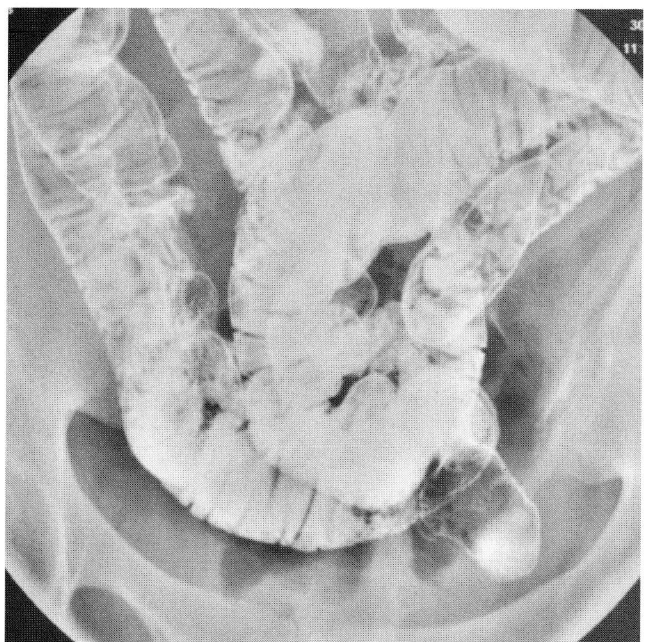

Figure 4–34 This middle-aged man underwent enteroclysis as part of a diagnostic workup for rectal bleeding. A spot view of the pelvis demonstrates a several-centimeter outpouching from the antimesenteric side of the distal ileum. Its mucosal border is irregular. This was a Meckel's diverticulum.

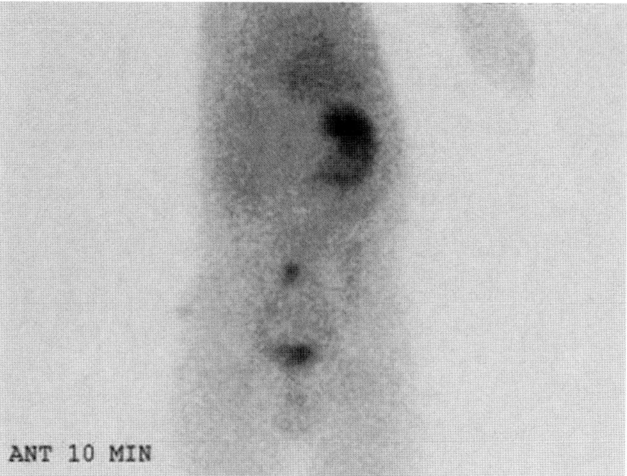

Figure 4–35 This technetium- (Tc-) 99m pertechnetate scan demonstrates an abnormal focus of radiotracer uptake in the lower abdomen, between the stomach and urinary bladder. This is a typical appearance of a Meckel's diverticulum with ectopic gastric mucosa.

the omphalomesenteric duct, which connects the primitive yolk sac to the bowel lumen through the umbilicus (**Fig. 4–34**), Meckel's diverticulum is characterized by the rule of 2s: it occurs in 2% of the population, it is usually located within 2 ft of the ileocecal valve, it usually measures ~2 inches in length, it usually presents with complications before 2 years of age, and ~20% of patients suffer complications. Complications stem from the presence of gastric mucosa within the diverticulum, the acidic secretions of which can produce inflammation, ulceration, and bleeding. Symptoms may mimic appendicitis, and the lesion may also serve as a lead point for intussusception, in which the segment of ileum containing the Meckel's diverticulum "telescopes" down into a more distal segment of ileum and/or colon. A Meckel's diverticulum is difficult to detect radiographically, because it usually does not fill with barium. The imaging study of choice is a nuclear medicine technetium- (Tc-) 99m pertechnetate scan, which will show accumulation of radiotracer in the ectopic gastric mucosa (**Fig. 4–35**). Another congenital abnormality is the enteric duplication cyst, which usually presents as a mass displacing adjacent bowel.

◇ Inflammatory

The most important inflammatory disease of the small bowel is Crohn's disease, with an incidence in the United States of ~3 per 100,000. It is 4 times more common in whites than nonwhites, and 4 times more common in Jews than non-Jews. It is characterized pathologically by transmural inflammation of the bowel and noncaseating granulomas. Because the entire wall is involved, there is a corresponding predilection to extraluminal manifestations, such as abscess and fistula formation. Crohn's disease most often affects young adults, who present with diarrhea, abdominal pain, lassitude, and weight loss—nonspecific symptoms that often lead to a long delay in diagnosis. Although Crohn's disease can involve the GI tract anywhere from the mouth to the anus, it involves the small bowel alone in 40% of cases, the large bowel alone in 30% of cases, and both in the remaining 30% of cases.

Imaging Radiographic findings in Crohn's disease include aphthoid lesions (tiny ulcerations up to several millimeters in diameter), cobblestoning (linear ulcerations with intact intervening mucosa), stricturing and rigidity (the "string sign" when severe), and fistula formation (**Fig. 4–36**). A fistula (from the Latin for "pipe") is an abnormal communication between two hollow viscuses or a viscus and the skin. Another

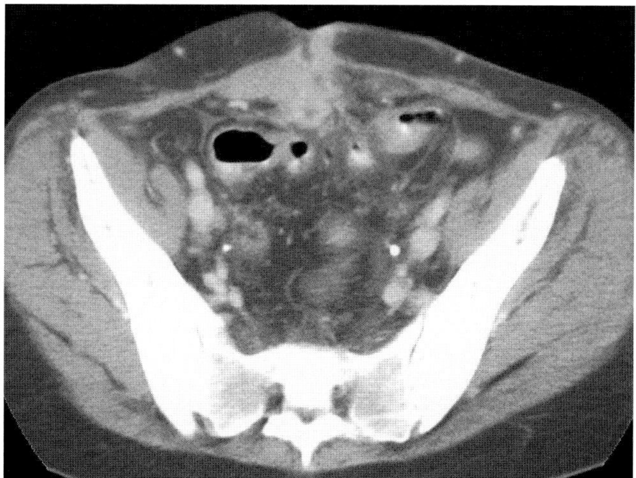

Figure 4–36 This axial CT image of the pelvis demonstrates a fistula with enhancing walls extending from the small bowel out to the skin surface in the Crohn's disease patient who has developed an enterocutaneous fistula.

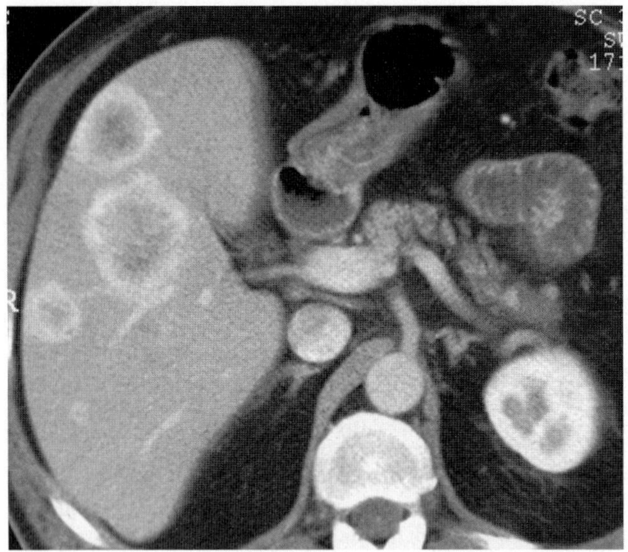

Figure 4–37 This postcontrast axial CT image of the upper abdomen in a patient with small bowel carcinoid tumor demonstrates three brightly ring-enhancing liver metastases. On other images at different levels of the liver (not shown), many additional metastatic lesions were identified.

characteristic finding is discontinuous involvement, or so-called skip lesions, which are separated from one another by normal bowel. Fistulization and skip lesions are not characteristic of ulcerative colitis, the other major type of inflammatory bowel disease. Unlike ulcerative colitis, surgery is not curative in Crohn's disease, and recurrences typically occur just distal to the site of anastomosis. Multiple bowel resections can result in malabsorption syndromes.

◇ Tumorous

The small bowel is the segment of the GI tract least often involved by neoplasms, despite the fact that it constitutes three quarters of its length. The most common primary small bowel neoplasm is carcinoid tumor, which arises from endocrine cells deep in the mucosa and secretes vasoactive substances such as serotonin. In some patients, this results in carcinoid syndrome, which consists of cutaneous flushing, cramps, and diarrhea, and is seen mainly in patients with liver metastases. In patients without liver metastases, such hormones are inactivated by the liver. The most common location of carcinoid tumor is the ileum, where serotonin induces an intense desmoplastic reaction that can cause strictures and fibrosis. Radiographic findings include small filling defects, kinking and stricture of bowel, and liver metastases that strongly enhance with contrast, due to the highly vascular nature of the tumor (**Fig. 4–37**).

Adenocarcinoma is the most prevalent primary malignancy of the proximal small bowel. It has a relatively poor prognosis, due to the high incidence of lymphatic and hematogenous spread at the time of diagnosis. Lymphoma is another important small bowel malignancy, and the small bowel is the most common site of primary GI tract lymphoma. Because it arises in and most often infiltrates the ample small bowel lymphoid tissues, especially in the terminal ileum, it often manifests radiographically with wall thickening, effacement of folds, and luminal widening.

Metastases occur either by intraperitoneal seeding from ovarian, gastric, or colon carcinoma, or by hematogenous spread, with implants of melanoma, breast, or lung carcinoma along the antimesenteric border.

◇ Infectious

Acute gastroenteritis is the most common infectious disease of the small bowel. Common pathogens include *Campylobacter jejuni* and *Staphylococcus aureus*. Imaging is rarely employed.

An uncommon systemic infectious disease that usually involves the GI tract is Whipple's disease, which is caused by a gram-positive actinomycete and is usually seen in middle-aged Caucasian males. It also involves the joints and the central nervous system in many patients. Radiographic findings include coarse, thickened bowel folds, predominantly in the proximal small bowel.

◇ Metabolic

Common metabolic diseases of the small bowel include lactase deficiency, amyloidosis, and sprue. Disaccharides such as lactose are not properly digested by the jejunum if sufficient quantities of lactase are not produced, a condition seen more commonly in blacks, Asians, and Arabs. Radiographic findings include bowel dilation without fold abnormalities.

Amyloidosis, a systemic condition, complicates inflammatory disorders such as rheumatoid arthritis and may also occur in primary form. It is associated with deposition of eosinophilic proteinaceous material that stains with Congo red. When the small bowel is involved, it demonstrates impaired motility and diffusely thickened folds.

Sprue comes in several forms, only one of which is discussed here. Nontropical sprue presents with steatorrhea and weight loss and is due to the toxic effect of gluten, a protein found in wheat and other grains, on the small bowel mucosa of susceptible individuals. Although the remainder of the bowel wall is normal, the mucosa becomes denuded and flattened. The radiographic picture is a dilated jejunum with a sparse fold pattern.

◇ Vascular

The most important vascular pathology of the small bowel is arterial ischemia, which is usually secondary to thrombosis or embolism of the superior mesenteric artery (SMA). The SMA supplies the bowel between the duodenal-jejunal junction at the ligament of Treitz and the splenic flexure of the colon. Venous thrombosis is also a possibility, most commonly due to low flow states such as congestive heart failure and portal hypertension or hypercoagulable states. Plain films show an ileus pattern with evidence of bowel wall thickening (separation of loops) and may show pneumatosis intestinalis (**Fig. 4–38**). On CT, a filling defect often can be visualized within the SMA or superior mesenteric vein.

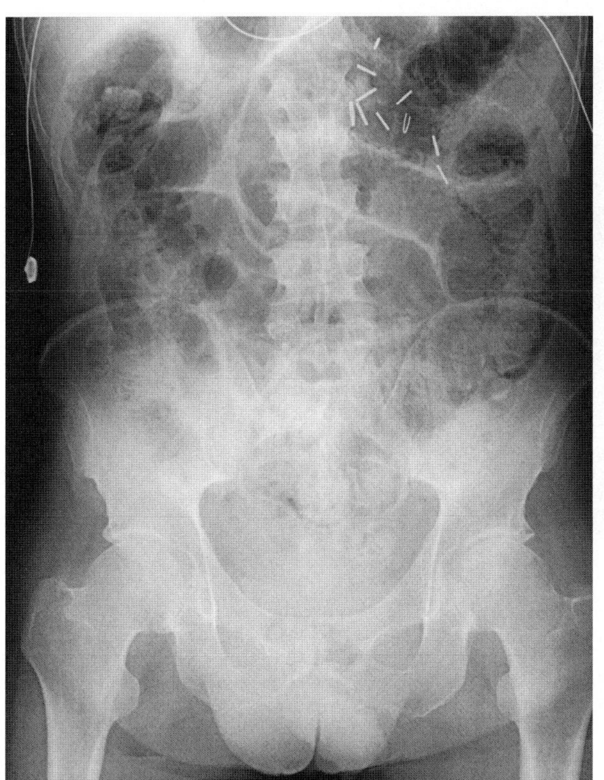
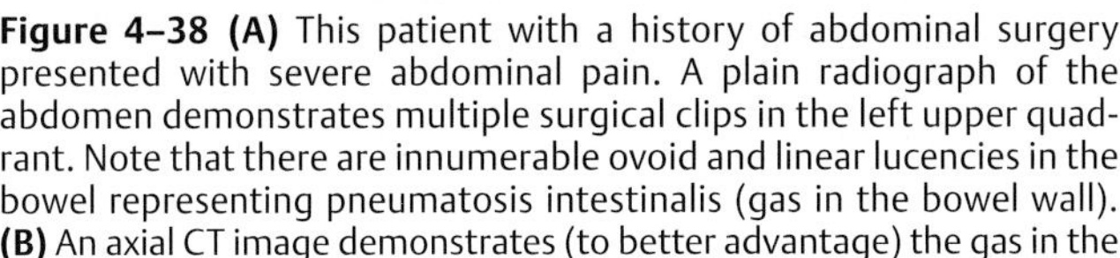
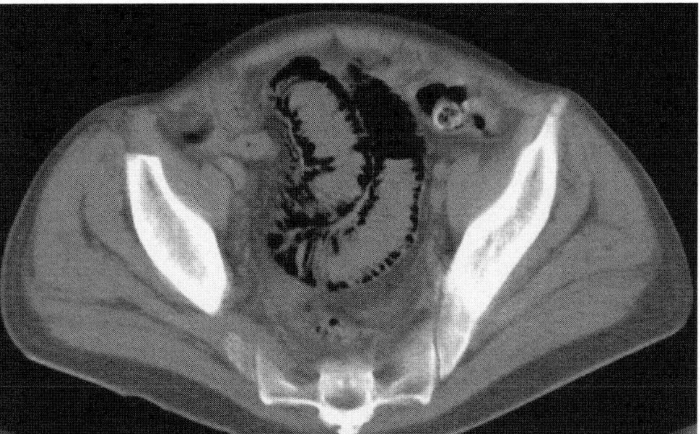
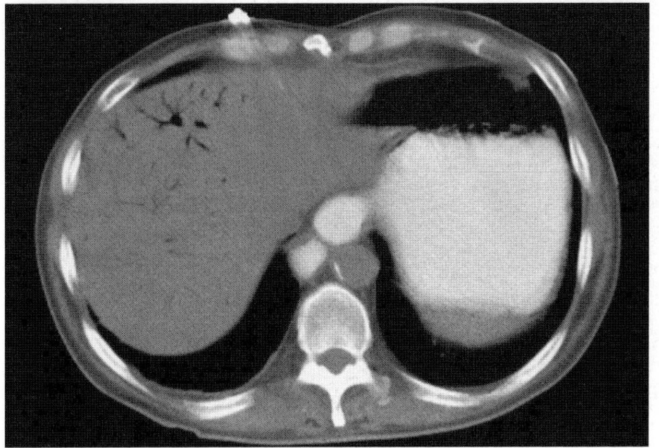

Figure 4–38 **(A)** This patient with a history of abdominal surgery presented with severe abdominal pain. A plain radiograph of the abdomen demonstrates multiple surgical clips in the left upper quadrant. Note that there are innumerable ovoid and linear lucencies in the bowel representing pneumatosis intestinalis (gas in the bowel wall). **(B)** An axial CT image demonstrates (to better advantage) the gas in the wall of a segment of small bowel. **(C)** A CT image of the liver demonstrates gas in the branches of the portal vein. Once intestinal mucosal integrity is sufficiently compromised, luminal gas enters the wall, gets into the tributaries of the superior mesenteric vein, then travels to the portal vein, where it branches out into the liver.

Colon and Rectum

◇ Inflammatory

Ulcerative colitis is the most important inflammatory disorder of the colon, with an incidence approximately twice that of Crohn's disease, 6 per 100,000. Peak incidence is in young adulthood, and it is more common in whites and females. Symptoms include bloody diarrhea and abdominal pain. When severe, systemic symptoms such as weight loss and anorexia may appear. Associated conditions include sclerosing cholangitis, arthritis, and ocular and dermatologic disorders. In contrast to Crohn's disease, ulcerative colitis is restricted to the mucosa, involves only the colon, virtually always begins in the rectum, does not involve the anus, does not produce skip lesions (i.e., involves the colon diffusely instead of in a discontinuous fashion), carries a 10- to 30-fold increased risk of malignancy, and can be cured with colectomy.

Imaging Radiographic findings include a granular-appearing mucosa, collar-button ulcers (due to undermining of the mucosa), foreshortening of the colon, and a lack of normal haustrations (**Fig. 4–39**). Pseudopolyps represent small areas of relatively normal mucosa surrounded by erosions. An acute life-threatening complication is toxic megacolon, which is caused by transmural colitis, loss of motor tone, and rapid dilation of the colonic lumen. Signs of toxic megacolon in a patient with ulcerative colitis include systemic toxicity and profuse bloody diarrhea associated with mucosal sloughing. Plain film findings include marked dilation of the colon, which normally manifests as a dilated (>6 cm), gas-filled transverse colon on supine radiographs (**Fig. 4–40**). Performance of a barium enema is contraindicated in toxic megacolon, due to the danger of perforation. Overall mortality is as high as 20%.

◇ Tumorous

Epidemiology Colorectal cancer is the second most common cause of cancer death in the United States, accounting for 10% of cancer mortality and ~60,000 deaths annually. Approximately 140,000 new cases are diagnosed each year. Most patients are between 50 and 70 years of age. An American's lifetime risk of developing colon cancer is 1 in 8, and once the diagnosis is made, the 5-year survival rate is ~40%. Early, small, and hence local disease enjoys the best prognosis. Surgical resection constitutes the only opportunity for cure, although surgery may also be performed for palliation (e.g., to relieve an obstruction) (**Fig. 4–41**).

Risk factors for colorectal cancer include a personal or family history of the disease, familial polyposis syndromes, multiple

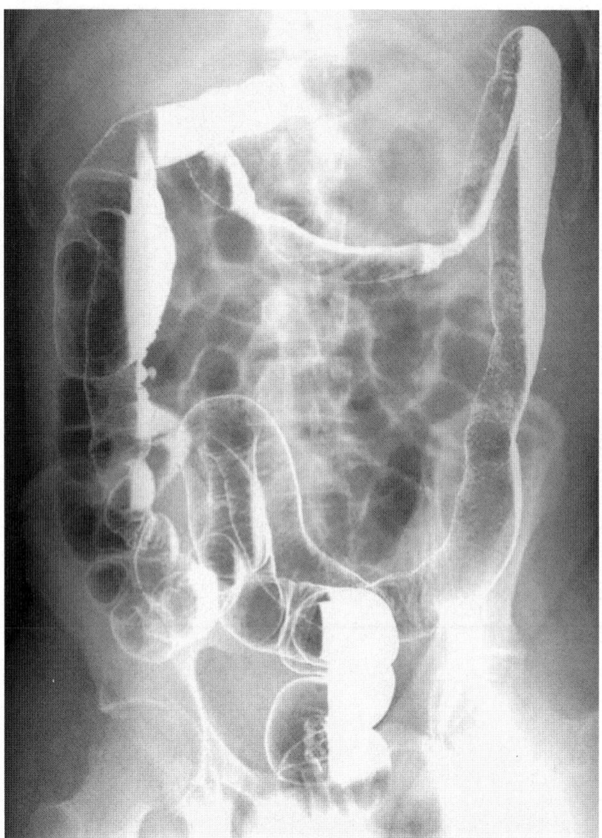

Figure 4–39 This left lateral decubitus radiograph from a double-contrast barium enema in a middle-aged man with a 2-month history of bloody diarrhea, weight loss, and anemia demonstrates loss of normal laustral markings and mucosal ulceration extending from the sigmoid colon to the hepatic flexure.

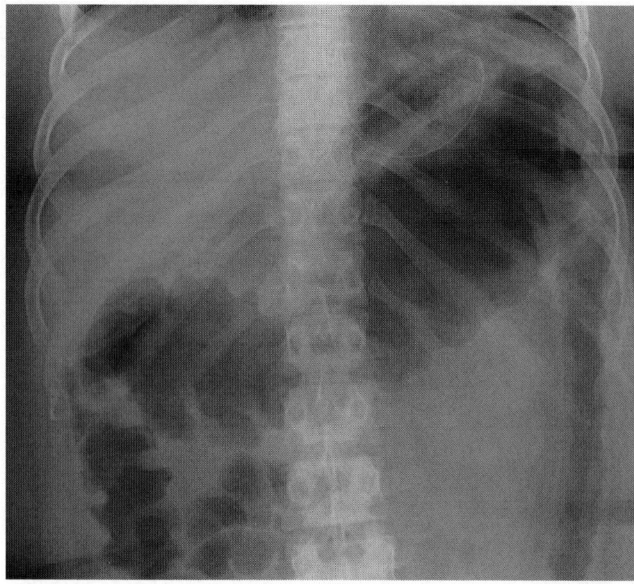

Figure 4–40 This young woman with known ulcerative colitis developed severe abdominal pain and bloody diarrhea. A plain radiograph demonstrates marked dilation of the transverse colon with "thumb-printing" most marked in the ascending and proximal transverse portions. "Thumb-printing" refers to the appearance that the colon wall has been impressed by thumbs, in reality reflecting severe inflammation of the wall. This appearance is consistent with toxic megacolon.

colonic polyps, and long-standing ulcerative colitis. Patients with familial polyposis syndromes or a long history of continuous ulcerative colitis are candidates for prophylactic colectomy.

Pathophysiology A variety of observations support the theory that carcinomas originate in adenomas, including the similar distribution of the two types of lesions in the colon, the parallel incidence rates of adenomas and carcinomas across different countries, the fact that endoscopic removal of adenomas reduces the incidence of carcinoma, and the finding of adenomas, carcinomas in situ, and invasive carcinomas together in some pathologic specimens. It probably takes at least 10 years for an adenoma to develop into a carcinoma, and the majority of adenomas appear never to realize their malignant potential.

Although numerous types of polyps, or mucosal elevations, may develop in the colon, including the most common hyperplastic variety (which has no malignant potential), the two types of adenomatous polyps of concern with regard to colorectal carcinoma are tubular adenomas and villous adenomas. Tubular polyps appear pedunculated (on a stalk), and villous polyps are often sessile (appearing to "bulge out" from the mucosa). When an adenoma is discovered, size is crucial in determining its probability of harboring a cancer. Those less than 1 cm in size have a less than 1% chance of malignancy, which increases to 10% for those between 1 and 2 cm and may be as high as 40% for those over 2 cm (**Fig. 4–42**).

When one adenoma is discovered, there is a 30% probability that the colon harbors another, and a 40% probability that another will develop in the future. The corresponding figures for synchronous ("same time") carcinomas are 1% and for metachronous ("later time") carcinomas, 10%. Hence, once an adenoma or carcinoma is discovered, it is vital that the remainder of the colon be examined, with regular follow-up.

Imaging The radiologist plays several roles in colorectal cancer. The barium enema, either single- or double-contrast, is the radiologic mainstay in screening and detection of new disease, as well as detection of recurrent disease. CT represents the primary modality for the staging of disease, in which MRI and endorectal ultrasound may also play a role.

The screening barium enema can detect polypoid lesions, masses, and strictures, and has a sensitivity of over 90% for lesions greater than 1 cm (**Fig. 4–43**). A challenge to the examiner is significant redundancy, which makes it more difficult to reflux barium all the way back to the cecum, and obscures visualization due to overlapping bowel. Another challenge is diverticular disease, which introduces significant mucosal distortion that can mask small polyps. Finally, a good examination may be impossible in patients whose bowel has not been prepped properly. Patients who do not follow the preparation regimen may exhibit significant amounts of fecal debris or a wet mucosal surface, to which barium will not adhere well.

Colonoscopy has advantages over the barium enema, including direct visualization, the ability to biopsy and

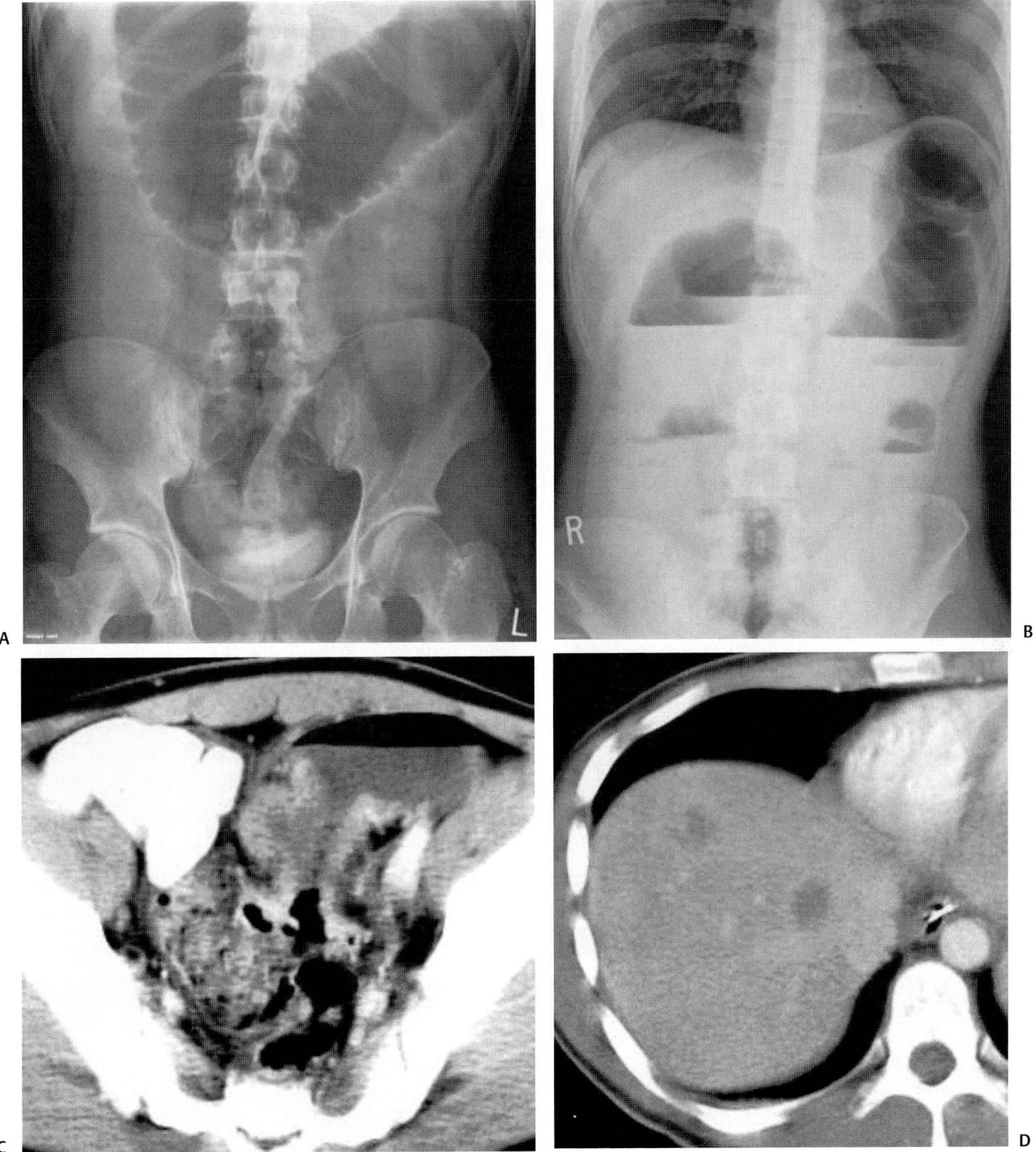

Figure 4–41 (A) This young man presented with 2 days of abdominal pain and distention. A supine abdominal radiograph demonstrates marked dilation of the ascending, transverse, and descending portions. **(B)** This upright abdominal radiograph demonstrates multiple air–fluid levels in the dilated colon, always an abnormal finding. **(C)** A CT image through the pelvis demonstrates an annular constricting lesion in the sigmoid colon, proximal to which the deleted portion of the colon (containing an air–fluid level) terminates. **(D)** This CT image demonstrates two hypodense lesions in the liver, indicating hematogenous metastatic disease.

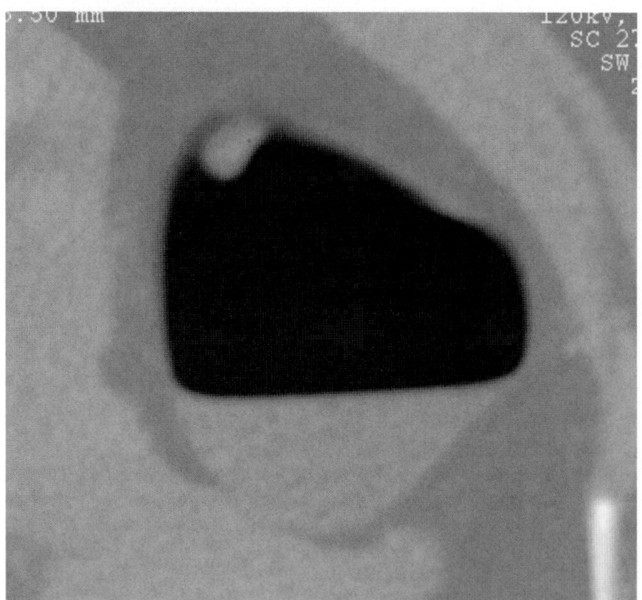

Figure 4–42 This close-up view of a source image from a CT colonography exam demonstrates a small sessile polyp on the nondependent wall of the descending colon.

remove lesions, and good performance in the sigmoid colon, an area of weakness for radiology due to the frequent presence of diverticula. On the other hand, endoscopy costs approximately 3 times as much as barium enema, often fails to reach the cecum (up to one third of examinations), and has ~10 times the risk of colonic perforation. Current screening recommendations call for flexible sigmoidoscopies or air-contrast barium enemas every 3 to 5 years in patients over 50 years of age.

◆ The Solid Organs of Digestion

Solid organs such as the liver and pancreas are better evaluated by cross-sectional imaging studies than fluoroscopic contrast studies, in which the presence of masses and the like can only be inferred indirectly. Cross-sectional imaging studies of the abdomen reveal a vast quantity of anatomy, and it is important to adopt an ordered approach to avoid missing important abnormalities.

Search Pattern

When faced with a CT or MRI study of the abdomen, the following represents a reasonable search strategy. First, examine each organ for size, shape, homogeneity, and abnormal areas of enhancement. Crucial parameters include the presence of masses or mass effects (e.g., displacement of blood vessels or adjacent organs), fluid collections, regions of altered brightness, and adenopathy. The organs and areas to be systematically inspected include the liver, gallbladder, spleen, pancreas, adrenal glands, kidneys, GI tract, mesentery,

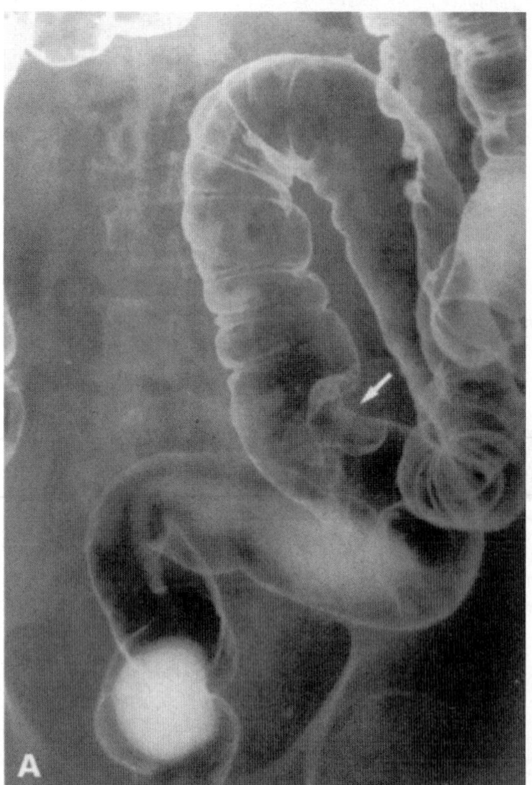

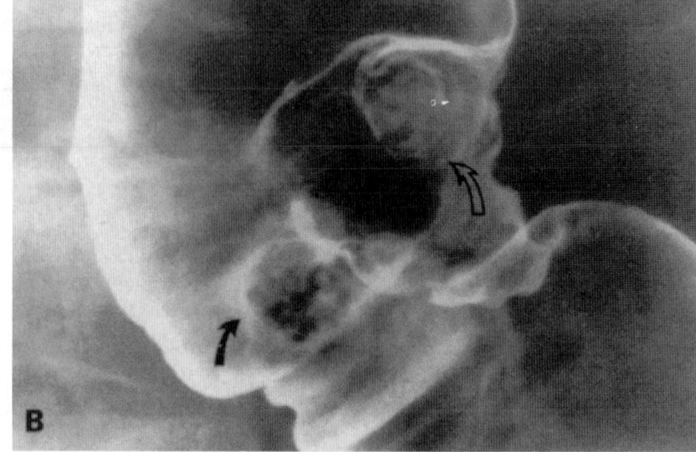

Figure 4–43 **(A)** Overhead and **(B)** magnified spot films from a double-contrast barium enema demonstrate a sessile mass in the proximal sigmoid colon (arrow). Interestingly, the mass exhibits both a sessile polypoid projection along its superior aspect (open arrow) and a pedunculated polypoid lesion (a villous adenoma) extending inferiorly (arrow). An adenocarcinoma was found at surgery.

retroperitoneum, and vessels (aorta and iliac branches, celiac axis, SMA, and the inferior vena cava and its iliac and femoral branches, as well as the portal vein and superior mesenteric vein). In addition, the bones and extra-abdominal soft tissues should be examined.

Select Pathologies

Liver

◇ Congenital

Hemochromatosis is one of the most common genetic diseases, which often presents due to its manifestations in the liver. The disease is inherited as an autosomal recessive trait and is found in heterozygous form in up to 10% of the white population. Although congenital, it rarely manifests before the third or fourth decade. It is characterized by a defect in intestinal iron absorption, which is normally down-regulated when systemic iron stores are sufficient. Secondary hemochromatosis occurs in individuals with hemolytic anemias who receive multiple blood transfusions.

Both primary and secondary forms result in iron deposition in such organs as the liver, the pancreas, and the skin, producing the classic triad of hepatic cirrhosis, diabetes, and bronze pigmentation ("bronze diabetes"). The definitive diagnosis is established by hepatic biopsy, but it can be suggested by elevated serum ferritin levels. Often, the diagnosis is not suspected, but it can be suggested in the appropriate clinical setting by such imaging findings as hyperechoic liver on ultrasound, a markedly increased density of the liver on noncontrast CT images (> 75 Hounsfield units [HU], and significantly denser than the spleen), and marked hypointensity of the liver on T2-weighted MR images (**Fig. 4–44**). Therapy usually consists of periodic phlebotomy.

◇ Inflammatory

A common "inflammatory" lesion of the liver is cirrhosis, which involves destruction of hepatocytes and hepatic lobular architecture, with replacement by scarring and regenerating hepatic nodules. Cirrhosis was so named by Laennec based on the yellowish appearance of the diseased liver, after the Greek *kirrhos*, meaning "tawny." The most common cause in the United States is alcoholism, although patients with viral hepatitis are also at considerably increased risk. Patients present with failure to thrive, jaundice (due to disordered bilirubin metabolism), ascites, signs of portal hypertension, and abnormal liver function tests.

Imaging Liver biopsy is the definitive test, but the presence of cirrhosis can be suggested by several imaging studies. Ultrasound signs include hepatomegaly and irregularity of the hepatic surface, ascites, and evidence of portal hypertension, including varices and splenomegaly. CT findings include heterogeneity of the hepatic parenchyma, nodularity of the liver surface, ascites, and signs of portal hypertension (**Fig. 4–45**). In sclerosing cholangitis, which is characterized by progressive fibrotic inflammation of the biliary tree leading to biliary obstruction and cirrhosis, percutaneous cholangiography demonstrates multiple focal strictures of the bile ducts.

◇ Tumorous

The liver and lung are the two visceral organs most often involved by metastatic malignancy, and hepatic metastases are 20 times more common than primary hepatic malignancies. Approximately one third of patients who die of malignancy demonstrate at least pathologic evidence of hepatic metastases. The liver is the most common site of metastatic disease in colorectal carcinoma, and other common sources of hepatic metastases include digestive system

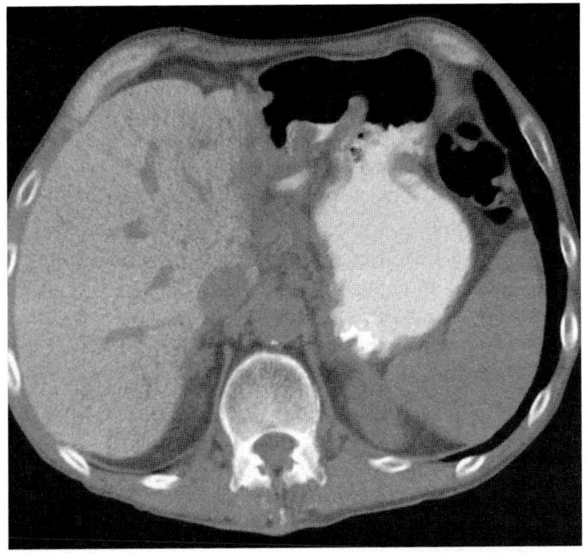

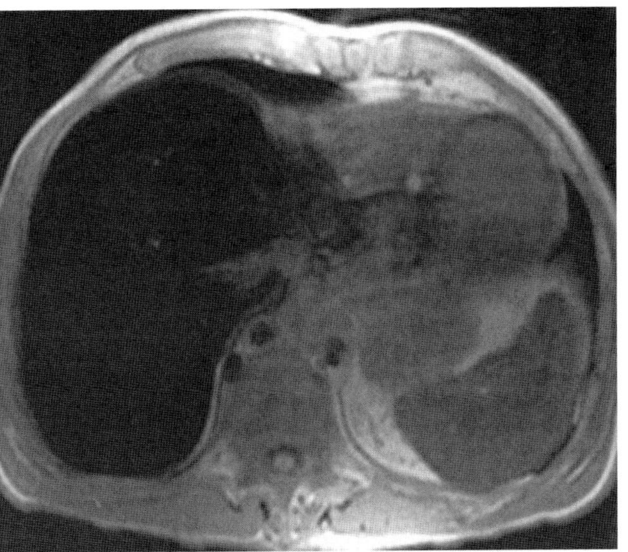

Figure 4–44 **(A)** This CT image of the upper abdomen without IV contrast demonstrates marked hyperdensity of the entire liver, which is much brighter than the spleen, and had a measured density of 100 Hounsfield units. **(B)** This T2-weighted MR image shows marked hypointensity of the liver compared with the spleen. These findings reflect marked iron deposition in this middle-aged man with primary hemochromatosis.

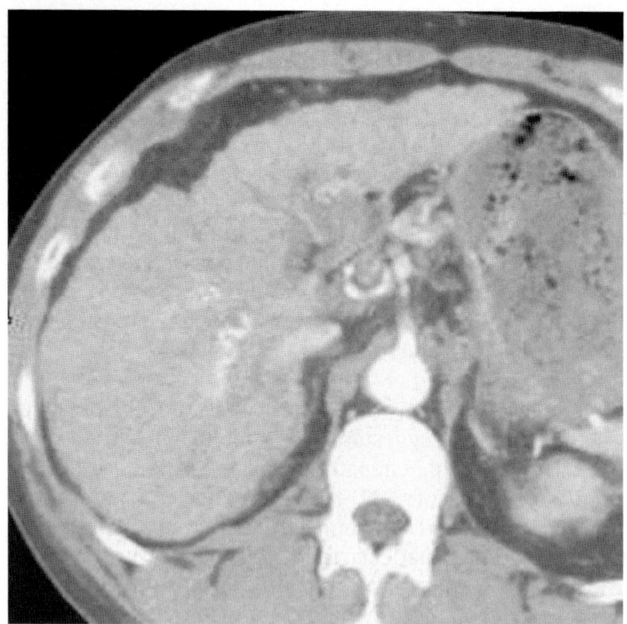

Figure 4–45 Note the small, heterogeneous, and nodular appearance of the liver on CT in this patient with alcoholic hepatic cirrhosis.

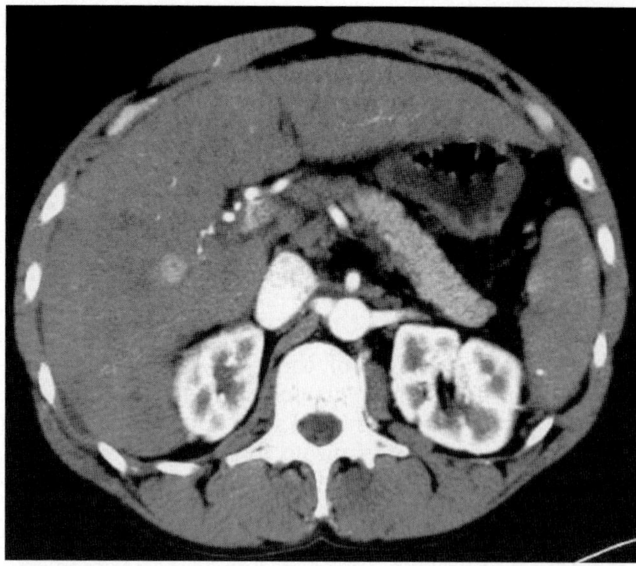

Figure 4–47 This postcontrast CT image in a patient with cirrhosis from long-standing hepatitis C infection demonstrates a 1 cm hyperdense nodule in the right lobe of the liver, very suspicious for hepatocellular carcinoma.

sites such as the stomach and pancreas, as well as the breast and lung (**Fig. 4–46**). As many as 15 to 20% of such patients actually die of hepatic disease, rather than their primary tumor.

Although several primary malignancies may develop in the liver, hepatocellular carcinoma is the most important, and constitutes the most common visceral malignancy worldwide. Risk factors include chronic hepatitis B and C, cirrhosis, and metabolic disorders such as glycogen storage diseases. Of the 6000 cases diagnosed each year in the United States, ~4800 occur in men. Patients present with a right upper quadrant mass and evidence of liver failure, including jaundice and ascites. Alpha-fetoprotein levels are elevated in two thirds of patients, and can be used to help distinguish hepatocellular carcinoma from metastatic carcinoma.

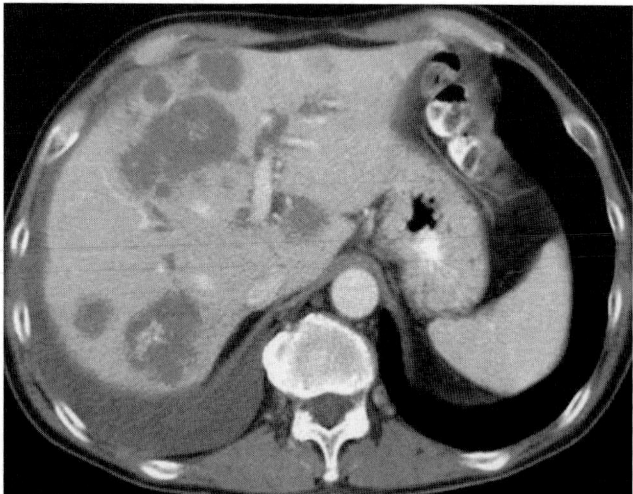

Figure 4–46 This postcontrast CT image of the upper abdomen demonstrates multiple hypodense liver lesions, some of which contain calcifications. Note also the presence of ascites behind the liver. The liver masses represented metastatic deposits from a mucin-producing adenocarcinoma of the rectum.

On CT, hepatocellular carcinoma appears as a contrast-enhancing lesion that often invades vascular structures such as the portal vein (**Fig. 4–47**). Ultrasound usually demonstrates a hypoechoic mass that may invade blood vessels and is associated with high velocity flow on Doppler imaging. Both CT and ultrasound provide excellent guidance for percutaneous biopsy.

Cavernous hemangioma is the most prevalent nonmalignant tumor, and is found in ~5% of the population (F:M = 4:1). These lesions consist of collections of large vascular channels containing slow-moving blood. The principal reason to be concerned about the presence of a hemangioma, which is nearly always asymptomatic, is to distinguish it from a more sinister process such as a hepatocellular carcinoma or metastasis. By ultrasound, hemangiomas are usually uniformly hyperechoic but demonstrate posterior acoustic enhancement. By CT or MR with contrast infusion and dynamic scanning (scanning the lesion multiple times over several minutes), they characteristically exhibit a pattern of enhancement that moves from the periphery to the center, eventually filling in completely (**Fig. 4–48**). On MRI, hemangiomas also demonstrate marked hyperintensity on heavily T2-weighted images (the "light bulb" sign).

◇ Infectious

From an imaging standpoint, infections of the liver usually take the form of abscesses. Enteric organisms such as *Escherichia coli* are most frequently responsible. On CT, they often appear hypodense with peripheral enhancement, but do not fill in centrally over time, in contrast to hemangiomas (**Fig. 4–49**). Many contain pockets of gas. Radiologists are frequently called upon

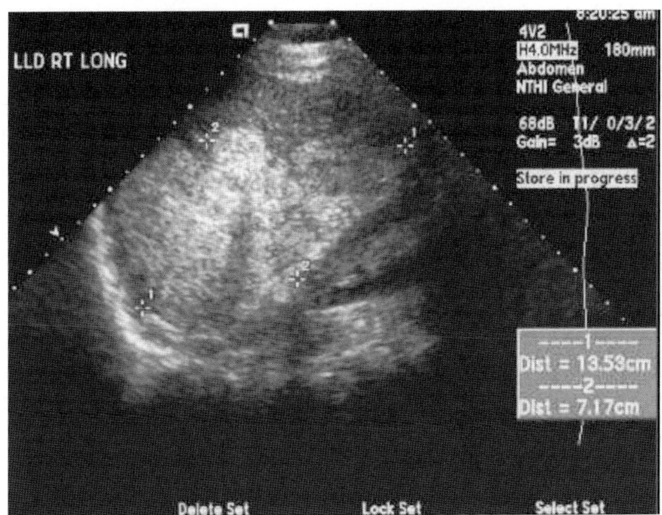

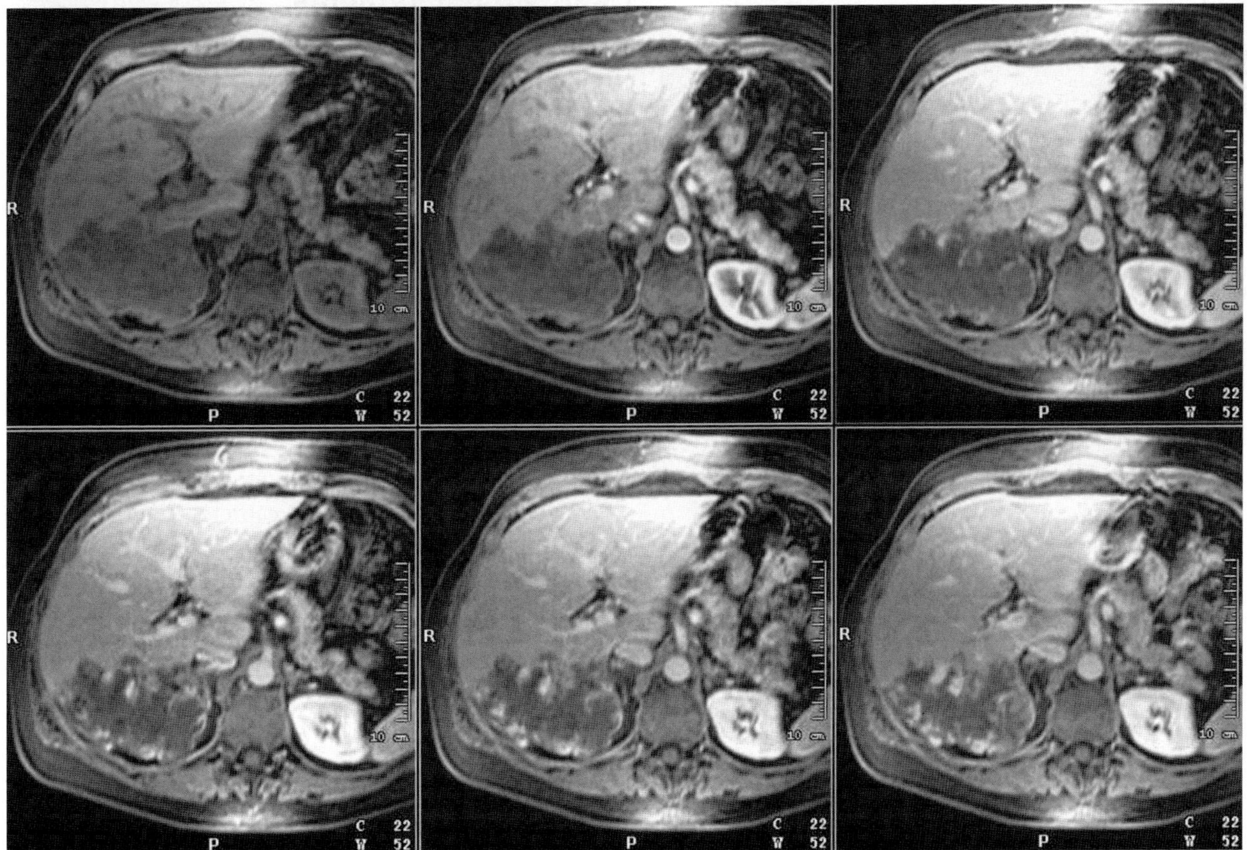

Figure 4–48 This middle-aged woman underwent an ultrasound exam for suspected gallbladder disease. **(A)** On ultrasound, large, hyperechoic mass was found in the posterior aspect of the right lobe of the liver. **(B)** Serial MR images after gadolinium contrast infusion show progressive peripheral-to-central enhancement of the lesion, consistent with a cavernous hemangioma.

to drain such lesions percutaneously. In combination with antibiotic therapy, this usually results in complete resolution.

Pancreas

◇ Congenital

The two most frequent congenital pancreatic anomalies are pancreas divisum and annular pancreas. Pancreas divisum results from lack of normal fusion of the dorsal and ventral pancreatic buds during embryogenesis, with the result that the main pancreatic drainage occurs through the minor papilla (located proximal to the papilla of Vater). It is thought that this orifice is often too small to accommodate the full volume of pancreatic exocrine secretions, resulting in obstruction and recurrent pancreatitis. Annular pancreas results from abnormal migration of the ventral pancreas, causing pancreatic encirclement of the duodenum and resultant obstruction. Both of these conditions are best imaged with magnetic resonance cholangiopancreatography (MRCP) or endoscopic retrograde cholangiopancreatography (ERCP),

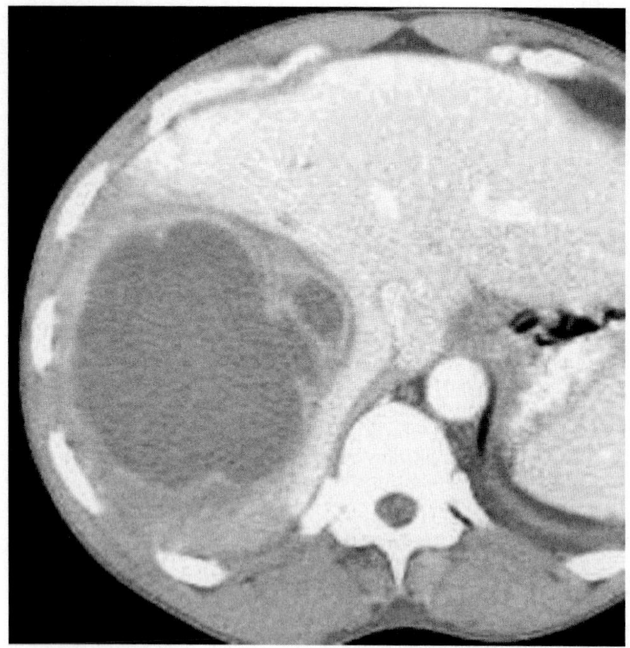

Figure 4–49 This postcontrast CT image of a middle-aged man with right upper quadrant pain, fever, and leukocytosis demonstrates a large hyperdense mass in the right lobe of the liver with enhancing walls. On ultrasound-guided aspiration, this proved to be a pyogenic abscess.

in which the pancreatic duct is cannulated and contrast is injected under fluoroscopic monitoring (**Fig. 4–50**).

◇ Inflammatory

A discussion of pancreatitis is found in Chapter 6.

◇ Tumorous

Ninety-five percent of all pancreatic malignancies are adenocarcinomas. The prognosis tends to be dismal, due to the high frequency of metastases at the time of diagnosis, resulting in ~29,000 deaths per year. Pancreatic malignancy is the fourth leading cause of cancer death among both men and women. Presenting signs and symptoms include jaundice, weight loss, and Courvoisier's sign (a palpable, nontender gallbladder). Imaging usually consists of contrast-enhanced CT or ultrasound, with CT demonstrating a hypodense mass (**Fig. 4–51**). On ultrasound, the mass appears hypoechoic relative to normal pancreatic parenchyma. Cure is possible only with surgical resection, but involvement of major vessels such as the celiac artery or SMA renders the tumor unresectable. Other pancreatic neoplasms include endocrine tumors such as insulinoma (most common) and gastrinoma, as well as cystic neoplasms such as macrocystic and microcystic adenomas.

◆ Abdominal Trauma

Trauma is the third leading cause of death in the United States, accounting for nearly 200,000 deaths per year. Because trauma constitutes the leading cause of death in persons under the age of 40 years, it exacts a particularly heavy toll in years of life lost. It also results in several million nonfatal injuries annually, many of which leave victims permanently disabled or disfigured.

Diagnosis

Diagnostic Peritoneal Lavage

Diagnostic peritoneal lavage (DPL) once represented the preferred means for detecting visceral injury, but CT scanning has now largely replaced this technique at most centers. Performed by inserting a catheter into the peritoneal space and first infusing and then withdrawing sterile fluid, peritoneal lavage is a highly sensitive technique for the

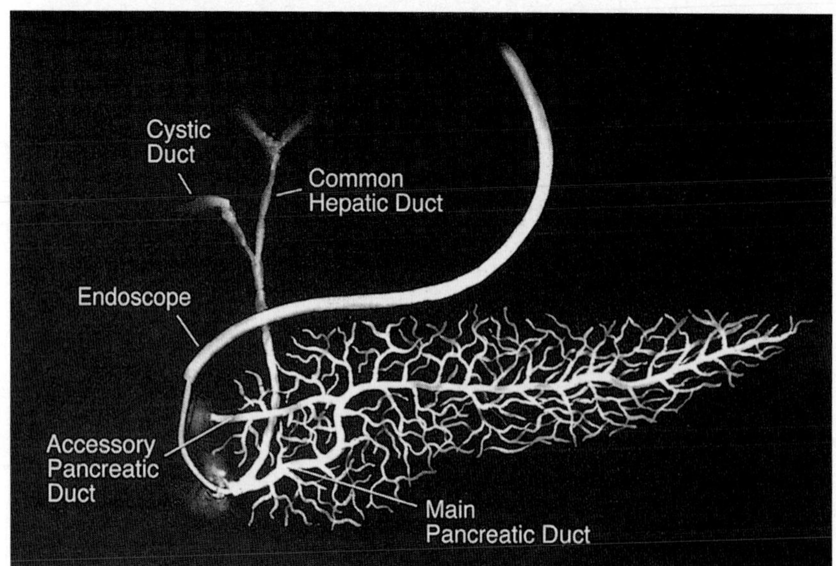

Figure 4–50 Illustration of an endoscopic retrograde cholangiopancreatogram, with the endoscope passing through the distal esophagus, stomach, and into the second portion of the duodenum, with injection of contrast via a cannula into the common bile duct, and filling of the biliary and pancreatic ductal systems. Under normal conditions, the pancreatic ductal system would not be filled so extensively with contrast, for fear of inciting or exacerbating pancreatitis.

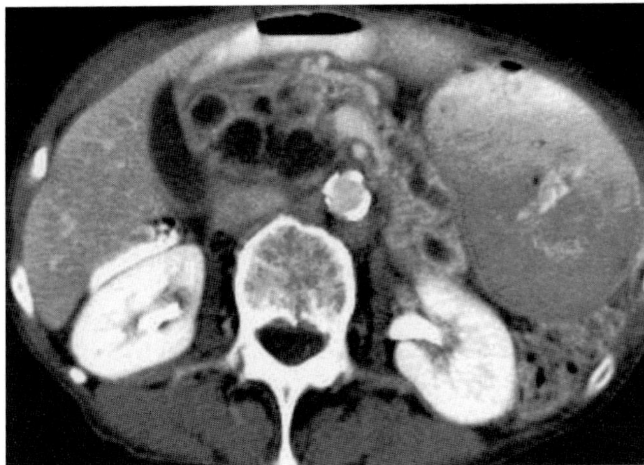

Figure 4–51 This elderly man presented with unexplained weight loss. An axial CT image of the upper abdomen demonstrates a large, multiloculated cystic mass of the head of the pancreas. There is dilation of the pancreatic duct to the left of the lesion, secondary to obstruction. Note also the calcific atherosclerotic plaque in the aorta. The pancreatic mass is consistent with a mucinous cystadenocarcinoma.

detection of hemoperitoneum. Occasionally, peritoneal lavage provides more specific information than CT, as when bile or a high amylase content is detected in the fluid (indicating biliary and pancreatic injury, respectively). DPL may also exhibit advantages over CT in the detection of bowel and mesenteric injury.

However, DPL is usually highly nonspecific, providing no information about the source of hemorrhage. Moreover, DPL cannot distinguish between inconsequential and serious injuries. Another difficulty with DPL is the fact that it cannot evaluate the retroperitoneum. Prior to the advent of CT scanning, laparotomy represented the only means of ascertaining the location and extent of the injury. Though not as sensitive in the detection of minute amounts of free fluid, CT yields highly organ-specific information in a noninvasive fashion (**Fig. 4–52**).

Computed Tomography

CT evaluation of abdominal trauma begins with the search for free intraperitoneal air (pneumoperitoneum), which tends to accumulate in the nondependent portion of the peritoneal cavity (in a supine patient, beneath the anterior abdominal wall). It is seen as an air-attenuation (black) collection or rim. In the absence of penetrating trauma, free air indicates rupture of a viscus. A second critical finding is that of free fluid. Free fluid tends to accumulate in the pelvis, the most dependent portion of the peritoneal cavity in both the upright and supine positions. Such fluid is most likely to represent extravasated blood, urine, bile, or enteric contents, or, later, a transudate or exudate secondary to post-traumatic inflammation. In evaluating abnormal fluid collections, it is important to recall that several important abdominal organs are in fact retroperitoneal, including most of the duodenum, the pancreas, the kidneys, and the great vessels. Fluid originating from these organs will therefore be found in a retroperitoneal location.

As a general principle, there is a linear relationship between the hematocrit of blood and its attenuation value, as

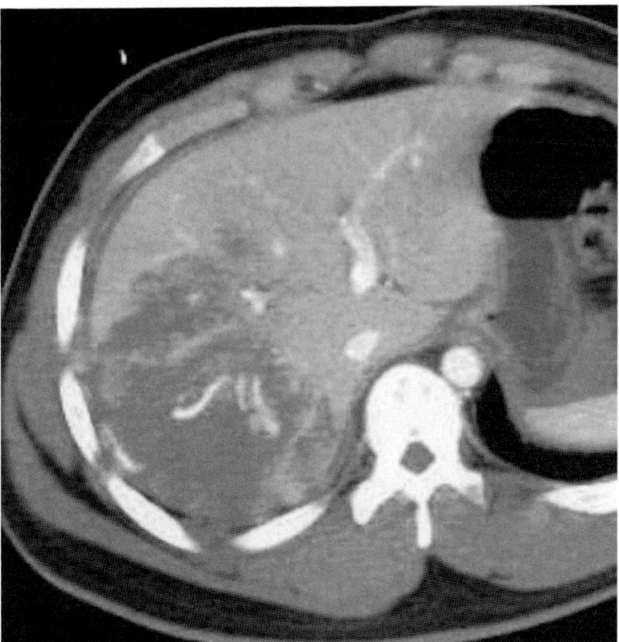

Figure 4–52 This young man complained of right upper quadrant pain and tenderness after a motor vehicle accident. A postcontrast CT image demonstrates irregular hypodensity in the right lobe of the liver, representing a hepatic laceration. The bright area in the hypodense hematoma represents active extravasation of contrast-opacified blood.

hemoglobin accounts for ~80% of total blood x-ray absorption. Consequently, hemorrhage in a severely anemic patient may appear surprisingly hypodense. The attenuation value of extravasated blood varies depending on the time at which it is imaged. In the first hour after hemorrhage, a hematoma will demonstrate attenuation values equivalent to intravascular blood, ~50 HU. With time, however, diffusion of serum into surrounding tissues and retraction of the fibrin clot

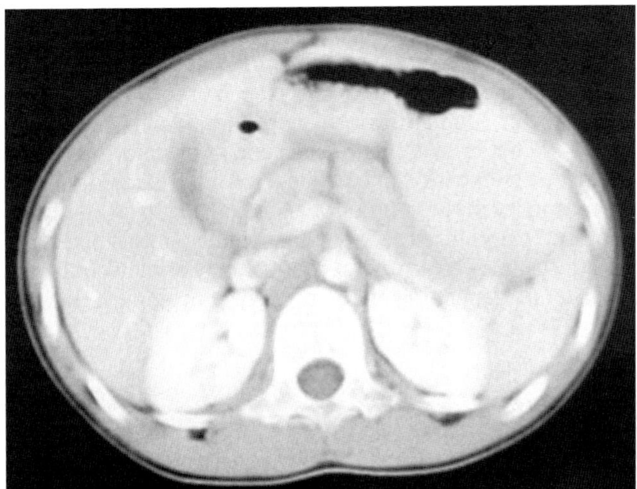

Figure 4–53 This young girl was struck in the epigastric region by a handlebar in a bicycle accident. The CT image demonstrates a pancreatic transaction with peripancreatic fluid. Without intravenous contrast administration, such an injury would be more difficult to detect.

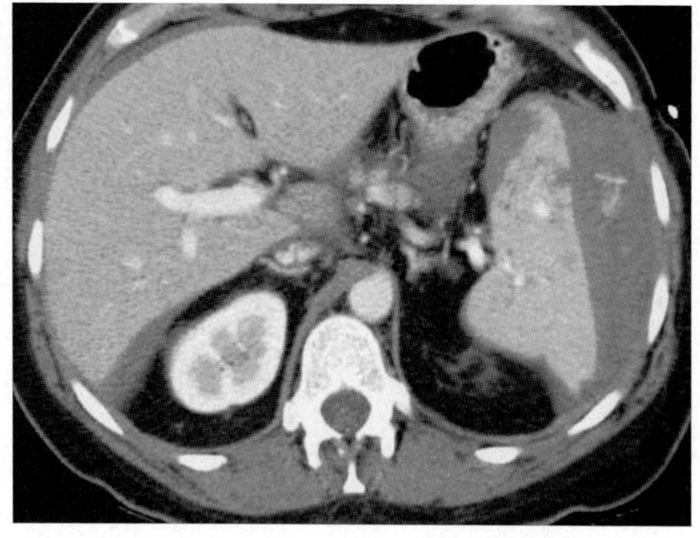

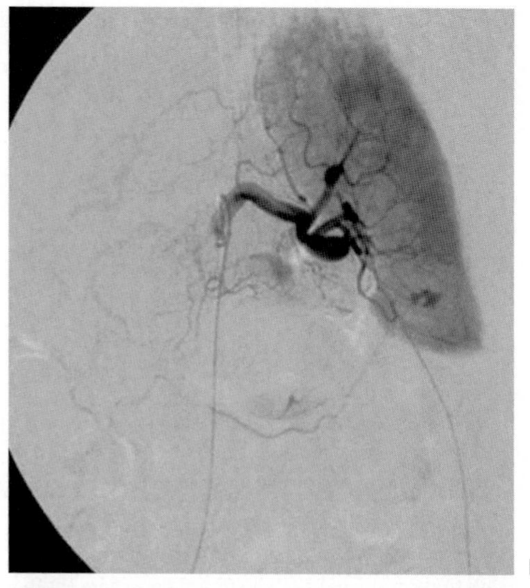

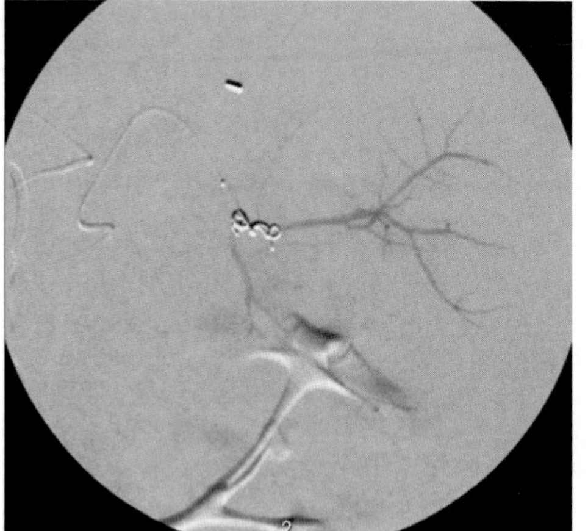

Figure 4–54 This middle-aged woman experienced severe left upper quadrant pain after an automobile accident. **(A)** The postcontrast CT image of the upper abdomen demonstrates areas of hypodensity within the normally enhancing splenic parenchyma, indicating splenic laceration. There is also a large hypodense fluid collection lateral to the spleen, a hematoma. The bright area within the hematoma represents active extravasation of contrast-opacified blood. **(B)** A selective splenic arteriogram shows the site of extravasation as an area of contrast pooling low in the spleen. **(C)** The splenic artery branch supplying the bleeding vessel was embolized with metallic coils, which stopped the bleeding.

results in an increase in attenuation, with values in the neighborhood of 80 HU. Over the ensuing days and weeks, hemoglobin is broken down, with a gradual decline in attenuation, eventually approaching that of water, 0 HU.

Other general signs of abdominal injury include an increase in the size of a normally shaped organ, reflecting hemorrhage or edema; intrinsic deformity of an organ due to direct impact or swelling; displacement or deformity of an organ due to extrinsic mass effect, as from a hematoma; and discontinuity in the contour of an organ, due to laceration or rupture. To optimize the detection of injury, intravenous contrast infusion is critical. Oral contrast may or may not be administered, depending on the urgency of imaging, because it can take several hours to opacify the whole bowel with oral contrast. Intravenous contrast improves lesion detection by delineating perfused and nonperfused tissues, which can be otherwise difficult to differentiate due to the isointensity of hyperacute blood (**Fig. 4–53**). Nonperfused areas within an organ indicate vascular injury, as in a laceration or fracture, and influence the decision whether or not to perform surgery. The focal accumulation of contrast suggests ongoing extravasation; a surgical emergency is a hypotensive patient (**Fig. 4–54**). In part because CT permits such detailed noninvasive assessment of the extent of injury, there has been a strong trend toward nonoperative management of blunt abdominal trauma over the past few decades.

5

The Urinary Tract

- **Anatomy and Physiology**
- **Imaging**
  - Intravenous Urography
  - Nuclear Medicine
    - *Blood Flow*
    - *Glomerular Filtration*
    - *Collecting System Drainage*
  - Other Modalities
- **Kidney**
  - Pathology
    - *Congenital*
    - *Infectious*
    - *Tumorous*
    - *Inflammatory*
    - *Traumatic*
    - *Vascular*
- **Ureter**
  - Pathology
    - *Congenital*
- **Bladder**
  - Pathology
    - *Infectious*
    - *Tumorous*
- **Common Clinical Problems**
  - Hematuria
  - Acute Renal Failure
  - Acute Flank Pain
    - *Urolithiasis*
- **Adrenal Glands**
  - Anatomy and Physiology
  - Pathology
    - *Tumorous*

◆ Anatomy and Physiology

The kidneys are paired retroperitoneal organs contained within the anterior and posterior renal (from the Latin *renes*, "kidneys") fasciae, also known as Gerota's fasciae. Between the anterior and posterior renal fasciae lies not only the kidney itself, but also the adrenal gland, the proximal portion of the collecting system and ureter, and the renal pedicle, including the renal artery, the renal vein, and lymphatics. Approximately two thirds of kidneys are supplied by a single renal artery, and multiple renal veins are seen in approximately one third of cases. Because the left renal vein must cross the midline to reach the inferior vena cava (IVC), it is approximately 3 times longer than the right renal vein, which makes the left kidney the preferred organ for renal transplantation. Moreover, because the left renal vein receives the left gonadal vein, a left renal cell carcinoma with ipsilateral renal vein thrombosis will commonly present with left scrotal swelling. The right renal vein typically drains directly into the IVC.

The adult kidneys normally measure ~3.5 lumbar vertebral body heights, or ~12 cm, in length. Plain radiography routinely overestimates their length due to magnification, whereas ultrasound often underestimates their length due to difficulties in imaging the kidney in its longest plane. The left kidney is normally positioned 1 to 2 cm higher than the right. The renal axes parallel those of the psoas muscles, with the lower poles positioned more laterally than the upper poles.

The kidneys excrete metabolic waste products, regulate salt and water balance, and modulate plasma pH through the production of urine. From the 1700 L of blood flowing through the kidneys every day, 1 L of urine is produced. The production of urine involves three processes: filtration, secretion, and reabsorption. These processes are performed by the nephron, the functional unit of the kidney (**Fig. 5–1**). Each kidney contains ~1 million nephrons. The nephron begins in the glomerulus (from the Latin *glomerule*, "a round knot"), a spherical tuft of capillaries 100 times more permeable than capillaries elsewhere, across which fluid is filtered into Bowman's capsule. From there, the filtrate passes through the proximal convoluted tubule, Henle's loop, the distal convoluted tubule, and into the collecting duct. In addition to forming urine, the kidney performs important endocrine functions. For example, the juxtaglomerular apparatus secretes renin in response to a fall in blood pressure, activating the renin–angiotensin–aldosterone system, which in turn increases sodium reabsorption in the distal tubules. Another important hormone secreted by the kidneys is erythropoietin, which stimulates red blood cell production. The kidneys also help to convert vitamin D to its active form. Consequences of renal failure include uremia, metabolic acidosis, hyperkalemia, disordered regulation of sodium, phosphate, and calcium balance, hypertension, anemia, and immune compromise.

Crucial urinary tract structures evaluated on imaging studies include the renal vasculature, the cortical and medullary portions of the parenchyma, the pyramids, the calyces, the pelvis, the ureters, the bladder, and the urethra (**Fig. 5–2**). The outer renal cortex (from the Latin for "bark of a tree") consists of the glomeruli and the proximal and distal convoluted tubules. The inner medulla (Latin for "marrow") consists of the collecting tubules and Henle's loops. The medulla is made up of several medullary pyramids, which are cradled by the cup-shaped calyces (Latin for "outer covering" or "pod") of the collecting system. Each kidney contains ~12 calyces. The calyces join together to form infundibula (Latin for "funnel"), which drain into the renal pelvis (Latin for "basin").

The pelvis joins the ureter (from the Greek *ourein*, "to urinate") at the ureteropelvic junction (UPJ), a common site of obstruction. The ureters contain circular and longitudinal layers of smooth muscle that actively propel urine toward the bladder by peristalsis. The bladder can accommodate between 300 and 600 mL in the normal adult. It is bounded

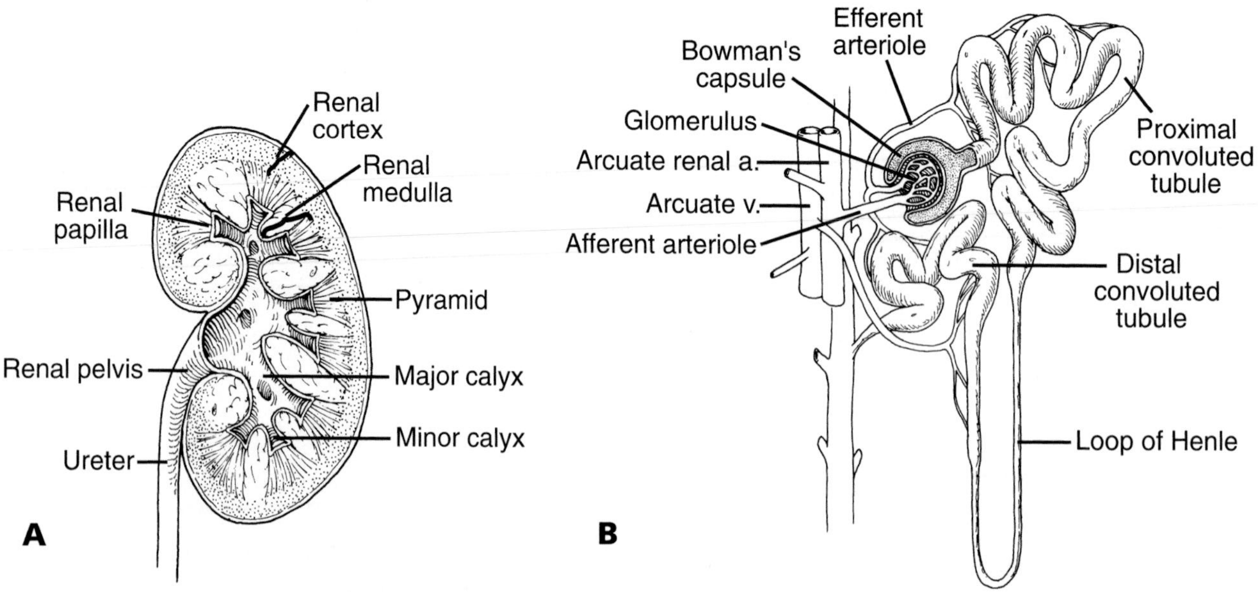

Figure 5–1 **(A)** The major structures of the kidney that are assessed on imaging studies. **(B)** The major structures of the nephron.

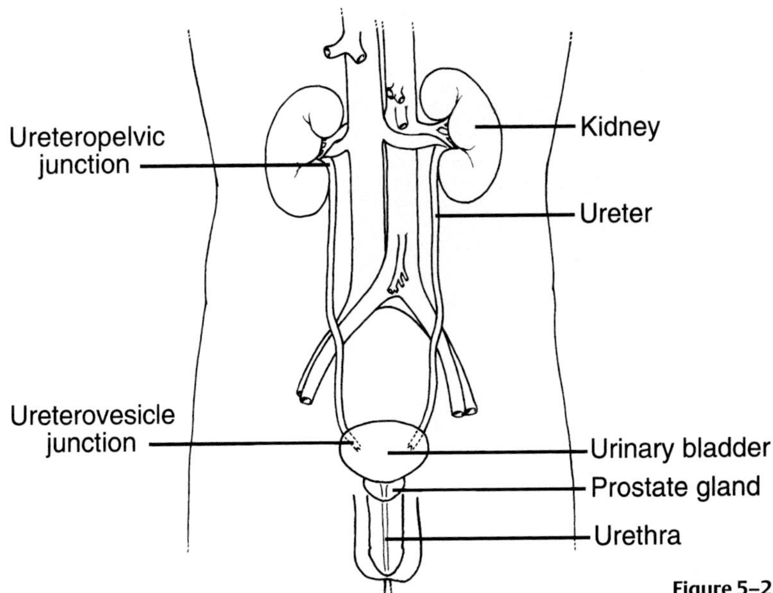

Figure 5–2 The major structures of the urinary system.

posteriorly by the uterus in females and by the rectum in males. The bladder and urethra meet at the trigone, a triangle formed at the bladder floor by the two ureteral orifices and the urethral orifice. The reproductive and urinary tracts are completely separate in the female but become joined at the base of the prostate gland in the male, where the ejaculatory ducts empty into the urethra. The female urethra is embedded in the anterior wall of the vagina and measures ~3 cm in length. The higher incidence of urinary tract infections (UTIs) in girls and young women, as opposed to young males, is often attributed in part to the relatively short female urethra, which may facilitate retrograde transit of bacteria.

◆ Imaging

Intravenous Urography

Urography was born of syphilology. The first urogram was performed in 1923 by physicians at the Mayo Clinic, who discovered that the sodium iodide they were investigating to treat syphilis possessed two intriguing properties: (1) it was excreted via the urinary system, and therefore passed through the kidneys, ureters, bladder, and urethra; and (2) the compound was radiopaque. However, sodium iodide produced relatively poor opacification, and displayed other shortcomings as well. The next crucial innovation occurred when German chemists, seeking to synthesize the "magic bullet" for syphilis, linked iodine to a pyridine ring. Although their invention proved not to be the magic bullet, their organic iodine compounds created a magic window on the urinary tract. By the early 1930s, physicians were relying on excretory urography to provide previously unimaginable images of the structure and function of the urinary system.

The intravenous urogram (IVU; often called an intravenous pyelogram, or IVP, a misnomer) has been largely supplanted by CT, but deserves discussion because of the urographic principles it embodies, which also apply in CT (**Fig. 5–3**). First, a preliminary frontal radiograph of the abdomen is obtained. This view may demonstrate stones or soft tissue masses, and provides a limited assessment of the morphology of the kidneys. Additional tomographic views of the kidneys are obtained to ensure that the technique will be optimal for obtaining nephrotomograms after contrast injection (**Fig. 5–4**). After verifying that the patient has no risk factors for an adverse contrast reaction, the technologist injects ~100 to 150 cc of iodinated contrast material into a peripheral vein, and films are obtained at several minute intervals until kidneys, ureters, and bladder have been well visualized. Tomographic views of the kidneys are also obtained, which provide optimal assessment of the morphology of the renal parenchyma. The study should be monitored by a radiologist, who can adapt the examination to various findings.

To understand the excretory urogram, it is necessary to view it in light of renal physiology. The principles of excretory urography apply equally well to other examinations that reveal renal anatomy and physiology, such as a CT scan of the abdomen and pelvis with intravenous contrast. Let us explore some potential findings on the urogram and attempt to understand their physiologic etiologies. First, suppose the patient receives an injection of contrast material, but initial films demonstrate no renal opacification. Several explanations are possible. The concentration of contrast material in the urine, or the urographic density achieved by the examination, can be analyzed according to the following formula:

$$[U] = ([P] \times GFR)/U_{vol},$$

where $[U]$ is urographic density, $[P]$ is the plasma concentration of contrast, GFR is glomerular filtration rate, and U_{vol} is the volume of urine produced. (The formula holds because nearly 99% of the contrast is filtered by the glomerulus, and there is virtually no distal tubular excretion or reabsorption.) If the kidneys are not seen at all, this formula

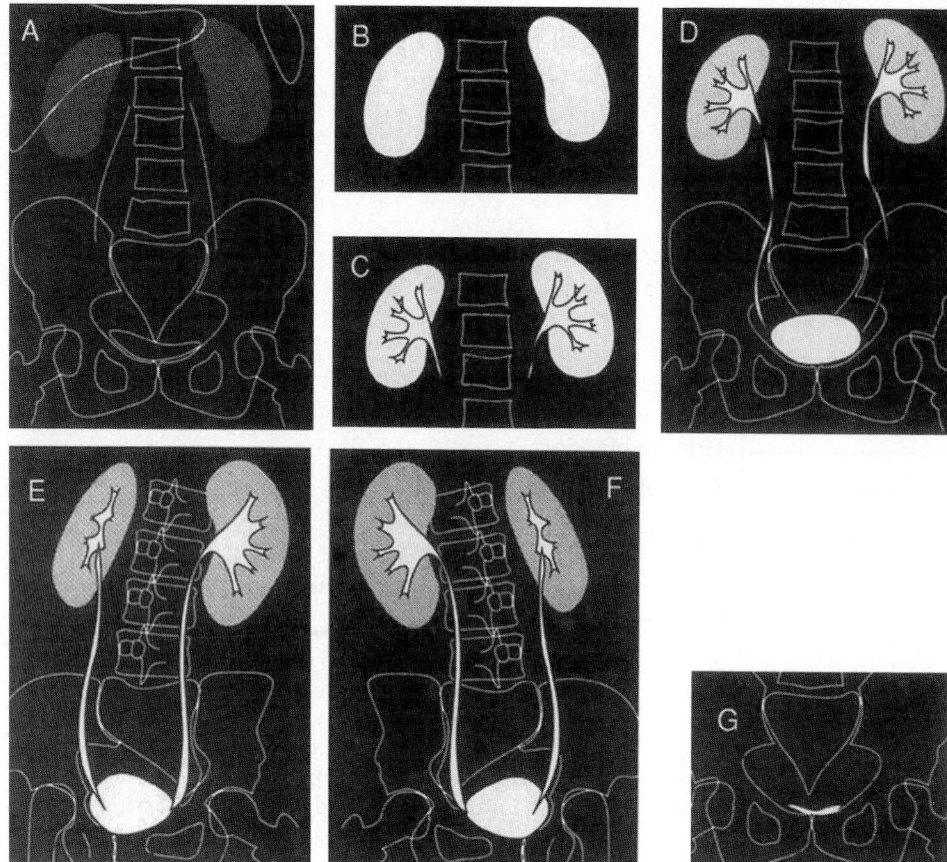

Figure 5–3 The intravenous urogram. Usual filming sequence for urography. **(A)** "Scout." **(B)** Early nephrogram phase when parenchyma is most radiopaque. **(C)** Five-minute radiograph to detect differential in function. **(D)** Large abdominal radiograph to visualize kidneys, ureters, and bladder obtained at 10 to 15 minutes. **(E,F)** Two oblique projections may be obtained over the kidneys only, or may include the ureter and bladder. **(G)** Postvoid radiograph may disclose unsuspected pathology in addition to providing information about residual urine. This sequence is by no means a rule and should be tailored to suit the individual patient.

indicates that there is either no contrast or no blood flow. The former would raise suspicion for extravasation of contrast at the injection site, which is why every injection must be monitored. The latter would suggest either that the blood is not circulating or that the glomeruli are not filtering (**Fig. 5–5**).

If the blood is not circulating, the patient requires urgent attention, as a full-blown contrast reaction with hypotension or even cardiopulmonary arrest may be under way, another reason why qualified personnel must be present while a patient is undergoing an examination using intravenous contrast

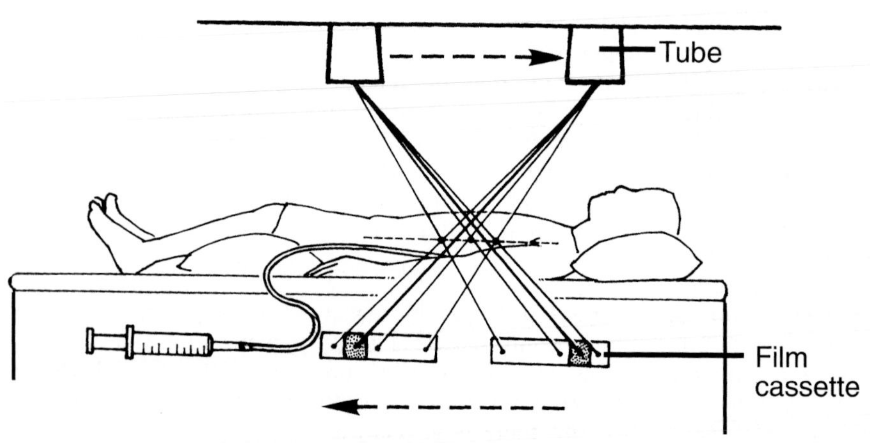

Figure 5–4 How tomograms are obtained during the intravenous urogram. The x-ray tube and film pivot around a focal plane in the abdomen centered on the kidneys, which produces clear images of the kidneys, with other abdominal structures anterior and posterior to them "blurred out" by motion.

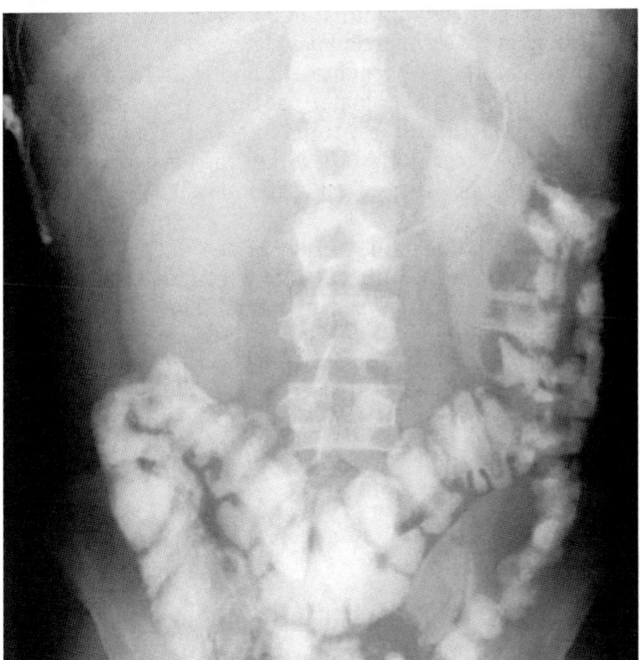

Figure 5–5 This abdominal radiograph was obtained 36 hours after a CT scan of the abdomen for which intravenous contrast was administered to this young man after a motor vehicle accident. The fact that the kidneys are still densely opacified likely indicates acute tubular necrosis. Note also a nasogastric tube in the stomach and residual oral contrast in the colon.

material. If the glomeruli are not filtering, it is likely that the renal tubular pressure distal to the glomeruli is elevated, as in acute obstruction (which would have to be bilateral), or the kidneys are no longer functional, as from chronic diabetes or hypertension. In the latter case, the patient would be in renal failure, and a urogram should not have been ordered.

A more likely scenario would be unilateral nonvisualization, failure to opacify one of the two kidneys. What could account for this? Again, obstruction, as from a stone in the ipsilateral ureter, would be the single most likely explanation. Other possibilities include unilateral renal agenesis, which is rare, or ectopia, such as a kidney unexpectedly located in the pelvis; complete renal artery obstruction due to thrombosis, embolus, or stenosis, which blocks inflow to the glomerulus; acute renal vein thrombosis, which blocks outflow from the glomerulus; and a disease process in the renal parenchyma, a congenital dysplasia, polycystic disease, or a tumor.

The change in the nephrogram over time is another valuable source of information. Normally, a peak plasma concentration of contrast is rapidly reached after contrast injection. Thereafter, both the plasma concentration and the density of the nephrogram fall linearly, with a half-time of ~1 hour. Hence the normal nephrogram exhibits a rapid peak in intensity followed by a linear decrease. The opposite pattern is the faint but gradually increasing nephrogram. Actually, the vascular causes of an "absent" nephrogram mentioned earlier typically produce a delayed nephrogram, which becomes increasingly dense over time. What appears initially to represent an absent nephrogram 3 minutes after injection usually turns out to be a delayed nephrogram, as the kidney slowly opacifies at 5, 15, or 60 minutes. This stems from the fact that, in vascular obstruction, GFR, though low, is not zero. The nephrogram becomes increasingly dense with time because what little iodine does make it into the renal tubule becomes increasingly concentrated as salt and water are reabsorbed. This same situation, the delayed but increasingly dense nephrogram, also typically occurs in the case of acute extrarenal obstruction (e.g., ureteral stone), where again, GFR is unlikely to be reduced all the way to zero (**Fig. 5–6**).

Another key nephrographic parameter is the parenchymal pattern. Suppose there is a single filling defect in the renal parenchyma; what might be the cause? A filling defect indicates a focal absence of functioning nephrons. Possible explanations would include a cyst, a space-occupying collection of

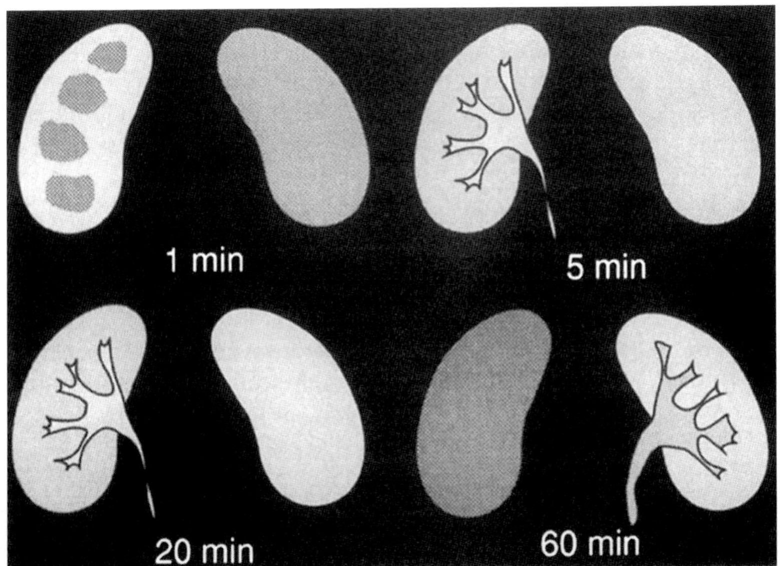

Figure 5–6 The expected urographic pattern in an acute left-sided ureteral obstruction. Note that while the right kidney passes almost completely through the nephrographic and excretory phases, the left kidney only becomes increasingly dense, with the eventual appearance of some contrast in the collecting system at 1 hour.

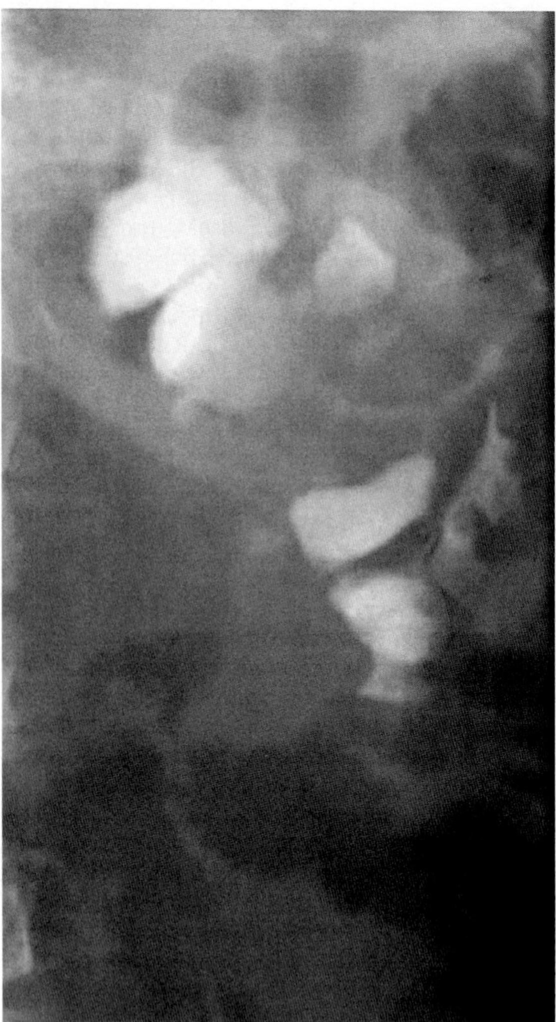

Figure 5–7 This view of the left kidney from an intravenous urogram demonstrates an unopacified central mass that is causing obstruction of the renal pelvis and resultant hydronephrosis, with dilation of the contrast-opacified renal calyces. This turned out to be a simple cyst.

fluid displacing adjacent nephrons; a tumor, such as a renal cell carcinoma; an abscess, which is sometimes surrounded by a rim of hypervascular granulation tissue; and trauma, such as a renal contusion (**Fig. 5–7**).

In the case of multiple filling defects, likely explanations include multiple idiopathic cysts (50% of patients older than 50 years have at least one), polycystic kidney disease, and multifocal pyelonephritis. A simple cyst will typically appear as a circular or oval defect occupying only a partial thickness of the renal parenchyma. Pyelonephritis, in contrast, extends from the innermost margin of the parenchyma, the papilla, to the outermost edge of the cortex, because the infection typically involves an entire lobe or lobule of the kidney.

The next phase of the urogram is the excretory phase, involving opacification of the pelvocalyceal system and the descending urinary pathways, including the bladder. Among the most important filling defects that may be detected in the excretory phase are stones, blood clots, cancer (especially transitional cell carcinoma), fungus, and papillary necrosis with sloughing of an infarcted papilla.

Another commonly encountered abnormality is a stricture, which is likely postinflammatory, as from previous impaction of a stone; infectious, most commonly from tuberculosis or schistosomiasis; or tumorous, either intrinsic (transitional cell carcinoma) or extrinsic (e.g., cervical cancer, with encasement of the ureter).

A common finding in the bladder aside from a filling defect is a thickened and/or trabeculated (irregular) bladder wall, indicating muscular hypertrophy or inflammation. Benign prostatic hypertrophy is the most common cause, which leads to compression of the prostatic urethra at the bladder base and resultant partial obstruction. Another common cause is cystitis, which may be secondary to infection (most commonly bacterial), drugs (especially cyclophosphamide), and radiation.

Nuclear Medicine

Although ultrasound, computed tomography, and magnetic resonance imaging have assumed an increasing role in the anatomic evaluation of the kidneys, nuclear medicine studies remain preeminent in the imaging evaluation of renal function. Examples of common clinical situations in which radionuclide imaging is used are renal artery stenosis, vesicoureteral reflux (discussed in Chapter 10), and collecting system obstruction. The four major renal parameters evaluated by radionuclide studies include renal blood flow, glomerular filtration, tubular function, and collecting system drainage.

Because the kidneys are positioned posteriorly in the abdomen, imaging is performed with the patient supine and the detector beneath the patient, producing images in the "posterior" projection. An exception is the post-transplant patient, whose kidney is typically located anteriorly in the pelvis and is therefore better evaluated with the detector positioned anteriorly. If ureteral drainage is of special concern, the patient may be imaged upright. In every case, immobilization of the patient is critical, because count acquisition takes place not over a period of milliseconds, but over seconds or even minutes. Over a period of 20 to 30 minutes, the movement of tracer from the blood to the renal cortex, from the renal cortex to the collecting system, and from the collecting system to the bladder can be assessed.

Blood Flow

An indication of the kidney's relative physiologic importance is the fact that at rest, the kidneys receive ~20% of the cardiac output, despite the fact that they represent only ~1% of body weight. The ideal agent for measuring renal blood flow (or plasma flow) would be one that is completely cleared from the blood during its passage through the kidney. In the laboratory, this is accomplished by the use of para-amino hippuric acid, the use of which yields an effective renal plasma flow of 500 to 600 mL/minute. The agents currently in use in nuclear medicine yield somewhat lower values of renal plasma flow and include technetium- (Tc-) 99m-DTPA and Tc-99m- MAG3. The measurement of renal plasma flow is based on the rate of disappearance of radiotracer from the blood. Typically, activity appears in the kidneys within several seconds of the time when the injected bolus of radiotracer reaches the abdominal aorta.

Renal plasma flow can be assessed using one of two fundamentally different techniques: the nonimaging serial quantitative assessment of radioactivity in the dose and plasma or by imaging methods. The former involves simply determining how much of the radioactivity has disappeared from the blood over a specified time interval. The latter involves the assessment of peak cortical activity, which can be compared from side to side to determine if one kidney is receiving more blood flow than the other. Such a determination is often critical, for example, in determining whether a patient with unilateral renal disease should undergo a nephrectomy. The greater the proportion of the patient's renal function supplied by the diseased kidney, the less attractive is nephrectomy.

Glomerular Filtration

Of the liter or so of blood flowing into the kidneys each minute, ~20% of the plasma (which constitutes 60% of the blood by volume) is filtered through the semipermeable membrane of the glomerulus, yielding an expected GFR of ~125 mL/minute. Filtration is not an active process, but occurs passively, based on differences in hydrostatic and oncotic pressures between the glomerular capillaries and the surrounding Bowman's capsule. Small molecular weight solutes pass freely across the glomerular basement membrane. Desirable agents for the assessment of glomerular filtration must be small enough to pass through the basement membrane, but not significantly protein bound (as plasma protein molecules are too large to be filtered). Tc-99m- DTPA is an excellent agent for the assessment of GFR, because it is small, only slightly protein bound, and undergoes no significant tubular reabsorption or secretion; thus, it only reaches the urine via glomerular filtration, and virtually all of the tracer that is filtered remains in the urine (**Fig. 5–8**).

Diseases that cause prerenal reductions in GFR include heart failure (with decreased cardiac output) and renal artery stenosis. Heart failure would be expected to cause bilaterally symmetrical reductions in GFR, whereas renal artery stenosis is usually asymmetrical in distribution. Causes of intrarenal reductions in GFR include chronic inflammatory conditions of the glomerulus, such as systemic lupus erythematosus, and hypertensive nephropathy. Examples of postrenal causes of decreased GFR include obstruction of the collecting system and descending urinary pathways.

◇ Renovascular Hypertension

A specific application of glomerular filtration imaging is the assessment of renovascular hypertension. More than 90% of cases of hypertension are primary or idiopathic; therefore, they cannot be traced to any anatomic abnormality; however, in a small percentage of cases, hypertension is secondary to diminished renal perfusion pressure, which causes production of renin by the cells of the juxtaglomerular apparatus. In the patient with renovascular hypertension, stenosis of one of the renal arteries results in diminished perfusion of the afferent arterioles, increased renin production, and resultant contraction of the smooth muscle cells surrounding the efferent arterioles, reducing the outflow of blood from the glomerulus and increasing intraglomerular hydrostatic pressure. Renin causes conversion of hepatically produced angiotensinogen to angiotensin I, which is then converted in the pulmonary capillaries to its active form, angiotensin II. Aside from causing constriction of the efferent arterioles, the active form of angiotensin also causes increased secretion of aldosterone by the adrenal cortex, promoting increased

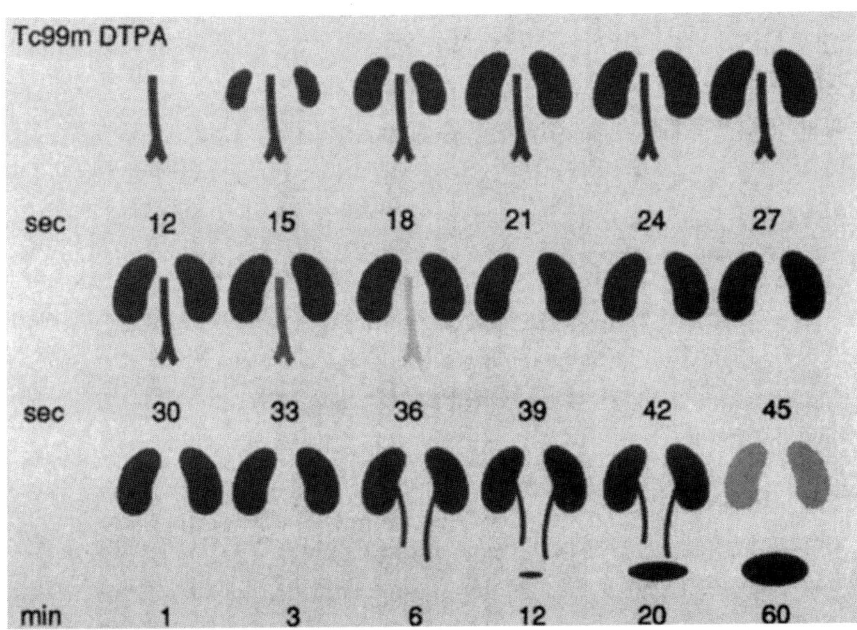

Figure 5–8 The expected distribution of radiotracer as a function of time elapsed after injection. Note that activity is first seen in the aorta, then the renal parenchyma, the renal collecting system, and finally in the bladder.

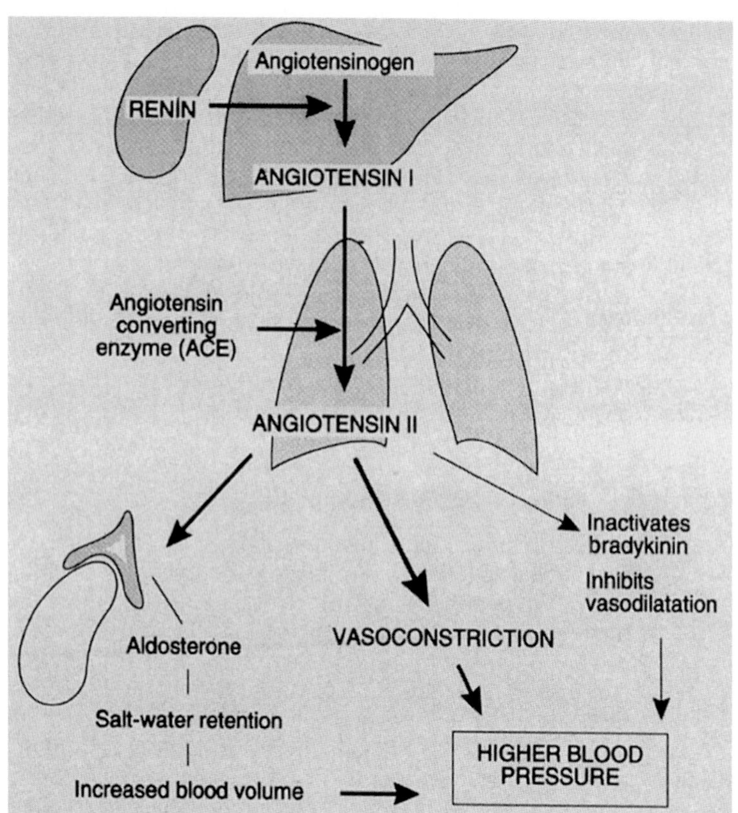

Figure 5–9 The renin–angiotensin axis, which provides the physiologic rationale for the use of an angiotensin-converting enzyme inhibitor in the diagnosis of renovascular hypertension.

systemic blood pressure, and thereby further augmenting renal perfusion (**Fig. 5–9**).

To determine whether one of the kidneys is affected by renal artery stenosis, renal perfusion can be assessed with and without the injection of an angiotensin converting enzyme (ACE) inhibitor, such as captopril. Absent ACE inhibitor injection, glomerular filtration in the affected kidney is relatively preserved, due to the increased glomerular hydrostatic pressure produced by efferent arteriolar constriction; however, when the ACE inhibitor is administered, glomerular filtration is reduced, due to a drop in glomerular perfusion pressure from relaxation of the efferent arteriole. Such a drop in the perfusion pressure of a kidney with ACE inhibitor administration is diagnostic of renal artery stenosis, which in many cases can be successfully treated by surgery.

Collecting System Drainage

Occasionally, the collecting system of a kidney is found to be dilated, but it is uncertain whether this represents obstruction. If attempts to drain the affected kidney by placing the patient upright are unsuccessful, a diuretic renogram may be performed. After the standard nuclear medicine renogram is performed, a dose of furosemide is administered. If activity promptly washes out of the dilated system, the dilatation of the collecting system is likely of little or no physiologic significance. On the other hand, if there is little or no washout of activity, the dilatation of the collecting system indicates a functionally significant obstruction (**Fig. 5–10**).

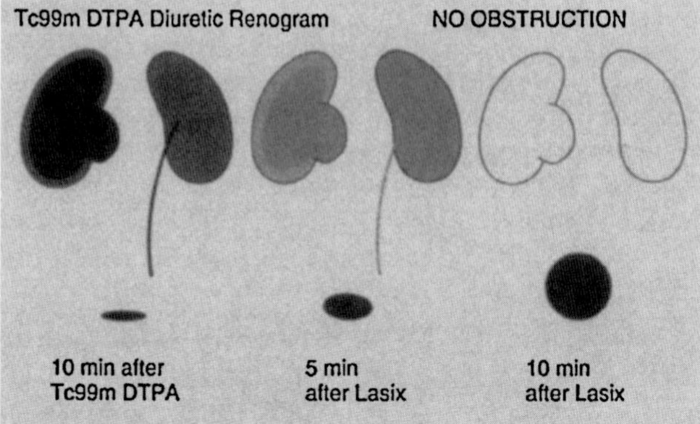

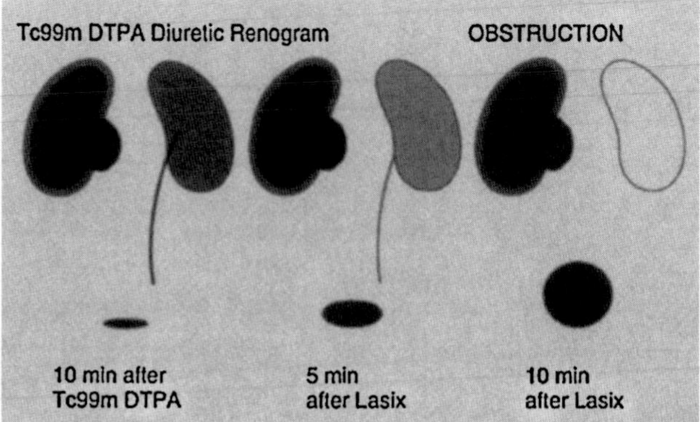

Figure 5–10 Diuretic renograms in two different patients demonstrate the expected appearance of a dilated collecting system **(A)** without obstruction and **(B)** with functionally significant obstruction of the left kidney.

Other Modalities

Renal imaging was dramatically enhanced by the introduction of the cross-sectional imaging modalities of ultrasound, CT, and MRI, which provide superior evaluation of the renal parenchyma compared with that of IVU and nuclear medicine. Ultrasound is the preferred modality to assess for urinary tract obstruction and evaluate the renal vasculature, whereas contrast-enhanced CT is best in detecting and evaluating renal tumor. Noncontrast CT is best for evaluating suspected urolithiasis. MRI is a good substitute for CT in patients who cannot tolerate iodinated contrast and provides superior tissue contrast. Both CT and ultrasound are commonly employed to guide renal biopsies. Both are also effective in guiding interventional procedures such as nephrostomy tube placement, where a catheter is placed percutaneously into a dilated renal collecting system to prevent permanent loss of renal function due to obstruction. Multidetector CT and MRI provide excellent assessment of renal vascular anatomy and tumor staging.

Excretory urography evaluates the collecting system and ureters, although obstruction may prevent sufficient opacification due to decreased renal contrast excretion. CT is generally superior to IVU. Pyelography (imaging of the collecting system and ureters) can be performed by either antegrade or retrograde techniques. Antegrade pyelography involves the placement of a nephrostomy catheter, followed by injection of iodinated contrast material. Retrograde pyelography is a urologic procedure performed by cystoscopic catheterization of the ureteral orifice, followed by retrograde contrast injection. CT and MRI also offer excellent visualization of the collecting system and ureters.

The bladder is commonly imaged during excretory urography, utilizing both pre- and postvoid views, and by CT, MRI, and ultrasound. Superior evaluation is provided by cystography, in which a Foley catheter is placed into the bladder via the urethra and used to instill iodinated contrast into the bladder lumen. Voiding cystourethrography evaluates the bladder outlet and urethra, and detects reflux into the ureters. Often, reflux may occur only during voiding, provoked by contraction of the bladder musculature and altered dynamics at the ureteral orifices. CT, MRI, and ultrasound can detect bladder neoplasms, and CT and MRI are commonly employed in staging. The urethra can be evaluated either by retrograde urethrography (after insertion of a catheter into the distal urethra) or during the voiding phase of a cystourethrogram, both of which utilize iodinated contrast material.

◆ Kidney

Pathology

Congenital

One of the most common congenital renal anomalies is a horseshoe kidney, so named because the lower poles of the kidneys are fused across the midline by an isthmus that may contain functional renal parenchyma or mere fibrous tissue (**Fig. 5–11**). It occurs in ~1 in 500 births and results from fusion of the inferior portions of the metanephric blastemas during embryogenesis. The isthmus causes incomplete ascent of the kidneys when they become "hooked" on the inferior mesenteric artery. It also causes rotational abnormalities, with the collecting systems positioned anteriorly instead of medially. The isthmus may interfere with normal urinary drainage, resulting in an increased risk of hydronephrosis and complications of stasis, such as infection and stone formation. The risk of renal malignancies is also increased. In general, the probability of finding reproductive tract anomalies in patients with congenital renal anomalies is relatively high. Imaging findings include an abnormal renal axis with the inferior poles located more medially than the upper poles, an abnormally anteroinferior location of the kidneys (predisposing them to injury in abdominal trauma), and demonstration of the isthmus, which may enhance with contrast administration.

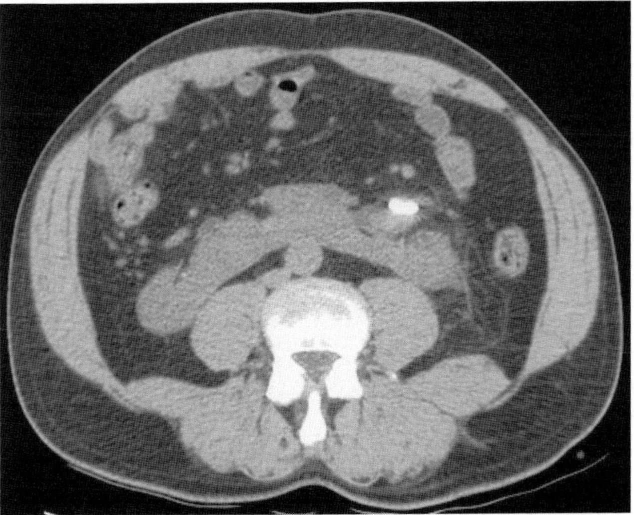

Figure 5–11 An axial image from a CT scan of the abdomen demonstrates an isthmus of tissue extending across the midline between the lower poles of the right and left kidneys, indicating a horseshoe kidney. Note also one of the complications of this condition, a stone in the left renal pelvis.

Polycystic kidney disease comes in two forms: autosomal recessive (infantile) and autosomal dominant (adult). Autosomal recessive polycystic kidney disease occurs in ~1 in 20,000 births and usually presents in the neonate or infant with enlarged and hyperechoic kidneys on ultrasound (**Fig. 5–12**). Death results from renal failure or hepatobiliary fibrosis. Autosomal dominant polycystic kidney disease has an incidence of 1 in 1000 and accounts for ~10% of patients on chronic hemodialysis. It results from cystic dilation of the nephrons and usually presents around the fourth decade of life with renal failure and enlarged kidneys. It is associated with hepatic cysts (75%) and intracranial berry aneurysms (10%). Common imaging findings include enlarged kidneys with a lobulated contour, innumerable renal cysts, some of which may be calcified, and stretching and deformity of the collecting system (**Fig. 5–13**).

Infectious

Pyelonephritis is the most common form of major urinary tract infection (UTI), with an annual incidence of ~5 cases in 10,000 persons, or 150,000 cases per year in the United States.

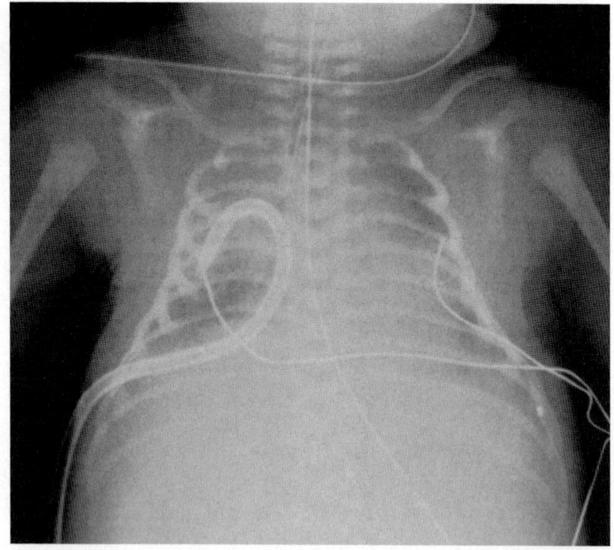

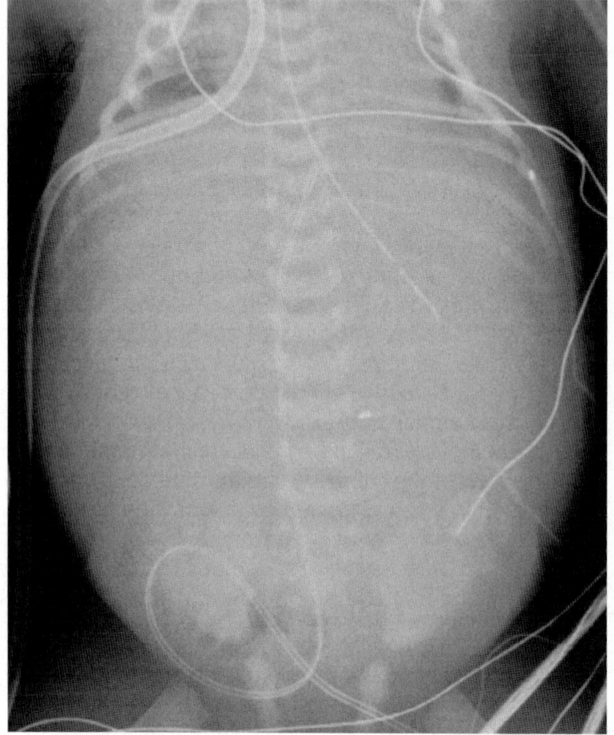

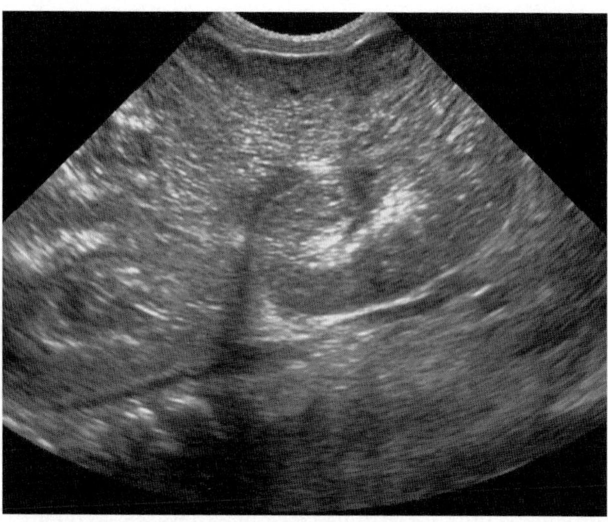

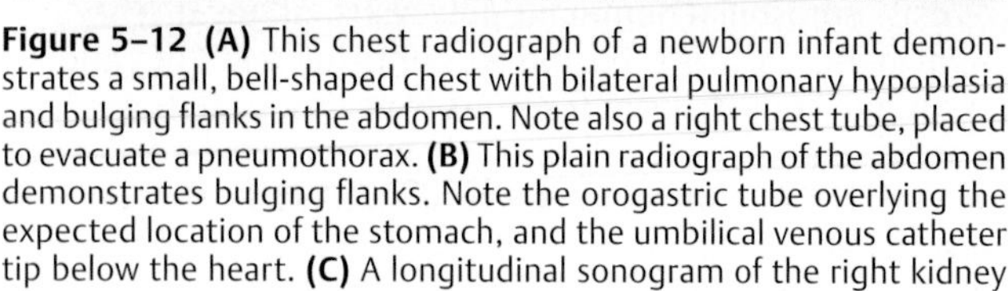

Figure 5–12 (A) This chest radiograph of a newborn infant demonstrates a small, bell-shaped chest with bilateral pulmonary hypoplasia and bulging flanks in the abdomen. Note also a right chest tube, placed to evacuate a pneumothorax. **(B)** This plain radiograph of the abdomen demonstrates bulging flanks. Note the orogastric tube overlying the expected location of the stomach, and the umbilical venous catheter tip below the heart. **(C)** A longitudinal sonogram of the right kidney (the left appeared quite similar) demonstrates marked nephromegaly, increased echogenicity, and lack of differentiation between renal cortex and medulla. Both the kidneys are twice as long as they should be, and because volume varies as the cube of length, each kidney is 8 times normal size. This patient has autosomal recessive polycystic disease, which caused oligohydraminos (most of the amniotic fluid being produced by the fetal kidneys), which in turn caused pulmonary hypoplasia.

Escherichia coli is the most common infecting organism. Most cases result from reflux of infected urine from the bladder into the kidney, so-called vesicoureteral reflux. Hematogenous seeding of the kidneys, in which *Staphylococcus aureus* is relatively more common, is another important route of infection. Pyelonephritis typically presents with the abrupt onset of fever, chills, and flank pain, with a predominantly neutrophilic leukocytosis. Urinalysis may show white cell casts, which are specific for pyelonephritis, and culture typically grows out the responsible organism. Xanthogranulomatous pyelonephritis is a more indolent form of renal infection that typically occurs in older women and simmers for months or even years prior to diagnosis. Patients may complain of low-grade constitutional symptoms such as fever and malaise,

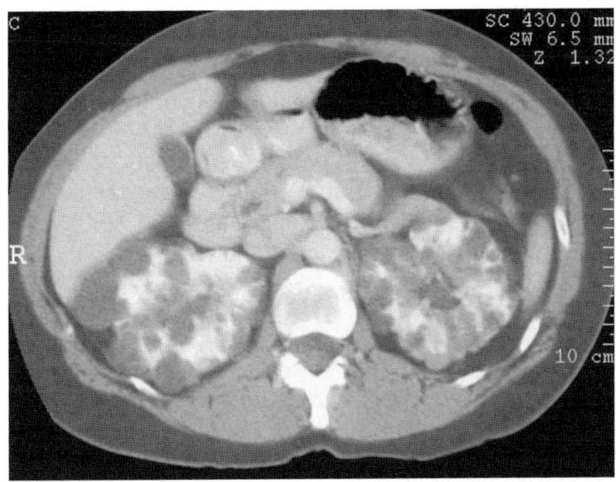

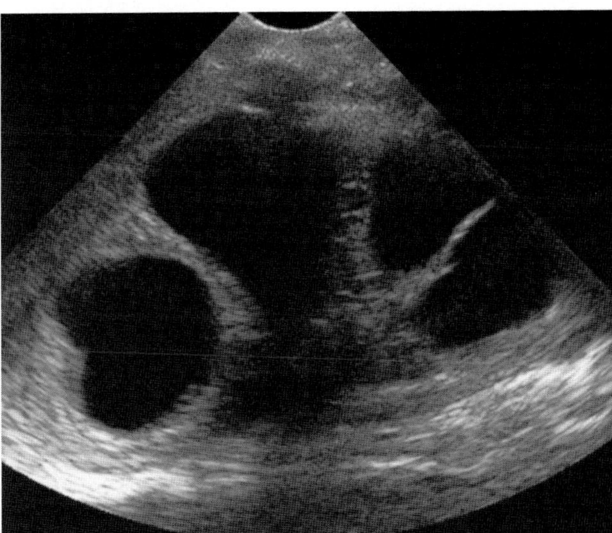

Figure 5–13 **(A)** This axial image from an abdominal CT scan after infusion of intravenous (IV) contrast demonstrates bilateral nephromegaly and innumerable bilateral renal cysts in this patient with autosomal dominant polycystic disease. **(B)** This longitudinal renal sonogram in another patient with autosomal dominant polycystic kidney disease demonstrates large cysts occupying much of the renal parenchyma.

and urinalysis is typically positive for white cells and proteinuria. There is a high incidence of large, branching "staghorn" calculi, and cultures usually grow out *E. coli* or *Proteus.*

Most patients with uncomplicated pyelonephritis do not require imaging and are treated with antibiotics based on their clinical presentation and laboratory findings; however, if a patient fails to respond within 3 days, or if an underlying condition such as diabetes or a known urinary tract stone is present, an imaging study is indicated to rule out predisposing conditions such as obstruction and complications such as abscess. Imaging studies are normal in many patients, although an especially suggestive finding is a striated nephrogram on IVU or CT (**Fig. 5–14**). CT with IV contrast is more sensitive than ultrasound in the detection of parenchymal inflammation, although sensitivity is approximately equal for the detection of abscesses, and ultrasound has the advantage that it requires no intravenous contrast material. MRI, which also requires no contrast material to demonstrate pyelonephritis and its complications, is playing a growing role.

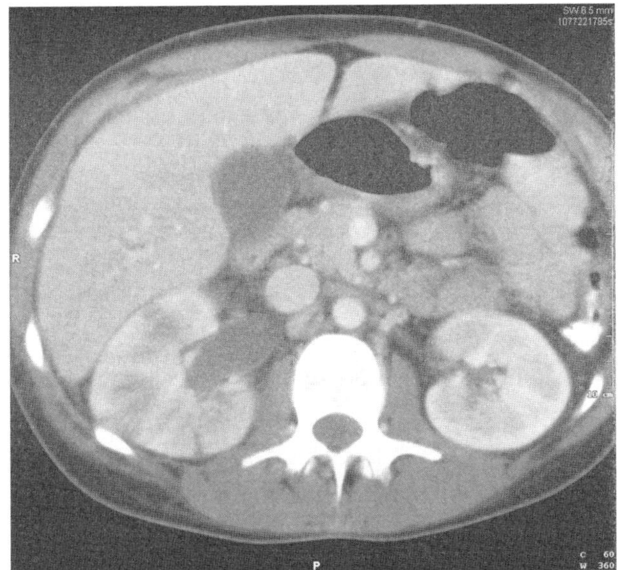

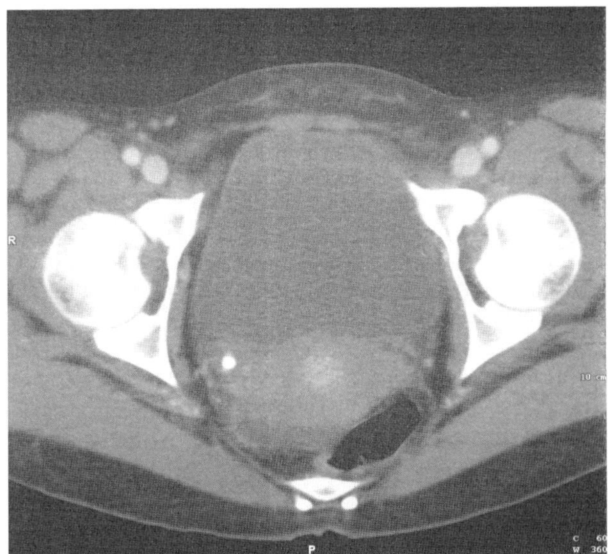

Figure 5–14 This patient presented with flank pain and high fever. **(A)** This axial image from an abdominal CT scan after IV contrast administration demonstrates a swollen right kidney with a striated pattern of contrast enhancement. Note the dilation of the right renal pelvis. **(B)** An image at the level of the bladder base demonstrates a calculus in the right ureterovesical junction, which was causing the right hydronephrosis and predisposed the right kidney to infection.

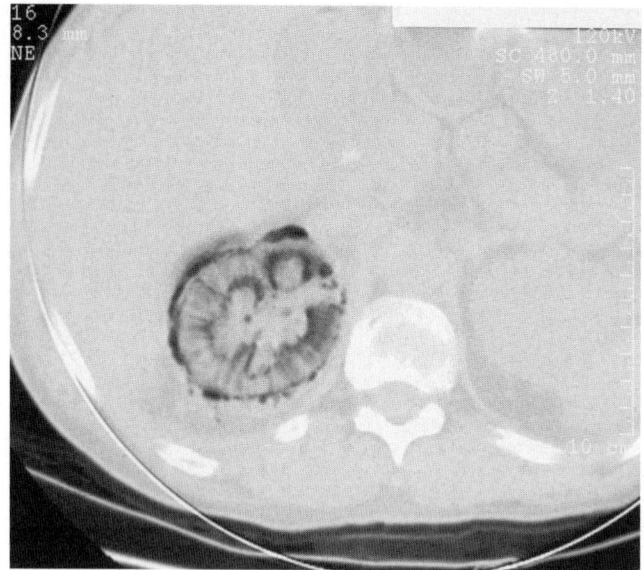

Figure 5–15 An axial image from an abdominal CT scan (viewed at lung windows to accentuate the finding) demonstrates gas throughout the tissue of the right kidney in this patient with emphysematous pyelonephritis.

Other than simple hydronephrosis indicating obstruction, a key imaging finding is the presence of pyonephrosis, which manifests as a pus–urine level in the collecting system on CT or ultrasound. Another key finding is the presence of gas within the renal parenchyma, so-called emphysematous pyelonephritis, which occurs with an especially high frequency in diabetic patients (90%) and women (70%) (**Fig. 5–15**). Emphysematous pyelonephritis represents a surgical emergency, due to its high mortality rate if untreated.

Tumorous

◇ Epidemiology

Approximately 30,000 cases of renal cell carcinoma are diagnosed each year in the United States, accounting for 12,000 deaths. The peak age of incidence is the sixth decade, and there is a male-to-female preponderance of 3:1. Most cases are idiopathic, but known risk factors include cigarette smoking, end-stage renal disease, and hereditary conditions such as von Hippel-Lindau disease. The latter, inherited as an autosomal dominant trait, includes cerebellar hemangioblastomas, retinal angiomas, and, in ~50% of patients, multiple renal cysts. The lifetime risk of developing renal cell carcinoma in these patients is nearly 100%, if they do not die first from other causes.

◇ Pathophysiology

Renal cell carcinomas are adenocarcinomas, most often of clear cell histology. They are usually hypervascular, and hemorrhage is a relatively frequent finding. Renal cell carcinoma, therefore, should be included in the differential diagnosis of hemorrhagic metastases elsewhere in the body. Typical sites of metastatic spread include the lungs, the skeleton (where lesions are characteristically lytic), the liver, and the brain. Central necrosis is also relatively common. One characteristic feature of renal cell carcinoma is its propensity to invade the renal veins, from which it may spread into the IVC, which is seen in ~5% of cases (**Fig. 5–16**). The tumor thrombus may even extend up the IVC and into the right atrium. This is an important preoperative finding, because it requires an operative approach that includes both the abdomen and the thorax.

◇ Clinical Presentation

About 10% of patients with renal cell carcinoma present with the classic triad of flank pain, gross hematuria, and a flank mass. Such a presentation implies advanced disease. Aside from hematuria, other common presenting symptoms and signs include constitutional complaints such as weight loss and fatigue, and more specific indications of renal pathology such as hypertension, secondary to hyperreninemia induced by vascular obstruction within the kidney. A small number of patients present with an enlarging left scrotal varicocele, a masslike collection of dilated veins around the testis. This results from the fact that the left gonadal vein drains into the left renal vein, which may be obstructed by tumor thrombus (**Fig. 5–17**). At least 30% of patients in whom renal cell carcinoma is detected are asymptomatic, their tumors detected incidentally on an ultrasound or CT performed for another reason. On laboratory evaluation, some patients may exhibit polycythemia secondary to increased erythropoietin production (again due to vascular obstruction by the tumor).

◇ Imaging

Imaging plays a crucial role in the detection and staging of these tumors. IVU still plays a role in the evaluation of hematuria in some institutions, and thus constitutes a gateway to the diagnosis of renal cell carcinoma. Diagnosis is based on the direct finding of a mass, which is often hypervascular, or based on indirect findings such as mass effect, with displacement of the pelvocalyceal system. CT is a more sensitive modality for the detection and staging of renal cell carcinoma. The mass is often hypervascular on contrast-enhanced images, and may also demonstrate areas of necrosis and hemorrhage. Sonography detects many tumors, but its primary role is in the differentiation of solid from cystic masses. Sonography also provides good assessment of vascular invasion, including the renal vein and IVC. Key staging criteria include the size of the mass, the presence or absence of extension beyond the renal capsule, lymph node involvement, vascular invasion, and the presence or absence of distant metastases.

The differential diagnosis of a renal mass is long. Aside from renal cell carcinoma, the diagnosis to be excluded in every case, several other masses merit brief discussion. The most common renal mass is a simple renal cyst. On CT, simple cysts should have an attenuation value near 0 Hounsfield

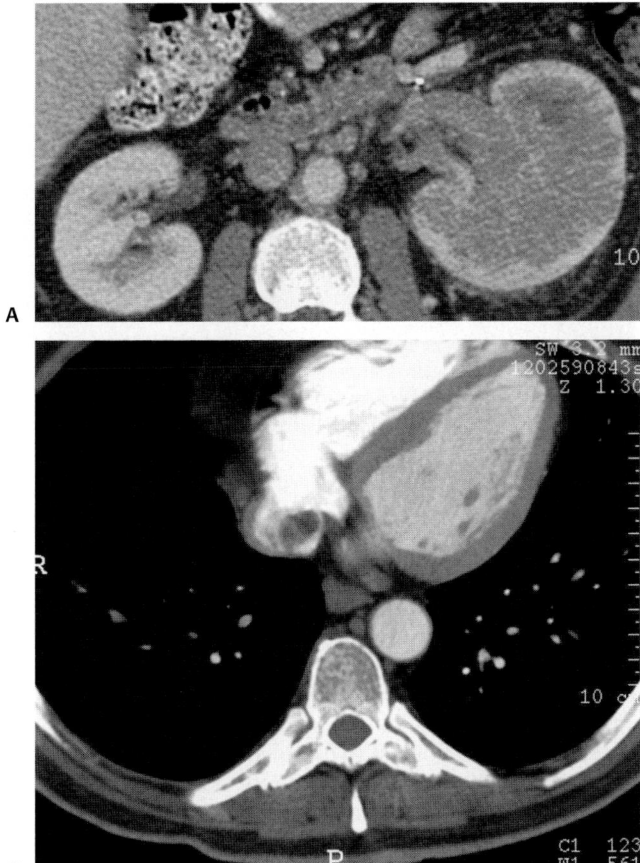

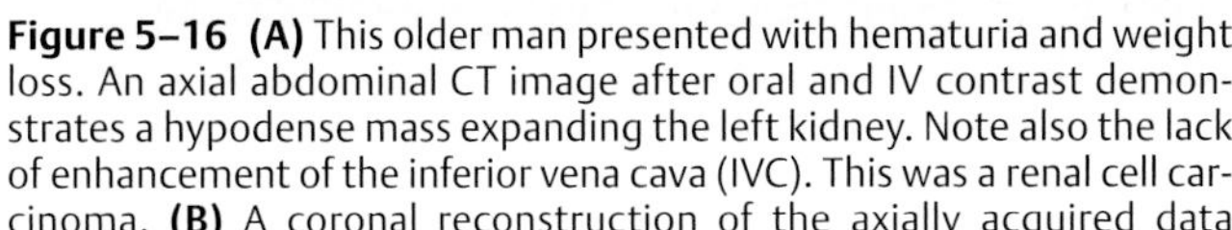

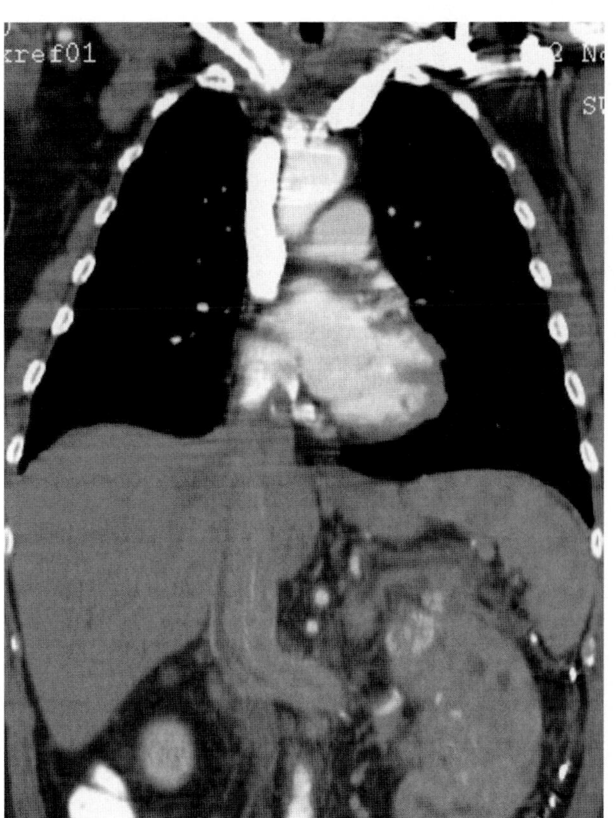

Figure 5–16 **(A)** This older man presented with hematuria and weight loss. An axial abdominal CT image after oral and IV contrast demonstrates a hypodense mass expanding the left kidney. Note also the lack of enhancement of the inferior vena cava (IVC). This was a renal cell carcinoma. **(B)** A coronal reconstruction of the axially acquired data demonstrates not only the heterogeneous left renal mass but also tumor thrombosis extending across the left renal vein and up the IVC. **(C)** This axial image at the level of the heart demonstrates that the tumor thrombus has extended all the way up to the right atrium, as shown by the filling defect.

units (HU) (the attenuation value of water) (**Fig. 5–18**). Characteristics of a simple cyst on ultrasound include anechoic luminal contents, an imperceptible wall, a distinct posterior border, and posterior acoustic enhancement. Posterior acoustic enhancement refers to the fact that the "water" in the cyst does not attenuate the beam, allowing structures posterior to it to produce stronger echoes. Moreover, the spherical shape of the cyst actually focuses the beam posterior to the cyst, likewise causing structures behind the cyst to appear more echogenic or "brighter" than they otherwise would.

Many cysts will contain blood or debris secondary to hemorrhage, in which case the diagnosis becomes more problematic. The situation is further complicated by the fact that a small percentage of renal cell carcinomas are cystic. The presence of a mural nodule within a cyst is suggestive of a malignancy. When imaging criteria of a benign cyst are not satisfied, ultrasound or CT may be used to guide aspiration or core-needle biopsy for tissue diagnosis, especially if the suspicion of malignancy is high (**Fig. 5–19**). Other lesions presenting as renal masses usually require biopsy or nephrectomy for diagnosis. Lesions typically undergoing nephrectomy include multilocular cystic nephroma, which presents as an intraparenchymal mass with multiple variably sized internal cysts, and oncocytoma, which often demonstrates a central scar on ultrasound or CT. Although both of these lesions are benign, nephrectomy remains the usual approach due to the inability to differentiate them preoperatively from a malignant tumor.

An exception to the general rule that tissue diagnosis is necessary is an angiomyolipoma, which, as its name implies, consists of vascular, muscular, and adipose tissue. It probably represents a hamartoma rather than a true neoplasm. These lesions are commonly found in middle-aged females, and in as many as 80% of patients with tuberous sclerosis. Tuberous sclerosis is a hereditary condition, inherited on an autosomal dominant basis, and is associated with a classic triad of mental retardation, seizures, and cutaneous lesions long referred to adenoma sebaceum (a misnomer). Central nervous system lesions include subependymal giant cell astrocytomas and cortical hamartomas. Most patients have renal involvement, with bilateral angiomyolipomas and perhaps cysts. The

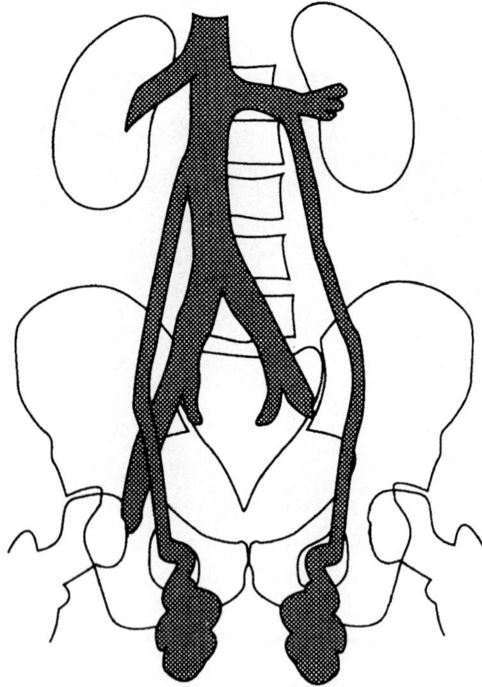

Figure 5–17 Bilateral varicoceles (palpable distention of the pampiniform venous plexus around the testis) and the venous drainage of each hemiscrotum. The fact that the left spermatic vein empties into the left renal vein, and the right empties directly into the inferior vena cava, explains the special tendency of left renal carcinomas with renal vein thrombosis to present with new-onset left-sided varicoceles.

angiomyolipoma is of interest because CT can definitively establish the diagnosis, based on the finding of fat attentuation tissue within the lesion (approximately -100 to -50 HU for fat; recall that water's attenuation value is 0 HU) (**Fig. 5–20**). The absence of fat does not prove that the lesion is not an angiomyolipoma, but its presence is highly reassuring.

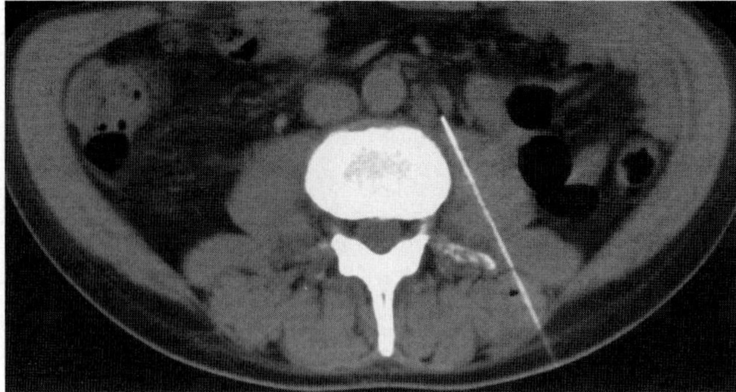

Figure 5–19 This axial CT image of a patient with a left renal mass (not shown) demonstrates a CT-guided biopsy of an enlarged periaortic lymph node. Note the biopsy needle tip in the node. The biopsy specimen contained renal cell carcinoma, indicating lymphatic spread of the tumor. Note that the biopsy was actually performed with the patient in the prone position, and the image has been inverted for ease of viewing.

Another important type of renal malignancy is a neoplasm arising in the collecting system, most often transitional cell carcinoma. Although these account for only ~10% of renal malignancies, they often present a distinctive imaging appearance, confined to the lumen of the collecting system. Moreover, it is important to establish that a renal tumor is a transitional cell carcinoma, due to the greatly increased risk of malignancy in the distal urinary tract. Often referred to as field carcinogenesis, this effect means that all portions of the urothelium are at increased risk of malignancy. Up to 80% of patients with transitional cell carcinomas will develop transitional cell carcinoma elsewhere in the urinary tract. Hence once a transitional cell carcinoma is detected, the remainder of the urinary tract must be carefully examined (**Fig. 5–21**). The differential diagnosis of a filling defect in the renal collecting system on excretory urography includes a transitional cell carcinoma, a blood clot, and a radiolucent

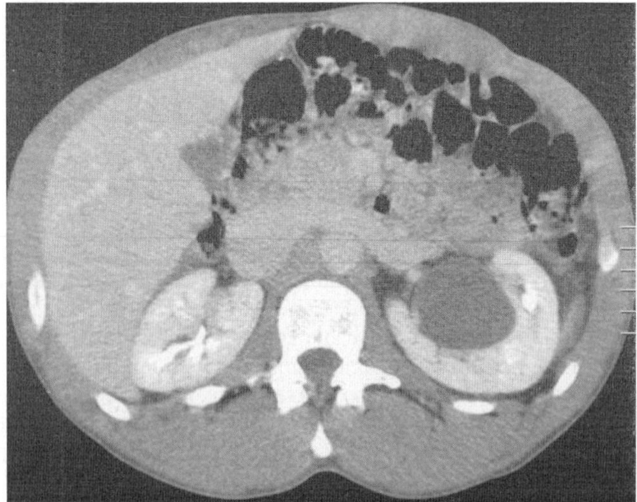

Figure 5–18 This axial image from an abdominal CT scan of the abdomen demonstrates a nonenhancing mass of the left kidney. Its walls are imperceptible, its borders are smooth, and its density was 0 Hounsfield unit, confirming a simple cyst of the renal pelvis.

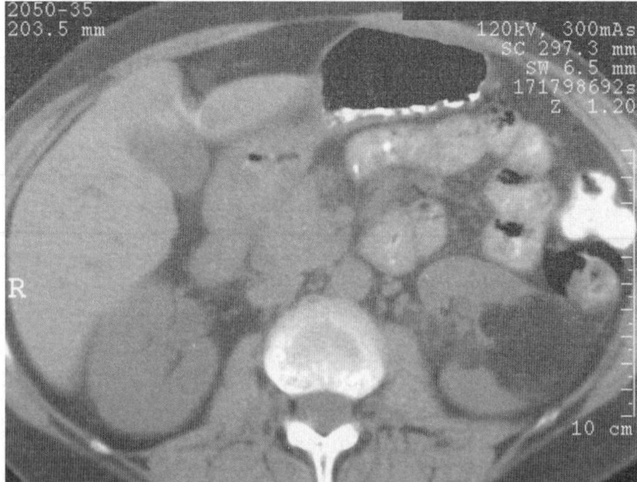

Figure 5–20 This axial image from an abdominal CT scan of the abdomen demonstrates a left renal mass with a density equal to that of intraperitoneal and subcutaneous fat, proving that the lesion represents an angiomyolipoma in this patient with tuberous sclerosis.

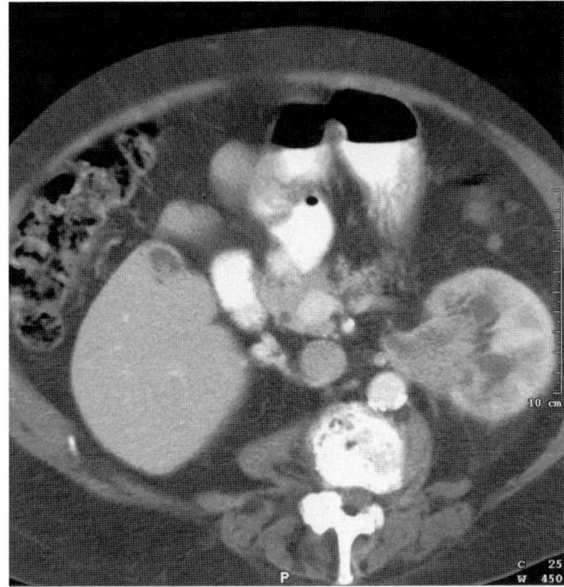

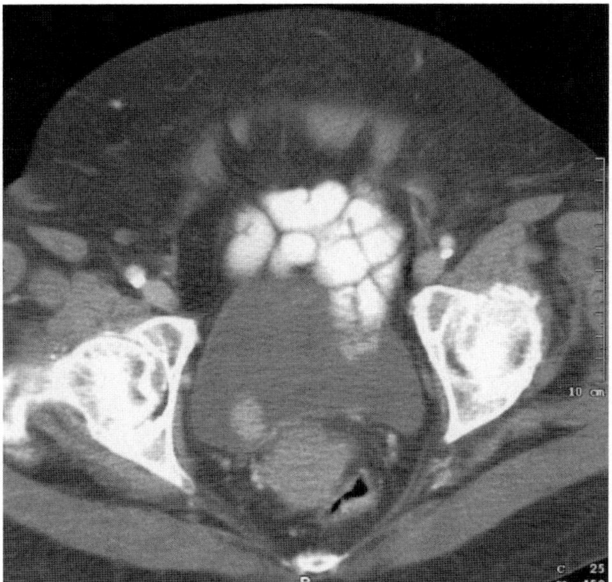

Figure 5–21 (A) This axial CT image demonstrates a heterogeneously enhancing mass of the left renal collecting system that is causing some hydronephrosis. **(B)** On an image of the pelvis, there is also an enhancing nodule of the posterior bladder wall. Both were transitional cell carcinomas in this 60-year-old woman with abdominal pain and microscopic hematuria.

calculus, although many other lesions, such as a sloughed renal papilla, are also possible.

Inflammatory

A wide variety of insults can, by the final common pathway of inflammation, produce the sonographic finding of diffusely hyperechoic kidneys. Common etiologies include glomerulosclerosis from hypertension or diabetes, infectious glomerulonephritis, infantile polycystic kidney disease, and acquired immunodeficiency syndrome (AIDS)–related nephropathy (**Fig. 5–22**). When the kidneys are not only echogenic but shrunken, the disease is chronic in nature, having had time to destroy renal tissue, and the patient will invariably suffer from some degree of chronic renal insufficiency. If the kidneys are asymmetrical in size and echogenicity, a unilateral process, such as reflux-related pyelonephritis or renal vein thrombosis, should be suspected.

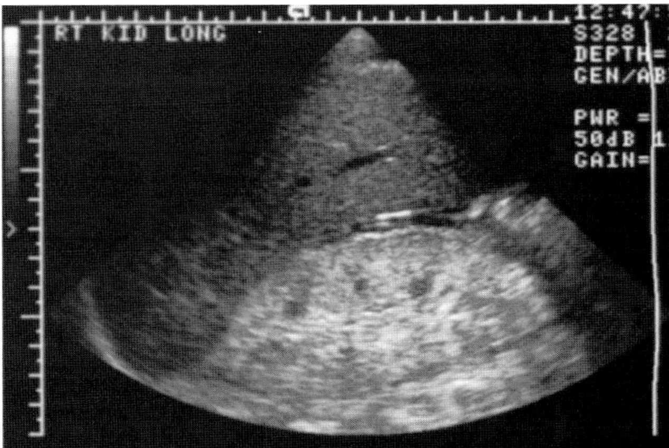

Figure 5–22 This longitudinal sonogram demonstrates a very echogenic right kidney behind the liver. Normally, except in infants, the kidneys should be less echogenic than the liver and spleen. In this case, both kidneys were much more echogenic, which was due to acquired immunodeficiency syndrome (AIDS) nephropathy.

Traumatic

Renal trauma is being managed in an increasingly conservative fashion. Imaging plays a crucial role in identifying the 80 to 90% of patients whose injuries do not require surgery. Minor injuries include hematomas, small lacerations, and small infarctions. Major injuries include renal rupture or masceration, vascular thrombosis, and renal pedicle avulsion. In the severely traumatized, unstable patient, a "one-shot" IVU is sometimes performed in the emergency room; contrast opacification of both kidneys rules out arterial thrombosis and pedicle avulsion. The study of choice to evaluate the trauma patient with possible renal injury is a contrast-enhanced CT scan, which evaluates not only the renal parenchyma and vasculature, but also the integrity of the collecting system and ureter (**Fig. 5–23**).

Vascular

Several renovascular disorders have been discussed in the nuclear medicine imaging section. Renal papillary necrosis is an additional vascular disorder that may be seen in patients with histories of flank pain, obstruction, or UTI. Papillary necrosis results from focal ischemia in the papillary portions of the renal pyramids, a region of relatively tenuous arterial supply. Common etiologic factors include diabetes mellitus, sickle-cell disease, infection, and heavy analgesic use.

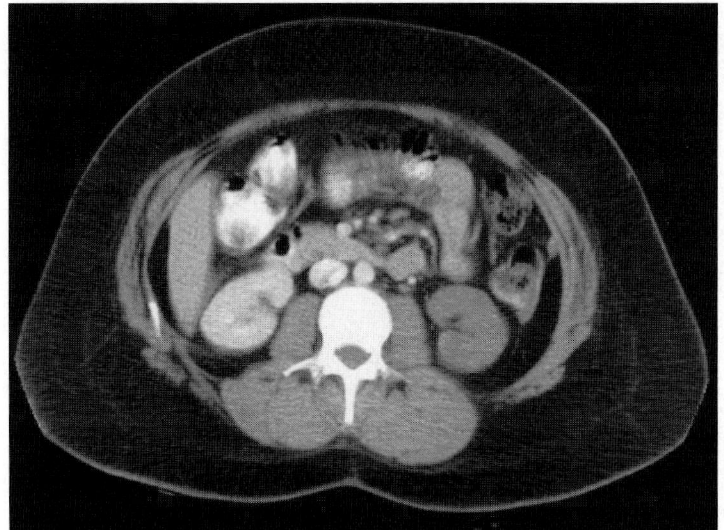

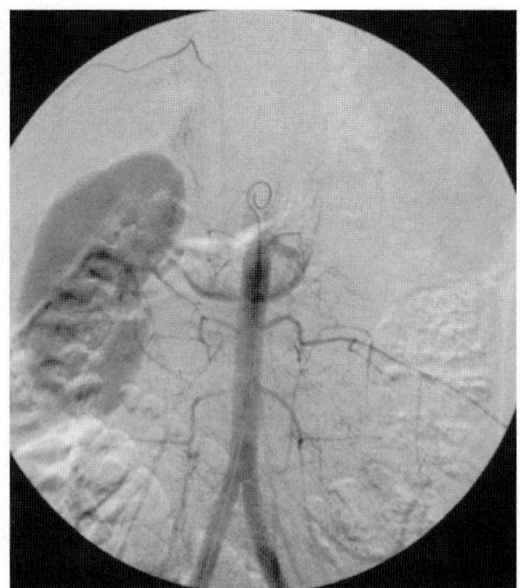

Figure 5–23 This 30-year-old man presented with hematuria and abdominal pain after a high-speed vehicular trauma. **(A)** An axial image from an abdominal CT scan with oral and IV contrast demonstrates normal-sized kidneys with no fluid collection, but the left kidney does not enhance. **(B)** A digital subtraction abdominal aortogram (note pigtail catheter tip just above renal arteries) demonstrates complete lack of enhancement of the left kidney. These findings indicate complete occlusion of the left renal artery, which prompted an emergent surgical procedure to restore blood flow.

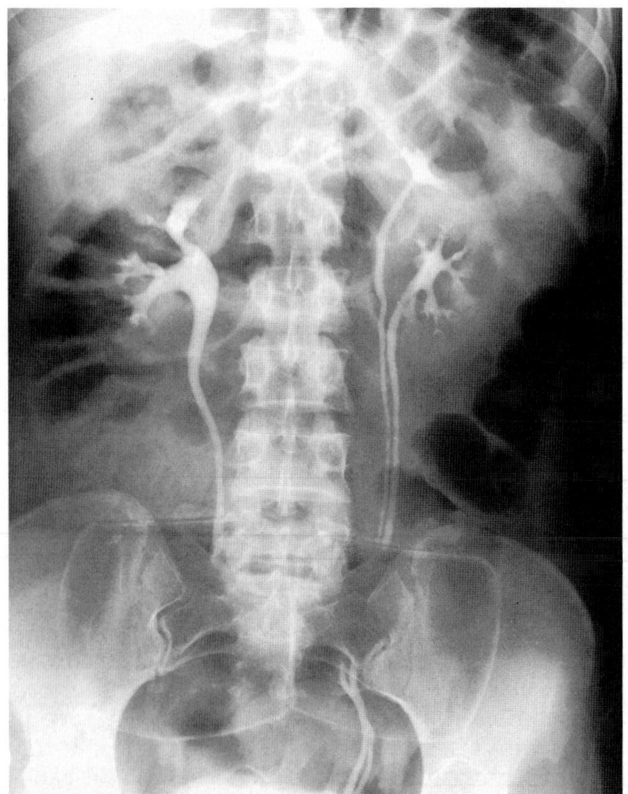

Figure 5–24 This abdominal radiograph from an intravenous urogram demonstrates a single right ureter but a complete left ureteral duplication, with the two left ureters extending down to the bladder, where their distal course was obscured by contrast in the bladder.

◆ Ureter

Pathology

Congenital

Ureteral duplication and congenital megaureter are two relatively common anomalies often detected in the adult. Ureteral duplication has an incidence of 1:200, and may be complete or incomplete (in the latter, the two ipsilateral ureters fuse before reaching the bladder) (**Fig. 5–24**). In complete duplication, the ureter arising from the lower pole joins the bladder at its normal location, while the upper pole ureter enters the bladder more inferomedially (ectopically), often resulting in obstruction and hydronephrosis. The incidence of ectopic ureter is approximately 6 times greater in females than males. Congenital megaureter results from a functional (not mechanical) obstruction of the distal ureter, somewhat analogous to achalasia in the esophagus. Both disorders are readily diagnosed by IVU or cross-sectional imaging.

◆ Bladder

Pathology

Infectious

Cystitis is an extremely common condition, with an annual incidence of 2 cases per 100 adults, or 5 million cases per year in the United States, although the incidence is even higher in the elderly. Run-of-the-mill acute cystitis most

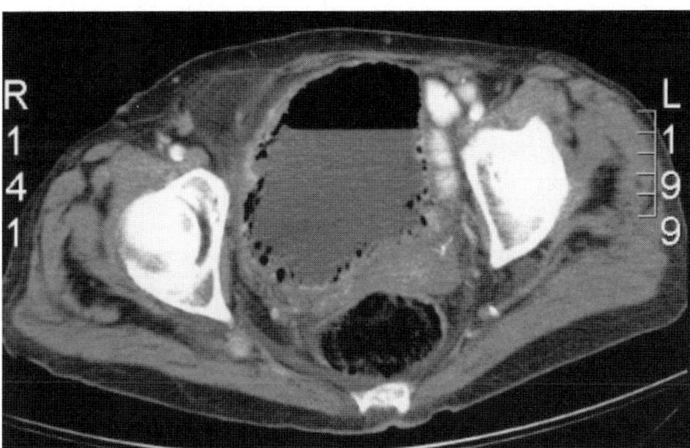

Figure 5–25 This elderly woman presented with severe dysuria. This axial image from a pelvic CT scan after IV contrast demonstrates an air–fluid level in the lumen of the urinary bladder, as well as gas bubbles throughout the bladder wall. The fact that these bubbles do not rise to the front of the bladder proves they are intramural, indicating emphysematous cystitis.

often results from infection by *E. coli*. Risk factors include instrumentation (commonly an indwelling Foley catheter), bladder outlet obstruction (commonly benign prostatic hypertrophy), calculi, and tumor. Patients present with complaints of abdominal pain, dysuria, frequency, and hematuria. Imaging findings include air within the bladder lumen (which can be a normal finding in patients with an indwelling bladder catheter), irregular bladder wall thickening, and stranding in the fat around the bladder. Gas in the bladder lumen may also indicate the presence of a fistula connecting to the vagina or rectum in patients who have undergone radiation therapy for cervical carcinoma. Emphysematous cystitis is a more dramatic form of cystitis, which causes gas within the bladder wall, and, like emphysematous pyelonephritis, is most commonly seen in diabetic women (**Fig. 5–25**). Fortunately, this condition responds readily to antibiotics and is not associated with significant mortality (in contrast to emphysematous pyelonephritis).

Tumorous

◇ Epidemiology

Bladder carcinoma is the fifth most common cancer diagnosis in the United States, with more than 50,000 cases and 10,000 deaths each year. The male:female ratio is ~3:1, and 90% of patients are over 50 years of age.

◇ Pathophysiology

Over 90% of bladder carcinoma is of the transitional cell type, with squamous cell carcinoma representing most of the remaining 10%. Recall that the normal epithelium of the bladder and ureter exhibits a transitional histology. Because transitional cell carcinoma is by far the most common type, it is the focus of this discussion.

Risk factors for transitional cell carcinoma include cigarette smoking (which increases risk 5 times), employment in the plastics industry, aniline dye exposure, previous pelvic radiation, cyclophosphamide therapy, and chronic infection. A patient with a history of previous transitional cell carcinoma of the upper urinary tract has an 80% probability of developing a tumor in the bladder, indicating that the carcinogenic effect is distributed throughout the urinary epithelium. The overall recurrence rate of the disease is greater than 50%.

◇ Clinical Presentation

Patients present with hematuria, increased urinary frequency (due in part to the reduction in bladder capacity produced by the space-occupying lesion), obstruction, and metastases. Cytology commonly discloses not only red cells but also malignant cells in the urine. The definitive diagnosis of bladder carcinoma is established via cystoscopy and biopsy, but radiology plays a major role in initially determining the presence or absence of a morphologic abnormality and in staging the disease.

◇ Imaging

Key imaging findings, whether on IVU, CT, ultrasound, or MRI, include a filling defect in the bladder lumen or irregularity or mass of the bladder wall (**Fig. 5–26**). When a filling defect is seen, other diagnostic possibilities include prostatic hypertrophy with a prominent impression on the base of the bladder, blood clot, calculus, and a ureterocele. Once the histologic diagnosis has been established, a key role of the radiologist is to stage the tumor. Aside from CT assessment of metastatic deposits in the lymph nodes, lung, liver, and bones, local tumor extent can be assessed according to tumor morphology. For example, the tumor may be pedunculated (on a stalk), which generally indicates a lower probability of bladder invasion. On the other hand, a sessile tumor associated with adjacent wall thickening is likely to have penetrated deep into the bladder wall. If the tumor is confined to the bladder, the integrity of the fat planes around the bladder should be preserved.

◆ Common Clinical Problems

Hematuria

◇ Epidemiology

Microscopic hematuria is a common clinical problem, found in 10 to 15% of men older than 35 years of age and women older than 55 years of age. Microscopic hematuria is defined as at least three to five red blood cells per high power field. From a strictly physiologic point of view, the finding of any red cells in the urine represents an abnormality, inasmuch as the vascular and urinary pathways should be completely separate; however, it is well known that vigorous exercise alone is sufficient to produce at least microscopic hematuria in otherwise healthy patients. As a screening test, chemical assays for hemoglobin are often substituted for microscopic examination, and more precise quantitation of the number of red blood cells per high power field is reserved for patients with chemical abnormalities.

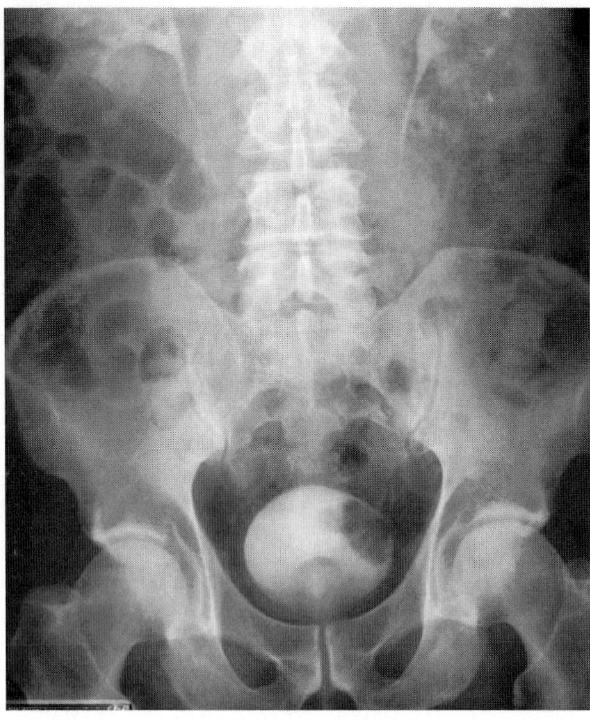

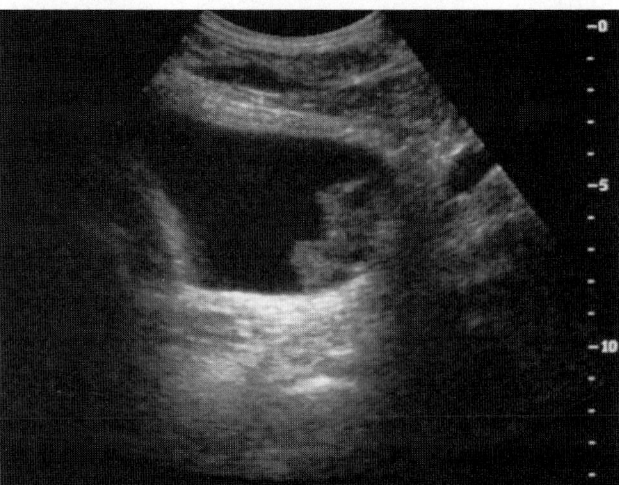

Figure 5–26 **(A)** This abdominal radiograph from an intravenous urogram demonstrates a large polypoid filling defect in the left side of the urinary bladder. **(B)** This transverse sonogram of the urinary bladder demonstrates the polypoid mass along the bladder wall. This was proven on cystoscopy to be a transitional cell carcinoma. The patient presented with hematuria.

◇ Pathophysiology

The distinction between gross and microscopic hematuria proves clinically useful, in that the frequency of various diseases varies between the two, as does the probability of serious disease. Gross hematuria is generally more serious than its microscopic counterpart, and nearly two thirds of patients will have a source in the bladder or prostate gland. Cystitis, bladder neoplasm, prostatic hypertrophy, prostatitis, and renal pathologies, including neoplasm, constitute the most common diagnoses. Almost 60% of patients with gross hematuria have marked abnormalities, and up to 20% have life-threatening disorders, such as carcinoma.

In the setting of microscopic hematuria, bladder disease is relatively less common, accounting for only 10% of cases. The prostate gland is the most common source, with the urethra (especially urethritis) second. In microscopic hematuria, no cause is found in over one third of patients, and only 20% of patients have a marked abnormality. The incidence of life-threatening pathology is only ~4%. Hence the key distinction between gross and microscopic hematuria is that a kidney or bladder neoplasm is many times more likely to be the source in gross hematuria.

◇ Clinical Presentation

A variety of laboratory tests can assist in the workup of hematuria. The finding of protein in the urine suggests glomerulonephritis with inflammation-associated increased capillary permeability as the etiology. Urine culture and microscopic examination for leukocytes may reveal a UTI. In concert with hematuria, pyuria often indicates hemorrhagic cystitis. Urine cytology may demonstrate sloughed malignant uroepithelial cells. Cystoscopy and retrograde endoscopic examination of the ureter and renal collecting system enable direct visualization and biopsy of lesions.

◇ Imaging

A young woman whose symptoms of hemorrhagic cystitis resolve after appropriate antibiotic therapy generally requires no further evaluation. In the workup of older patients with unexplained hematuria, imaging is a logical first step, because the pretest probability of a serious disorder such as malignancy is elevated. As a general rule, in patients younger than 40 years of age, the incidental finding of microscopic hematuria probably does not warrant further urologic investigation; however, over age 50, when the incidence of a serious disease such as bladder cancer has increased nearly 100 times, a more aggressive approach to diagnostic evaluation is warranted. When imaging is undertaken, its principle goal is to detect, localize, and if possible, characterize any morphologic abnormality. Many abnormalities, such as urinary tract calculi and simple cysts, can be characterized as benign based on imaging criteria alone. When a lesion's features are equivocal in terms of benignity, imaging localization may direct further urologic examination (such as cystoscopy) and also provide guidance for biopsy.

The preferred tests in the radiologic evaluation of hematuria, discussed earlier, are ultrasound, CT, and MRI

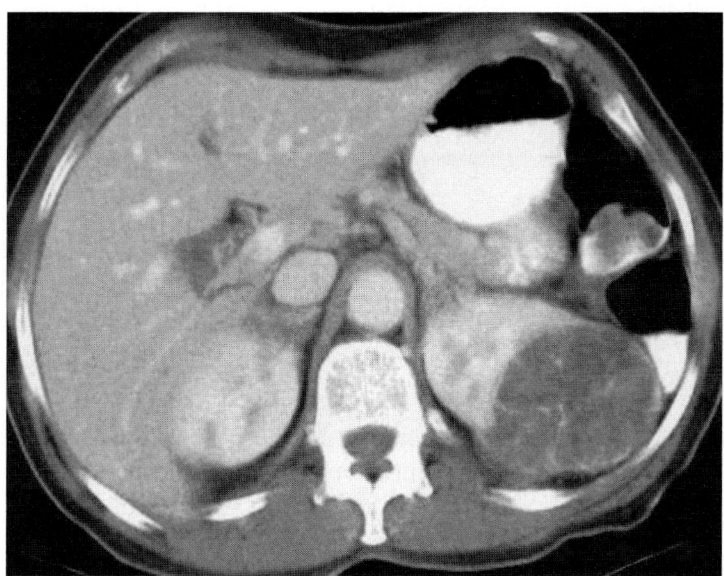

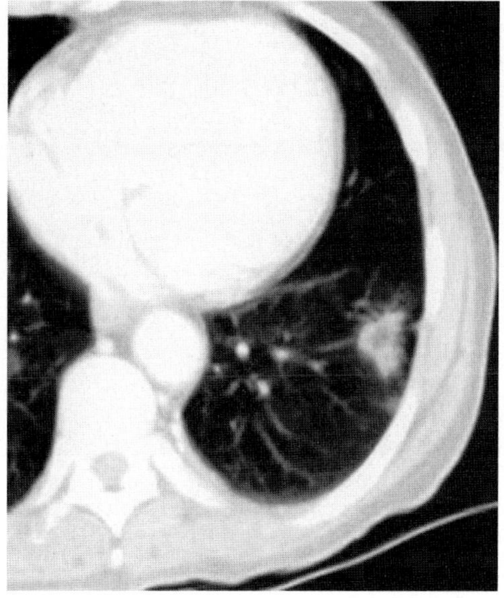

Figure 5–27 This older patient presented with gross hematuria. **(A)** An axial image from an abdominal CT scan with oral and IV contrast demonstrates a large, heterogeneous left renal mass that was proven at surgery to be a renal cell carcinoma. **(B)** Staging lung CT demonstrated this cavitary left lung nodule. Biopsy demonstrated not metastatic renal cell carcinoma, but bronchogenic carcinoma, reminding us that cigarette smoking is a risk factor for both.

(**Fig. 5–27**). In general, ultrasound or MRI will be preferred in patients in whom the use of intravenous contrast material is contraindicated due to renal disease, heart disease, a history of adverse contrast reactions, or other factors.

Acute Renal Failure

◇ Epidemiology

Acute renal failure has an incidence of ~3 per 10,000 patients admitted to hospitals. Chronic renal failure, by contrast, has an incidence of 2 per 10,000 population, and over 300,000 people in the United States are afflicted.

◇ Pathophysiology

Classically, acute renal failure is divided into three categories: prerenal causes, renal causes, and postrenal causes. Prerenal causes of acute renal failure center on a diminished flow of blood to the nephron, and include decreased circulating blood volume due to hemorrhage, congestive heart failure (CHF), hypotension, and renal artery stenosis. A clue to the prerenal nature of the failure is contained in the ratio of serum blood-urea nitrogen (BUN) to creatinine. Both substances, major metabolic waste products excreted by the nephron, are freely filtered at the glomerulus, but urea is reabsorbed by the peritubular capillaries. Decreased peritubular perfusion causes impaired urea reabsorption, and BUN increases disproportionately to creatinine. Generally, it is possible to determine if a patient is suffering from prerenal causes of acute renal failure based on clinical grounds, including not only the BUN/creatinine ratio, but a history of hypotension or CHF, including accumulation of excess fluid within body tissues.

Intrinsic renal causes of acute renal failure include acute tubular necrosis (ATN) and acute glomerulonephritis. In hospitalized patients, ATN accounts for the majority of cases. In community-acquired acute renal failure, acute glomerulonephritis is relatively more common. In all types of intrinsic renal disease, there will be a decline in the kidney's ability to concentrate urine. Hence the patient with intrinsic acute renal failure will excrete a relatively dilute urine, while the patient with prerenal disease (whose concentrating ability is relatively unimpaired) will excrete a highly concentrated urine.

From the point of view of diagnostic imaging, the most important causes of acute renal failure are postrenal. Up to 25% of patients with acute renal failure suffer from urinary tract obstruction. To cause a significant alteration in BUN and creatinine, the output of both kidneys must be obstructed. In rare cases, this may result from bilateral ureteral obstruction, as seen in diffuse retroperitoneal processes such as lymphoma or retroperitoneal fibrosis; however, a far more common cause is urethral obstruction, especially that secondary to prostatic enlargement. This diagnosis can be readily confirmed by ultrasound examination to determine if the bladder is distended, or even more readily, by passing a Foley catheter into the bladder, which should promptly restore normal urine output. In the case of a patient with an indwelling bladder catheter who becomes anuric, the catheter may be obstructed, often secondary to blood clot.

◇ Clinical Presentation

Acute renal failure typically manifests first by oliguria (the production of <400 mL of urine per day), followed by a rise in the BUN and creatinine. It should be noted, however, that patients in renal failure may continue to produce normal or even increased volumes of urine; however, most will have lost the ability to concentrate urine to the normal degree.

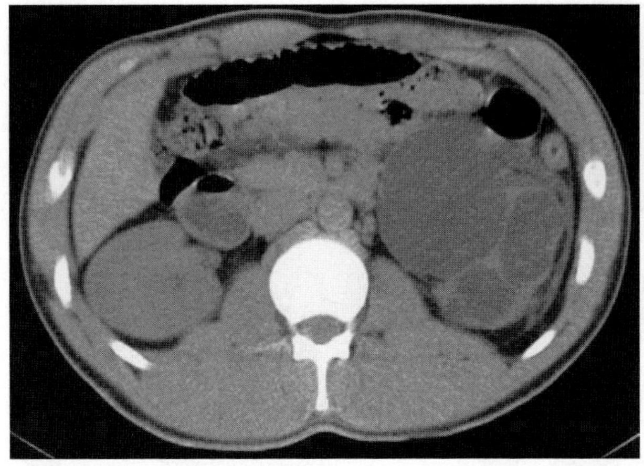

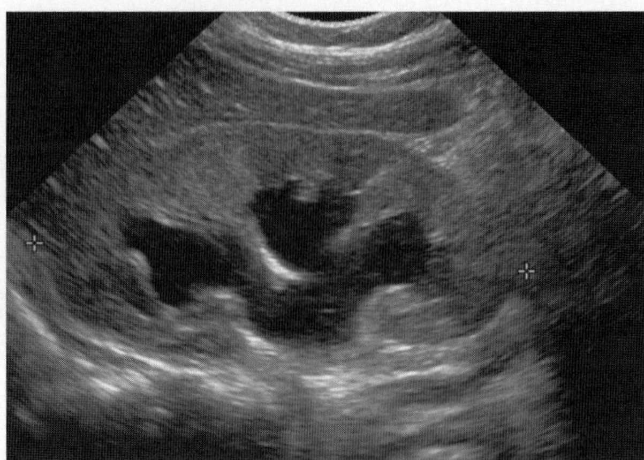

Figure 5–28 (A) This axial image from an abdominal CT scan demonstrates severe left hydronephrosis, due to a left ureteropelvic junction stenosis. If such findings were present bilaterally, the patient might well be in renal failure. **(B)** This longitudinal renal sonogram in another patient demonstrates moderate hydronephrosis, with dilation of the renal pelvis and calyces.

◇ Imaging

The principal reason that ultrasound examinations are routinely obtained in patients presenting in acute renal failure is to exclude the possibility of a postrenal (obstructive) cause. Ruling out obstruction is critical for two reasons. First, obstruction, as distinct from prerenal and intrinsic renal disorders, is generally a surgical problem, as opposed to a medical problem. Moreover, postrenal pathologies are often readily and completely reversible through relief or correction of the anatomic lesion. In all cases of postrenal acute renal failure of sufficient duration, ultrasound examination should reveal signs of hydronephrosis, with dilatation of the renal collecting system secondary to increased pressure proximal to the obstruction (**Fig. 5–28**). When the ureters are also dilated, it is called hydroureteronephrosis.

Assessment of renal echogenicity is important, because the finding of echogenic kidneys tends to indicate intrinsic renal disease. The size of the kidneys is also important. Normal-sized or enlarged kidneys indicate a good probability that the disorder may still be reversible. If the kidneys are small and echogenic, the condition is likely to be irreversible.

Acute Flank Pain

The patient presenting with acute flank pain is generally evaluated for the presence of urolithiasis and pyelonephritis; however, another relatively common cause of acute flank pain is the back itself, including muscle strain and degenerative disease of the spine. Additional differential diagnostic considerations include appendicitis, dissecting or ruptured aortic aneurysm, bowel obstruction or ischemia, and retroperitoneal fibrosis, among numerous other possibilities. True urinary tract pain is generally associated with symptoms such as dysuria, urinary frequency, and urgency. Like all colicky pain, discomfort tends to wax and wane, and patients move about, complaining that they cannot get comfortable. The key to differentiating renal pathology from other causes of abdominal and back pain is the urinalysis. If hematuria or pyuria is not present, the pain is less likely to be of urinary tract origin.

Urolithiasis

◇ Epidemiology

The formation of renal calculi is an extremely common problem in the United States, affecting at least 1 of every 20 persons at some time during their lives. There is a definite male preponderance, and the condition becomes more prevalent with age. Once a patient has suffered a bout of urolithiasis, the lifetime probability of recurrence is 50 to 70%, making prior urolithiasis one of the most important elements in a good history of the suspected stone patient. Conditions predisposing to stone formation include infection, hypercalcemia, renal tubular acidosis, and hyperoxaluria, among others.

◇ Pathophysiology

Approximately 70% of kidney stones are formed of calcium oxalate, 15% of struvite (magnesium ammonium phosphate), 10% of uric acid, and 5% of calcium phosphate. The vast majority of calcium oxalate stones are considered idiopathic. Crohn's disease is an example of a condition that predisposes patients to form oxalate stones. Dietary oxalate is normally complexed with calcium in the gut, but the fat malabsorption associated with Crohn's disease causes lipid saponification of calcium, meaning that oxalate passes unbound into the colon, where it is absorbed into the blood. The oxalate is then excreted in large amounts in the urine, where it causes stone formation.

Any condition that increases urinary calcium concentration will contribute to calcium stone formation. An example is type I renal tubular acidosis, in which urine pH remains fixed above 5.5 and there is a leak of calcium into the urine, with an associated deficiency of one of the most important stone inhibitors, citrate. Struvite stones are associated with infection by urea-splitting organisms such as *Proteus* and

Pseudomonas, with an increase in urine pH. Struvite stones may become particularly large, forming a cast of the collecting system, and are then referred to as staghorn calculi. As distinct from the other major types of stones, uric acid stones are often radiolucent. They are associated with low urine pH, which decreases the solubility of uric acid. Common predisposing conditions include gout, hemolytic anemia, and myeloproliferative disorders, the latter two secondary to cell lysis.

The management of urolithiasis begins with adequate hydration and analgesia, generally employing narcotics. At least 80% of stones will pass spontaneously, and no further intervention is required. Virtually all stones less than 0.5 cm in diameter pass without any medical or surgical assistance. Those larger than 1 cm usually require surgical removal. This is often accomplished via ureteroscopically guided crushing and extraction of the stone. Extracorporeal shock-wave lithotripsy relies on the use of focused shock waves to pulverize stones without surgery. Complications of stones include infection due to stasis, calyceal perforation, and the development of chronic obstruction, with associated loss of nephrons and irreversible loss of renal function.

◇ Clinical Presentation

Urolithiasis is the most common cause of both acute urinary tract obstruction and acute flank pain. Renal colic refers to spasms of intense pain that begin in the region of the flank and radiate into the groin. The pain results from spasms of ureteral smooth muscle, generated by the ureter's attempt to overcome the distention and increased intraluminal pressure caused by obstruction. Other common presenting symptoms include urinary urgency and frequency. The differential diagnosis of an obstructing lesion in the urinary tract includes blood clot, tumor, sloughed papilla, and extrinsic compression.

◇ Imaging

Imaging may begin with a high-quality abdominal plain film, which will often reveal a calculus (**Fig. 5–29**). Stones must generally measure at least 2 mm in diameter and contain some calcium to be visible by plain film. Ureteral calculi tend to lodge at one of three positions: the uteropelvic junction (UPJ; the pelvic brim), and the ureterovesical junction (UVJ), the latter being the most frequent (**Fig. 5–30**). In the appropriate clinical setting, the finding of a calculus in the distribution of the urinary tract, particularly at one of these locations, is strongly suggestive of urolithiasis. Mimics of urinary calculi include gallstones, phleboliths, and calcified mesenteric lymph nodes.

Intravenous urography is still employed in some centers in the evaluation of stones, and in such settings many stones are first detected on the "scout" film (precontrast administration)

A

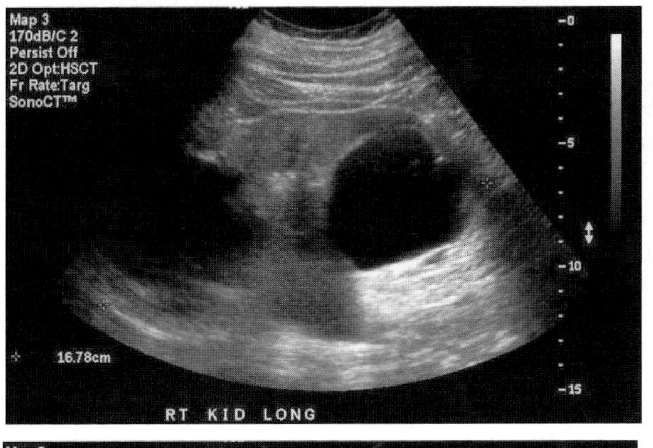

B

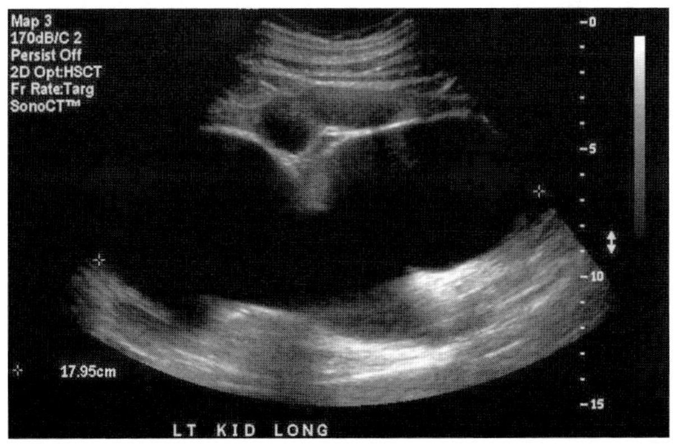

C

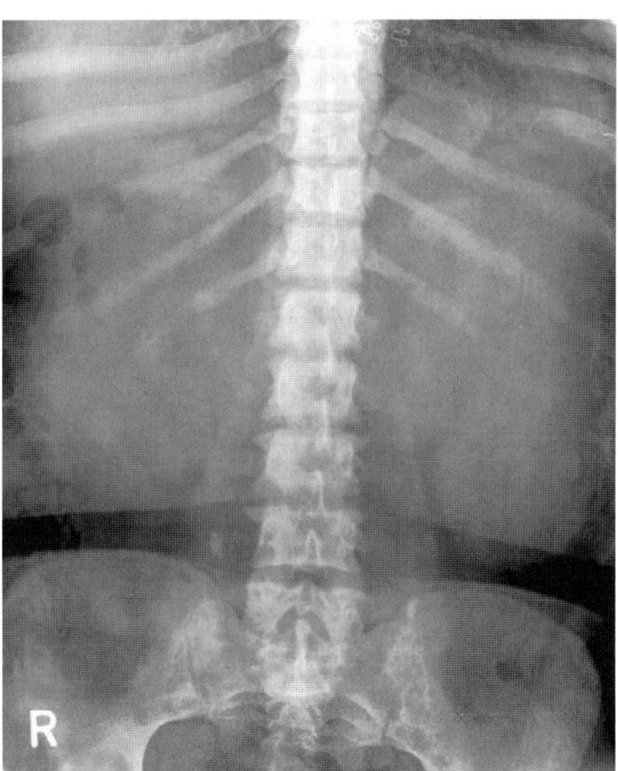

Figure 5–29 This middle-aged woman presented with several months of low back pain. **(A)** A longitudinal sonogram of the right kidney demonstrates severe hydronephrosis. **(B)** A longitudinal sonogram of the left kidney demonstrates even more severe hydronephrosis. What is the most common cause of bilateral hydronephrosis? In men, the answer would be a prostatic mass causing bladder outlet obstruction, most often benign prostatic hyperplasia. In women, a pelvic mass would be more likely, but in this case urolithiasis was the culprit. **(C)** This plain radiograph demonstrates bilateral stones in the expected locations of the ureters. The one on the right is just lateral to the fourth lumbar vertebra, and the one on the left is just above the sacroiliac joint.

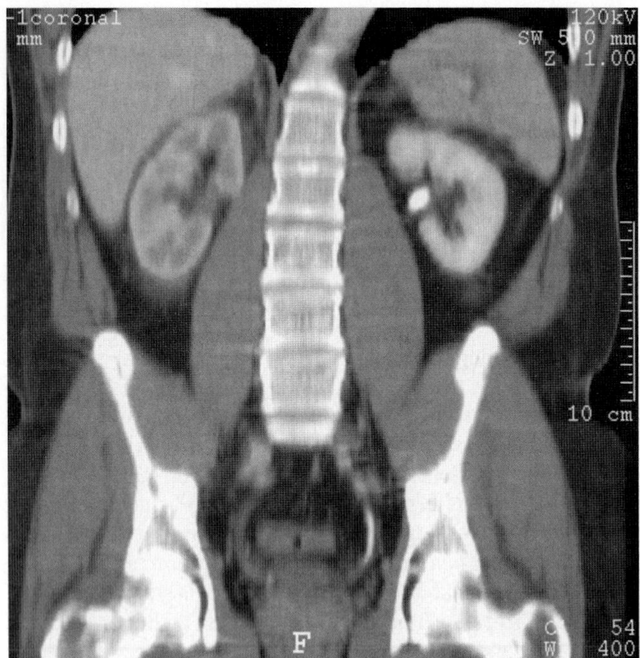

Figure 5–30 Axially acquired data reformatted in the coronal plane from an abdomen–pelvis CT on this patient with left flank pain demonstrates a stone in the left ureteropelvic junction with no evidence of hydronephrosis.

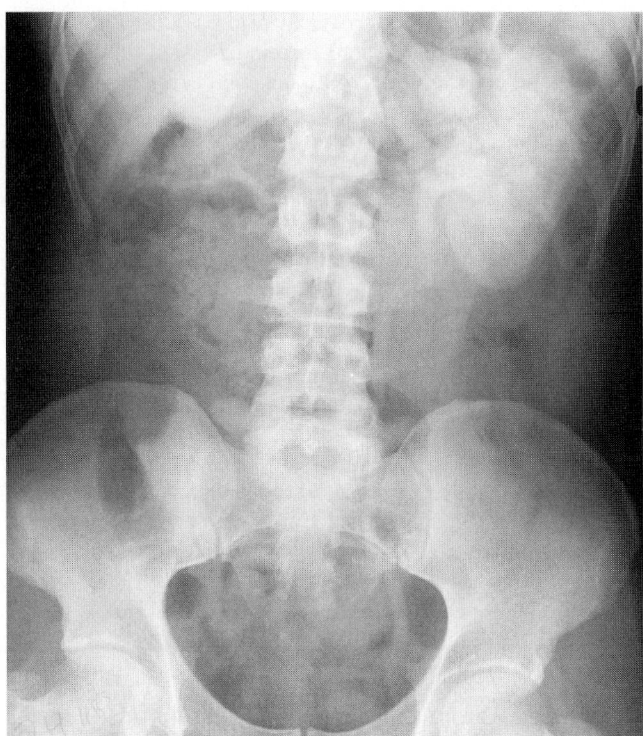

Figure 5–31 This 30-year-old male with gout presented with acute onset left flank pain. An intravenous urogram was performed, which demonstrated normal excretion of contrast by the right kidney. However, this abdominal radiograph obtained 24 hours later demonstrates a persistent left nephrogram and dilated left ureter, as well as vicarious excretion of contrast by the liver into the contrast-opacified gallbladder. The patient was found to have an obstructing distal left ureteral uric acid stone.

of an IVU. A scout film should be obtained at the beginning of every urogram to optimize patient positioning and radiographic technique, to detect calculi (which will become invisible once surrounded by contrast material), and to determine if bowel preparation is adequate. Indirect signs of a radiolucent obstructing calculus include an ipsilateral delayed nephrogram, delayed excretion, and dilation of the collecting system (**Fig. 5–31**). A contrast-filled, dilated ureter may eventually be followed down to the level of the obstruction.

Sonography is particularly useful in the evaluation of patients with mild or repetitive attacks, pregnant women, and patients with a contraindication to IVU. Stones are seen as hyperechoic, often shadowing foci within the collecting system or ureter. The uterovesical junctions can be visualized using the urinary bladder as an acoustic window. The presence of a “jet” of urine flowing from the ureter on the affected side argues against the presence of a complete obstruction. If the patient is well hydrated and the uterovesical junction is continuously monitored for a sufficient length of time, the absence of a jet is essentially diagnostic of complete obstruction. If obstruction has been present for a length of time sufficient to produce hydronephrosis, ultrasound is quite sensitive in its detection. Mild hydronephrosis refers to slight distention of the collecting system, with multiple anechoic spaces that conform to the expected configuration of the renal collecting system and communicate with a dilated renal pelvis. Severe hydronephrosis includes not only greater dilatation, but thinning of the renal cortex as well.

Thin-section noncontrast CT examination has supplanted IVU as the study of choice in most centers. This study provides several important advantages. First, the study is performed without intravenous contrast material, eliminating the risk of adverse reaction. Second, the patient requires no bowel preparation to eliminate overlying fecal material and gas. Third, the superior contrast sensitivity of CT over plain radiography means that even noncalcified calculi, such as uric acid stones, are usually visible. Other findings easily detected on CT include hydronephrosis and hydroureter. By using a collimation that is narrower than the usual 1 cm, even small stones can be reliably detected. A major role of interventional radiology in the management of obstruction is the placement of percutaneous nephrostomy and nephroureterostomy catheters (**Fig. 5–32**) to provide drainage of an obstructed collecting system. This represents an emergent procedure in a patient with urosepsis.

◆ Adrenal Glands

Anatomy and Physiology

Although the adrenal glands belong to the endocrine system and not the excretory system, they are often discussed in conjunction with the kidneys. In fact, the adrenal glands are named for their close renal proximity (*ad-*, “near,” and *renal*, “kidney”). The adrenal glands are paired structures lying within the perirenal space, superior or anteromedial to the upper poles of the kidneys. On axial cross-sectional images, they appear as inverted Y- or V-shaped structures with limbs measuring less than 1 cm in width.

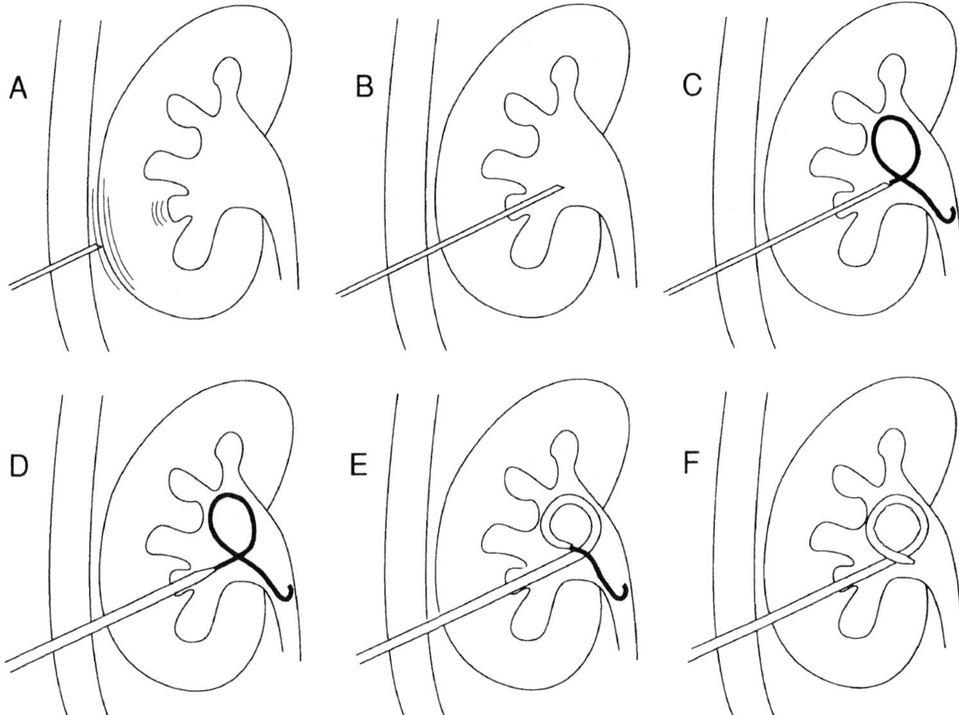

Figure 5–32 Percutaneous nephrostomy tube (PNT) placement. **(A)** After local anesthesia is instilled, the introductory needle is directed toward the kidney. Slight deflecting motion of the kidney assures the operator that he or she is in the appropriate plane. **(B)** Puncture is made into the posterior calyx. **(C)** Proper position is confirmed by obtaining urine. Needle obdurator is exchanged for a guidewire. **(D)** Tract is dilated using progressively larger dilators. **(E)** Finally, PNT is placed over the guidewire, coiled in the collecting system, and **(F)** locked in place.

About 80% of the mass of the adrenal gland is composed of adrenal cortex, which consists of three layers or zones (**Fig. 5–33**). These zones produce steroid hormones from a cholesterol precursor. The outer zona glomerulosa produces the mineralocorticoid aldosterone, which acts on the distal convoluted tubules of the nephrons to enhance sodium retention and potassium excretion. Aldosterone is absolutely essential for life, and its absence rapidly produces a state of circulatory shock due to hypovolemia. The glucocorticoids such as cortisol are produced in the middle zona fasciculata and the inner zona reticularis. Cortisol functions in gluconeogenesis, in stress adaptation, and in suppressing the inflammatory and immune responses. The adrenal cortex also produces sex hormones, including the androgens that are responsible for the growth of pubic and axillary hair, enhancement of the pubertal growth spurt, and sex drive in women.

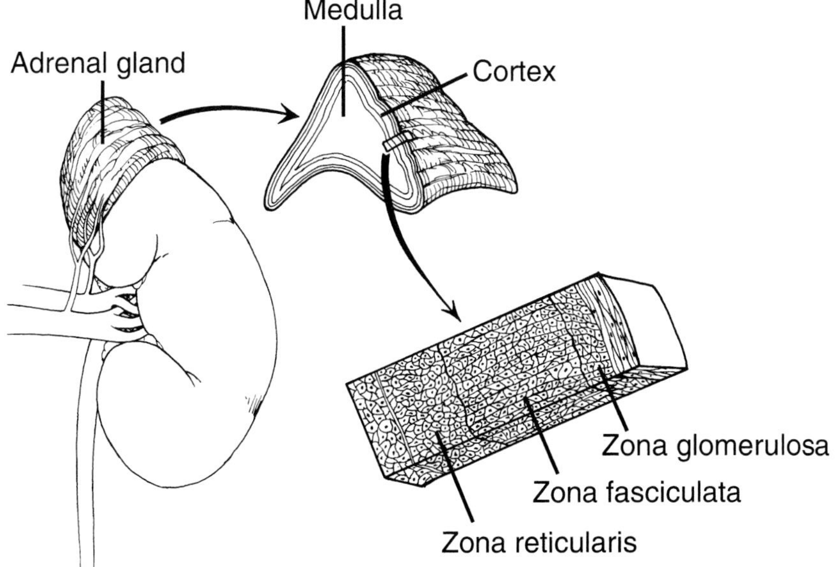

Figure 5–33 The anatomic relationship between the kidneys and adrenal glands, as well as the structure of the adrenal cortex and medulla.

Global adrenal cortical hypofunction is called Addison's disease and is associated with hyperkalemia and hyponatremia, hypoglycemia, and poor response to stress. Most cases are thought to be autoimmune in etiology, although bilateral infarction or hemorrhage may also be responsible. Conn's syndrome refers to hyperaldosteronism. It manifests with hypertension and hypokalemia, and most often results from an isolated, hormonally active adrenal adenoma (**Fig. 5–34**). Cushing's syndrome refers to excess glucocorticoid secretion and manifests with truncal obesity, hypertension, muscle atrophy, cutaneous striae, and amenorrhea. Most cases result from bilateral adrenal hyperplasia, which in 90% of cases is due to a corticotropin-secreting pituitary adenoma (Cushing's disease); 10% of cases are due to an adrenocortical carcinoma.

The adrenal medulla is composed of modified postganglionic sympathetic neurons, which release their "neurotransmitter" directly into the circulation under sympathetic stimulation. Its greatest product is epinephrine. Levels of epinephrine in the blood may rise by as much as 300 times under severe stress, preparing the patient for the so-called fight-or-flight response.

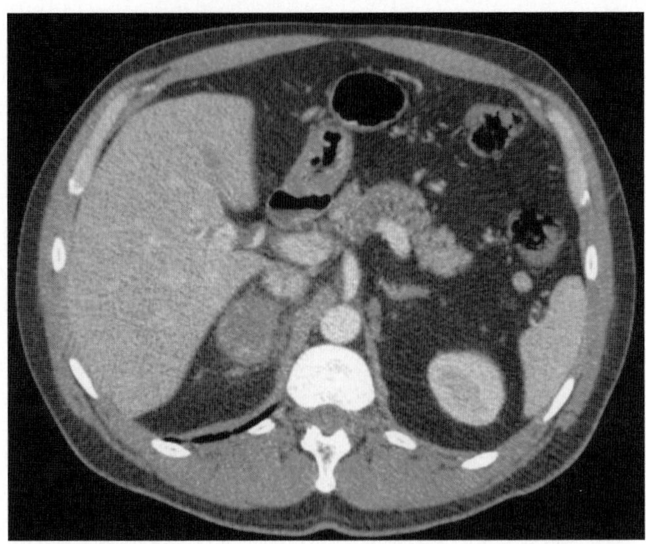

Figure 5–34 This patient presented with hypertension and hypokalemia. An axial CT image of the abdomen demonstrates a 4 cm heterogeneous right adrenal mass, an aldosteronoma.

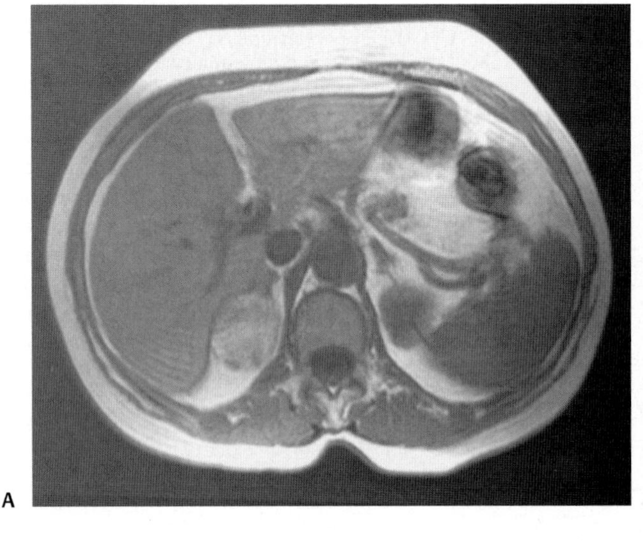

A

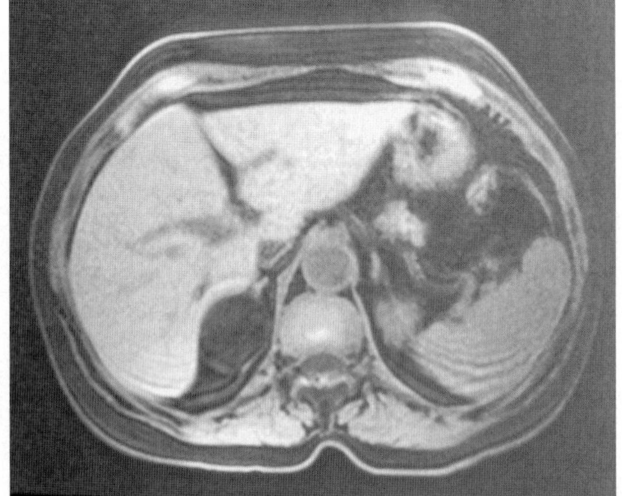

B

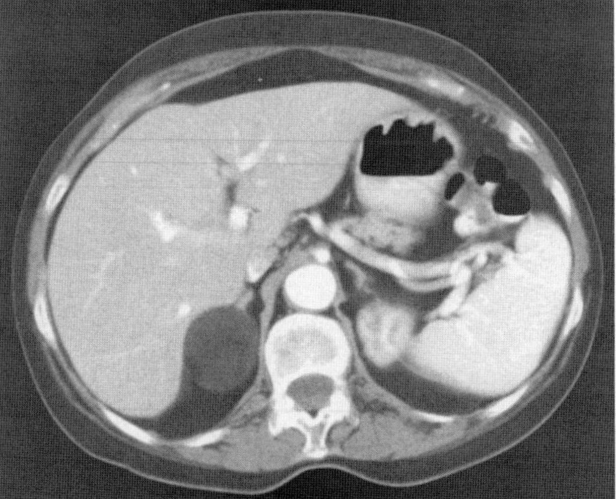

C

Figure 5–35 Axial T1 **(A)** and T1 fat-suppression **(B)** images of a right adrenal mass demonstrate high signal on T1 that drops on the fat-suppression image, indicating a fat-containing adrenal myelipoma. **(C)** An axial CT image demonstrates that the lesion is fat density.

Pathology

By far the most important role of imaging in the evaluation of the adrenal glands lies in the detection, characterization, and staging of adrenal tumors.

Tumorous

Adrenal cortical tumors include both benign and malignant varieties. A benign adrenal adenoma is the most prevalent tumor, frequently detected as an incidental finding on imaging studies performed for other reasons. These tumors characteristically produce no endocrine abnormalities, measure 3 cm or less in diameter, exhibit slight uniform enhancement, and have a CT attenuation value of less than 10 HU, due to the presence of a considerable amount of lipid material. This lipid material can also prove useful in characterizing these lesions by MRI, where fat suppression techniques will demonstrate a dramatic drop-off in signal intensity in an adenoma (**Fig. 5–35**).

The most common adrenal cortical malignancy is a metastasis, found at autopsy in approximately one quarter of patients who die from malignancy. Common sources of adrenal metastases include lung cancer (especially small cell carcinoma), breast cancer, and melanoma. Unfortunately, small metastases often appear homogeneous and well defined on CT, proving indistinguishable from adenomas. On MRI, however, metastases will be hyperintense on T2-weighted images. CT or ultrasound-guided needle biopsy can easily resolve equivocal cases.

Adrenocortical carcinoma is the most common primary adrenal-cortical malignancy. Approximately 50% of these tumors exhibit clinically significant endocrine function, usually Cushing's syndrome. The masses are usually 5 cm or greater in size, demonstrate areas of necrosis, hemorrhage, or calcification, and typically have a poor prognosis due to their large size (and high probability of metastasis) at the time of diagnosis.

Pheochromocytoma is the most important adrenal medullary tumor. These tumors follow the so-called rule of 10s: 10% are extra-adrenal, 10% are bilateral, and 10% are malignant. Pheochromocytomas are associated with the multiple endocrine neoplasia syndrome type II (medullary thyroid cancer, pheochromocytoma, and parathyroid or other soft tissue tumors). Patients often present with symptoms of sustained or episodic catecholamine excess, including hypertension, tachycardia, and headaches. Imaging studies include nuclear medicine radioactive iodine labeled meta-iodobenzylguanidine (MIBG) scans (especially useful for localizing extra-adrenal tumors or metastatic lesions), ultrasound, and CT or MRI (**Fig. 5–36**). Pheochromocytomas enhance strongly and demonstrate extremely high signal on T2-weighted MR images. Because manipulation of these tumors can precipitate a hypertensive crisis, pharmacologic adrenergic blockade is warranted before biopsy.

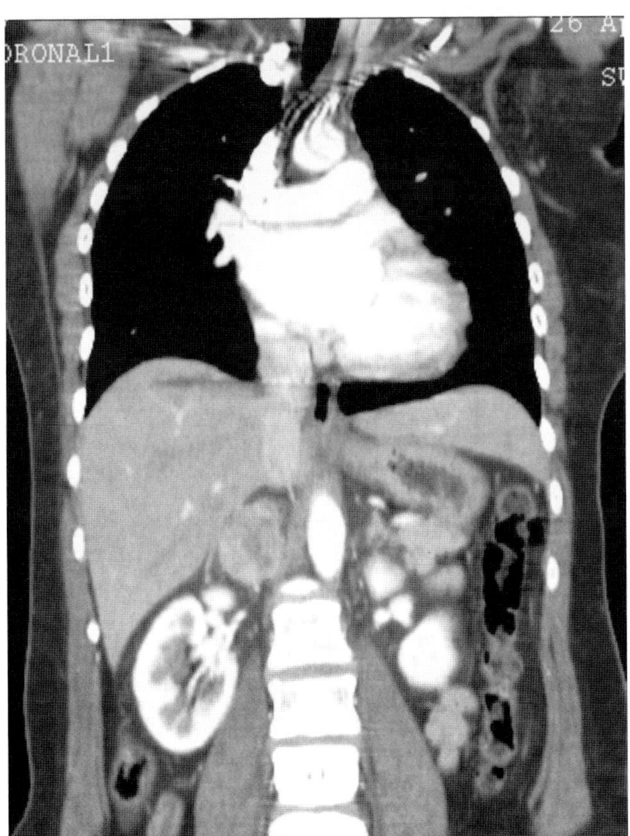

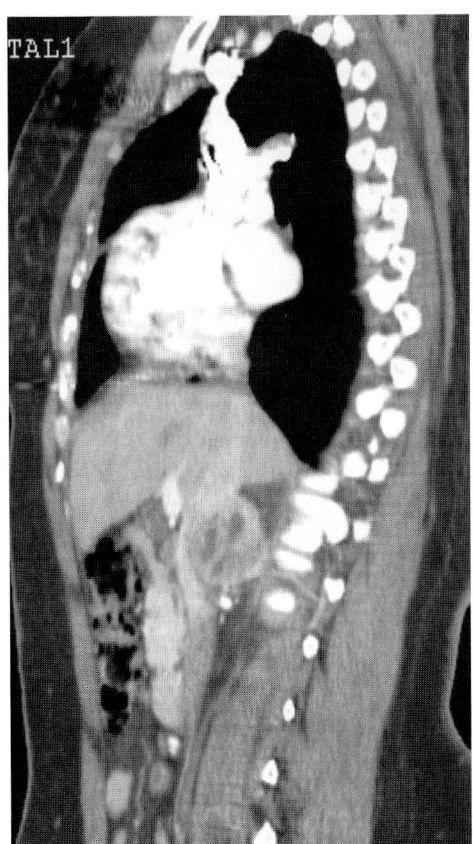

Figure 5–36 Reformatted coronal **(A)** and sagittal **(B)** images from a CT scan of the chest and abdomen in a patient with hypertension and elevated catecholamines demonstrate a heterogeneous right adrenal mass, a pheochromocytoma.

6

The Acute Abdomen

- **Critical Radiographic Signs**
  - Pneumoperitoneum
  - Pneumatosis Intestinalis
  - Hepatic Gas
- **Pathology**
  - Abscess
  - Peptic Ulcer Disease
    - *Epidemiology*
    - *Pathophysiology*
    - *Clinical Presentation*
    - *Imaging*
  - Acute Cholecystitis
    - *Epidemiology*
    - *Pathophysiology*
    - *Clinical Presentation*
    - *Imaging*
  - Pancreatitis
    - *Epidemiology*
    - *Pathophysiology*
    - *Clinical Presentation*
    - *Imaging*
  - Diverticular Disease
    - *Epidemiology*
    - *Pathophysiology*
    - *Clinical Presentation*
    - *Imaging*
  - Appendicitis
    - *Epidemiology*
    - *Pathophysiology*
    - *Clinical Presentation*
    - *Imaging*
  - Bowel Obstruction
    - *Epidemiology*
    - *Pathophysiology*
    - *Clinical Presentation*
    - *Imaging*

Acute abdominal pain is one of the three or four most common complaints of patients presenting to emergency rooms and admitted to hospitals. The goal of this chapter is not to provide a comprehensive review of this complex topic, but to present a general imaging approach to the problem and to discuss seven of the most frequently encountered and illustrative etiologies. The single most common etiology of acute abdominal pain is functional and has no specific therapy; however, other conditions do warrant urgent medical or surgical therapy; these include peptic ulcer disease, cholecystitis, pancreatitis, intestinal obstruction, appendicitis, diverticular disease, urinary tract infection (considered in Chapter 5), and diseases of the female reproductive tract (considered in Chapter 7). Before discussing these entities, let us briefly examine several important radiographic findings that may be present in patients presenting with an acute abdomen.

◆ Critical Radiographic Signs

Pneumoperitoneum

A key finding to rule out on every abdominal plain film is pneumoperitoneum, or free intraperitoneal air (**Fig. 6–1**). Absent trauma or recent surgery, free air most often indicates perforation of a duodenal or gastric ulcer, although rupture of any hollow viscus may produce this sign. In the setting of obstruction, free air generally indicates a bowel perforation. In hospitalized patients, pneumoperitoneum is most often iatrogenic, secondary to surgery or peritoneal dialysis. Air may also be introduced into the peritoneal cavity via the female genital tract. In the postsurgical setting, free air should resolve within 3 to 6 days. Failure to resolve or an increase in the amount of gas should prompt evaluation for a leak at the surgical site. Pneumoperitoneum generally resolves more slowly in thin patients than in obese patients. The finding of free air in a patient with an acute abdomen warrants emergent surgical consultation.

Free air is best detected on upright chest radiographs, where it will usually be seen as a rim of lucency immediately below one or both hemidiaphragms (**Fig. 6–2**). In the patient who cannot be placed upright, a left-side-down decubitus view will cause air to appear between the liver and the lateral abdominal wall (**Fig. 6–3**). On supine films, often the only films obtainable in very ill patients, free air may manifest as a double-wall sign (gas on both sides of the bowel wall, causing unusually good visualization) or the "football sign," which appears as a large central lucency in the abdomen (**Fig. 6–4**). Free air may also outline both sides of the falciform ligament, which connects the liver to the anterior abdominal wall.

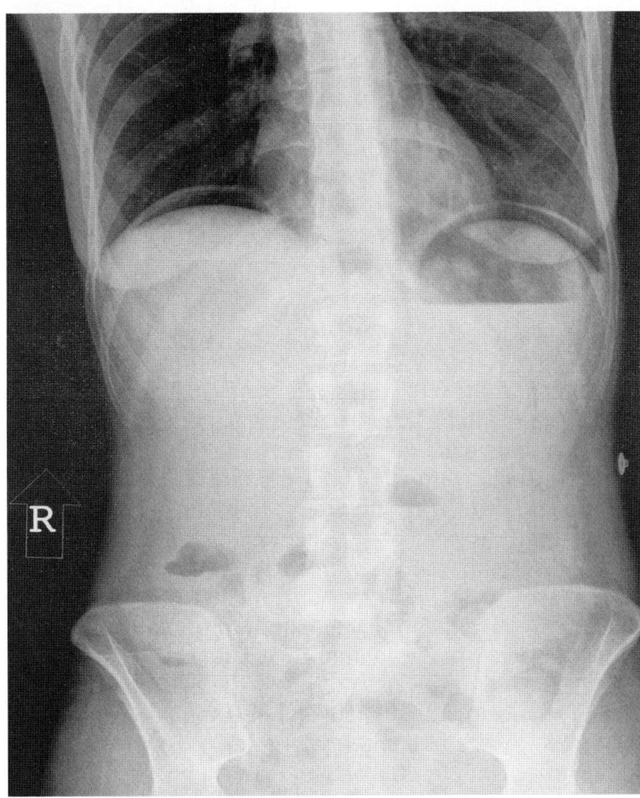

Figure 6–1 This upright view of the abdomen demonstrates crescents of gas underneath the patient's hemidiaphragms, indicating pneumoperitoneum. When possible, upright positioning is helpful, because it causes free intraperitoneal gas to rise up to the top of the peritoneal cavity.

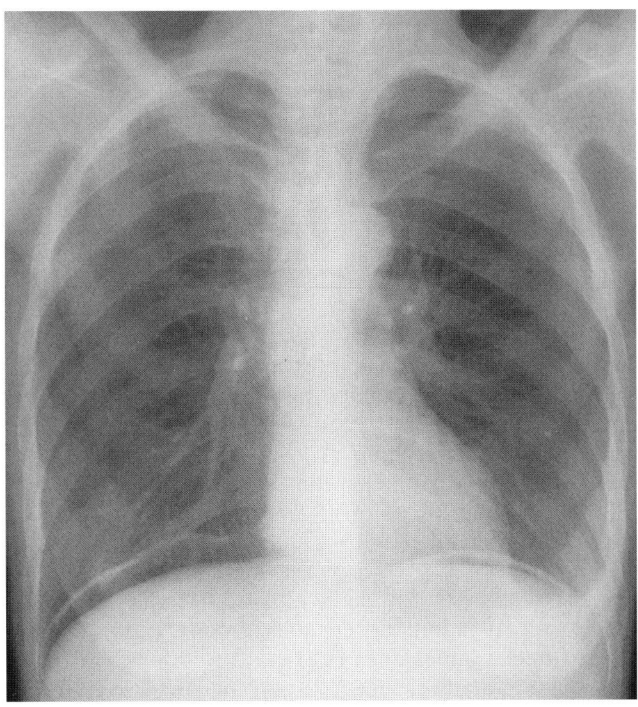

Figure 6–2 This upright chest radiograph demonstrates free peritoneal air, manifesting as crescents of lucency under both hemidiaphragms.

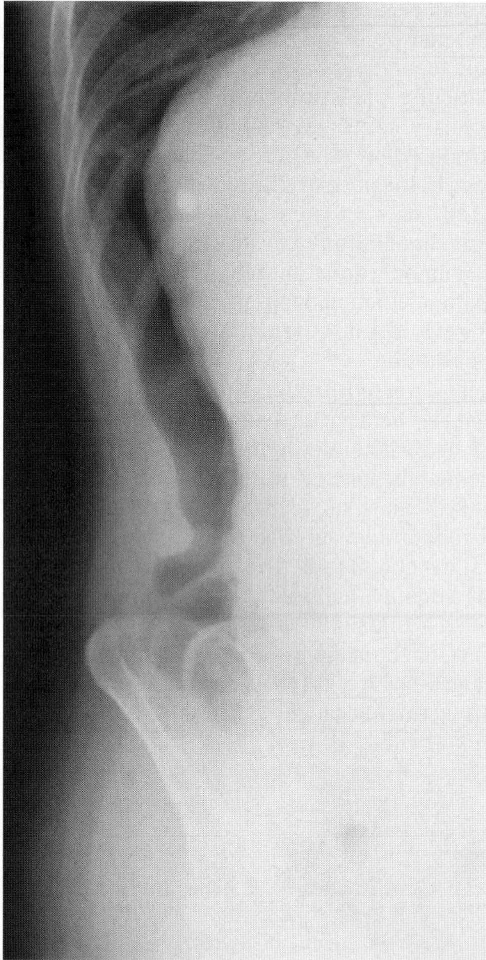

Figure 6–3 This left lateral decubitus view of the right side of the abdomen (patient lying left side down with the x-ray beam parallel to the floor) demonstrates a crescent of free intraperitoneal air between the liver edge and lateral abdominal wall. Some patients who are too ill to stand or sit upright may tolerate being positioned on their side.

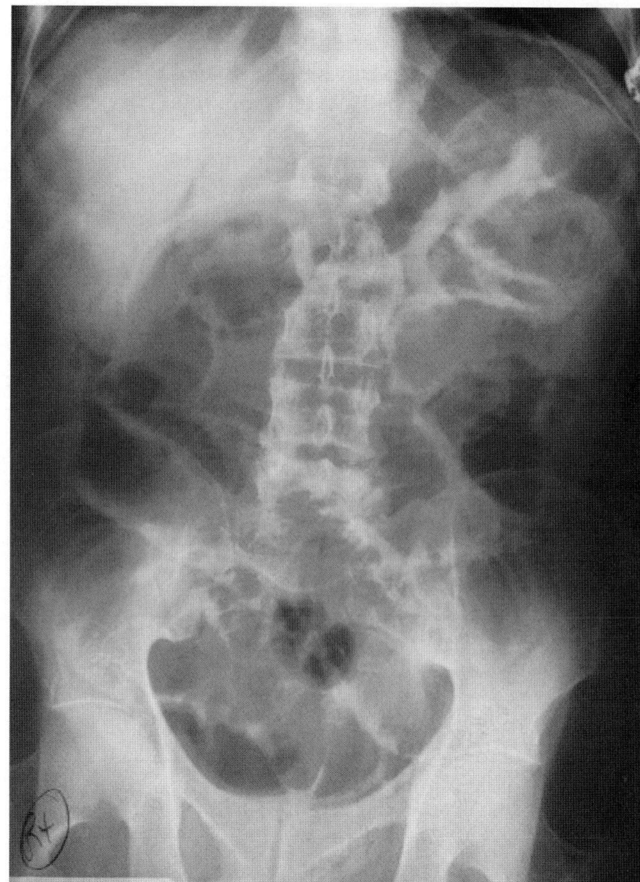

Figure 6–4 The inner wall of the bowel is usually sharply defined where the lumen is filled with gas. When the outer wall is also sharply defined, it indicates gas in the peritoneal cavity, the so-called double-wall sign. Note the inverted U-shaped dilated bowel in the right upper quadrant/epigastric region, which demonstrates the double-wall sign.

Pneumatosis Intestinalis

Another important plain radiographic finding in the acute abdomen is pneumatosis intestinalis, or gas within the bowel wall, which usually signifies severely ischemic bowel. It appears as linear gas, either encircling the gas-containing bowel lumen when viewed on end or paralleling the bowel lumen when viewed from the side (**Fig. 6–5**). Pneumatosis must be distinguished from the normal layering out of air over luminal contents in the nondependent (upper) portion of a segment of bowel. In pneumatosis intestinalis, the gas extends all the way around the bowel wall, including its dependent (lower) portion. Every case of pneumatosis does not herald an abdominal catastrophe, and many cases turn out to be benign, related to such factors as obstruction, ileus, and medications. In the setting of an acute abdomen, however, it naturally heightens concern.

Hepatic Gas

The finding of gas collections over the liver shadow, particularly if they exhibit a linear, branching pattern, should arouse suspicion for one of two processes: portal venous gas (pneumoportia) or gas within the biliary tree (pneumobilia). Portal venous gas typically results from severe intestinal ischemia and is usually associated with pneumatosis intestinalis. Gas in the bowel wall tracks up through the superior mesenteric vein into the portal venous system. Portal venous gas is usually peripheral in the liver, extending out from the main portal vein into its smaller branches. Biliary gas, in contrast, is usually located in the central biliary ducts at the porta hepatis. The most common cause of pneumobilia is previous surgery, such as a papillotomy to relieve obstruction at the sphincter of Oddi or choledochojejunostomy performed in conjunction with a Billroth II procedure for pancreatic cancer. Other causes include a fistula from the gallbladder into the bowel, as in gallstone ileus, and a peptic ulcer eroding into the common bile duct.

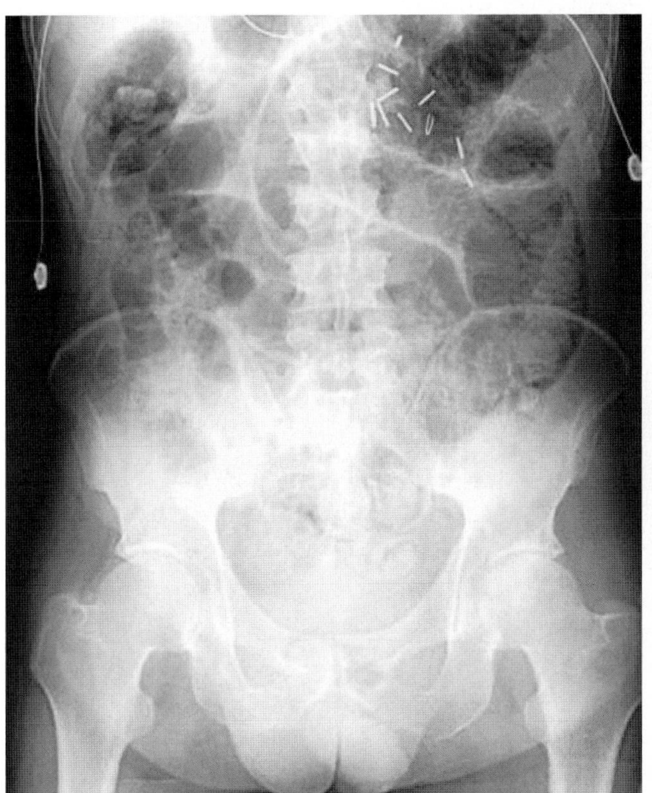
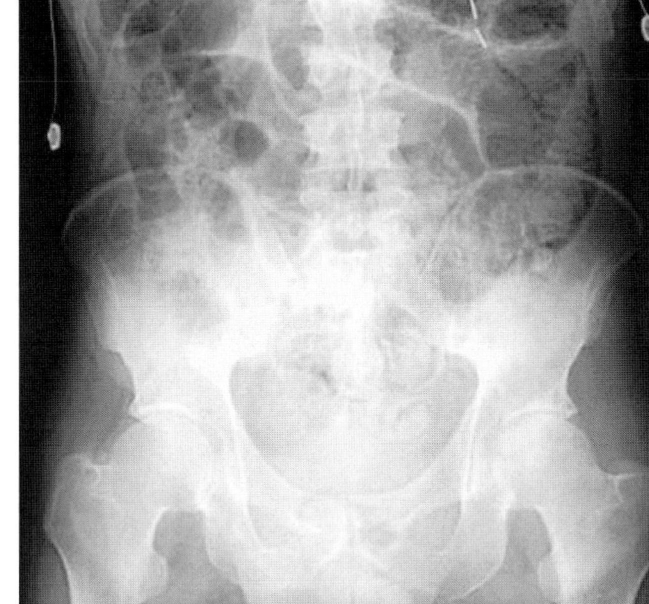
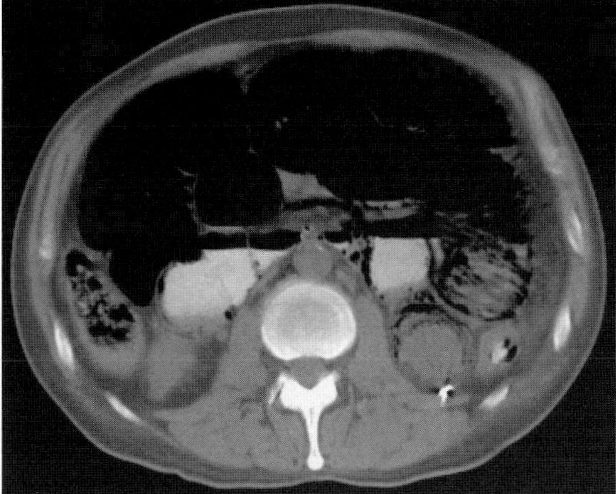
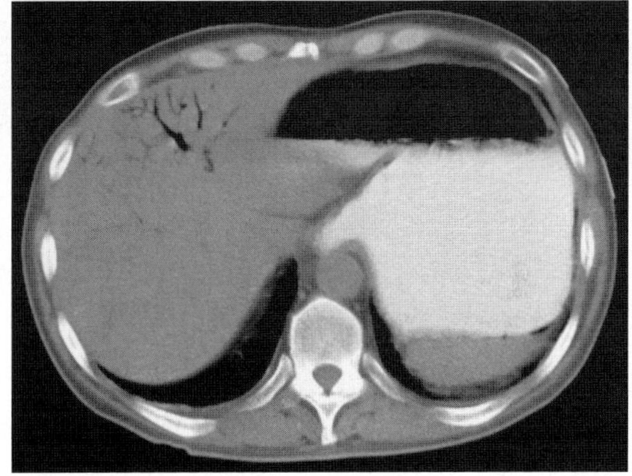

Figure 6–5 This 55-year-old man presented with crampy abdominal pain that was worse after meals, a classic history for mesenteric ischemia. **(A)** The abdominal plain film shows gas in the bowel wall (pneumatosis intestinalis), best seen on the left. **(B)** Axial CT shows the pneumatosis more clearly. **(C)** An axial CT image at a more cranial level demonstrates gas in the portal vein branches of the liver.

◆ Pathology

Abscess

The annual incidence of abdominal abscess in the United States is approximately 1 in 10,000, amounting to 30,000 cases per year. Over three quarters of abdominal abscesses occur in postoperative patients; other causes include perforated appendicitis, diverticulitis, and inflammatory bowel disease. Abdominal abscesses can be difficult to diagnose by plain film, but they should be suspected whenever an abnormal gas collection is seen outside the expected distribution of the bowel in a patient with fever and leukocytosis. Other signs of abdominal abscess include a soft tissue mass displacing air-filled bowel (which will often exhibit focal dilation), pleural effusion (especially when the abscess involves the subdiaphragmatic space), and effacement of normal tissue planes, such as the psoas muscle shadow. On computed tomography, it is much easier definitively to ascertain the presence of a loculated fluid collection outside the alimentary canal, where abscesses may contain gas and demonstrate a rim of peripheral enhancement (**Fig. 6–6**). Recently, the role of the radiologist has expanded beyond the diagnosis of abscesses to include their treatment; a discussion of percutaneous catheter drainage is found in Chapter 1.

Peptic Ulcer Disease

Epidemiology

Approximately 350,000 cases of peptic ulcer disease are diagnosed each year in the United States, with 100,000 hospitalizations. Risk factors for peptic ulcer disease include male sex (M:F = 3:1), use of nonsteroidal anti-inflammatory drugs or corticosteroids, severe illness, and bacterial infection.

Pathophysiology

Duodenal ulcers are much more common than gastric ulcers (discussed in Chapter 4), but each represents a manifestation of the same disease. Peptic ulcer disease is characterized by a breakdown in the intrinsic protective mechanisms of the mucosa, with subsequent acid-induced mucosal and submucosal erosions. An important role in the pathogenesis of peptic ulcer disease has been attributed to the spiral gram-negative

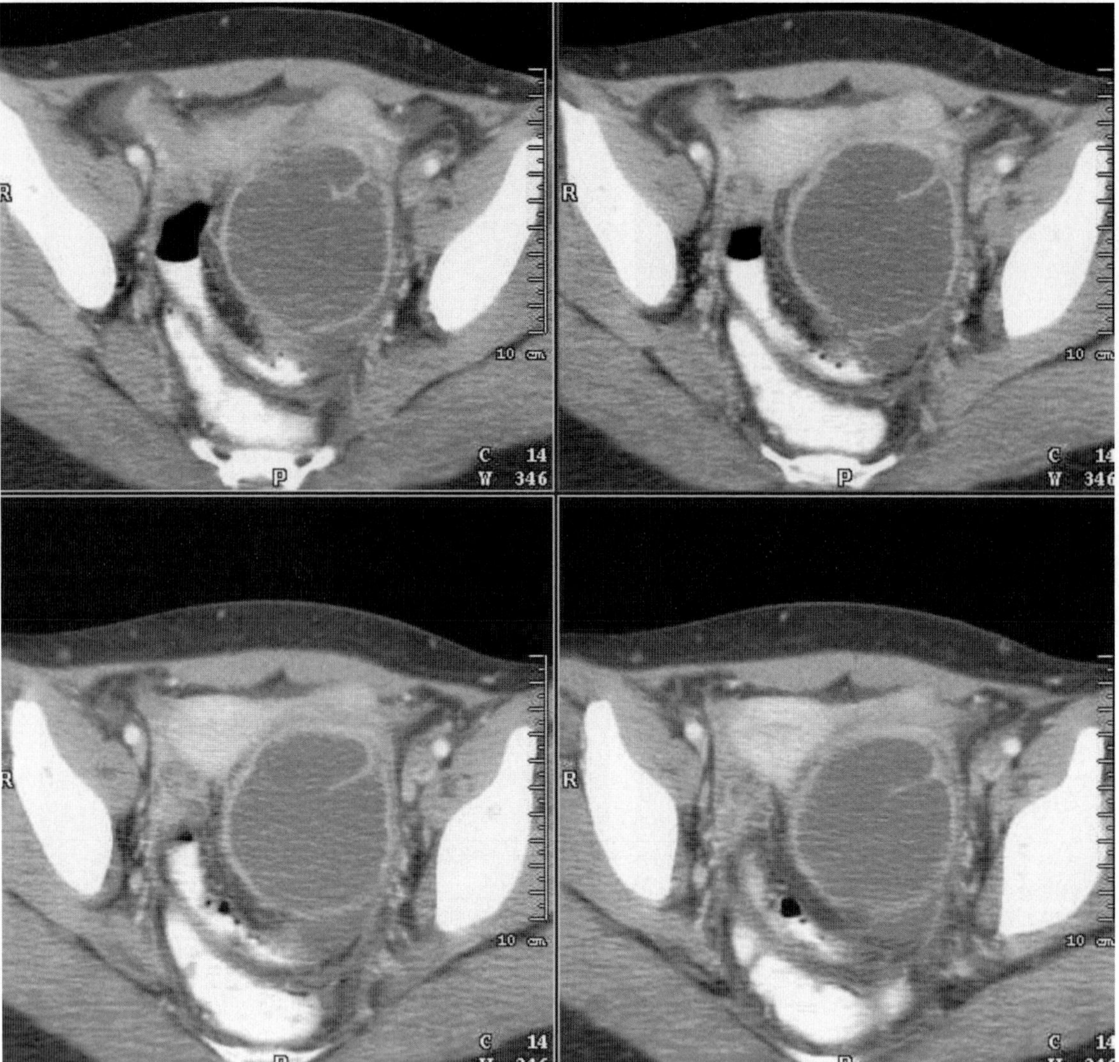

Figure 6–6 These contiguous axial CT images demonstrate a fluid collection in the pelvis, representing a tubo-ovarian abscess secondary to pelvic inflammatory disease. Note the peripheral rim of enhancing tissue, a typical finding in abscesses. There is also enhancement of a partial septation.

bacterium *Helicobacter pylori.* This bacterium is present in approximately one quarter of the general population and has been found to inhabit the gastric mucosal epithelium of nearly all patients with duodenal ulcers and most with gastric ulcers; its eradication is associated with a dramatic reduction in ulcer recurrence. The presence of *H. pylori* can be diagnosed by endoscopic biopsy or breath test, due to the organism's urea-splitting capabilities. In contrast to gastric ulcers, duodenal ulcers are virtually never malignant.

Clinical Presentation

The patient with uncomplicated peptic ulcer disease presents with burning or gnawing epigastric pain that tends to occur before meals and is relieved with food. When peptic ulcer disease presents acutely, it is due to deeper penetration of the ulcer crater into the submucosa, which may result in perforation and an abdominal catastrophe (**Fig. 6–7**). Perforated duodenal ulcers present with severe abdominal pain that often radiates to the back and right shoulder. Leakage of enteric fluid into the peritoneal cavity may cause hypotension, peritonitis, and shock. Nearly all perforations involve the posterior aspect of the duodenum.

Imaging

In young patients with uncomplicated symptoms, the initial diagnostic study for peptic ulcer disease is often an empirical trial of antisecretory therapy.

◇ Uncomplicated Ulcer

Both younger patients in whom empirical therapy is not successful and older patients in whom the possibility of a gastric malignancy must be considered should undergo imaging. Although endoscopy is more sensitive and specific than

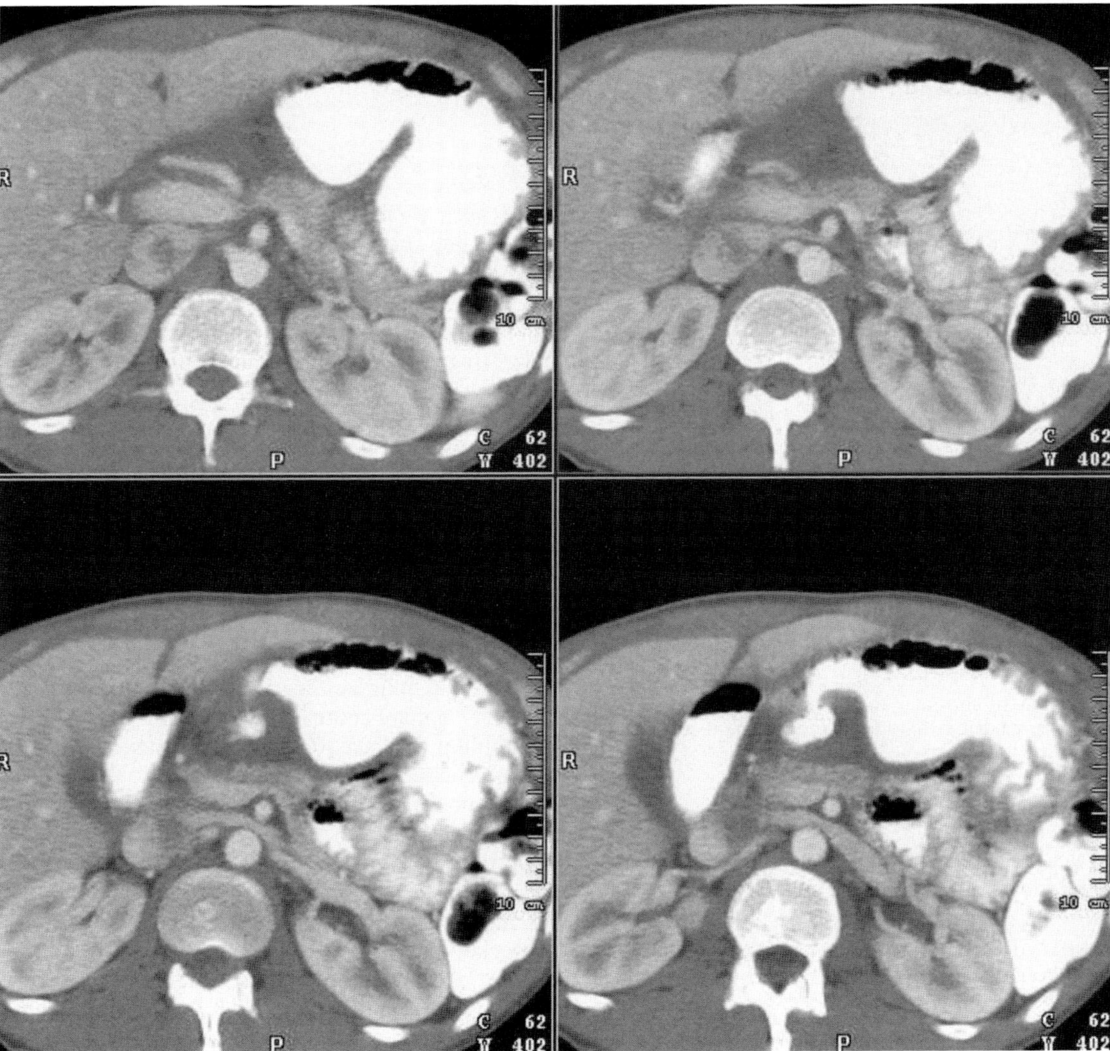

Figure 6–7 These contiguous axial CT images after oral and intravenous (IV) contrast administration demonstrate a large penetrating ulcer extending posteriorly from the gastric antrum, filled with contrast. It would not be much longer before the ulcer erodes completely through the gastric wall, with free spillage of gastric contents into the peritoneal cavity.

barium studies in detecting small or superficial ulcers, a barium study is a significantly more comfortable and less costly procedure for the patient (between one quarter and one third the cost). Endoscopy may be reserved for the small percentage of patients in whom radiology is equivocal or tissue biopsy is required (e.g., when an ulcer has failed to heal completely with 6 weeks of antisecretory therapy or when an underlying malignancy must be excluded).

Findings of peptic ulcer disease on upper gastrointestinal (GI) examination include an ulcer crater (a fixed pocket of barium) and associated deformities, such as an edematous collar around the ulcer, radiating folds of mucosa, and scarring (**Fig. 6–8**).

Patients whose duodenal ulcers are refractory to therapy should be evaluated for Zollinger-Ellison syndrome, which is related to the presence of a gastrinoma, a gastrin-producing tumor. Serum gastrin levels should be obtained for diagnosis. Unfortunately, a high percentage of these lesions are malignant (60%), and surgery offers the only hope for cure. Formerly, symptomatic relief could often be achieved only by gastrectomy, but now many patients can be palliated with proton pump blockers, such as omeprazole, which block acid secretion by gastric parietal cells. Because the typical gastrinoma is a relatively small tumor, with a mean size of 3 cm, detection can be difficult. Techniques include ultrasound, CT, and nuclear medicine studies. The nuclear medicine In-111-octreotide study exploits the fact that pancreatic islet cell tumors such as gastrinomas arise from cells in the amine precursor uptake and decarboxylation (APUD) system. These cells, like those of carcinoid tumors and small cell lung carcinomas, selectively take up this somatostatin analogue, and neoplasms comprised of such cells appear "hot" on scintigraphy.

◇ Suspected Perforation

In contrast to the patient with symptoms of an uncomplicated duodenal ulcer, the first imaging study in every case of

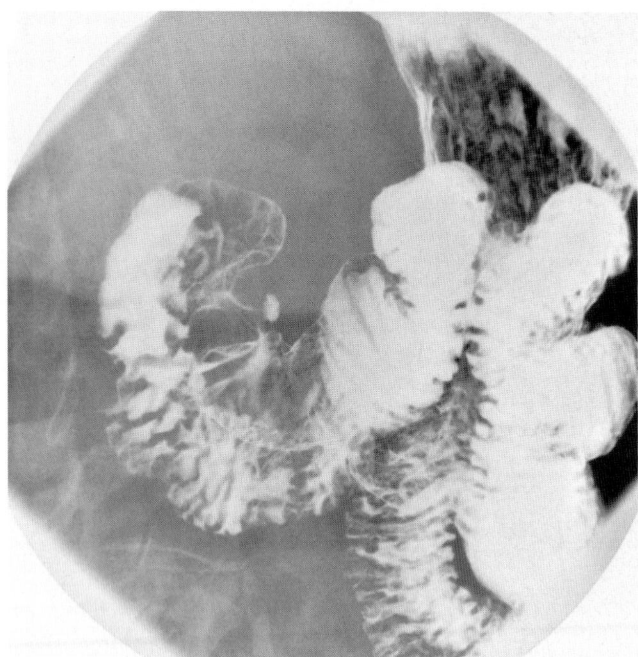

Figure 6–8 This spot image from a barium upper gastrointestinal exam demonstrates a peptic ulcer in the antrum of the stomach, manifesting as a barium-containing outpouching extending beyond the expected margin of the gastric mucosa.

suspected perforation should be plain films of the abdomen. These are obtained to look for evidence of free air under the diaphragm on upright views or adjacent to the liver on left-side-down decubitus views. If perforation is suspected but no free air is seen, an upper GI examination with a water-soluble contrast agent or a CT scan of the abdomen should be performed, looking for extravasation of contrast (**Fig. 6-9**). Endoscopy is contraindicated, because insufflation of large amounts of air required to adequately open the lumen for visualization is likely to exacerbate the problem. Definitive treatment consists of surgical repair.

Acute Cholecystitis

Epidemiology

Gallstones are present in approximately 15% of persons between the ages of 40 and 60 years, four out of five of whom are asymptomatic (**Fig. 6–10**). Prevalence increases with age. There is an extremely high incidence of gallstones among the Navajo and other groups of Native Americans. Cholecystitis constitutes the most common cause of acute abdominal surgery in women, and the second most common cause in men. One-half million cholecystectomies are performed each year in the United States, most in the nonacute setting for patients with recurrent bouts of biliary colic.

There are two types of gallstones: cholesterol stones (85%) and bilirubin stones (15%). Risk factors for the formation of bilirubin stones relate to hemolytic anemia, and include hemoglobinopathies, especially sickle-cell disease, a prosthetic heart valve, and hypersplenism. Risk factors for the formation of more common cholesterol stones include female sex (F:M = 4:1), diabetes, and cirrhosis. Ileal disease, such as Crohn's disease, is another risk factor, as it disrupts the normal enterohepatic circulation of bile salts, which solubilize cholesterol.

Pathophysiology

Gallstones as such are harmless, but they can become symptomatic when they obstruct some portion of the biliary tree, most commonly the cystic duct. Obstruction of the cystic duct causes stasis of bile within the gallbladder, which may permit the proliferation of bacteria, or incite inflammation due to direct irritation of the gallbladder by bile salts themselves, resulting in acute cholecystitis.

Clinical Presentation

The typical patient with biliary colic presents with the acute onset of right upper quadrant or epigastric pain that increases in intensity over minutes to hours. Like all colicky pain, it tends to wax and wane to some degree, in relation to smooth muscle spasm. Some patients experience nausea and vomiting. Acute cholecystitis is suspected once the pain has persisted beyond 6 hours, indicating persistent biliary tract obstruction. The pain of acute cholecystitis often radiates to the right shoulder and is associated with nausea, vomiting, low-grade fever, and chills.

Laboratory analysis is often helpful in the diagnosis of acute cholecystitis. Alkaline phosphatase, which also is produced in bone and other tissues, derives primarily from the biliary tract. Hence a normal alkaline phosphatase level usually excludes biliary tract disease, and high levels are classically associated with extrahepatic biliary obstruction. Hepatitis may also produce increased alkaline phosphatase levels, but these are typically not as high as in biliary obstruction and are accompanied by elevated transaminases (aspartate aminotransferase [AST] and alanine aminotransferase [ALT]), which are produced by the hepatocytes themselves. Pancreatitis usually produces an elevation of pancreatic amylase and lipase. In suspected pyelonephritis, white blood cells and bacteria should be sought in the urine.

A potentially worrisome sign in a patient with acute or chronic cholecystitis is the sudden resolution of pain. If the patient then develops peritoneal signs such as guarding and rebound tenderness, this suggests perforation of the gallbladder, which may prove rapidly fatal. Although there is a risk of perforation in every patient, surgeons typically prefer to delay surgery for several days in cases of acute cholecystitis, to give antibiotics an opportunity to calm the inflammation. The patient is treated with narcotic analgesia (*not* morphine, which induces spasm of the sphincter of Oddi, but meperidine). However, if there is evidence of perforation, or the patient does not respond within hours to medical management, urgent surgery is required. Patients at highest risk of perforation include diabetic patients and patients with debilitating illnesses.

Imaging

Only approximately one third of patients presenting with acute right upper quadrant pain suffer from acute cholecystitis.

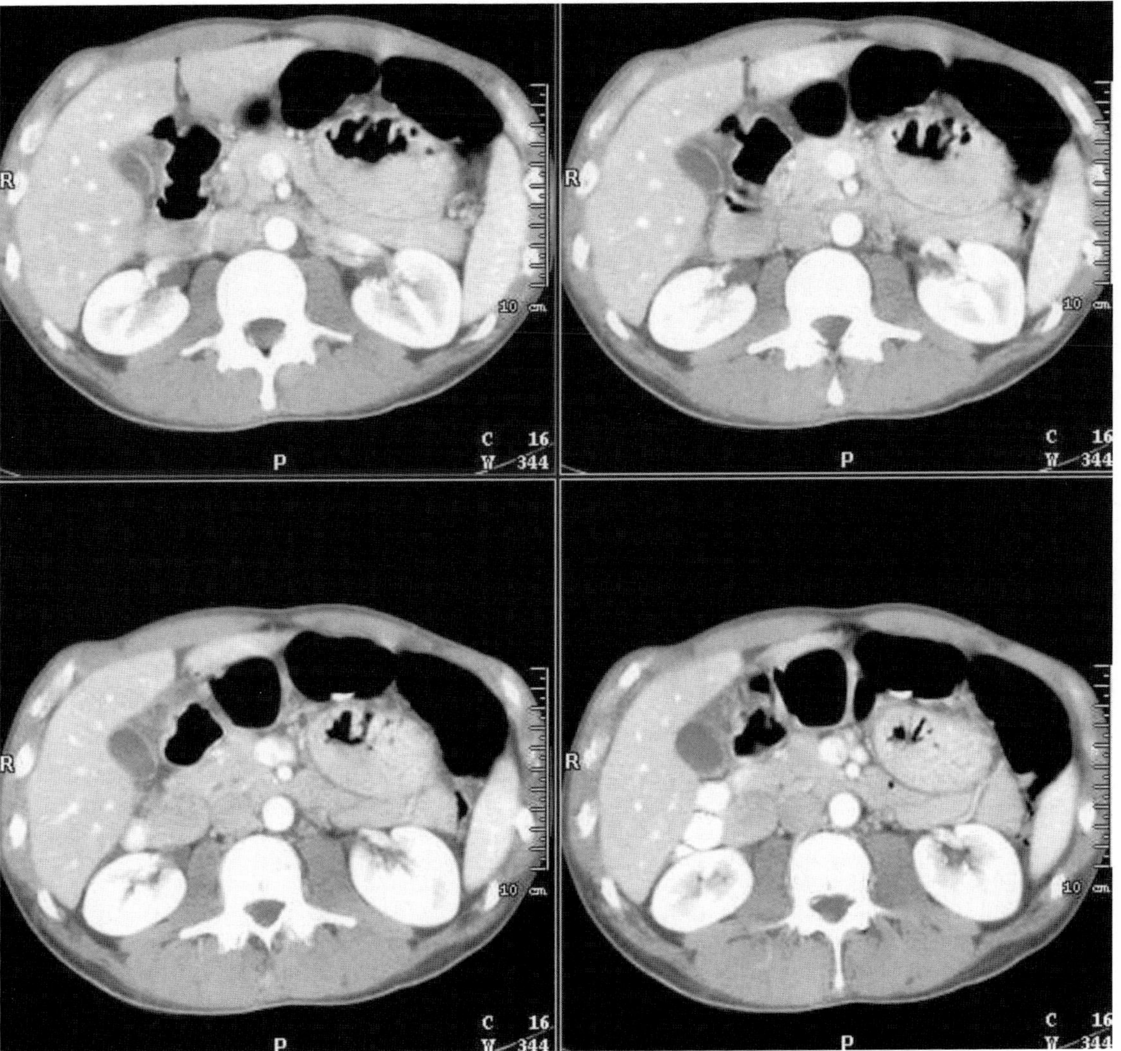

Figure 6–9 These contiguous axial CT images demonstrate an air-filled duodenal lumen with an air-containing outpouching representing a perforated duodenal ulcer. This is one of the more serious complications of peptic duodenitis.

A patient with right upper quadrant pain and a history consistent with acute cholecystitis may be suffering from any one of several common conditions. The differential diagnosis includes hepatitis, pancreatitis, peptic ulcer disease, and even pyelonephritis or pneumonia. It is important to ascertain the source of the patient's pain because, although acute cholecystitis is often managed surgically, the usual treatments for these other conditions are nonsurgical.

Plain films of the chest and abdomen are often helpful. First, they help to rule out pneumonia or evidence of free intraperitoneal air, which would indicate perforation of a viscus and a surgical emergency. Second, the plain film will demonstrate gallstones in approximately 15% of cases; when stones are found, the probability of a biliary etiology increases.

◇ Ultrasound

The imaging study of first choice in suspected acute cholecystitis is ultrasonography, which is more than 95% sensitive and specific for the detection of gallstones. Stones are found in 90 to 95% of patients with acute cholecystitis. Although the presence of gallstones does not prove that the patient has inflammation secondary to obstruction, the absence of stones is strong evidence against it. Stones appear rounded and echogenic, casting acoustic shadows, and, if lying in the gallbladder lumen, move with changes in patient position (because they are suspended in bile) (**Fig. 6–11**). Stones lodged in the bile duct are not mobile. Another corroborative finding is biliary dilatation, either intra- or extrahepatic, which occurs once the biliary tract has been obstructed for a period of hours. The finding of an impacted stone in a dilated cystic duct or common bile duct virtually assures the diagnosis.

To increase the specificity of ultrasound for the detection of acute cholecystitis, two additional findings should be present: a positive sonographic Murphy's sign (maximum tenderness is elicited directly over the gallbladder) and thickening of the gallbladder wall, indicating edema. The thickness of the wall of a normal gallbladder should measure 3 mm or less (**Fig. 6–12**).

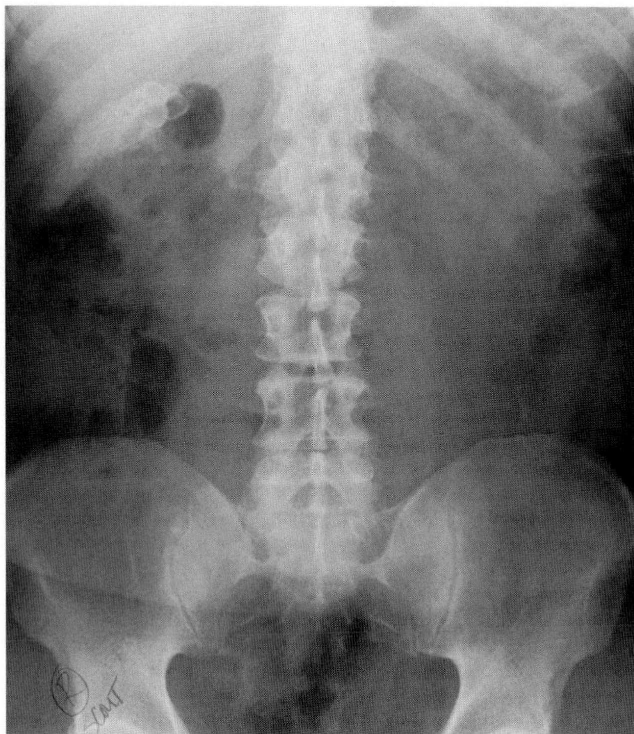

Figure 6–10 This abdominal radiograph reveals multiple calcium-containing gallstones in the right upper quadrant, presumably virtually filling the gallbladder lumen.

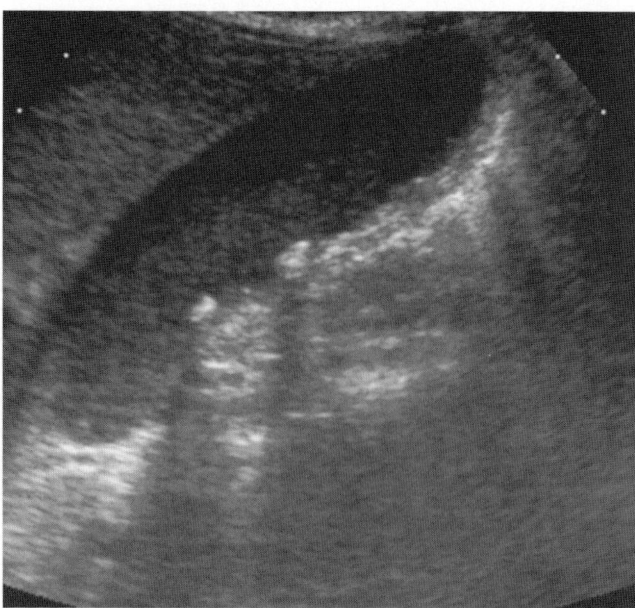

Figure 6–11 This longitudinal sonographic view of the gallbladder demonstrates anechoic (black) bile up closest to the transducer, with biliary sludge layering out below it, as well as two echogenic foci that cast acoustic shadows at the bottom. These moved with changes in patient position and represented gallstones.

Additional findings that further increase the specificity of ultrasound in the diagnosis of acute cholecystitis stem from its complications. If fluid is visible around the gallbladder in the gallbladder fossa (pericholecystic fluid), this may indicate perforation of the gallbladder, with bile extravasation. A discrete, heterogeneous fluid collection in the region of the gallbladder may represent an abscess, also secondary to perforation. When such a collection contains gas, it is almost certainly an abscess. Similarly, air in the gallbladder lumen or its wall (emphysematous cholecystitis) strongly suggests complicated cholecystitis (**Fig. 6–13**).

◇ Nuclear Medicine

A second test that is equally sensitive for the detection of acute cholecystitis, and actually demonstrates physiologically the cystic duct obstruction, is cholescintigraphy. The most important disadvantage of cholescintigraphy as compared to ultrasound (and CT) is the latter's ability to evaluate other

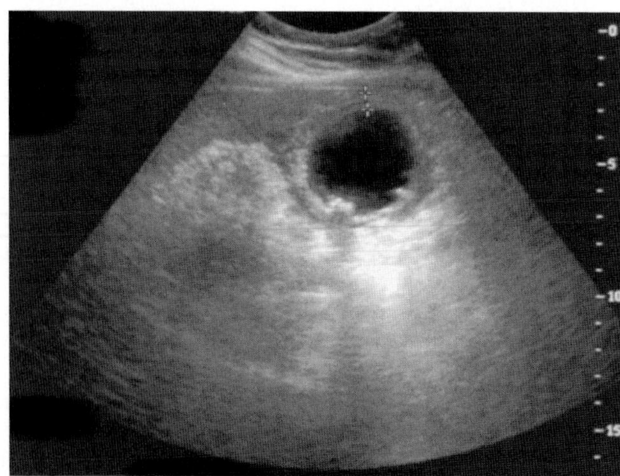

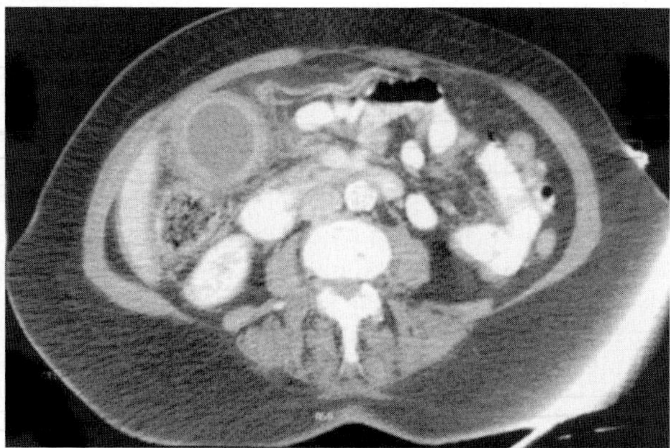

Figure 6–12 This 50-year-old woman presented with right upper quadrant pain, and on ultrasonography, a sonographic Murphy's sign was present. **(A)** A transverse image of the gallbladder demonstrates echogenic, shadowing foci in the lumen, indicating stones, as well as wall thickening (> 6 mm), consistent with cholecystitis. **(B)** Axial CT images in the same patient demonstrate gallbladder wall thickening and pericholecystic inflammation (vague increased density in the pericholecystic fat).

right upper quadrant sources of pain. The hepatobiliary scan is at least as good as any other imaging modality in detecting acute cholecystitis, but if the patient's pain has some other etiology, it is far less likely than other studies to reveal it. In an era when laparoscopy has become the preferred means of surgically removing the gallbladder, ultrasound's ability to provide preoperative information about the size and position of the gallbladder, the presence or absence of wall thickening and pericholecystic fluid, and the size, number, and location of stones is especially beneficial to the surgeon.

Mechanism of Localization The cholescintigram relies on the avid hepatic uptake and biliary excretion of technetium- (Tc-) 99m–labeled iminodiacetic acid compounds into the biliary system by the liver, even in the presence of an elevated serum bilirubin. Normally, the radiopharmaceutical begins to accumulate in the liver promptly after injection. Activity appears within minutes in the gallbladder, and soon thereafter in the small bowel, as bile is ejected out the common bile duct through the ampulla of Vater. Acute cholecystitis is diagnosed when there is no activity in the gallbladder 30 minutes after injection (**Fig. 6–14**). The absence of activity in the small bowel indicates a common duct obstruction, which would eventually produce jaundice and perhaps pancreatitis.

Pharmacologic Maneuvers Two pharmacologic maneuvers may be employed to enhance the specificity of the hepatobiliary scan. The first involves the administration of morphine, which causes contraction of the sphincter of Oddi, and thereby tends to shunt bile into the gallbladder. If the patient's gallbladder was contracting at the time of the study, perhaps under the influence of a recent meal, bile might not enter the gallbladder; however, morphine-induced sphincter of Oddi contraction helps to ensure that excreted bile is shunted into the gallbladder.

The second maneuver is to provoke secretion of cholecystokinin (CCK). Cholecystokinin is the hormone secreted by the duodenal epithelium in response to intraluminal protein and lipid content, and causes contraction of the gallbladder and ejection of bile. In a patient who has been fasting for a long period of time, the gallbladder may be full, and thus not fill during the examination. In this case, certain foods can be administered to provoke CCK secretion, followed by repeat radiopharmaceutical injection. The absence of gallbladder filling after one or both of these maneuvers further increases the radiologist's confidence in the diagnosis of acute cholecystitis.

Perhaps 5 to 10% of patients with acute cholecystitis may exhibit no stones and no evidence of biliary obstruction.

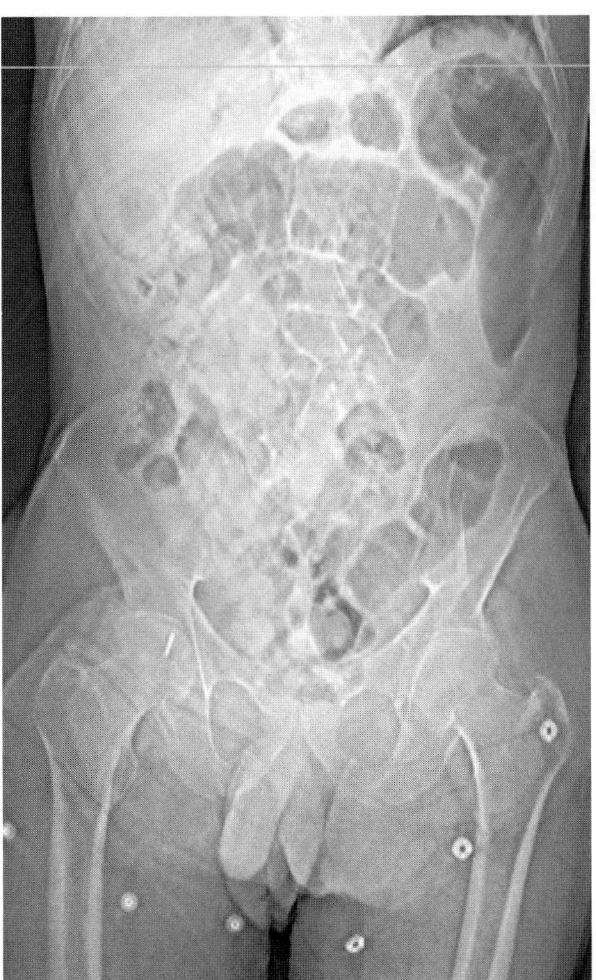

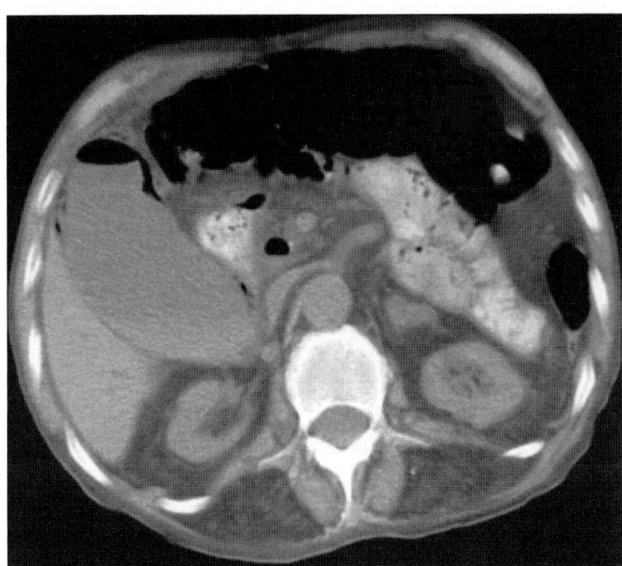

Figure 6–13 **(A)** "Scout" image from an abdominal CT exam demonstrates a ringlike lucency in the right upper quadrant, representing gas in the gallbladder wall in this patient with emphysematous cholecystitis. **(B)** Axial CT image in the same patient demonstrates a distended gallbladder with linear gas collections in its wall.

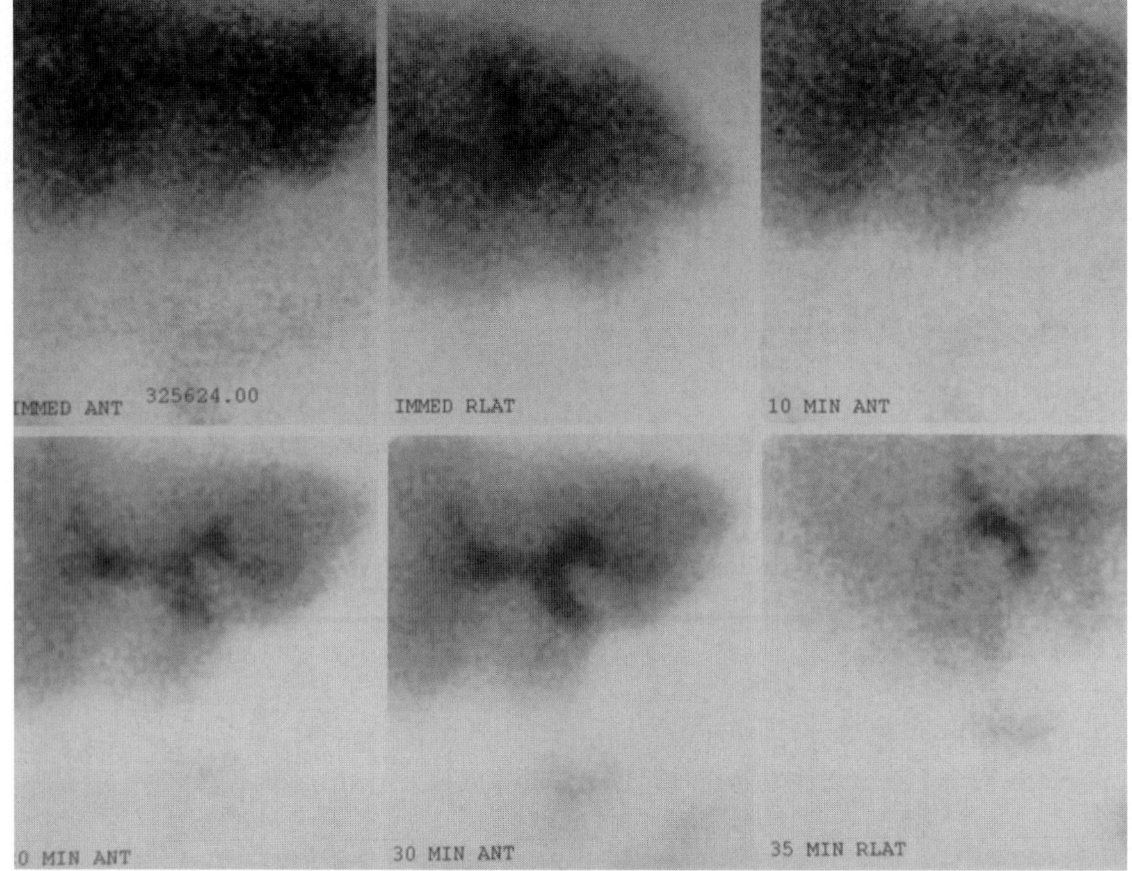

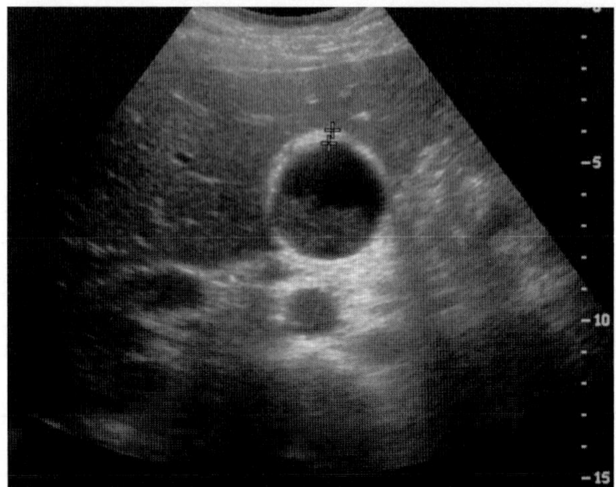

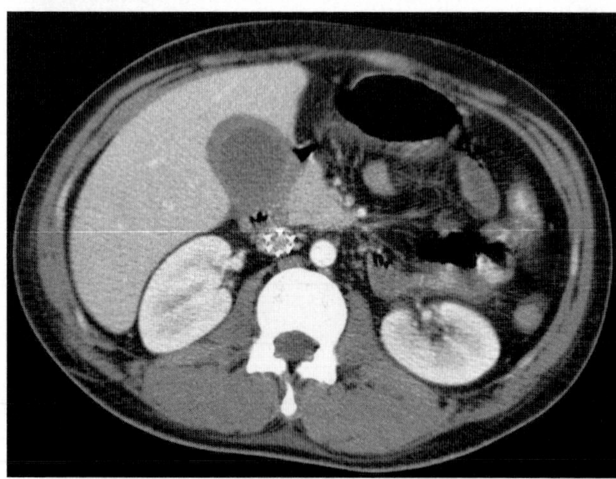

Figure 6–14 **(A)** Six images obtained over 35 minutes from a nuclear medicine hepatobiliary scan demonstrate radiotracer in the liver and inter- and extrahepatic bile duct, but no activity in the gallbladder, indicating cholecystitis. **(B)** Transverse ultrasound image shows sludge in the gallbladder and a thickened gallbladder wall (> 4 mm). **(C)** Axial CT image demonstrates gallbladder wall thickening. Note the metallic filter in the patient's inferior vena cava, which had been placed to prevent pulmonary thromboembolism. **(D)** Spot fluoroscopic image from a cholecystostomy procedure shows a pigtail catheter in the gallbladder lumen, which is opacified with contrast. **(E)** Spot fluoroscopic image after drainage of the gallbladder lumen demonstrates contrast in the bile ducts and extending into the duodenum, indicating that the cholecystitis was not due to an obstructing stone in the cystitic duct or common bile duct. The diagnosis was acalculous (without stone) cholecystitis.

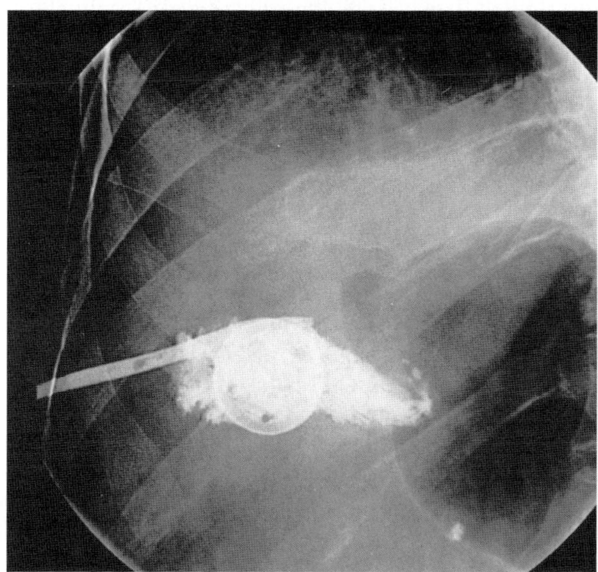

D

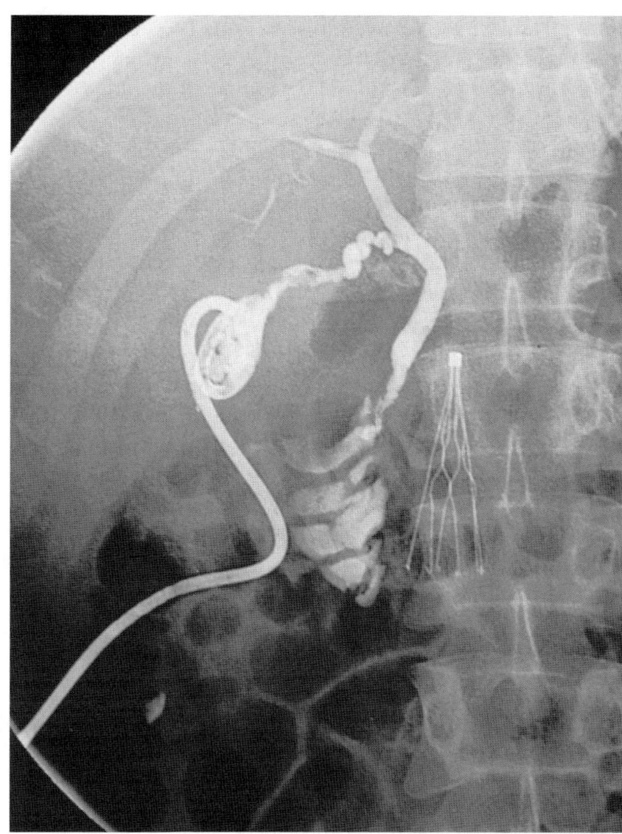

E

Figure 6–14 (*Continued*)

These patients suffer from a condition termed acalculous cholecystitis, which may be caused by ischemia or infection of static bile. Patients at risk include patients on total parenteral nutrition, burn patients, trauma patients, and patients with acquired immunodeficiency syndrome (AIDS). Although ultrasound will demonstrate no stones in these cases, the hepatobiliary scan will still demonstrate nonfilling of the gallbladder in the vast majority of cases; specificity, however, is much lower than in the typical "calculous" cholecystitis.

◇ Interventional Procedures

The interventional radiologist may be called upon to treat acute biliary obstruction. In severely ill patients who are poor surgical candidates, the gallbladder may be decompressed percutaneously under ultrasound guidance, with a drainage catheter left in place, in a procedure known as percutaneous cholecystostomy. The biliary system may be directly visualized by percutaneous transhepatic cholangiography, in which a catheter is placed into the biliary tree and contrast injected. If an obstruction in the common duct is found, a stent can be placed across it, typically extending from the common hepatic duct into the small bowel, permitting internal drainage of the biliary system. The latter procedure is most commonly performed in patients with neoplasms obstructing the bile duct, such as cholangiocarcinoma and carcinoma of the pancreas.

Pancreatitis

Pancreatitis comes in two presentations: acute and chronic. Acute pancreatitis is defined as inflammation of the pancreas with the potential for complete healing, and chronic pancreatitis is associated with permanent sequelae, including altered structure and impaired function. In chronic pancreatitis, the loss of both endocrine function (insulin and glucagon secretion) and exocrine function (secretion of digestive enzymes, including amylases, proteases, and lipases) may play a role in the clinical course. It should be emphasized that chronic pancreatitis is not equivalent to repeated episodes of acute pancreatitis, and both types may be associated with episodes of acute exacerbation.

Epidemiology

There are approximately 40,000 cases of acute pancreatitis per year in the United States, with a peak incidence in the sixth decade of life. The two most important risk factors are cholelithiasis and alcoholism.

Pathophysiology

The pathophysiology of pancreatitis is multifaceted and complex, but all mechanisms have in common the end point of pancreatic autodigestion, with activated pancreatic enzymes escaping from the ductal system and lysing the tissue of the pancreas and adjacent structures. The fact that the pancreas lacks a capsule tends to facilitate the spread of the inflammatory process.

Alcohol ingestion is a more common factor in men, whereas cholelithiasis is more common in women. Gallstone pancreatitis results from impaction of a gallstone in the distal common bile duct, after the point of entry of the pancreatic duct, with resultant obstruction of pancreatic secretion. Alcoholic pancreatitis may stem from inspissation of secretions in the pancreatic ductal system, secondary to the increased concentration of secretions associated with alcohol consumption. It is also known that alcohol causes activation of intracellular digestive enzymes in the pancreatic acini. Other causes include pancreas divisum, trauma (including iatrogenic), penetrating ulcer, hyperlipoproteinemia, and various drugs. Alcoholism is the most prominent cause of chronic pancreatitis.

Clinical Presentation

Patients experiencing an acute attack present with severe abdominal pain that radiates through to the back, peritoneal signs, and fever. They may exhibit respiratory distress with atelectasis and effusions, subcutaneous fat necrosis (manifesting as purple skin lesions), and saponification of serum calcium (precipitation of calcium soaps in fat necrosis), with resultant signs and symptoms of hypocalcemia. In severe cases, patients may present in shock, with renal failure and disseminated intravascular coagulation.

The diagnosis of acute pancreatitis is best made clinically, based on the constellation of history, physical signs, and laboratory findings. Classic laboratory findings include elevations of serum amylase and lipase, with the latter being the more specific of the two, because the salivary glands, fallopian tubes, and lungs also synthesize amylase.

Imaging

◇ Acute Pancreatitis

Imaging is usually performed in cases where the diagnosis is uncertain or to detect complications and assess prognosis. In the acute setting, CT is the study of choice, providing a comprehensive assessment of the gland itself and the surrounding tissues (**Fig. 6-15**). In many cases, the gland appears normal, which does not exclude the diagnosis. Common findings include diffuse or focal swelling of the gland, heterogeneity, poor definition, fluid collections, and thickening of the pararenal fascia.

One of the most important complications of acute pancreatitis, seen in 10% of cases, is a pancreatic pseudocyst. A pancreatic pseudocyst is a fluid collection surrounded by a fibrous capsule (**Fig. 6–16**). It is not a true cyst because it does not have an epithelial lining. A significant percentage of pseudocysts will not resolve spontaneously. Pseudocysts are often seen not only within the pancreas but also in the lesser sac (between the pancreas and stomach) and in the left pararenal space, potential spaces with which the gland itself is continuous.

Abscess, a rarer but more serious condition, develops in approximately 1 in 20 cases and increases the risk of mortality. Abscesses are often recognized by the presence of gas and require urgent drainage. Patients whose hematocrits are falling should be suspected of an even rarer condition, hemorrhagic pancreatitis. Pseudoaneurysm formation or rupture may present in a similar way. Ultrasound is useful in following up on complications and in guiding therapeutic interventions, such as the drainage of fluid collections.

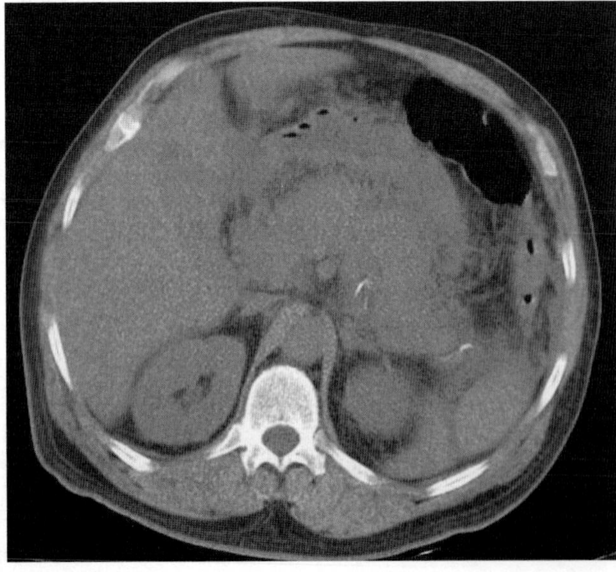

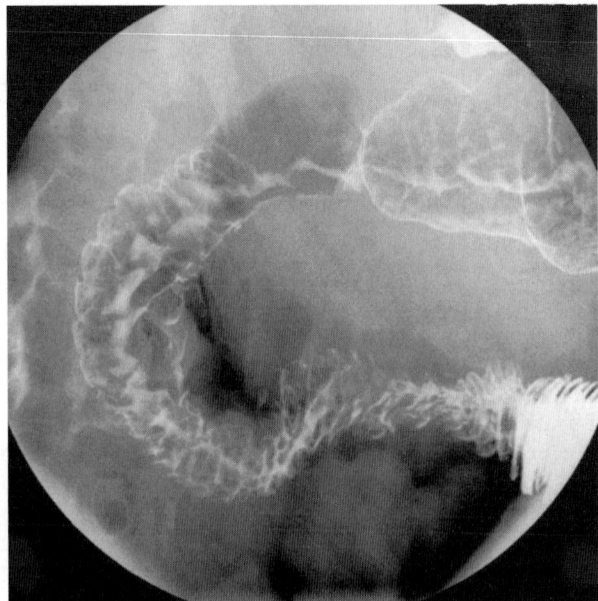

Figure 6–15 **(A)** Axial CT image demonstrates severe inflammation of the pancreas, which is enlarged and shows very indistinct margins. **(B)** Double-contrast view of the gastric antrum and duodenum demonstrates marked irregular spiculation of the mucosal folds in the third and fourth portion of the duodenum, secondary to the adjacent pancreatitis.

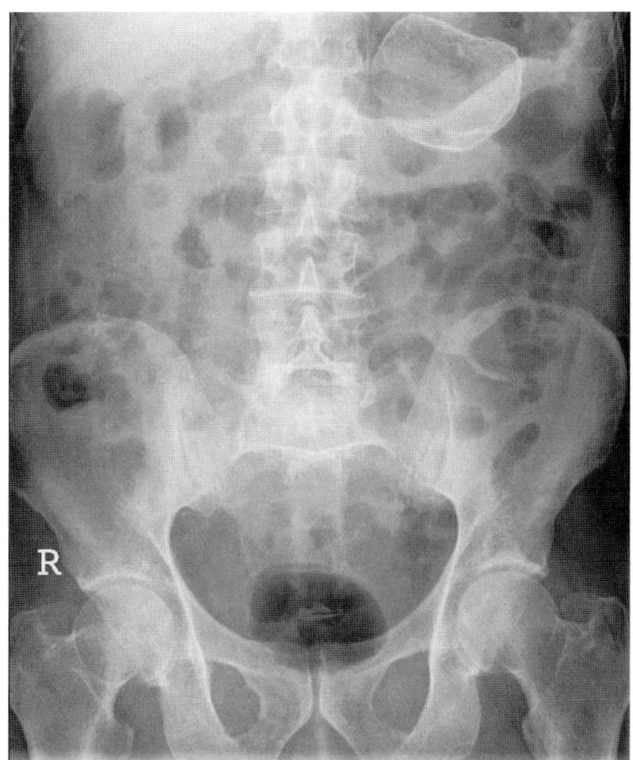

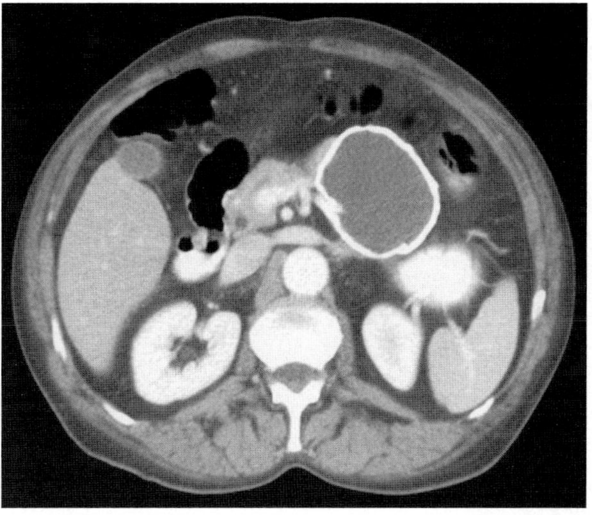

Figure 6–16 **(A)** Abdominal radiograph demonstrates a calcified mass in the left upper quadrant. **(B)** Axial CT image after IV and oral contrast administration shows that the mass is a cyst with a calcified wall. This represented an old pancreatic pseudocyst. Most pseudocysts do not have calcified walls.

◇ Chronic Pancreatitis

Chronic pancreatitis more often requires imaging to confirm the diagnosis, as symptoms may be vague. Some of the most common manifestations of chronic pancreatitis are the presence of calcifications in the pancreatic parenchyma (which are often visible on plain films), a dilated or irregular pancreatic duct, and generalized atrophy of the gland (**Fig. 6–17**). The presence of calcification is not an indicator of disease severity, whereas ductal abnormalities usually indicate more severe insufficiency. It is not possible to state with certainty that a pancreatic mass represents inflammatory tissue, and a small percentage of patients with chronic pancreatitis will also harbor a carcinoma. In some cases, image-directed biopsy (with CT or ultrasound guidance) is necessary.

Diverticular Disease

Epidemiology

Half of Americans over the age of 60 years have colonic diverticula, and the condition becomes increasingly common with advancing age. Although most of those affected never suffer symptoms, approximately 20% suffer at least one episode of diverticular inflammation during their lifetime. The spectrum of diverticular disease ranges from simple diverticulosis (the presence of multiple diverticula) to diverticular disease (multiple diverticula and evidence of colonic muscular hypertrophy), to frank diverticulitis (inflammation of a diverticulum, which may lead to perforation and abscess) (**Fig. 6–18**). Nearly 0.1% of Americans are admitted to the hospital each year for this disease, and nearly one fifth of these require an emergency operation.

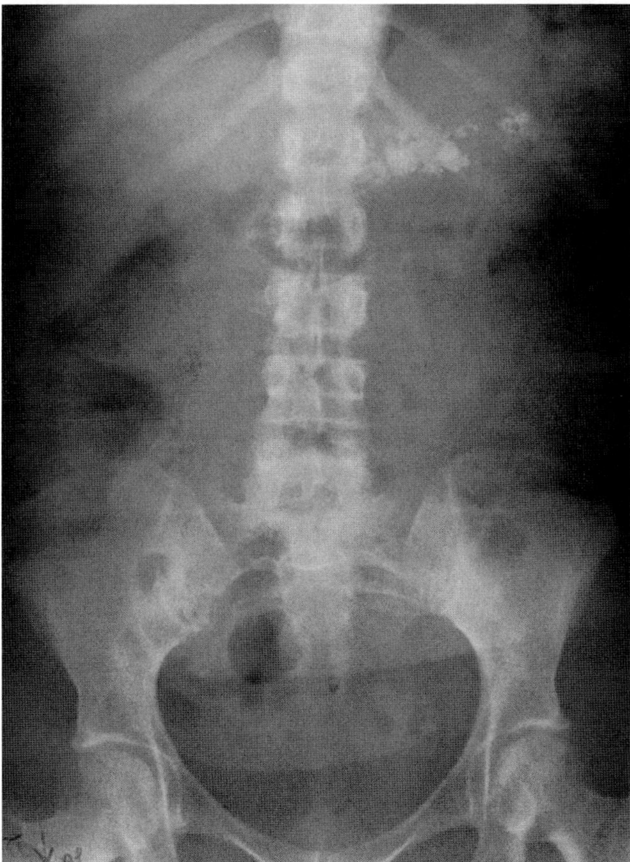

Figure 6–17 This plain radiograph of the abdomen demonstrates a swath of calcification extending across the epigastric area, classic for chronic calcific pancreatitis.

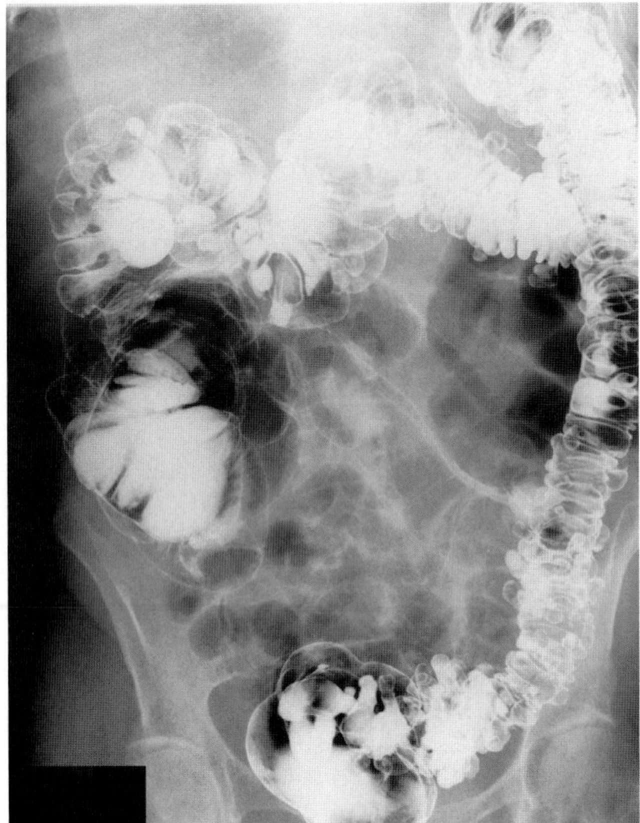

Figure 6–18 This radiograph of the abdomen in a patient undergoing a double-contrast barium enema demonstrates innumerable diverticula, luminal outpouchings filled with barium and air, most numerous in the descending and sigmoid portions of the colon. This established the diagnosis of diverticulosis.

Pathophysiology

Diverticula are thought to result from decreased stool bulk, with impaired colonic motility, overactivity of the bowel musculature, and herniation of mucosa through defects in the muscle layers. Although this is by far the most common condition of the colon in the United States, it is virtually unheard of in many developing nations, where diets are higher in dietary fiber that promotes colonic motility. As one would expect, the distribution of diverticula within the colon is highest in the sigmoid region, which is the narrowest segment and generates the highest pressures. The outpouchings of the wall are often associated with hypertrophy of the longitudinal and circular smooth muscle layers, which causes the mucosal folds to become bunched together and limits luminal distensibility, diagnosed on barium enema as diverticular disease.

Diverticulitis results from inspissation of luminal contents within a diverticulum, which may abrade the mucosa and incite inflammation. As the inflammatory process within the thin wall of the diverticulum progresses, it may cause tiny perforations, with extraluminal leakage of contents (including feces and bacteria) into the surrounding fat. This results in the formation of an abscess within the wall or external to the colon.

Clinical Presentation

Patients with uncomplicated diverticulosis may experience spasmodic pain and mild rectal bleeding. Once diverticulitis develops, patients typically present with pain, tenderness, and/or a mass in the left lower quadrant. Fever is also present in many patients, as is leukocytosis.

Imaging

The radiologist plays several roles in the setting of suspected diverticulitis. First, the diagnosis must be made: Is there or is there not imaging evidence of diverticulitis? Second, the extent of the disease must be assessed: Is the process confined to the wall of the bowel, or how far has the inflammatory process spread within the abdomen? Third, there may be a role for radiologic intervention: Is percutaneous or transrectal drainage of an abscess necessary? If the disease is mild, the patient is likely to be managed with antibiotics. If inflammation is more widespread, or an abscess has formed, surgical or radiologic intervention is likely to be required. The radiologic approach to percutaneous abscess drainage is discussed in the interventional section of Chapter 1. The definitive treatment, typically delayed if possible until the inflammatory process has subsided, is resection of the diseased segment of the bowel.

Radiologic findings vary by modality. Plain films of the abdomen may demonstrate a left lower quadrant soft tissue mass, a focal ileus, or even a gas collection suggestive of an abscess. One of the main functions of the plain film is to rule out free air, which would indicate perforation. If there is no evidence of perforation, a water-soluble contrast enema may be performed to look for evidence of an abscess and extravasation of contrast through a fistula, which virtually establishes the diagnosis. In advanced cases, fistulae may develop to the bladder, vagina, and small bowel. CT is the examination of choice and should be performed with oral and, if necessary, rectal contrast to ensure good bowel opacification. Findings include diverticulosis, inflammation in the pericolic fat, a pericolic fluid collection that may contain air (indicating abscess), and perhaps fistulae (**Fig 6-19**). The possibility of a perforated colonic neoplasm cannot be absolutely ruled out on the basis of any of these studies.

Appendicitis

Epidemiology

Acute appendicitis constitutes the most common abdominal surgical emergency, affecting approximately 1 in 14 Americans at some point in their lives, and 0.1% of the U.S. population per year. Approximately 250,000 appendectomies are performed each year in the United States.

Pathophysiology

The appendix arises from the cecum 1 to 2 cm below the ileocecal valve and demonstrates considerable lymphoid tissue when sectioned. Though highly variable in size, it typically measures approximately 8 cm in length, and its diameter is 6 mm or less. Acute appendicitis results from

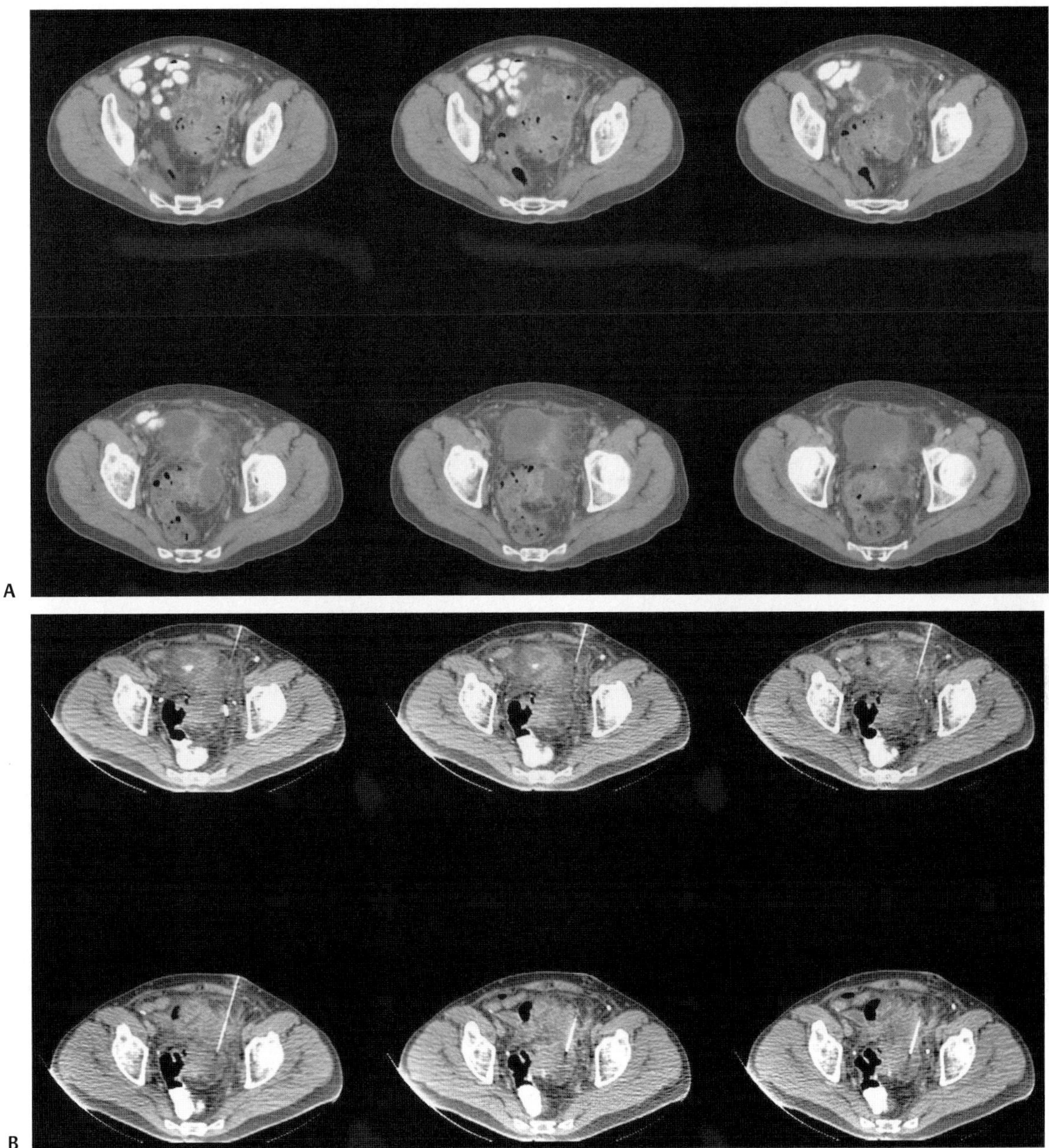

Figure 6–19 **(A)** Six axial CT images demonstrate multiple air-containing diverticula of the sigmoid colon and a perisigmoidal fluid collection with an enhancing wall, an abscess secondary to diverticulitis with perforation. **(B)** Six axial CT images demonstrate that a needle has been placed percutaneously into the fluid collection under CT guidance.

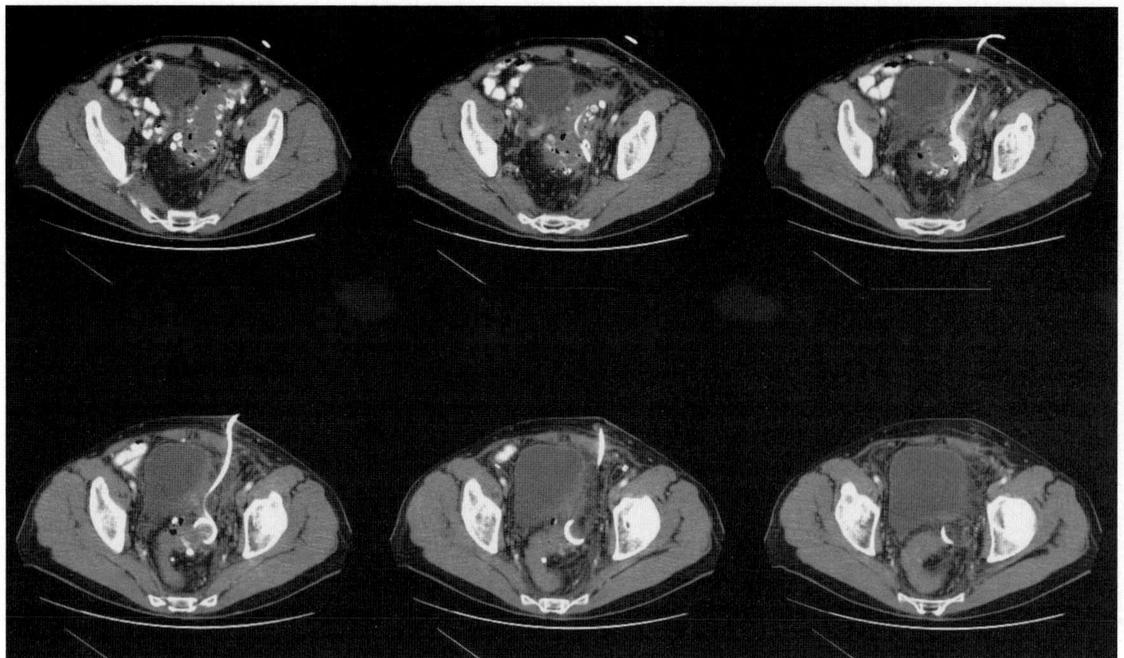

Figure 6–19 (C) Six axial CT images demonstrate placement of a catheter into the now drained fluid collection. Note contrast in many of the diverticula.

obstruction of the appendiceal lumen, which is secondary to lymphoid hyperplasia in the majority of cases, and secondary to a fecalith in approximately one third of cases. Continued mucus secretion results in increased intraluminal pressure, which may eventually compromise venous drainage, resulting in ischemia and breakdown of the mucosa. Bacterial superinfection may also result. The major danger in appendicitis is perforation, which occurs in approximately one quarter of patients, and can result in abscess formation, peritonitis, and life-threatening sepsis. The hazards associated with these complications render acute appendicitis a surgical emergency.

Clinical Presentation

The typical patient presents with abdominal pain, nausea, and vomiting. At onset, the pain is usually periumbilical and diffuse because only visceral pain receptors are involved, but as inflammation of the appendix spreads to the peritoneum, the pain becomes sharper and localized to the right lower quadrant. Additional findings in many patients include fever and leukocytosis of around 15,000 cells/mm^3. In the majority of patients, the clinical diagnosis is relatively straightforward; however, acute appendicitis presents atypically in approximately one in four patients, and even in the best of hands, appendectomy discloses a normal appendix approximately 20% of the time. The single most difficult clinical situation is a young woman, in whom a ruptured ovarian cyst, ectopic pregnancy, or pelvic inflammatory disease could produce virtually identical symptoms and signs. Judicious use of imaging resources should make it possible to reduce the rate of negative appendectomy in the subgroup of patients in whom the diagnosis is uncertain.

Imaging

The initial radiologic study obtained in many patients with suspected appendicitis is supine and upright radiographs of the abdomen. This is abnormal in most patients, although the findings may be nonspecific. The only specific finding is a calcified appendicolith, which is seen 10% of the time but is associated with a nearly 50% probability of perforation. An appendicolith is usually approximately 1 cm in diameter, is round or oval in shape, and demonstrates concentric rings of calcification, called lamellation. If an appendicolith is detected, appendectomy is warranted. Nonspecific plain film findings in the right lower quadrant include a soft tissue mass, a dilated segment of bowel with an air–fluid level, and obscuration of the psoas muscle margin by adjacent inflammation.

Barium enema, once a mainstay of imaging, is rarely used for suspected appendicitis, looking for failure of the appendix to fill due to luminal obstruction, as well as mass effect on the cecum by the inflammatory mass. Ultrasound has received considerable attention as a means of diagnosing appendicitis. In skilled hands, it has a sensitivity greater than 90%, and an even higher specificity. The examination is performed by gradually pressing the transducer down on the skin of the right lower quadrant, thereby displacing gas-filled bowel loops and minimizing the distance between the transducer and the appendix. The diagnosis is made when a tubular, noncompressible structure measuring 6 mm or more in diameter and demonstrating no peristalsis, representing the inflamed appendix, is identified (**Fig. 6-20**). Confidence is further increased when an appendicolith, an echogenic focus with posterior shadowing seen in approximately one third of patients, is identified. Difficulties with the sonographic approach include a retrocecal appendix and obese or

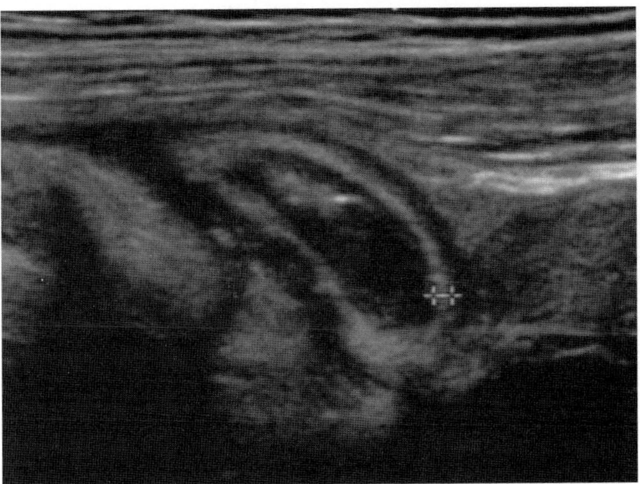

Figure 6–20 A sonographic image of the right lower quadrant demonstrates a tubular, noncompressible structure in the right lower quadrant. The patient was tender to pressure from the transducer at this point. There is echogenic material in the lumen. Surgery confirmed the diagnosis of acute appendicitis.

uncooperative patients. Moreover, the examination is highly operator dependent.

CT represents perhaps the best radiologic modality, because it not only directly visualizes the appendix and surrounding structures, but also provides the most help in evaluating other abdominal and pelvic pathologies. Accuracy is well more than 95% in the diagnosis of acute appendicitis. Noncontrast scanning offers improved visualization of appendicoliths, but both intravenous and oral contrast should be administered to enhance differentiation of the bowel from other structures and to assess enhancement patterns. The inflamed appendix appears as a fluid-filled tube with wall thickening of several millimeters, and is surrounded by periappendiceal inflammation that appears as ill-defined stranding in the fat, which may extend to involve adjacent bowel (**Fig. 6–21**). If perforation has occurred, an abscess may be seen.

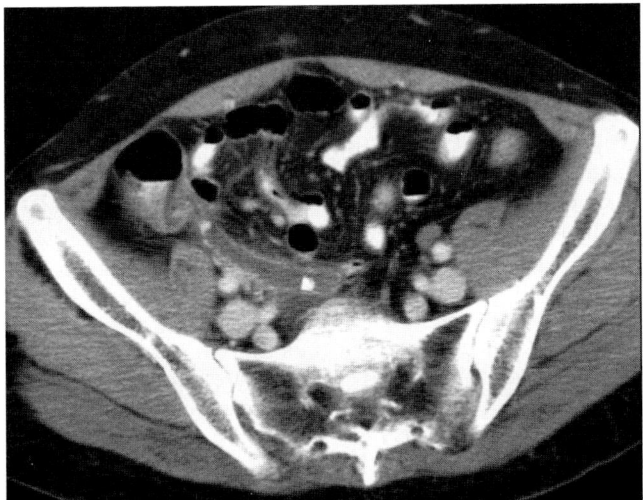

Figure 6–21 Axial CT image demonstrates the fluid-filled, dilated appendix with inflammatory stranding in the periappendiceal fat. Note the bright appendicolith in the lumen. Surgery confirmed acute appendicitis.

Bowel Obstruction

Epidemiology

Approximately 300,000 cases of bowel obstruction are diagnosed each year in the United States. At least three quarters of small bowel obstructions in the United States and other industrialized nations result from postsurgical adhesions, making prior surgery one of the most common reasons for acute abdominal surgery. Other causes of small bowel obstruction in adults are incarcerated hernia, malignancy, intussusception, and volvulus (**Fig. 6–22**).

Pathophysiology

In general, bowel obstruction results from one of three causes: an endoluminal mass, thickening or inflammation of the bowel wall, or extraluminal compression. Small bowel obstructions account for approximately four of five cases of adult GI tract obstruction.

Although it is obvious why a bowel obstruction will produce serious consequences over a period of days to weeks, the reasons why suspected obstructions warrant urgent diagnostic evaluation may be less clear. One reason for urgency is the effects of obstruction on the bowel proximal to it. Swallowed air, saliva, and GI secretions (succus entericus) progressively accumulate proximal to the point of obstruction, and stasis allows bacterial proliferation and the production of toxins that directly injure the bowel.

Moreover, increasing distention of the bowel increases intramural tension, as described by the law of Laplace, which states that for a constant intraluminal pressure, increasing the radius of a viscus by a factor of 2 will double its intramural tension. This increased intramural tension may eventually overcome capillary perfusion pressure and result in ischemic injury, with subsequent tissue necrosis, perforation, and peritonitis. The law of Laplace also explains why the cecum is the segment of colon most likely to perforate. The cecum is relatively thin walled and has the greatest initial luminal diameter; thus, for a given colonic pressure, it will experience the greatest intramural tension and hence distend the most.

For these reasons—stasis and distention—one of the first and most important therapeutic interventions in suspected bowel obstruction is to make the patient NPO (nothing by mouth) and to pass a nasogastric tube and place it on suction, in an attempt to decompress the bowel.

Mechanical obstruction may be classified according to several categories. The first is simple obstruction, which simply refers to blockage of the intestinal lumen without compromise of blood supply. A closed-loop obstruction refers to blockage of both afferent and efferent limbs of an obstructed segment, with a higher risk of bowel ischemia. This is often seen in volvulus or incarcerated hernias (**Fig. 6–23**). A strangulated obstruction refers to obstruction with impairment of blood supply, which usually affects venous outflow before arterial inflow.

Clinical Presentation

Clinical indicators of small bowel obstruction include nausea and vomiting, hyperactive followed by absent bowel sounds,

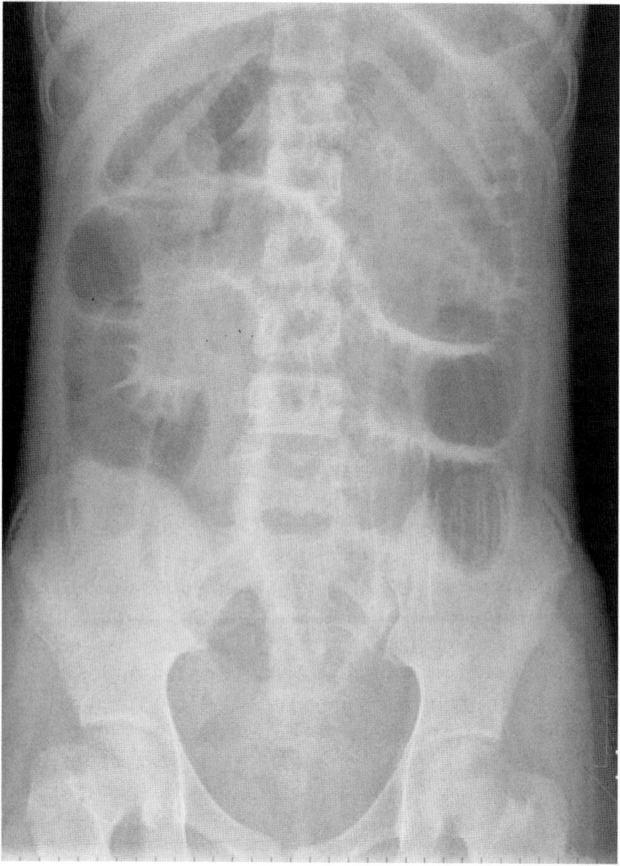
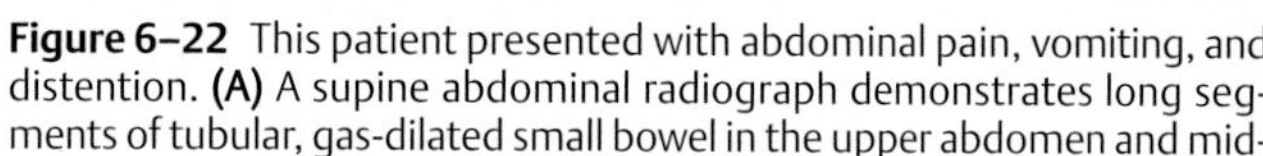
A

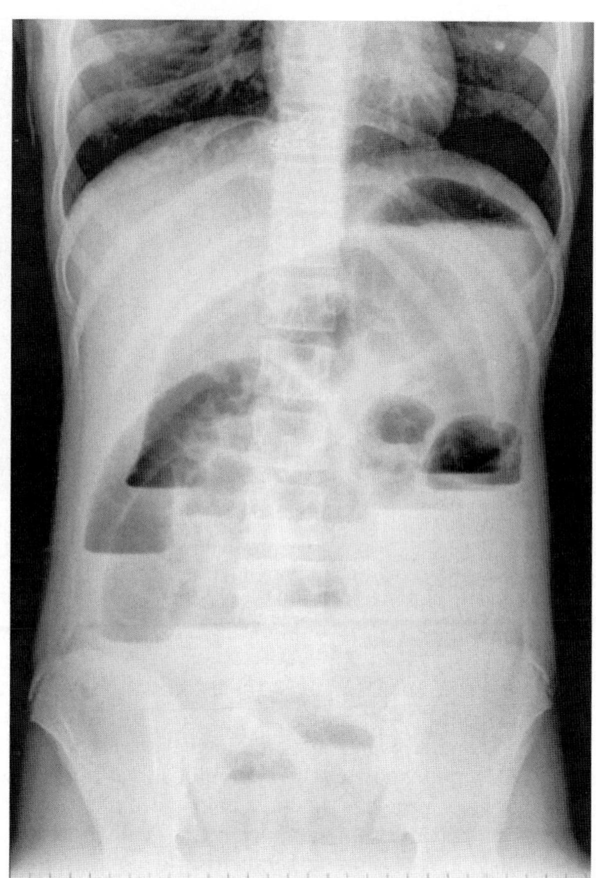
B

Figure 6–22 This patient presented with abdominal pain, vomiting, and distention. **(A)** A supine abdominal radiograph demonstrates long segments of tubular, gas-dilated small bowel in the upper abdomen and midabdomen. At surgery, there was a complete distal small bowel obstruction. **(B)** An upright view demonstrates multiple air–fluid levels in the dilated small bowel.

progressive abdominal distention and pain, and absence of flatus and bowel movements.

Imaging

Radiology plays a major role in the evaluation of intestinal obstruction. Abdominal radiographs can detect obstruction many hours before the diagnosis becomes clinically obvious, delineate the level and often the etiology of obstruction, and can be used to follow the course of obstruction over time. CT is even better at determining etiology.

◇ Small Bowel Obstruction

The most common radiographic sign of small bowel obstruction is distention, which is visualized as dilated, air-containing segments of small bowel (measuring more than 3 cm in diameter), with or without air–fluid levels (**Fig 6-24**). The most common causes of functional ileus include medication (opiate analgesics and anticholinergics), metabolic derangements (diabetes mellitus, hypokalemia, and hypercalcemia), and the postoperative state (which usually resolves within several days to a week).

The level of mechanical obstruction can be estimated by assessing the number of dilated segments of bowel and the location at which the dilated segments terminate. A proximal small bowel obstruction will produce relatively few dilated segments, which will be located predominantly in the left upper quadrant. A distal small bowel obstruction will produce a greater number of dilated segments, extending down into the right lower quadrant. How does one determine whether segments of air-filled bowel are enteric or colonic? Generally, small bowel segments will exhibit thin valvulae conniventes extending all the way across their lumen, whereas the thicker haustral markings of large bowel do not extend all the way to the luminal midline.

A common cause of small bowel obstruction in elderly women is gallstone ileus, caused by erosion of a large gallstone through the gallbladder wall and into the duodenum, with passage into the distal small bowel and eventual impaction, usually in the ileocecal region. In the majority of cases, gallstone ileus will manifest radiographically as one or more of the findings of Rigler's triad, including dilated small bowel loops, air in the biliary tree (secondary to choledochoduodenal fistulae), and a calcified gallstone outside the gallbladder fossa.

Signs of intestinal ischemia include bowel wall thickening, effacement of folds, and, eventually, the appearance of intramural air (pneumatosis intestinalis), which may travel via the mesenteric and portal veins into the biliary tree. Pneumatosis intestinalis raises concern that frank bowel necrosis is under way.

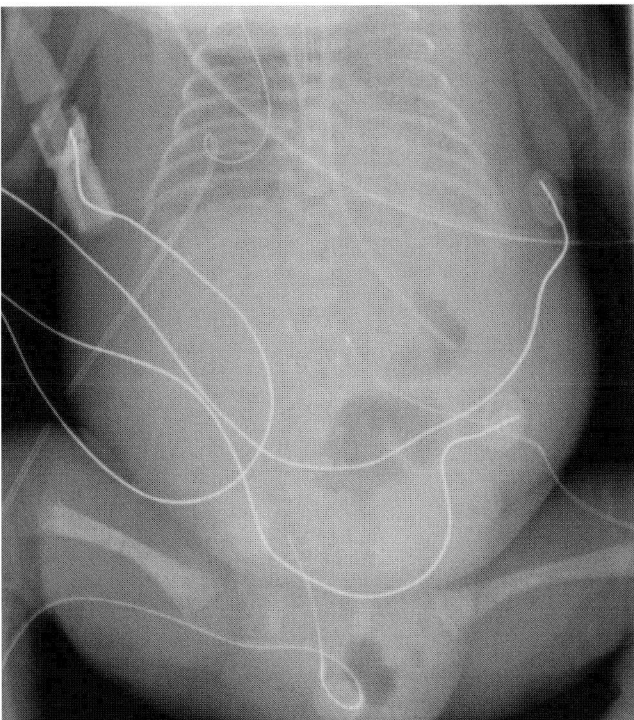

Figure 6–23 An abdominal radiograph in an infant with vomiting and abdominal distention demonstrates dilated, gas-filled bowel in the lower abdomen and a collection of gas in the scrotum. The scrotal gas is in the small bowel that had herniated down through the inguinal canal and became entrapped, an incarcerated hernia.

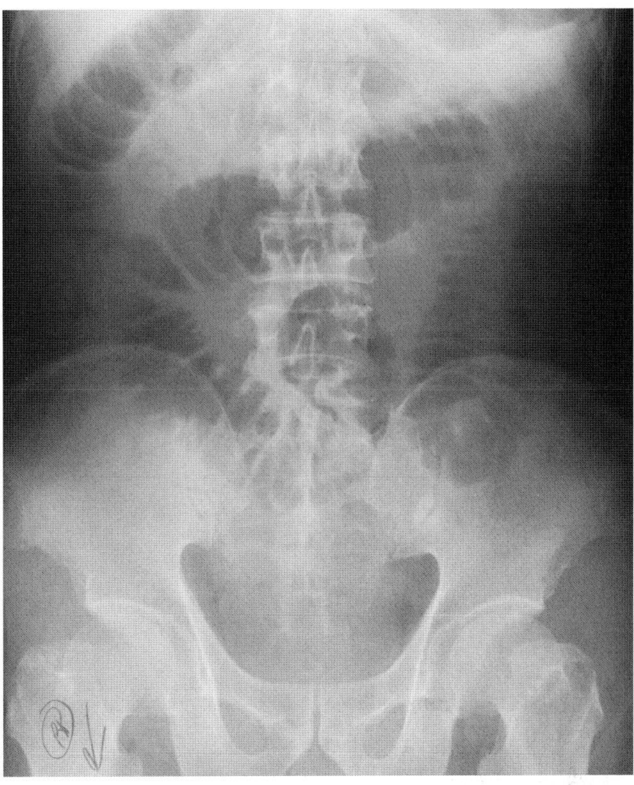

Figure 6–24 A supine abdominal radiograph demonstrates dilated small bowel in the upper abdomen and midabdomen in this patient with a mechanical small bowel obstruction. Note that the folds extend all the way across the lumen, indicating that it is the small bowel.

◇ Large Bowel Obstruction

Large bowel obstructions are generally more ominous than small bowel obstructions, because they tend to occur in older age groups and reflect more serious pathologies, such as malignancy. Nearly two thirds of adult large bowel obstructions reflect the presence of a colon carcinoma, and pelvic malignancies such as cervical and ovarian carcinoma constitute the second most frequent offender (**Fig. 6–25**). A more benign process, diverticulitis, is the third most common cause. Other causes include sigmoid volvulus, in which the colon twists around its mesentery, fecal impaction, and ischemia.

The findings in colonic obstruction depend on whether the ileocecal valve is incompetent. If it is competent, distention will be confined to the colon, which cannot decompress into the small bowel. If it is not competent, reflux of luminal contents into the small bowel will produce both colonic and distal small bowel distention. Regardless of the level of colonic obstruction, the cecum is the segment that dilates most, and when its diameter exceeds 10 cm, it is at risk for perforation. Although plain films are often diagnostic, barium enema or CT may be used to precisely localize and characterize the obstructing lesion prior to surgery.

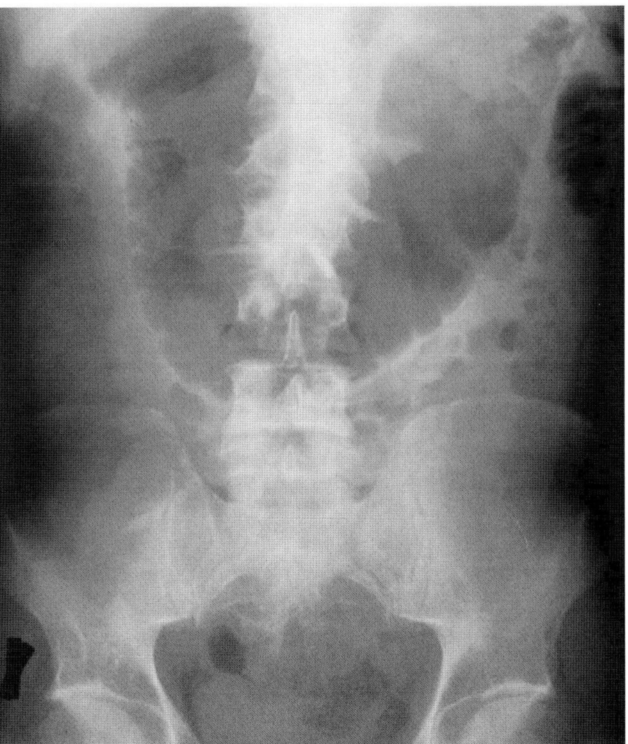

Figure 6–25 A supine abdominal radiograph demonstrates dilated ascending and transverse colon in a patient with an annular adenocarcinoma obstructing the proximal descending colon. Note that the haustral folds do not extend all the way across the colonic lumen.

7

The Reproductive System

◆ Female Reproductive System: Breasts

Anatomy and Physiology

Anatomically, the breast is a relatively simple structure, consisting primarily of skin, supportive elements (Cooper's ligaments), fat, the nipple-areolar complex, and ductal and lobular tissue (**Fig. 7–1**). The network of lactiferous (from the Latin *lac,* "milk") ducts branches out from the nipple and terminates in lobules, each of which is made up of saclike alveoli, where milk production occurs. The duct system remains rudimentary in the nongravid breast, but it proliferates under the stimulation of high levels of estrogen (from the Latin *oestrus,* "frenzy") during pregnancy.

Mammary gland function depends on the secretion of prolactin-releasing hormone by the hypothalamus, which induces secretion of prolactin by the anterior lobe of the pituitary gland, as well as the secretion of oxytocin (from the Greek *oxys,* "quick," and *tokos,* "birth") from the hypothalamus, by way of the posterior pituitary. The word *mammary* is derived from the Latin *mamma* (breast), from which the term *mammal* is derived. Prolactin stimulates milk production, and oxytocin stimulates milk letdown, by inducing contraction of the myoepithelial cells surrounding the alveoli. Recall that oxytocin also stimulates uterine contractions during labor. Both prolactin and oxytocin are secreted in response to the nipple stimulation of suckling. The estrogen-dependent proliferation of tissue in the nonlactating breast also functions in sexual dimorphism, conferring a distinctively female appearance.

Pathology

Breast Cancer

Although all categories of pathology may manifest in the breast, the imaging diagnosis of breast disease is almost completely focused on a single pathologic entity: breast cancer. Interest in other types of lesions, including a variety of benign processes, stems largely from their ability to mimic cancer and the need to reliably distinguish benign from malignant disease.

◇ Epidemiology

The importance of breast imaging is conveyed by the fact that breast cancer is the most common cancer in U.S. women, with ~185,000 new cases per year. It is second only to lung cancer as a cause of cancer death among women, resulting in 45,000 deaths annually (**Fig. 7–2**). It has been estimated that as many as one in nine women in the United States will develop the disease during their lifetime, should they live long enough. The risk of breast cancer increases with age; very few cases are diagnosed in women under age 30, and the vast majority of patients are over age 50. The average age of diagnosis is 65. Female gender is the greatest risk factor for breast carcinoma, as only 1% of cases occur in men (**Fig. 7–3**). In women, the single strongest risk factor for the development of breast cancer is a personal history of previous breast cancer. Additional risk factors include a first-degree relative with the disease, nulliparity or late parity, and exposure to

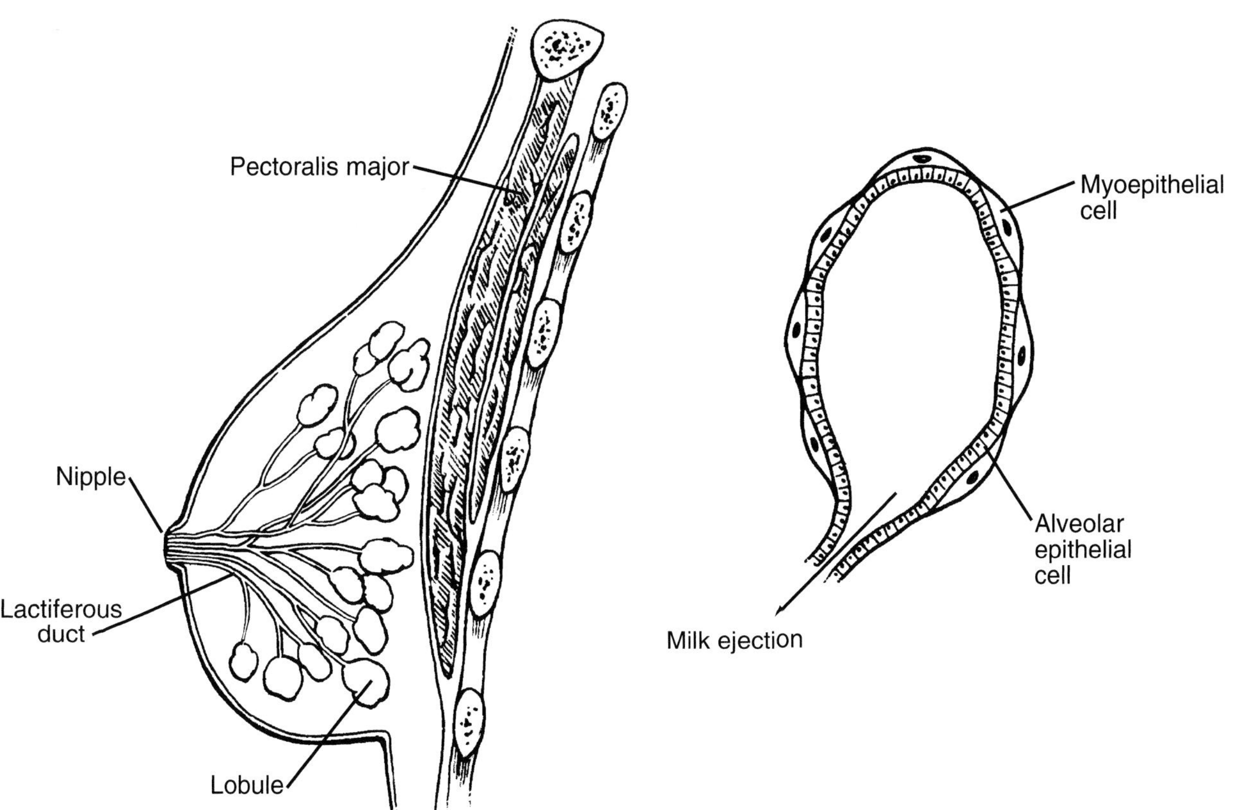

Figure 7–1 Anatomy of the breast and the terminal lobule. The lobule and its duct constitute the terminal lobular-ductular unit, from which the vast majority of breast cancers arise.

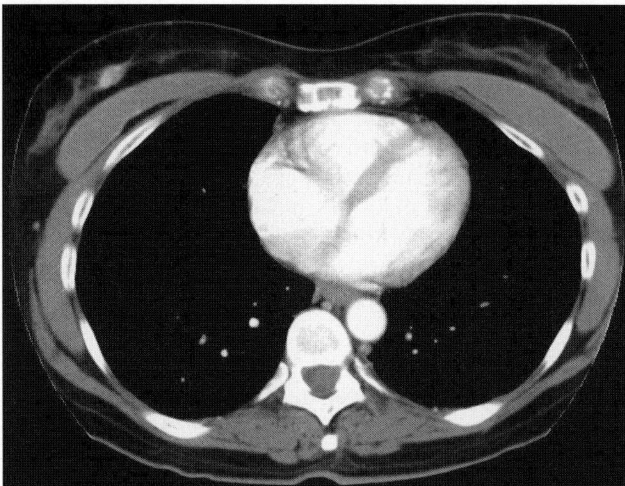

Figure 7–2 This axial CT image of the chest in a 57-year-old woman undergoing staging for ovarian carcinoma demonstrates an enhancing mass in the right breast. This proved to be a ductal carcinoma in situ. Note also that the patient had bilateral breast implants, which had been placed for cosmetic reasons. CT is not a sensitive technique for the detection of breast cancer, but it is important to inspect all of the anatomy visible on radiologic images. Fortunately, the radiologists interpreting this study did not restrict their attention to the lung, where the referring physician had intended to rule out hematogenous metastases.

large amounts of ionizing radiation, as in radiotherapy for lymphoma.; however, ~70% of women diagnosed with breast cancer have no significant risk factors.

◇ Pathophysiology

Infiltrating ductal carcinoma, accounting for ~80% of cases, is the most common type of breast cancer. These cancers arise from the epithelial cells that line the breast ducts (**Fig. 7–4**). Approximately 10% of breast cancers arise from the terminal lobules and are called lobular carcinomas. Medullary breast carcinoma arises from the supporting stromal cells of the breast; mucinous carcinoma is associated with large amounts of cytoplasmic mucin. The latter two are generally larger than ductal and lobular carcinomas at the time of diagnosis, but they enjoy a better prognosis, due to their lower propensity to metastasize. Paget's disease, a ductal carcinoma that has invaded the skin of the nipple, tends to be detected early and therefore also has a somewhat better prognosis. A prognostically less favorable type of breast cancer is inflammatory carcinoma, which represents an aggressive tumor that has invaded the dermal lymphatics and presents clinically with prominent breast inflammation.

An important prognostic indicator in breast cancer is the level of estrogen and progesterone receptors expressed by the tumor. Tumors expressing higher levels of hormone receptors tend to be both more differentiated and more responsive to hormone deprivation. This explains the widespread use of tamoxifen (an antiestrogen agent) in this disease, which is generally used in postmenopausal patients whose tumors express estrogen receptors.

A ductal carcinoma in situ is a tumor whose cells have not yet penetrated the basement membrane of the ducts. It is thought that nearly all breast cancers arise in the terminal duct-lobular unit, beginning as ductal or lobular carcinoma in situ, which at some point becomes invasive. When a carcinoma in situ is detected, local treatment to the breast is generally considered adequate. In contrast, local therapy generally does not suffice for invasive ductal carcinoma, which has a propensity to metastasize hematogenously and via the lymphatics. Invasive carcinoma is treated with a combination of local and systemic therapy.

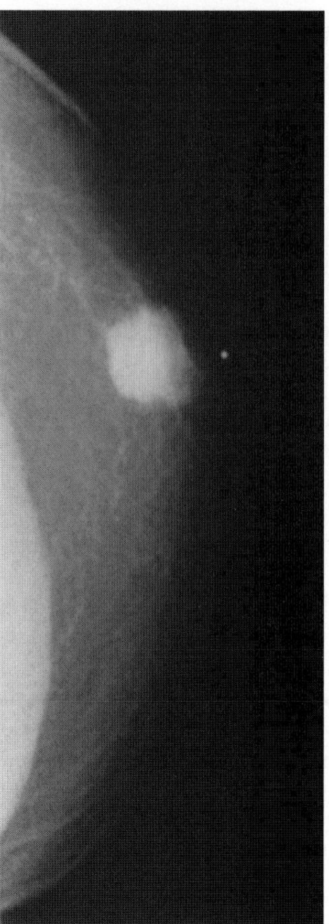

Figure7–3 This 55-year-old man presented with a mildly tender left breast lump. The craniocaudal mammogram demonstrates a 2 cm mass with irregular borders that turned out to be a carcinoma. Note the paucity of breast tissue compared with mammograms of women's breasts.

Local therapy may consist of mastectomy alone or lumpectomy with radiation. Both generally involve an axillary nodal dissection for staging. In patients with large tumors and small breasts, conservative therapy (lumpectomy) is less likely to produce an acceptable cosmetic result. Adjuvant therapy is intended to irradicate micrometastases and is employed in most premenopausal patients and in those postmenopausal patients whose tumors do not exhibit estrogen receptors.

◇ Clinical Presentation

The goal of breast cancer screening is to diagnose breast cancer in patients who have not yet developed clinical signs or symptoms of the disease. By the time symptoms and signs have developed, the tumor has usually become invasive, and the prognosis is less favorable. The most typical clinical presentation of breast cancer is a painless breast mass. Many

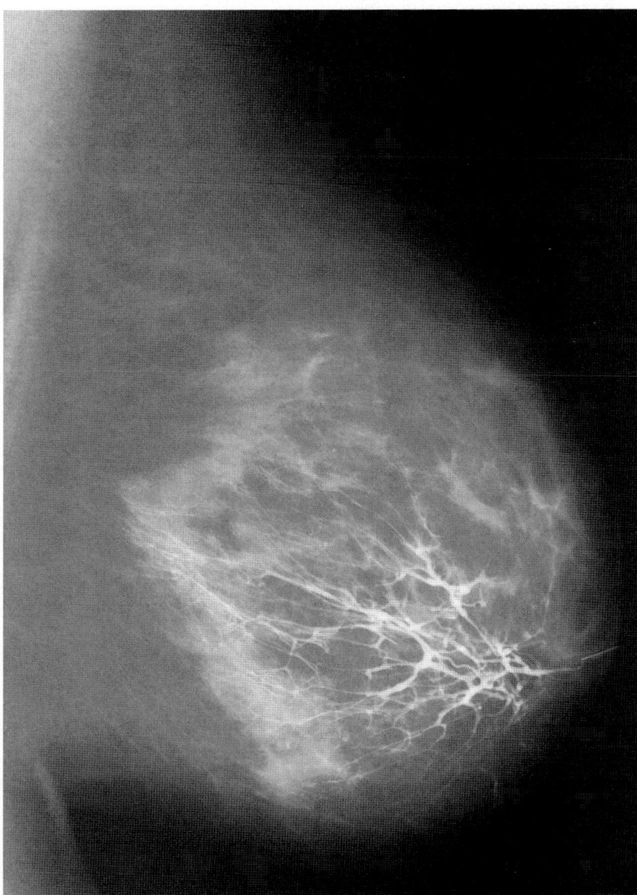

Figure 7–4 A ductogram, performed by cannulating the lactiferous sinuses at the nipple and injecting iodinated contrast material, demonstrates opacification of a portion of the ductal system. The procedure may be part of the workup for patients presenting with a nonmilky or bloody discharge, which can result from an intraductal mass.

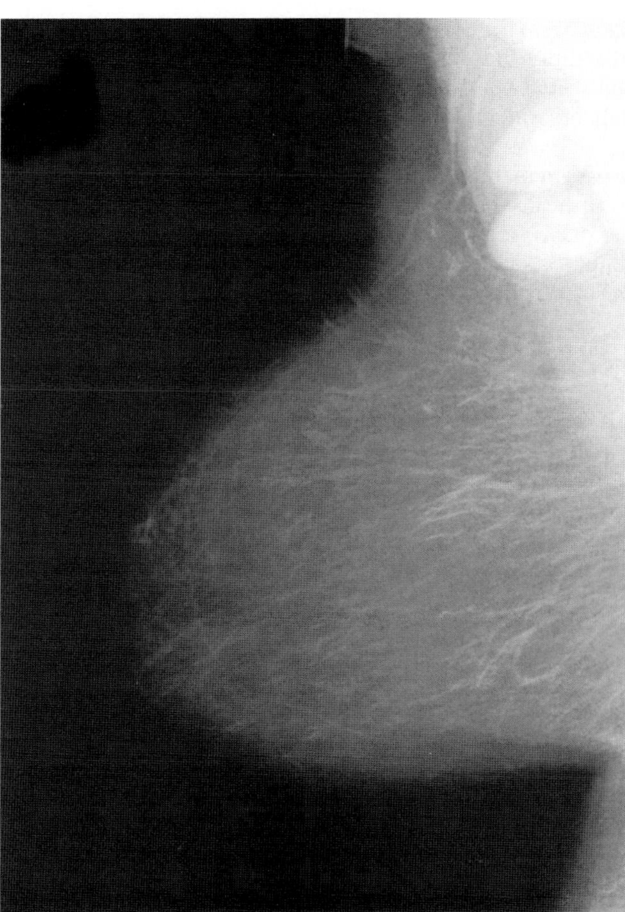

Figure 7–5 This mediolateral oblique (MLO) view of the right breast demonstrates large ovoid masses in the axilla. These represent pathologically dense and enlarged lymph nodes. If they contained metastatic breast carcinoma, the disease would be at an undesirably advanced stage. In this case, however, there is no breast cancer. Instead, the patient turned out to be suffering from non-Hodgkin's lymphoma.

women feel soft lumps within their breasts, which are sometimes painful and may wax and wane with the menstrual cycle; such findings are almost always benign. A hard, nontender, unchanging or slowly growing mass is of concern. Other clinical findings of breast cancer include changes in the contour of the breast, skin thickening, a new bloody nipple discharge, and axillary or supraclavicular adenopathy.

The trend toward conservative, breast-sparing therapy has increased the importance of the radiologist in the detection and management of breast cancer, for two reasons. First, this option is only available when the disease is detected at an early stage (**Fig. 7–5**). Second, prior to therapy, the remainder of the involved breast and the contralateral breast must be exonerated. A patient with multicentric breast cancer (multiple lesions more than 2 cm apart) is a poor candidate for conservative therapy.

◇ Imaging

Although no effective means of preventing breast cancer is at hand, the prospects for patient survival can be dramatically improved by detecting the disease early in its course through screening. Ten-year survival rates in women whose lesions are small (<2 cm), and therefore likely not to have spread at the time of diagnosis, are better than 90%, whereas larger cancers, which are more likely to have metastasized, fare relatively poorly. The number of cells in a breast cancer typically doubles every 3 to 6 months.

Mammography Mammography is the most widely employed form of radiological screening. As with any form of screening, its goal is to detect disease at a presymptomatic and therefore more curable stage. Mammography consists of highly tailored plain radiographs of the breast. It detects 90% of breast cancers, many before they become palpable. Large trials of annual screening mammography indicate that breast cancer mortality can be decreased by as much as 70%. Current guidelines of the American Cancer Society call for every woman age 40 or over to undergo annual mammography. Nearly 10% of breast cancers are detected not by mammography but by palpation; hence, monthly self-examination and annual clinical examination are also recommended. Lesions must be at least 1.5 to 2 cm in diameter to be palpable.

Mammography is also indicated as a diagnostic tool in symptomatic patients presenting with a bloody nipple discharge or a palpable mass, to find and characterize the responsible lesion. In addition, it is important to search both breasts for other lesions. Conservative therapy is contraindicated, for example, in patients with cancers in multiple quadrants of the breast.

The risk of cancer due to the ionizing radiation dose to the breast in mammography appears to be negligible in women over the age of 40. It is estimated that the risk of breast cancer death from a mammogram may be as high as 1 to 2 per million, and the risk of death from spontaneous breast cancer is between 700 and 1000 per million. The risk of radiation-induced breast cancer is inversely correlated with age, whereas the risk of death from spontaneous breast cancer is directly correlated with age—hence, the recommendation that annual screening commence at age 40.

The standard screening mammogram includes two views of each breast: the craniocaudal view and the mediolateral oblique (MLO) view (**Fig. 7–6**). In both cases, the name of the view describes the course of the x-ray beam through the breast; for example, the MLO view is angled from superomedial to inferolateral. To obtain optimal visualization, the

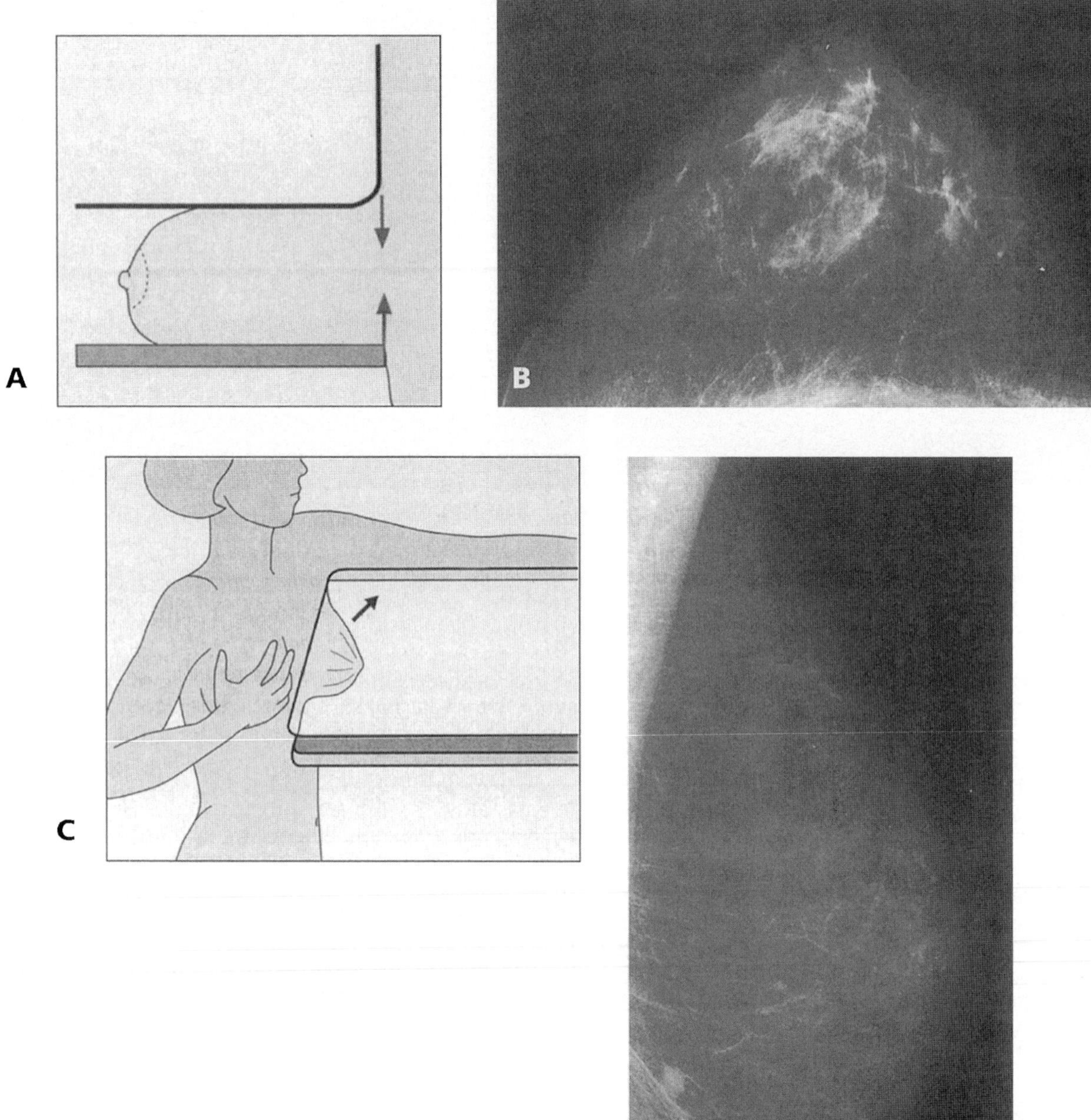

Figure7–6 Normal positioning of the **(A,B)** craniocaudal and **(C,D)** mediolateral oblique views of the breast, as well as representative images in each projection. Note the use of a compression paddle in both positions.

technologist must mobilize, elevate, and pull the breast forward to place as much of the breast as possible over the detector; any portions of the breast not visualized on the film constitute "blind spots" for cancer detection. Compression of the breast spreads apart otherwise overlapping structures, reduces motion artifact (produced when the patient moves during the 1- to 2-second interval during which the exposure is made), minimizes unsharpness by placing breast structures as close as possible to the detector, and minimizes radiation dose.

Once a possible abnormality is detected, additional views, including other projections (e.g., a lateral view), spot compression views, and magnification views may be obtained. Palpable abnormalities are often marked with a radiopaque BB to facilitate correlation with the physical findings. Comparison with previous images is highly valuable, because stability tends to imply benignity, whereas lesions that increase in size or the aggressiveness of their appearance are generally worrisome. The principles of mammographic interpretation are relatively straightforward, although practice is considerably more complex. The mammographer seeks to identify such abnormalities as masses, calcifications, architectural distortions, and adenopathy.

Signs of Malignancy Although the size and number of masses are important, the critical characteristic of a mass is its margins, which represent the radiologic signature of a lesion's biologic behavior. Ill-defined and irregular margins indicate infiltrative behavior and likely represent malignancy, whereas well-defined, regular margins suggest benignity. The margins of a classic breast cancer are spiculated, meaning that strands of tissue are seen to radiate outward in a stellate (starlike) pattern from the mass (**Fig. 7–7**). Histologically, spiculation represents a combination of tumor cells infiltrating out into surrounding tissue and fibrotic reaction to the tumor's presence; however, all spiculated masses are not malignant, and this appearance may also be seen in areas of scarring due to previous trauma or surgery. Before imaging is performed, sites of previous biopsies or lumpectomies should be marked with radiopaque BBs. In young and middle-aged patients, multiplicity of masses tends to indicate benignity (either cysts or fibroadenomas); in older patients, metastases must be considered (**Fig. 7–8**).

The other primary mammographic sign of malignancy is calcification, and approximately one half of all mammographically detected malignancies are found through the presence of suspicious microcalcifications. Calcification as such is not usually worrisome. Most breasts contain some type of calcification, and only certain types of microcalcifications tend to suggest malignancy (**Fig. 7–9**). Microcalcifications associated with carcinoma form a "cast" of the inner walls of the ductules and lobules of the tumor. The most worrisome types of calcification are fine, granular or branching, and pleomorphic (heterogeneous) in morphology (**Fig. 7–10**). They invariably measure less than 2 mm in diameter, and most are less than 0.5 mm. This is why mammographic technique has been developed to provide the highest spatial resolution of any radiologic examination, up to 20 or more line pairs per millimeter. When a suspicious cluster of microcalcifications is identified on standard views, additional spot magnification views are often obtained to provide better assessment of their number and morphology. In general, a mass containing suspicious microcalcifications has a 25 to 30% chance on biopsy of proving to be malignant, although the probability varies widely depending on the morphologic characteristics of the particular lesion.

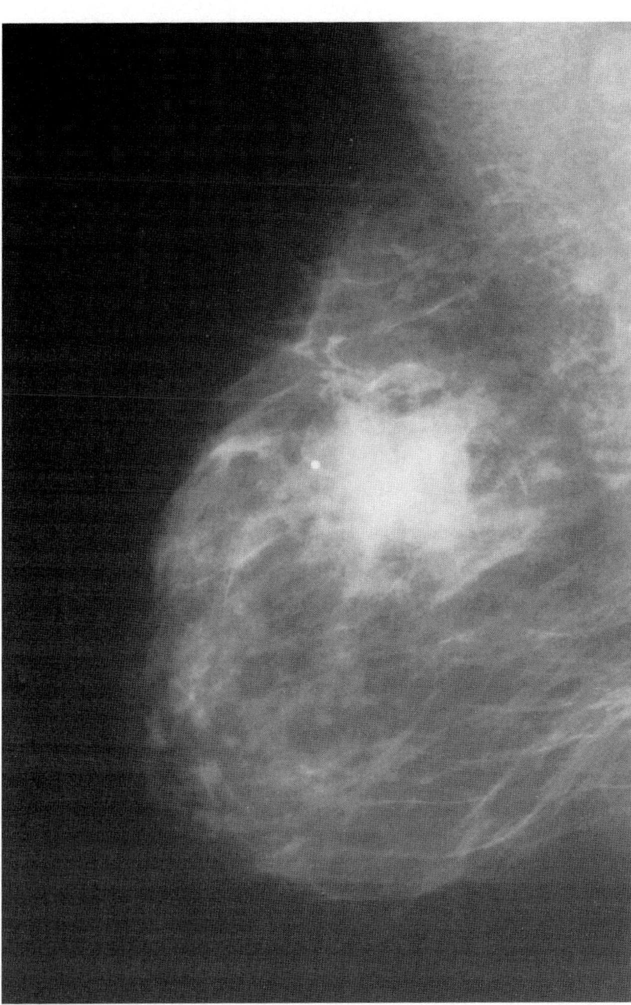

Figure 7–7 This MLO view of the right breast demonstrates a large spiculated mass in the upper outer quadrant, which represented an invasive ductal carcinoma. Note the BB overlying the mass, which was placed at the site of a palpable lump, indicating that the mammogram and physical examination correspond to the same abnormality.

Secondary signs of malignancy include distortion of breast architecture, thickening or retraction of the skin or nipple, and asymmetry of breast tissue. Other than malignancy, a common cause of architectural distortion is previous trauma or surgery. Skin thickening and nipple retraction may be caused by tumor-related fibrosis, but they can also be seen in benign conditions such as infection or disorders associated with edema, such as congestive heart failure. Asymmetric dense tissue is seen in up to 5% of breasts. What is the difference between a mass and an asymmetric density? A mass does not change shape on different views, whereas an asymmetric density does. An asymmetry generally raises concern only if it is associated with a palpable abnormality or other mammographic abnormalities, especially if they are progressing over time.

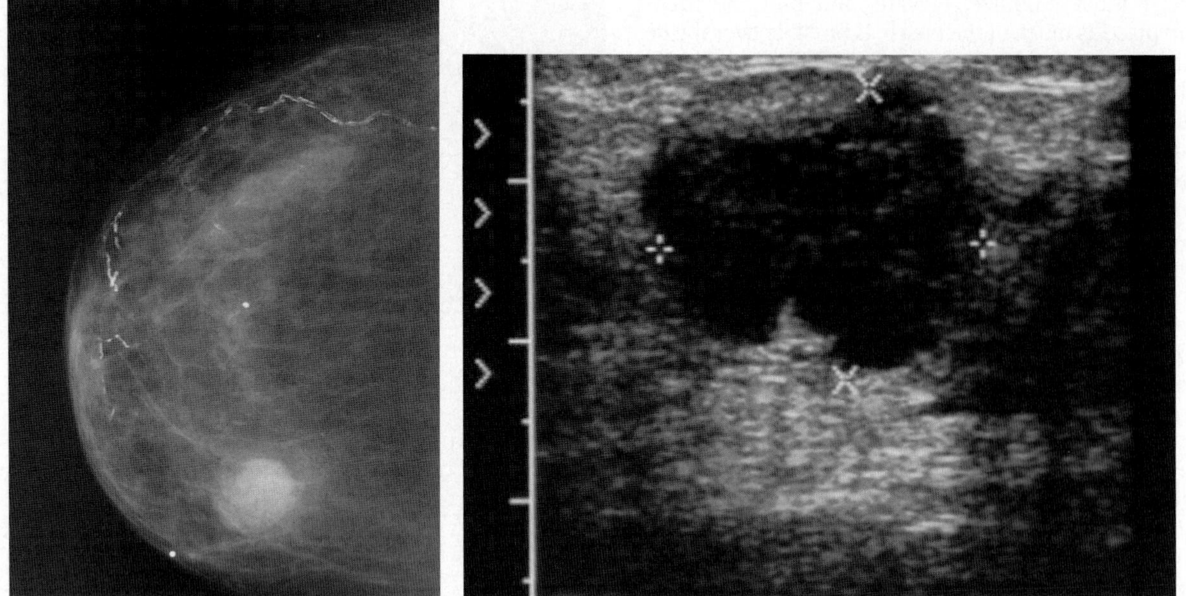

Figure 7–8 (A) This elderly woman with a history of malignant melanoma presented with a palpable right breast mass. The craniocaudal view demonstrates an irregular high-density mass in the inner aspect of the breast. Note also the benign vascular calcifications. **(B)** Sonographic evaluation revealed a hypochoic irregular mass, which was needle biopsied under sonographic guidance and proved to be a metastasis from melanoma.

Benign Lesions The relatively simple structures within the breast can give rise to numerous benign abnormalities, which can sometimes be proved only by tissue biopsy. The most common benign lesion is a simple cyst, which may be seen in up to one half of examinations. These appear as rounded, sometimes lobulated lesions, and are usually multiple in number (**Fig. 7–11**). When a worrisome lesion that could represent a cyst is identified mammographically, the diagnosis of simple cyst usually can be definitively established by ultrasound. As elsewhere in the body, a simple cyst will appear as an anechoic structure with sharply defined margins, round or oval in shape, and will demonstrate posterior acoustic enhancement (tissue directly behind it will appear somewhat brighter than adjacent tissue) (**Fig. 7–12**). If the appearance of

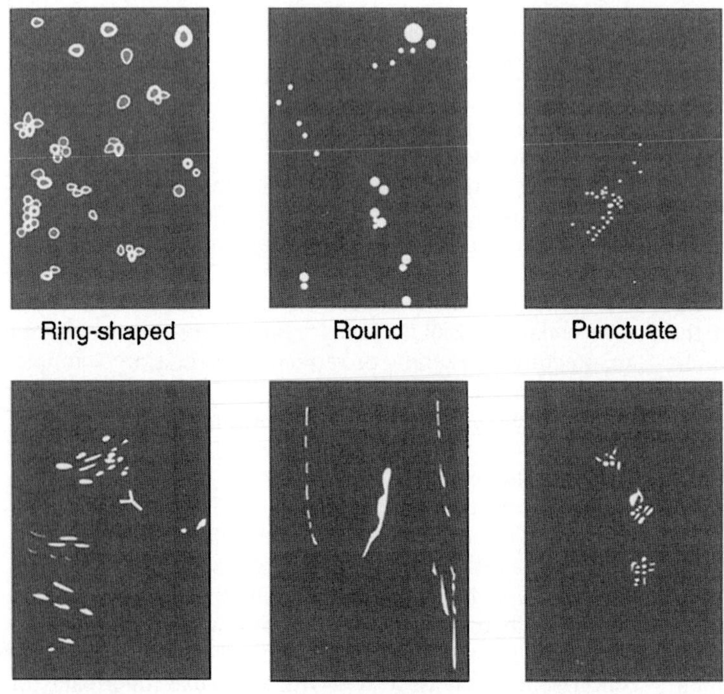

Figure 7–9 The types of microcalcifications commonly seen on mammographic studies. Of these types, only linear and branching or pleomorphic are strongly suggestive of malignancy.

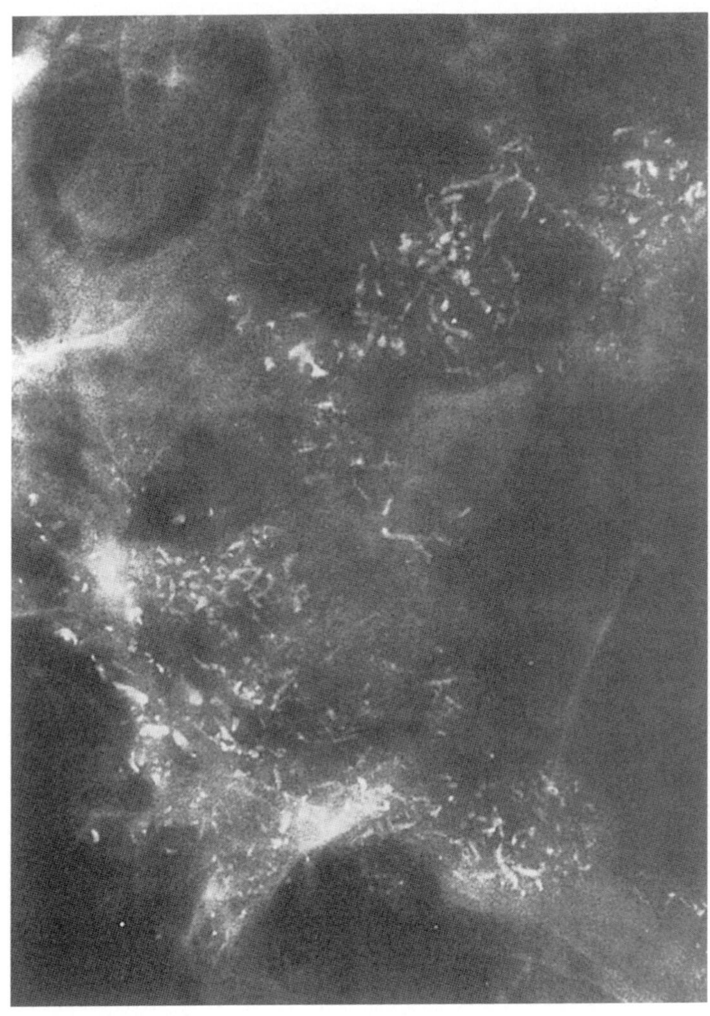

Figure 7–10 This magnified view demonstrates a dramatic appearance of malignant microcalcifications, with innumerable pleomorphic linear and branching forms.

the cyst is not classic, it may be aspirated under ultrasound guidance; complete disappearance with aspiration is also diagnostic, because it indicates that no solid tissue was present.

The most common solid benign lesion of the breast is a fibroadenoma, which probably represents estrogen-induced proliferation of normal lobular connective tissue. These masses occur during the reproductive years, often enlarging during pregnancy and involuting after menopause. In contrast to malignancies, fibroadenomas usually exhibit smooth, regular margins and are often round or oval in shape. One classic mammographic sign of a fibroadenoma is the presence of internal "popcorn" dystrophic calcification (**Fig. 7–13**).

Mammographic reporting has been standardized according to a useful classification scheme, called BI-RADS (Breast Imaging Reporting and Data System). Category 0 means that the mammographic assessment is incomplete, and further imaging is needed; category 1 means the patient has no significant findings, and routine screening is recommended; category 2 means there is a benign finding, such as an intramammary lymph node; category 3 means that the finding is probably benign, such as asymmetric parenchymal densities that are not palpable, but shorter-term follow-up is warranted; category 4 means that there is a suspicious lesion warranting biopsy; and category 5 means that the findings, such as a cluster of pleomorphic calcifications, are highly suggestive of malignancy.

Biopsy and Staging Once a suspicious mass is identified and a tissue diagnosis is needed, the radiologist plays several additional roles. First, mammographically or ultrasonographically guided fine-needle aspiration and/or core-needle biopsy can be performed to obtain tissue for pathologic analysis. These procedures offer a high rate of success, low cost, and low rate of complications. When a surgical approach to biopsy is chosen, the radiologist may perform a needle localization to guide the surgeon to nonpalpable lesions such as a suspicious cluster of microcalcifications. In the needle localization procedure, mammographic or ultrasonographic guidance is used to place a hooked wire within the lesion, which the surgeon then follows by palpation to locate the area of breast tissue to excise.

Once a cancer is discovered, several factors affect prognosis. These include not only size but also evidence of lymph node spread (especially involving the axilla) and distant metastases (often involving the lung, liver, skeleton, or central nervous system [CNS]). One of imaging's most

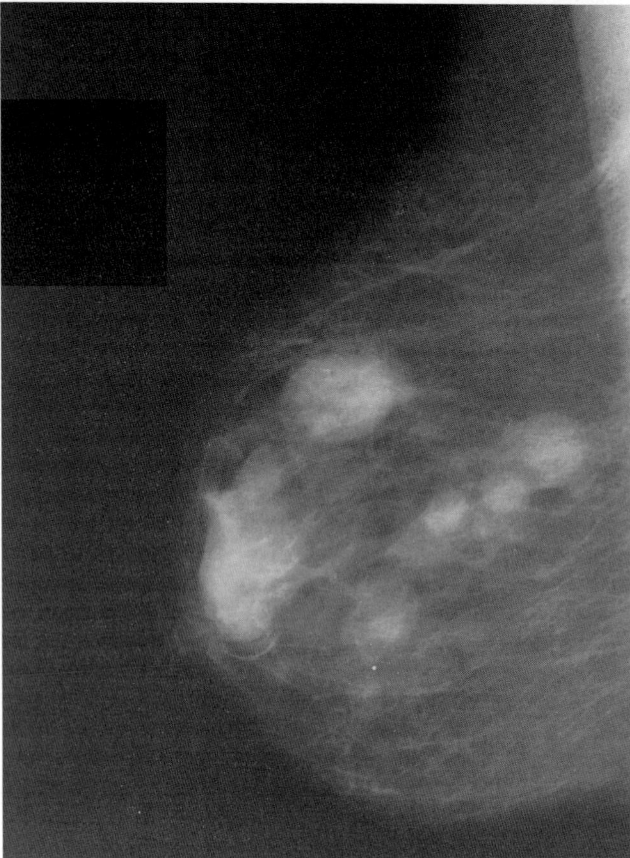

Figure 7–11 This MLO view of the right breast demonstrates multiple well-circumscribed ovoid masses with smooth borders. Similar lesions were seen in the left breast; these masses had been present and fluctuated in size between previous mammograms. They were not palpable and represented benign cysts in this premenopausal patient.

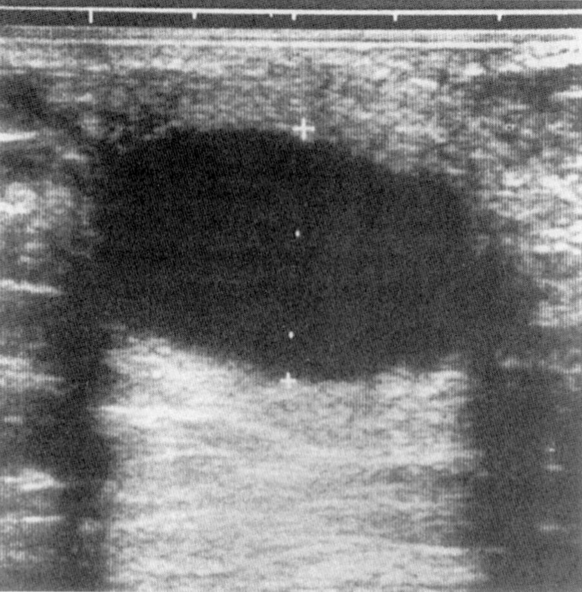

Figure7–12 A 48-year-old woman had noticed enlargement of a mass in her left breast, which was readily palpable on physical examination. This sonographic image of the palpable lesion demonstrates the sonographic characteristics of a simple cyst: no internal echoes; a smooth, oval shape; sharp margins; and posterior acoustic enhancement. The lesion was undetectable after aspiration, which yielded clear fluid.

important roles in the management of breast cancer lies in the staging of disease (looking for metastases in organs such as the liver, lungs, and skeleton), and in monitoring response to therapy (e.g., assessing the change in size of metastatic lesions after a course of chemotherapy). Plain radiographs of the chest and bones, nuclear medicine bone scans, and computed tomography of the head, chest, and abdomen constitute the most frequently employed modalities (**Fig. 7–14**). Magnetic resonance imaging is playing a greater role in cancer detection and staging and in the evaluation of breast implants.

◆ Female Reproductive System: Pelvis

Any time an imaging study of the pelvis is reviewed, it is important to follow an ordered search pattern to ensure that all major structures are dependably evaluated. The aortic bifurcation and iliac vessels should be traced out to rule out aneurysms, and their accompanying nodal chains should be inspected for adenopathy. Their venous counterparts should be inspected for the presence of thrombus. The distal gastrointestinal (GI) tract should be inspected for

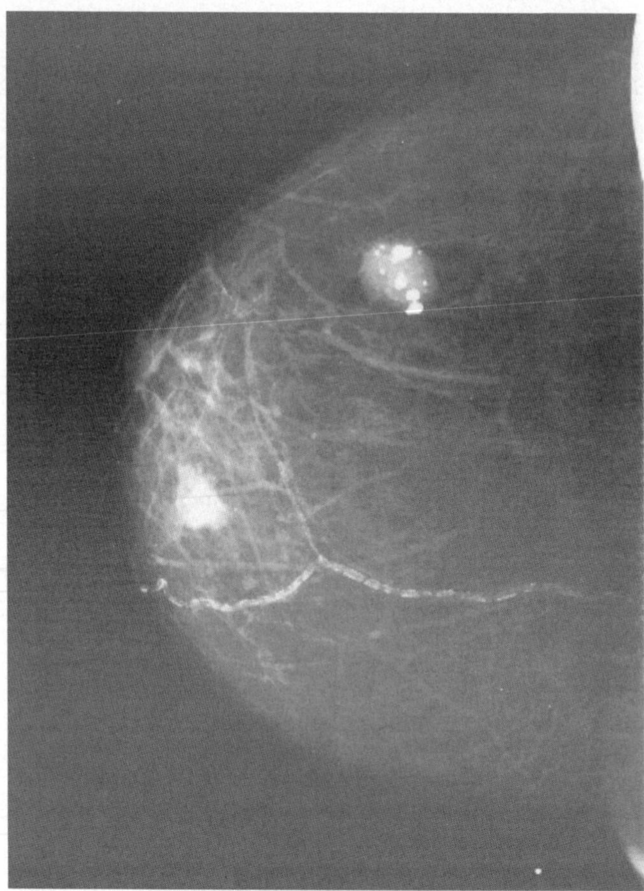

Figure 7–13 A craniocaudal view of the right breast demonstrates benign vascular calcifications as well as two well-circumscribed masses containing "popcorn" calcifications classic for involuting fibroadenomas.

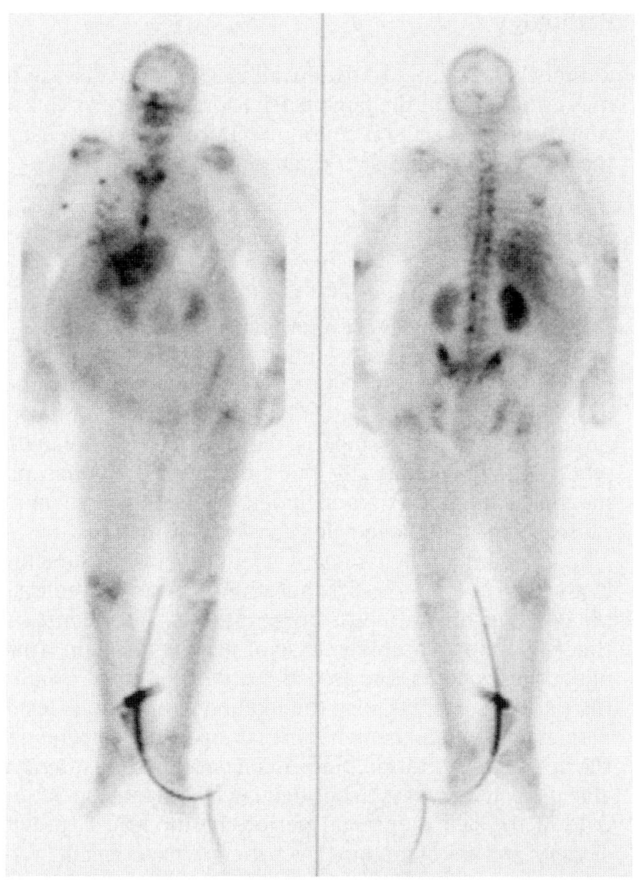

A

Figure 7–14 This elderly woman with a history of breast cancer presented with back pain and increasing abdominal girth. **(A)** The anterior and posterior images from a nuclear medicine bone scan demonstrate multiple abnormal areas of radiotracer accumulation in the spine, ribs, and liver, with radiotracer in the peritoneum raising concern for malignant ascites. **(B)** These six images from an abdominal CT scan with oral and intravenous (IV) contrast demonstrate that the liver is diffusely involved with hypodense hematogenous metastases. More caudal images confirmed ascites.

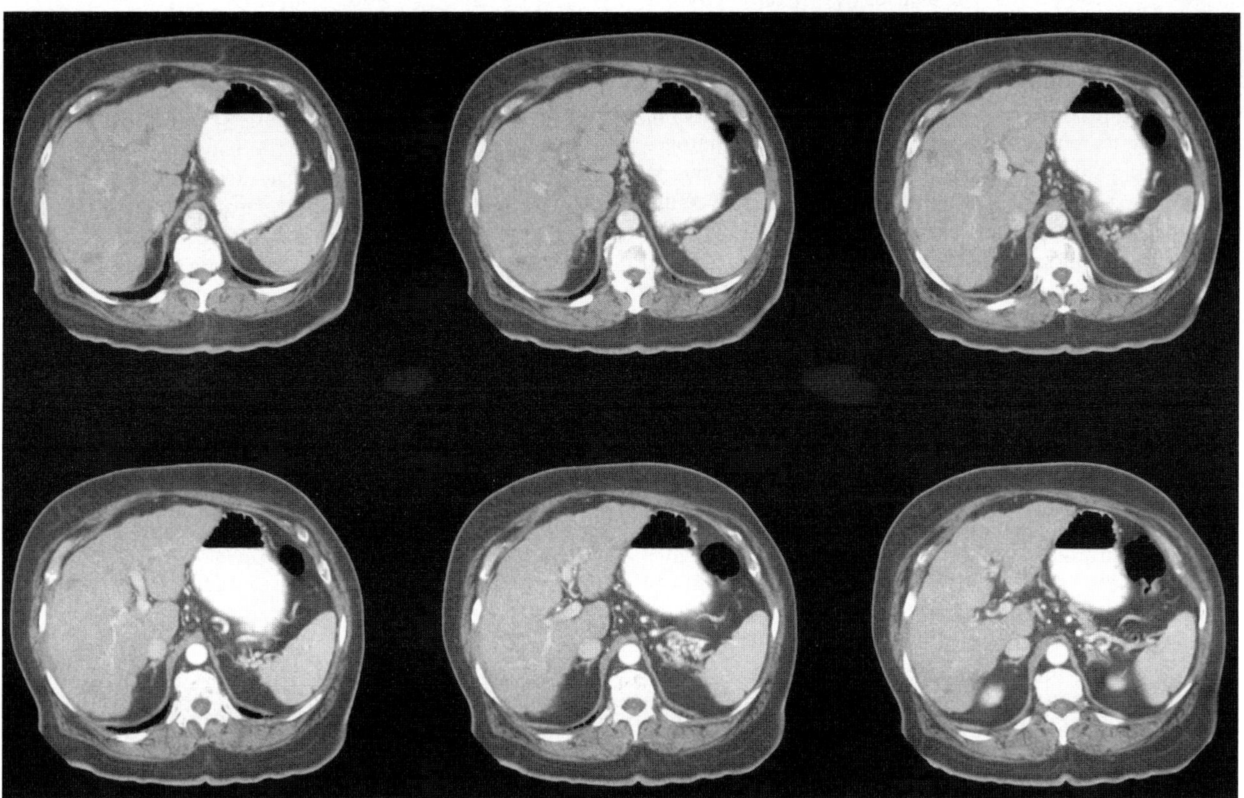

B

masses and mural abnormalities, as well as for the presence of surrounding ascites. The urinary tract, including the distal ureters and bladder, should be evaluated for masses, mural abnormalities, and evidence of obstruction. As always, bones and soft tissues should be inspected. In a male patient, special areas of attention include the size, shape, and tissue characteristics of the prostate gland, as well as the condition of periprostatic tissues. In a female patient, attention should be directed to the size, shape, and position of the uterus, cervix, and adnexa (from the Latin for "appended to").

Anatomy and Physiology

The female pelvis contains the vagina, the cervix, the uterus, and the paired oviducts and ovaries (**Fig. 7–15**). The muscular, expansile vagina (from the Latin for "sheath") serves both as the female organ of copulation and the birth canal. The cervix (from the Latin for "neck") is the distal portion of the uterus that projects into the vagina and represents the site from which cells are scraped in a "Pap test" (after George Papanicolaou) in an effort to detect cervical cancer at an early stage. The muscular, thick-walled uterus is responsible both for housing the developing embryo/fetus during gestation and for expelling it during parturition (from the Latin *parere*, "to bring forth," from which the word *parity* is derived). The oviducts function to collect the ovum (from the Latin for "egg") from the ovary at ovulation, as the site of fertilization, and as the conveyors of the fertilized egg to the uterus. The ovaries perform the two expected gonadal (from the Greek *gone*, "seed") functions, gametogenesis (ovum production) and the secretion of sex hormones.

The female reproductive tract performs a greater variety of functions than its male counterpart. These include gametogenesis, receiving sperm, transporting both sperm and ova to the site of fertilization, transporting the fertilized ovum (zygote) to its endometrial site of implantation, sheltering and nourishing the developing fetus (with the aid of the placenta) until it can survive outside the mother's body, and parturition.

Female reproductive anatomy and physiology exhibit a notable cyclicity. In the male, gonadotropin secretion and spermatogenesis are pulsatile over hours but otherwise essentially constant, whereas female sex hormones display wide swings, and normally only one ovum is produced each menstrual cycle. In the first half of the menstrual cycle, the ovarian follicle secretes estrogens and low levels of progesterone; in the second half, after a surge in leutinizing hormone levels stimulates ovulation, the corpus luteum (Latin for "yellow body") secretes estrogen and high amounts of progesterone to prepare the uterus for implantation. If fertilization does not occur, the corpus luteum involutes, and the thickened uterine lining is sloughed at menstruation. Imaging findings such as the number and size of follicles in the ovaries, the presence of free fluid in the pelvic cul-de-sac (the peritoneal extension into the space between the uterus and rectum), and the thickness of the endometrial stripe are all hormonally mediated and markedly variable, depending on the phase of the menstrual cycle.

Pathology

Rather than attempt to review all categories of disease that may afflict each of the female pelvic organs in turn, this section focuses on several common clinical presentations and the role of imaging in their evaluation.

Pelvic Masses

◇ Clinical Data

Palpable pelvic masses are a common clinical problem. In hospitalized patients of both genders, a distended urinary bladder is the most common culprit. In women, the most common cause of a pelvic mass is an enlarged uterus. In women of reproductive age, pregnancy is the most likely explanation, whereas leiomyomata are the most prevalent when postmenopausal patients are included. The next most common cause of a mass in the female pelvis is an ovarian cyst.

To evaluate a pelvic mass, certain aspects of the clinical history are crucial. The first question to be answered is simply whether the patient is pregnant. Pregnancy constitutes the single most common cause of pelvic masses in women under the age of 35. The second crucial bit of clinical data are the patient's age, because the likelihood of various lesions, both malignant and benign, varies dramatically depending on the age at presentation. Additional data that must be available if a pelvic mass is to be adequately evaluated include the date of the last menstrual period, hormone use, previous surgery, and any symptoms the patient is experiencing.

◇ Imaging

Ultrasound is by far the most important radiologic modality in the evaluation of the pelvis, and alone is adequate to characterize more than 90% of lesions (**Fig. 7–16**). The crucial questions to be addressed by the sonographer include the following: Which anatomic structure is involved? What are the imaging characteristics of the lesion? How is it changing over time? The most common pelvic masses, aside from pregnancy, include uterine leiomyomata ("fibroids"), ovarian cysts, pelvic inflammatory disease, endometriosis, and cancers of the ovary and uterus (**Fig. 7–17**). This discussion is organized around the different anatomic points of origin of pelvic masses.

◇ Adnexal Masses

A variety of benign processes may produce adnexal masses. The two most important categories of disease are "medical" (nonsurgical) conditions such as physiologic cysts and infectious and inflammatory processes and "surgical" processes, for which urgent surgical intervention should be considered.

"Medical" Adnexal Masses Among the physiologic cysts, the most common are the follicular cysts. These typically arise either from failure of a follicle to involute after ovulation or an anovulatory cycle. Follicular cysts also represent the most common cause of an ovarian mass in the neonate and can be traced to maternal estrogen stimulation. In most cases, they appear round and anechoic, fulfilling the sonographic criteria

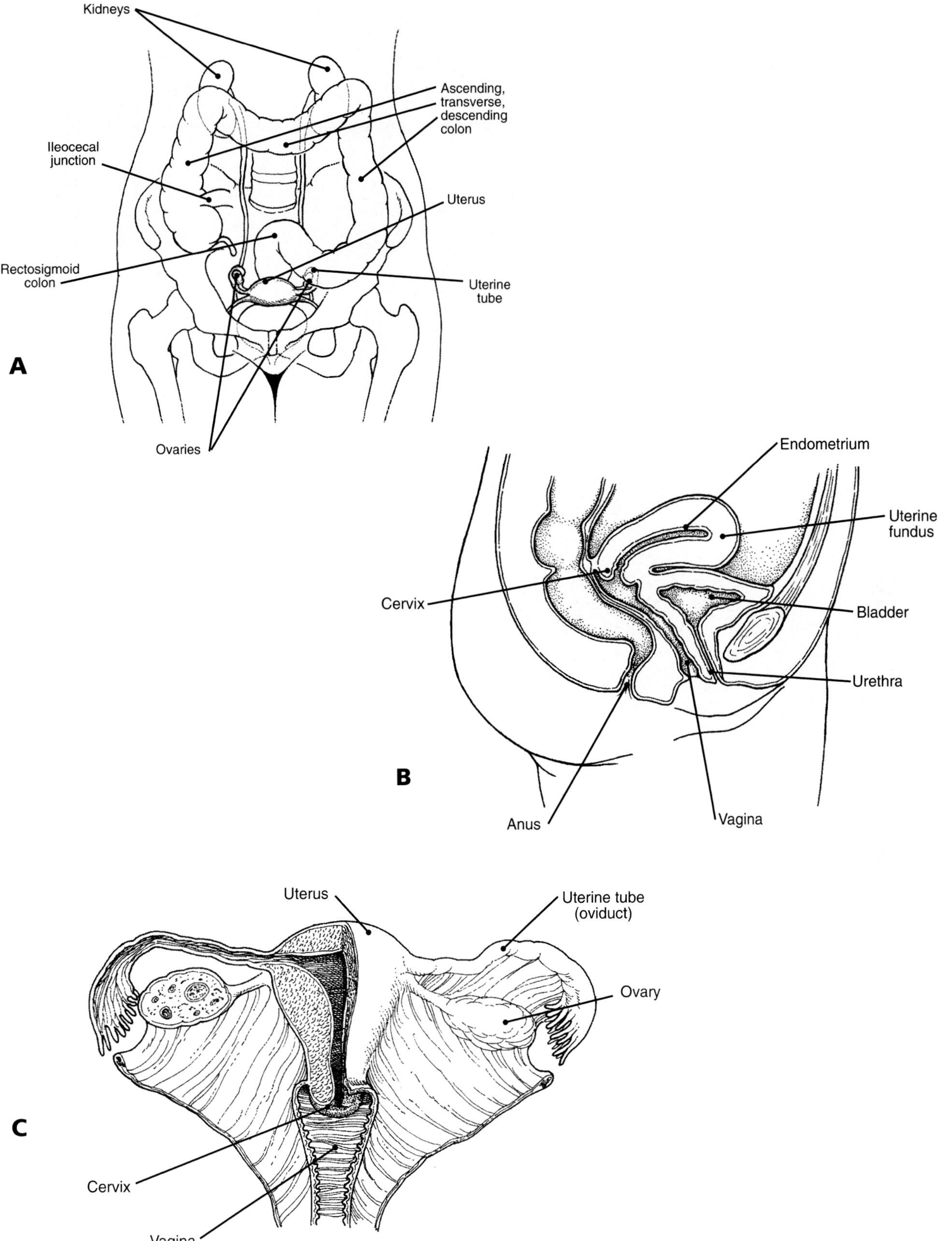

Figure 7–15 **(A)** Diagram depicting the close proximity of other physiologic systems (e.g., urinary and digestive systems) to the female reproductive organs. Multiple systems must be borne in mind when a patient presents with pelvic symptoms. **(B)** Sagittal and **(C)** coronal views of the key anatomic structures of the female reproductive system.

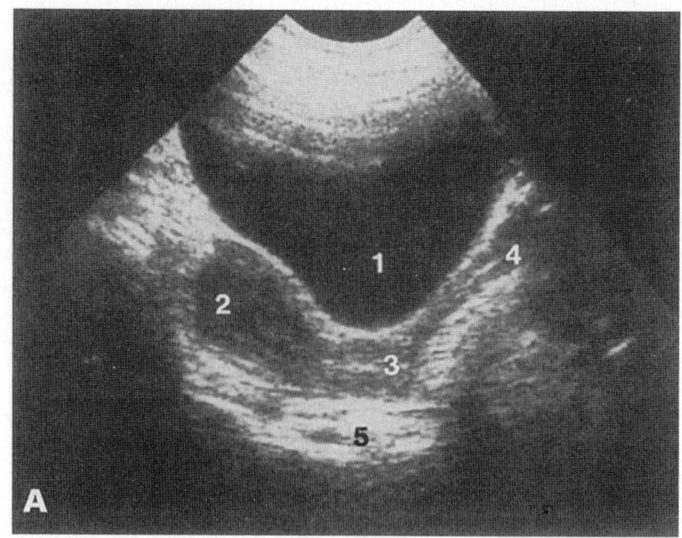

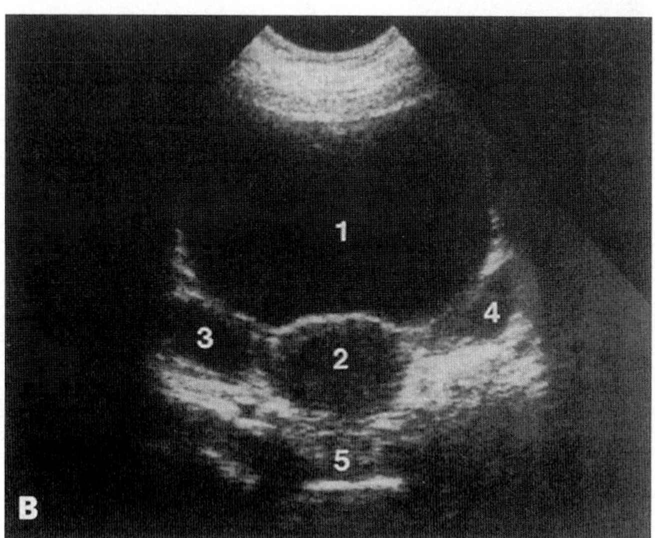

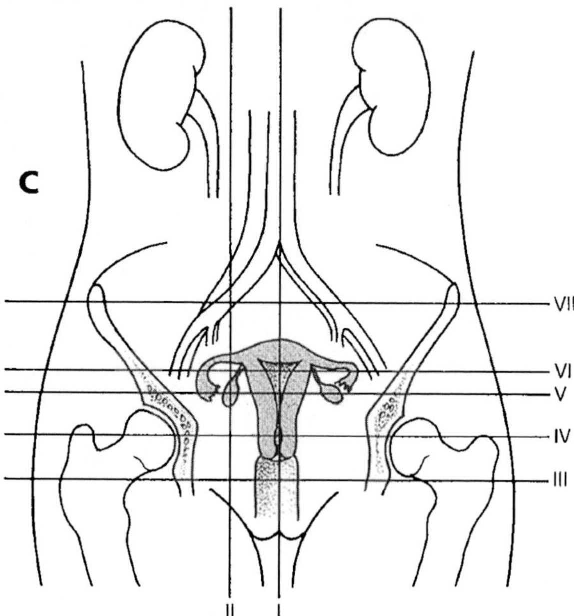

Figure 7–16 These **(A)** longitudinal and **(B)** transverse ultrasound images of the pelvis demonstrate the normal sonographic appearance of the pelvic structures. **(A)** 1, filled urinary bladder; 2, uterus; 3, cervix; 4, vagina; 5, rectum. **(B)** 1, filled urinary bladder; 2, uterus; 3, right ovary; 4, left ovary; 5, colon. **(C)** The planes in which images are normally obtained. Image **A** was obtained in plane I, and image **B** was obtained in plane V.

of a simple cyst; however, they may be complicated at any age by hemorrhage and commonly present with pain. The presence of internal hemorrhage gives them a heterogeneous echotexture on ultrasound. The next most prevalent physiologic cyst is a corpus luteum cyst, typically formed by hemorrhage into the corpus luteum after ovulation. These are usually larger than follicular cysts and often measure 5 to 10 cm in diameter. They are most common in the first months of pregnancy. High levels of human chorionic gonadotropin (HCG) may produce a theca lutein cyst, which is the largest of all ovarian cysts and may measure up to 20 cm in diameter. The finding of a theca lutein cyst should raise suspicion for either multiple gestations or gestational trophoblastic disease (hydatidiform mole or choriocarcinoma). Each of these lesions may have the appearance of a simple or complex cyst, and the differentiation must be based on clinical grounds (**Fig. 7–18**).

Infectious causes of pelvic masses include nongynecologic processes such as appendicitis and diverticulitis, which can sometimes be distinguished from gynecologic processes on the basis of absence of both cervical motion tenderness and purulent vaginal discharge. Pelvic inflammatory disease is the most common gynecologic cause. Risk factors include young age, history of previous salpingitis, and use of an intrauterine device. Patients may present with pain, vaginal discharge, abnormal bleeding, or peritoneal signs, depending on the stage of infection. Ultrasound is used primarily in assessing for signs of advanced disease. Visible oviducts are abnormal, and in hy-

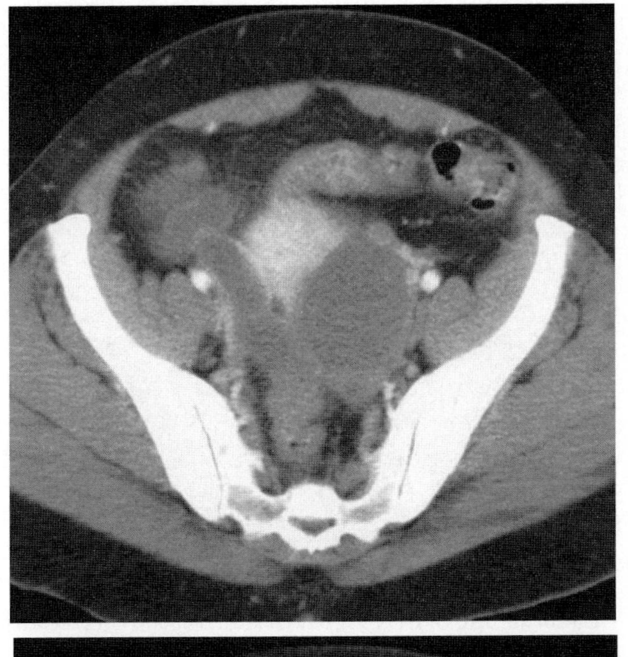

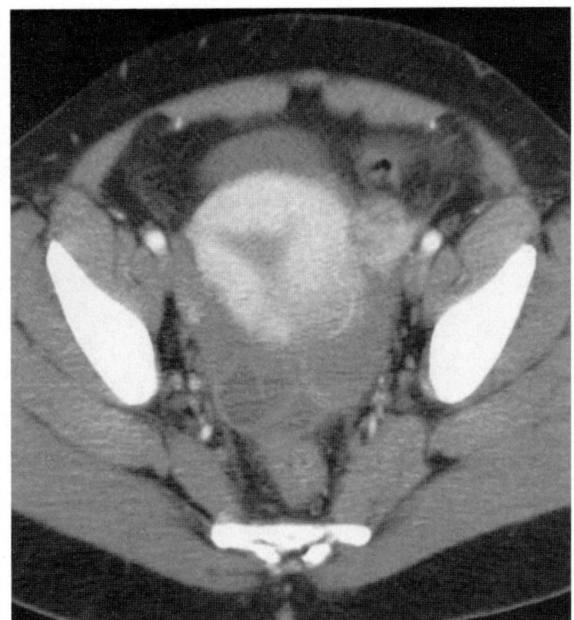

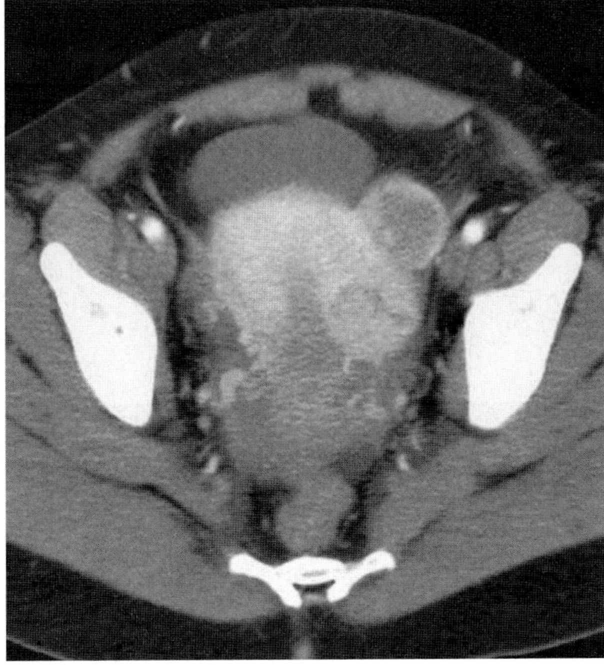

Figure 7–17 **(A)** An axial CT image after IV contrast demonstrates the top of the enhancing uterus centrally, as well as a dilated, fluid-filled right fallopian tube (hydrosalpinx) and large left ovarian cyst. **(B)** A more caudal image demonstrates the brightly enhancing myometrium with fluid in the endometrial canal. **(C)** A still more caudal image demonstrates heterogeneous enhancement in mural and exophytic leiomyomas.

drosalpinx one or both oviducts have a characteristic folded, tubular shape. A tubo-ovarian abscess usually appears as an ill-defined mass with heterogeneous echotexture. Fluid is often seen in the cul-de-sac. The most common organisms are *Neisseria gonorrhoreae* and *Chlamydia trachomatis* (**Fig. 7–19**).

By far the most common inflammatory condition causing an adnexal mass is endometriosis, the presence of functional endometrial tissue outside the uterine cavity. Seen in 5% of premenopausal women, the incidence is much higher in series of infertility patients. The endometrial implants undergo expected changes with the menstrual cycle, with hemorrhage producing local inflammation and adhesions. Endometriosis usually presents with dysmenorrhea, chronic pelvic pain, dyspareunia, or infertility. In patients with minor disease, the lesions are often undetectable by imaging. In more severe cases, the ultrasound appearance is typically that of a cystic, hyperechoic mass, and it often proves indistinguishable from a hemorrhagic ovarian cyst.

"Surgical" Adnexal Masses Ectopic pregnancy, the implantation of the fertilized egg outside the uterine cavity, occurs in ~1% of all pregnancies, with a peak incidence in the teens and twenties. Approximately 75,000 cases are diagnosed in the United States each year. The principal risk factor is a history of previous salpingitis, and 95% of ectopic pregnancies occur in the oviducts. Ectopic pregnancy has a 10% risk of

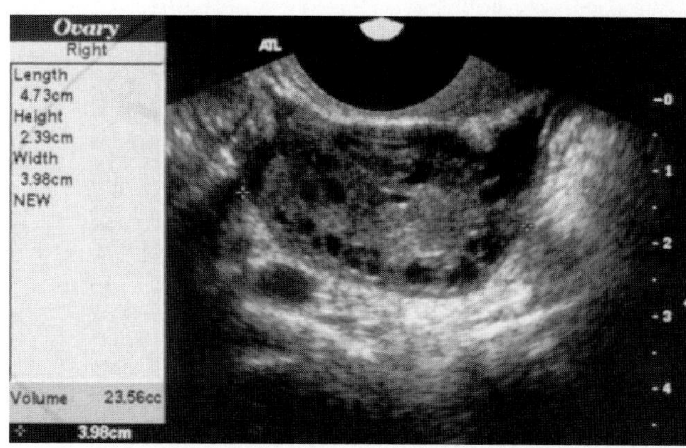

Figure 7–18 This young woman presented with dysfunctional uterine bleeding. The sonographic image of the right ovary demonstrates multiple abnormalities. First, the ovary is enlarged, with a volume of 24 cc. Second, it is hyperechoic. Third, it contains many peripherally located follicles. The left ovary had a similar appearance. These findings are typical of polycystic ovary disease.

recurrence. It accounts for 15% of all maternal deaths, and the risk of maternal death in ectopic pregnancy is 10 times greater than that of natural childbirth. Death results from massive hemorrhage following tubal rupture. Patients present with a classic picture of abnormal vaginal bleeding, pelvic pain, amenorrhea, and a palpable adnexal mass in only a minority of cases. Diagnostically, two critical questions must be answered, one clinical and one ultrasonographic: (1) Is the patient pregnant? and (2) Is there an intrauterine pregnancy? If the answer to question 1 is yes, and to question 2 no, then the diagnosis of ectopic pregnancy must be strongly considered, and emergent surgery may be indicated.

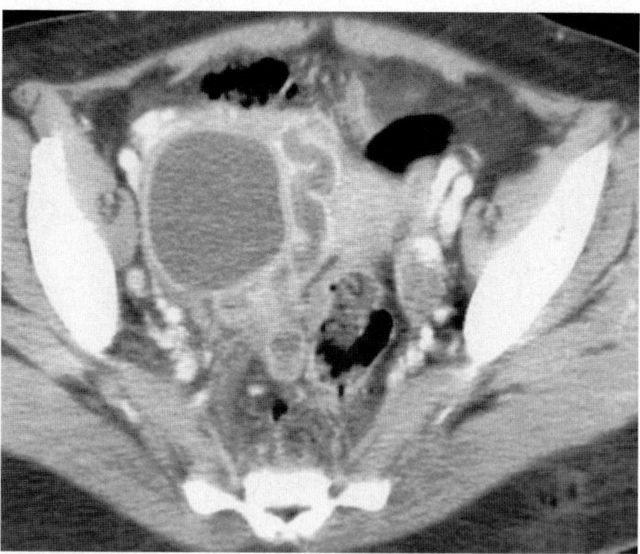

Figure 7–19 This young woman presented with abdominal pain, fever, tachycardia, and an elevated white blood cell (WBC) count. The axial CT image of the pelvis after oral and IV contrast demonstrates the dilated and tortuous fluid-filled right oviduct just medial to a large cystic right adnexal mass, both of which show thickened and enhancing walls. This represented a pyosalpinx and tubo-ovarian abscess.

Another important diagnostic tool in suspected ectopic pregnancy is the levels of HCG. Low levels of HCG are strongly suggestive of an ectopic pregnancy, which is corroborated on ultrasound by such features as a normal uterus with no gestational sac, free fluid in the cul-de-sac (from tubal bleeding), a complex adnexal mass, and the finding of a live embryo outside the uterus (diagnostic) (**Fig. 7–20**). A live extrauterine embryo is seen in ~25% of

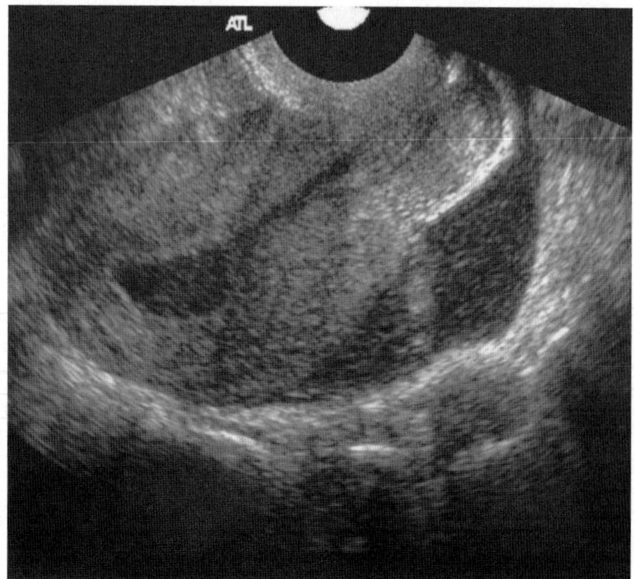

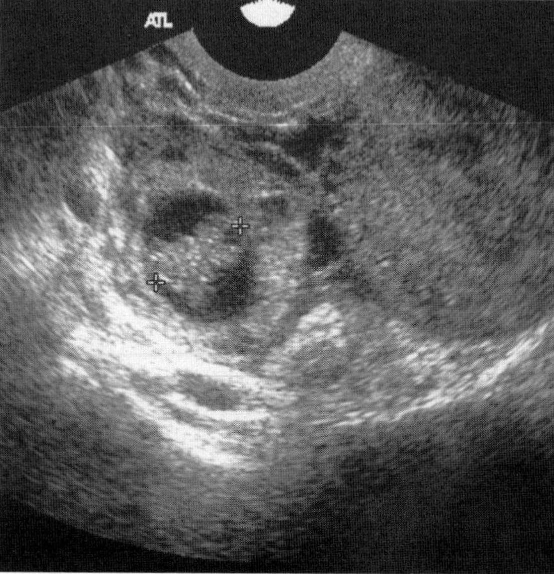

Figure 7–20 This young woman presented with pelvic pain and last menstrual period 8 weeks ago. She was found to be pregnant with a β-human chorionic gonadotropin (HCG) of 75,000. **(A)** The transvaginal longitudinal sonogram of the uterus demonstrates fluid in the endometrial canal but no products of conception. Note the complex fluid collectors in the cul-de-sac behind the uterus. **(B)** A right adnexal image demonstrates a 3 cm mass containing a fetal pole with a length corresponding to 8-week gestational age and a heart rate of 167 beats/minute. This represented an ectopic pregnancy in the right fallopian tube.

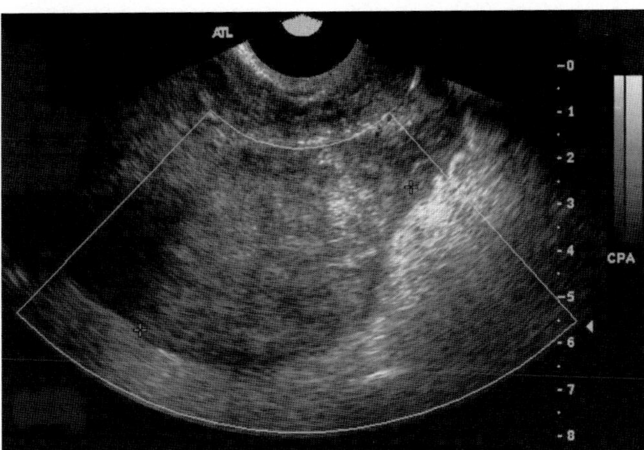

Figure 7–21 This 30-year-old woman presented with several hours of excruciating right lower quadrant abdominal pain. Transvaginal sonography was performed. The left ovary (not shown) appeared normal, with a volume of 6 cc. This image of the right ovary is markedly abnormal. The ovary has a volume of 50 cc and demonstrates heterogeneously increased echogenicity. Doppler imaging shows no internal blood flow. This represented an ovarian torsion.

cases. If an intrauterine pregnancy is seen, and the patient is not on fertility drugs (which increase the probability of multiple gestations), the diagnosis of ectopic pregnancy is essentially excluded, because concomitant intra- and extrauterine pregnancies are seen in only 1 in 7000 cases, even in patients with risk factors for multiple gestation.

Ovarian torsion may occur in a normal ovary, but more often occurs in an ovary enlarged by the presence of a cystic or solid mass. Torsion results from rotation of the ovary on its vascular pedicle, with venous and then arterial obstruction. It most commonly occurs in children and adolescents, and presents with pain and a palpable mass in half of all patients. Ultrasound demonstrates an enlarged, heterogeneous ovary, and free fluid is often seen in the cul-de-sac (**Fig. 7–21**). As in suspected testicular torsion, Doppler examination may be useful in demonstrating decreased or absent blood flow on the affected side.

Benign versus Malignant Adrenal Masses Pregnancy excluded, the essential distinction to be made in the diagnostic workup of most adult adnexal masses is whether they are likely to represent malignancy. The case in which this question can be answered firmly in the negative is that of the simple cyst. Physiologic cysts may measure up to 3 cm in diameter and demonstrate cyclical change in size with the menstrual cycle. No follow-up is required, so long as the cyst measures less than 3 cm and the patient is premenopausal. If the patient is postmenopausal, follow-up in 2 to 3 months is indicated. The premenopausal patient requires such follow-up only for cysts measuring between 3 and 5 cm. When the finding represents a cyst measuring more than 5 cm, or a solid mass of any size, tissue will need to be obtained. Many of these lesions will turn out to be pedunculated benign uterine leiomyomata simulating an adnexal mass, but there is no way to make this determination without histology. Tissue is obtained surgically, either by laparoscopy or, if the probability of malignancy is considered higher, by laparotomy.

At least 80% of adnexal tumors are benign and usually present in women between the third and fifth decades. Although numerous types of lesions are known, the most interesting from a radiologic point of view is the dermoid cyst, also sometimes referred to as a benign cystic teratoma. These tumors generally appear in a somewhat lower age range, in the teens and twenties. Fortunately, they represent the most common ovarian neoplasm in the reproductive years. Strictly speaking, a teratoma represents a tumor containing all three cell types—ectoderm, mesoderm, and endoderm—whereas a dermoid contains only ectodermal elements. Depending on the maturity of the ectodermal elements in these tumors, they often contain structures such as hair, bone, and teeth. Calcified elements including teeth are sometimes visible on abdominal plain films, and the finding of fat within the lesion on CT is also virtually diagnostic (**Fig. 7–22**). A common ultrasound appearance is that of a cystic lesion with a mural nodule, which often contains fluid–fluid levels.

Ovarian carcinoma is the fifth leading cause of cancer death among American women, resulting in ~25,000 new cases and 15,000 deaths per year. This translates to a lifetime risk of ~1 in 70 women, although the risk is increased in patients with a positive family history or a history of prior breast cancer. Symptoms are relatively uncommon prior to dissemination, rendering regular pelvic examination with palpation of the adnexa a key to early diagnosis. Because epithelial cells on the surface of the ovary are the source of 90% of malignant ovarian tumors, and these cells are readily shed into the peritoneal cavity, approximately three quarters of patients present with disseminated disease. Symptoms and signs of dissemination include constipation, edema, invasion of adjacent structures such as the uterus or rectum, ascites, and pleural effusions. CA 125 levels are elevated in ~80% of patients.

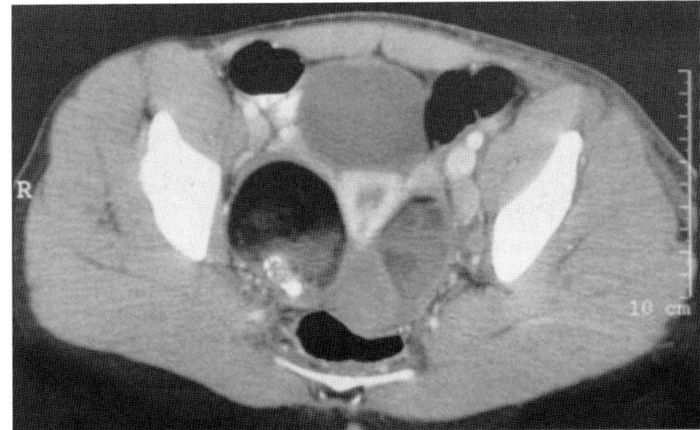

Figure 7–22 This 18-year-old woman presented with a pelvic mass. Axial CT of the pelvis after IV contrast demonstrates bilateral heterogeneous adnexal masses flanking the uterus, both of which contain fat. These represented ovarian teratomas.

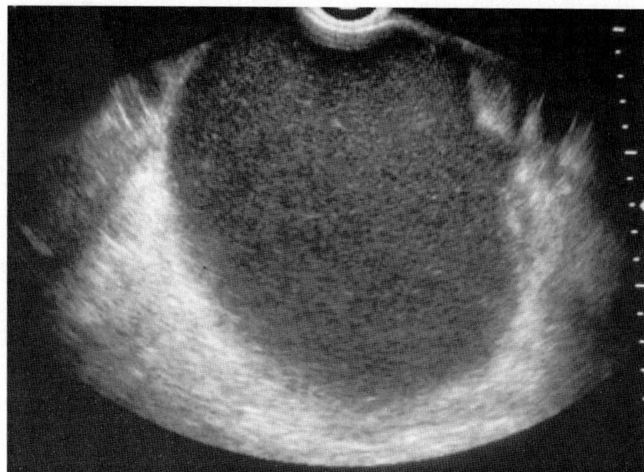

Figure 7–23 A transvaginal sonogram of the right adnexa in a patient with a pelvic mass demonstrates a very large cystic mass that exhibits considerable internal echogenicity and therefore does not qualify as a simple cyst. At surgery this was found to be an ovarian cystadenoma.

Common types of epithelial ovarian malignancies include mucinous and serous cystadenocarcinomas. The principal roles of imaging are to identify lesions warranting surgery for histologic characterization and to stage known carcinoma. On ultrasound, carcinomas typically exhibit a cystic appearance, ranging from simple unilocular cysts to complex multilocular cystic lesions containing considerable solid elements (**Fig. 7–23**). In general, the more solid tissue visualized, the more likely the lesion is to prove malignant. A significant percentage of tumors are bilateral. The primary route of spread is peritoneal seeding, with implants on the omentum producing a characteristic pattern of "omental caking." The presence of ascites argues strongly in favor of implants on the omentum, bowel mesentery, or peritoneal membrane. Hematogenous spread to lungs and liver tends to occur late.

◇ Uterine Masses

The three most important masses involving the uterus are leiomyomata, endometrial carcinoma, and cervical carcinoma. Leiomyomata ("fibroids") represent the most common uterine tumors, seen in more than one quarter of women over the age of 35. Most are located within the myometrium, although they may also arise from the submucosa (in which case they are very likely to produce symptoms) or the subserosa (which often results in a pedunculated tumor). Due to their estrogen sensitivity, they often enlarge during pregnancy and tend to regress at menopause. Most lesions are asymptomatic, although patients may present with abnormal bleeding, pain, and infertility. On ultrasound, most leiomyomata tend to be hypoechoic, multiple, and may deform the uterine contour. On plain film and CT, they often contain coarse calcifications (**Fig. 7–24**). On MRI, they tend to be hypodense relative to the uterus on T2-weighted images, although cystic degeneration may produce areas of hyperintensity.

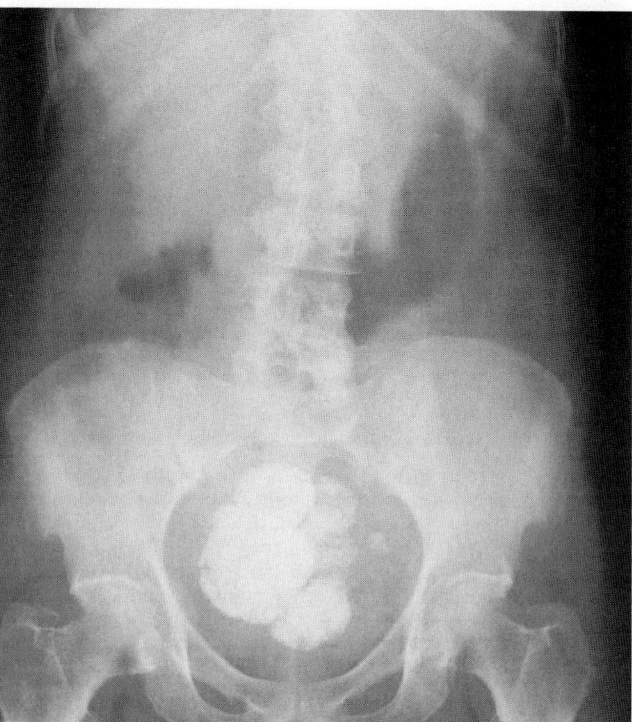

Figure 7–24 The large, lobulated, coarsely calcified masses in this elderly woman's pelvis represent involuted uterine leiomyomas. Calcified fibroid tumors are not an uncommon finding on plain radiographs in older women.

Endometrial hyperplasia is a precursor to endometrial carcinoma. Hyperplasia occurs with unopposed estrogen stimulation, as seen in exogenous estrogen therapy, anovulation, and estrogen-producing tumors. Tamoxifen, which is often employed in breast cancer therapy, possesses weak estrogenic activity and is therefore associated with endometrial hyperplasia. Risk factors for endometrial carcinoma are similar to those of breast cancer, and include nulliparity, early menarche and late menopause, and ovulatory failure. The histology of endometrial carcinoma is adenocarcinoma. On ultrasound, endometrial hyperplasia appears as thickening of the echogenic endometrial stripe. In a premenopausal woman, a thickness of 15 mm is sufficient to warrant biopsy; in the postmenopausal patient, the same recommendation would follow for a thickness greater than 5 mm. Findings of endometrial carcinoma include a thickened endometrial stripe and the presence of fluid within the endometrial cavity (hydrometria) due to cervical obstruction.

Deaths due to cervical carcinoma have been dramatically reduced due to the widespread practice of annual Pap tests. Risk factors include multiple sex partners and a history of sexually transmitted diseases. Human papilloma virus is implicated as an etiologic factor. In contrast to endometrial carcinoma, cervical carcinoma is of squamous cell histology. Findings include endometrial fluid collections and masses arising from the cervix (**Fig. 7–25**). CT is commonly employed in staging.

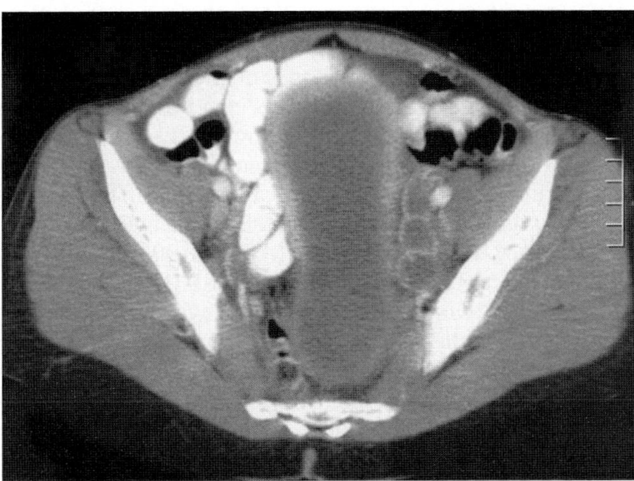

Figure 7–25 An axial CT image of the pelvis after IV contrast demonstrates a markedly dilated endometrial cavity and left fallopian tube in this middle-aged woman with abnormal vaginal bleeding. The patient was found to have cervical carcinoma, which was obstructing the cervical os.

◆ Pregnancy

Anatomy and Physiology

After ovulation, an egg requires ~4 to 5 days to travel through the oviduct into the uterine cavity. It remains fertile for only 24 hours, meaning that fertilization must take place in the ampullary (most lateral) portion of the tube. Once fertilized, the zygote begins to divide, reaching the blastocyst stage by the time it implants in the endometrial lining of the uterus, ~7 days after ovulation. During this time, the ruptured graafian follicle in the ovary gives rise to the corpus luteum, which produces the estrogen and progesterone (from the Latin *pro*, "before," *gestatio*, "carry," and the chemical terms *sterol*, "from cholesterol," and *one*, "ketone"), necessary for the maintenance of pregnancy during the first 10 weeks. The corpus luteum requires the stimulation of HCG, which is synthesized by the chorion. HCG is the hormone detected by most pregnancy tests, and its levels double approximately every 2 to 3 days. After 10 weeks, the placenta (from the Greek *plakos*, "flat cake") takes over the production of estrogens and progesterones, and the corpus luteum involutes. After that point, castration is compatible with a normal pregnancy outcome.

At implantation, the outermost layer of the blastocyst, the trophoblast, releases proteolytic enzymes that allow it to burrow into the endometrium. In response, the surrounding endometrial tissue becomes increasingly vascular (corresponding to increased echogenicity on ultrasound) and is called the decidua (**Fig. 7–26**). The digestion of decidual cells by the trophoblast supplies energy to the growing embryo until the formation of the placenta. Important membranes in the developing products of conception include the amnion, the fluid-filled cavity that cushions the embryo; the chorion, with which the enlarging amnion eventually fuses; and the yolk sac, which is located outside the amniotic cavity but within the chorionic cavity and is connected to the primitive gut by the omphalomesenteric duct (which may persist into postnatal life as a Meckel's diverticulum). The yolk sac is involved in early hematopoiesis, and a portion of it is incorporated into the primitive gut. The placenta becomes well established and operational by ~5 weeks after implantation, interlocking the fetal (chorionic) and maternal (decidual) circulations, and allowing for the exchange of nutrients and waste products. The umbilical cord normally contains two arteries and one vein and inserts centrally on the placenta. Two-vessel cords are associated with fetal anomalies.

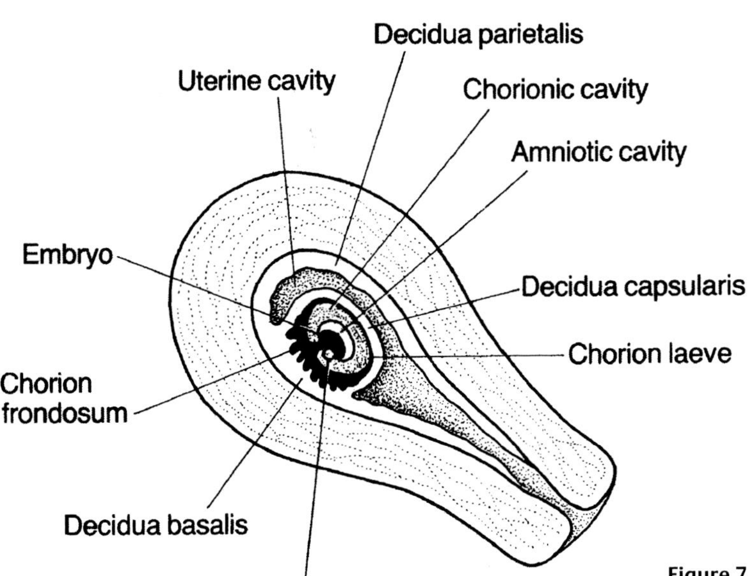

Figure 7–26 The state of the embryo, membranes, and uterus at the seventh week of gestation.

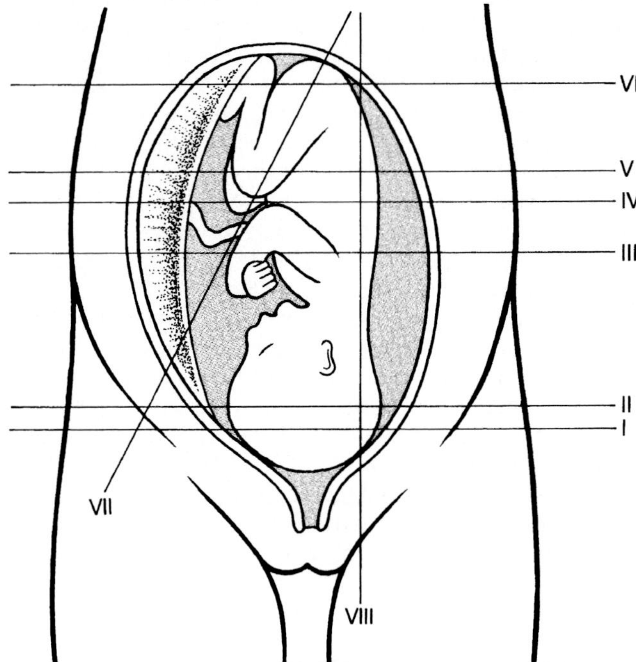

Figure 7–27 The scan planes for evaluating various parameters of a fetus in cephalic presentation. I, lateral ventricles; II, head circumference; III, chest circumference; IV, abdominal circumference; V, fetal kidneys; VI, urinary bladder; VII, femur length; VIII, spine.

Imaging

Because ultrasound involves no ionizing radiation and allows real-time assessment of several obstetrical parameters, it constitutes the preferred imaging technique of pregnancy (**Fig. 7–27**). Most patients can be examined transabdominally. Patients early in pregnancy are encouraged to drink several glasses of water prior to the examination to fill the urinary bladder, which provides an excellent acoustic window on the pelvis. In patients with a retroverted uterus, a transvaginal approach may be necessary, at least early in pregnancy. Generally, the rationale for the examination differs depending on whether it is performed in the first trimester of pregnancy or thereafter.

First Trimester

Indications for imaging in the first trimester include to confirm an intrauterine pregnancy, to evaluate a suspected ectopic pregnancy, to define the cause of vaginal bleeding of uncertain etiology, to estimate gestational age, to assess the number of gestations, to confirm embryonic life, to aid in the performance of chorionic villus sampling or amniocentesis, and to evaluate the uterus and any pelvic masses. The key determination to be made in the first trimester is the presence or absence of an intrauterine pregnancy. The determination of gestational age is another important consideration, in part because up to one quarter of patients, especially those with irregular menstrual cycles, are uncertain about the date of their last menstrual period. In general, the embryo should be detectable by transabdominal scanning by the sixth or seventh week of gestation. If the embryo is seen, it should be possible to detect heart motion, which indicates viability.

The earliest finding of pregnancy on prenatal ultrasound is the presence of a gestational sac, which normally becomes visible by ultrasound when it is 2 mm in diameter, at ~28 to 30 days of pregnancy. Though not as accurate as the crown–rump length, the length of pregnancy can be approximated by the mean sac diameter (MSD). The number of days of pregnancy roughly equals the MSD plus 30 days. The yolk sac and fetal heartbeat both become visible near week 5.

The key questions to be answered in every first trimester examination include the location of the gestational sac, the presence of an embryo, and the crown–rump length, which allows the most accurate estimation of gestational age. When the embryo is first detectable, it is not possible to determine which end is the crown and which the rump, but the measurement of the longest axis is sufficient. The first-trimester crown–rump length measurement provides an accurate measure of gestational age to within 5 to 7 days and is used in conjunction with the last menstrual period to calculate the expected date of confinement (**Fig. 7–28**). It can be compared with the diameter of the gestational sac, which can be identified by 5 weeks. Other important data include the number of gestations and the presence or absence of heart activity. The maternal pelvis should also be examined, including the size of any uterine fibroids or other pelvic masses. Extensive fibroids may contribute to spontaneous abortion.

◇ Vaginal Bleeding

An important indication for prenatal ultrasound is vaginal bleeding. Threatened abortion refers to vaginal bleeding in the presence of a closed cervical os during the first 20 weeks

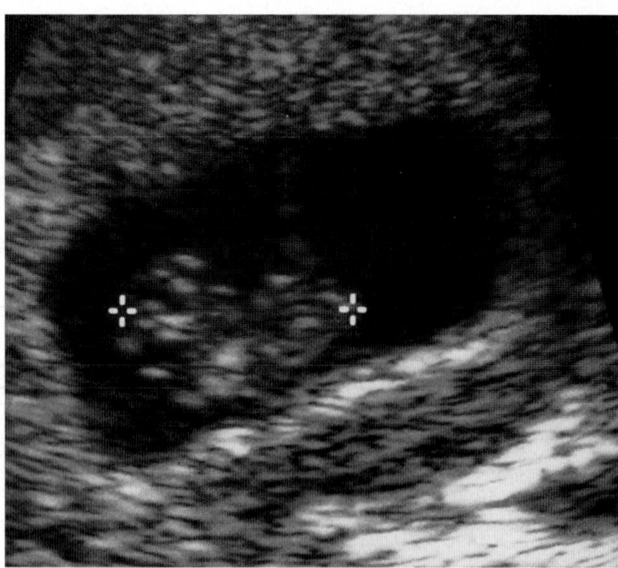

Figure 7–28 The crown–rump length of this embryo on transabdominal sonography was 21 mm, corresponding to a gestational age of ~9 weeks. (Reprinted with permission from Bluth, et al, eds. Bluth-Ultrasound: A Practical Approach to Clinical Problems. New York: Thieme; 2000:305, fig. 26–4B).

of pregnancy. Approximately one half of these pregnancies will end in spontaneous abortion. Spontaneous abortion refers to vaginal bleeding with the passage of tissue; in a high percentage of cases, the fetal tissues are found to harbor chromosomal abnormalities. An inevitable abortion is diagnosed when there is vaginal bleeding and an open cervical os. Incomplete abortion refers to continued vaginal bleeding due to retained products of conception and is often an indication for dilation and curettage. Finally, missed abortion refers to embryonic death with no spontaneous abortion. The most important criterion of fetal death is the absence of cardiac activity in an embryo of at least 5 mm crown–rump length.

The differential diagnosis of vaginal bleeding includes several possibilities. By far the most important diagnosis to exclude in threatened abortion is ectopic pregnancy, which has been discussed in the section on pelvic masses. It is worth reiterating that a normal (nongravid) transvaginal ultrasound does not exclude the diagnosis of ectopic pregnancy, but the finding of a normal intrauterine pregnancy virtually does, unless the mother is taking fertility drugs. Other differential possibilities in vaginal bleeding include inevitable abortion, incomplete abortion, and missed abortion, as well as a blighted ovum (an anembryonic pregnancy).

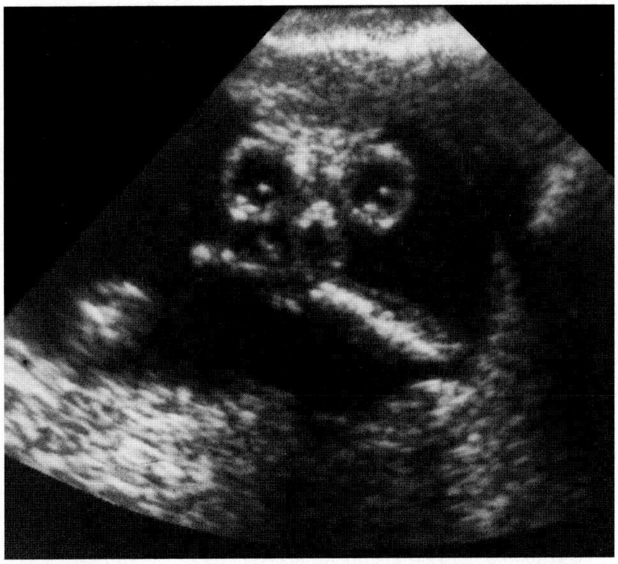

Figure 7–29 The transvaginal view of the fetal head demonstrates the absence of any brain in the skull above the level of the orbits. This fetus was diagnosed with anencephaly. (Reprinted with permission from Bluth, et al, eds. Bluth-Ultrasound: A Practical Approach to Clinical Problems. New York: Thieme; 2000:317, fig. 27–13A.)

◇ Genetic Screening

Under certain circumstances, imaging may be employed to assist in the acquisition of tissue for genetic screening. Indications include maternal age over 35 years, a history of other children with genetic defects, certain metabolic disorders such as diabetes, and exposure to teratogens or toxins. Another indication for genetic screening is an abnormality in maternal serum α-fetoprotein (AFP) levels. AFP is formed by the fetal liver, and levels in the maternal blood may be elevated when there is increased diffusion of AFP into the maternal blood, as in an open neural tube defect (**Fig. 7–29**). Tissue can be obtained via amniocentesis (aspiration of amniotic fluid and culture of desquamated fetal cells), transcervical chorionic villus sampling, and fetal blood sampling, which allows the most rapid analysis of the fetal karyotype. Ultrasound is used to guide the biopsy needle.

Genetic screening may also be indicated by certain findings on obstetrical ultrasound. For example, the finding of a cystic hygroma in the cervical region has a high association with a variety of chromosomal abnormalities, including Turner's syndrome, trisomies 13, 18, and 21, and Noonan's syndrome ("male Turner's syndrome"). Cystic hygroma is found in 1 in 6000 pregnancies and carries a poor prognosis.

Second and Third Trimesters

In the second and third trimesters, assessment of fetal viability and number of gestations remains important, but new parameters come into play as well. An assessment of fetal presentation is helpful to the obstetrician, a cephalic (head down) presentation being the most common and most favorable for vaginal delivery; however, it must be borne in mind that many breech and transverse presentations will correct themselves by the time of delivery, at which point such presentations are seen in only a small percentage of cases (**Fig. 7–30**).

The amount of amniotic fluid can be an important parameter of fetal well-being. Amniotic fluid volume is a dynamic quantity, with complete turnover every 3 to 4 hours, in part because the fetus can swallow up to 0.5 L per day. One means of determining the amount of amniotic fluid is the so-called four-quadrant method, in which the largest fluid pocket in each of the four uterine quadrants is measured; a total between 5 and 20 cm is generally regarded as within normal limits. An excess of amniotic fluid is called polyhydramnios and is associated with fetal conditions that interfere with normal swallowing and absorption of amniotic fluid, such as CNS abnormalities and GI atresias (**Fig. 7–31**). Additional and more common associations include maternal diabetes and hypertension. Oligohydramnios, too little amniotic fluid, is associated with decreased fetal urine output, as seen in renal agenesis, multicystic dysplastic kidney, and urinary tract obstruction. Obstruction of the urinary tract is seen most commonly at the ureteropelvic junction, although ureterovesical junction obstruction and posterior urethral valves are also important differential considerations (the latter in males). Oligohydramnios is associated with the Potter sequence, in which the paucity of amniotic fluid causes pulmonary hypoplasia and a characteristic facies (low-set ears, beaked nose, receding chin, etc.). Other causes of oligohydramnios include fetal demise, intrauterine growth retardation (IUGR), and premature rupture of membranes (**Fig. 7–32**).

The character of the placenta must be noted. The finding of a retroplacental hemorrhage represents a significant threat to fetal well-being, and proliferation of trophoblastic tissue beyond the normal endometrium can be associated with severe maternal hemorrhage at delivery. The location of the placenta

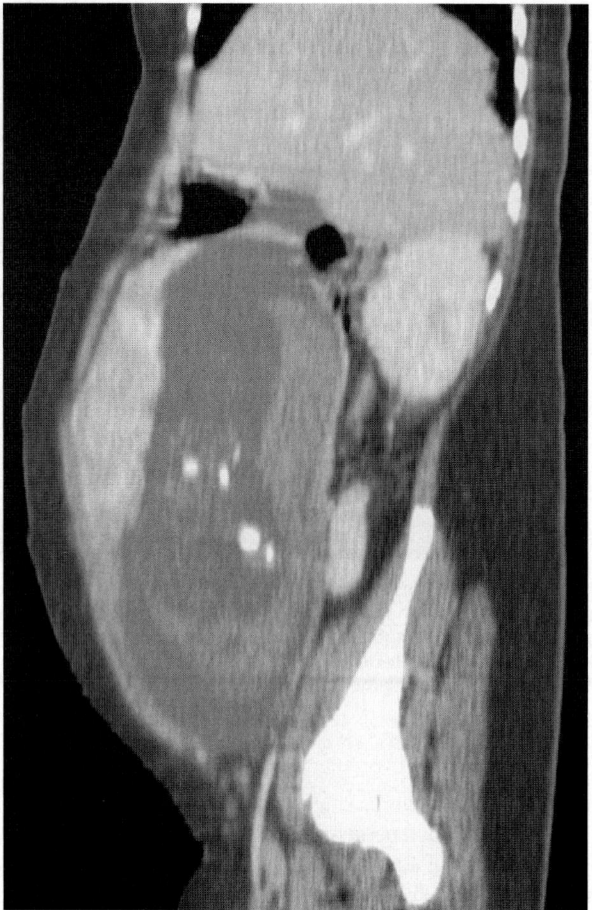

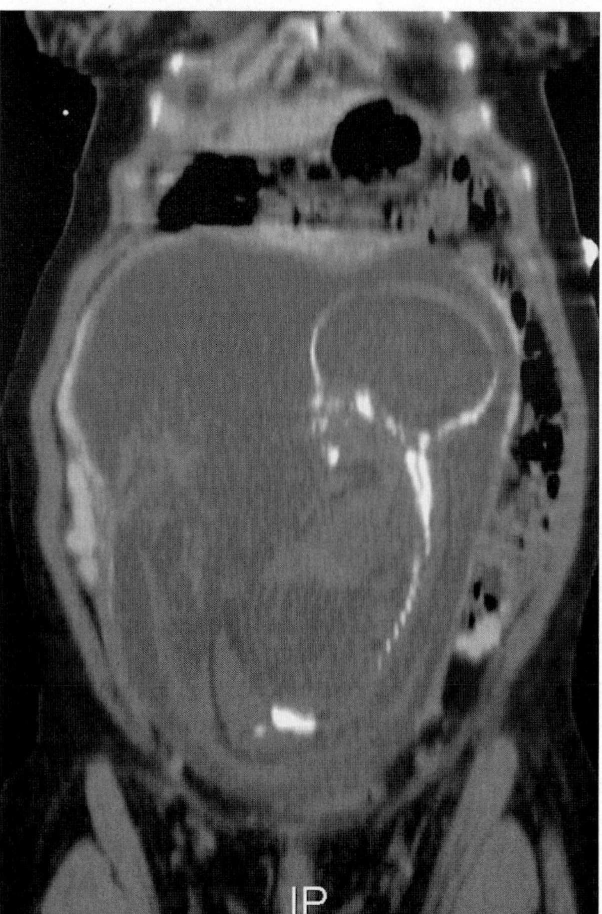

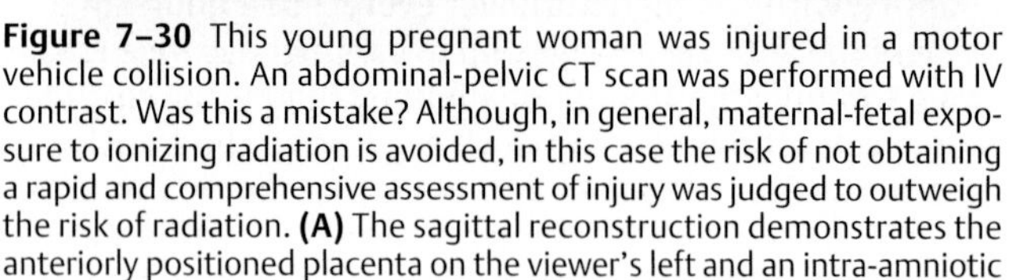

Figure 7–30 This young pregnant woman was injured in a motor vehicle collision. An abdominal-pelvic CT scan was performed with IV contrast. Was this a mistake? Although, in general, maternal-fetal exposure to ionizing radiation is avoided, in this case the risk of not obtaining a rapid and comprehensive assessment of injury was judged to outweigh the risk of radiation. **(A)** The sagittal reconstruction demonstrates the anteriorly positioned placenta on the viewer's left and an intra-amniotic hematoma on the right, with the fetus in between. The patient is facing to the viewer's left. Why is the hematoma on the right? Because the patient was supine during scanning. Note the hypodense rim beneath a portion of the placenta, likely representing a partial abruption. **(B)** This coronal reconstruction clearly demonstrates that this third-trimester fetus is in breech position.

must be determined, particularly as regards its relationship to the internal cervical os. When the placenta overlies the os, a placenta previa may be diagnosed. Placenta previa is associated with an increased risk of hemorrhage and fetal demise; however, such a diagnosis should not be entertained prior to 20 weeks' gestation, as many apparent previas resolve spontaneously prior to that time. In some cases, emptying the bladder will reveal that an apparent placenta previa is in fact merely a low-lying placenta, which is not as hazardous.

◇ Central Nervous System

The assessment of the fetal CNS begins with a search for neural tube defects, seen in 1 in 600 U.S. births. The two most common neural tube defects are anencephaly and myelomeningocele. Anencephaly (Latin, "without head"), absence of the cranial vault, is an invariably lethal condition, and is recognized as an absence of the cranium above the level of the orbits. Myelomeningocele is more common in the British Isles and in women over 35 years of age. Like anencephaly, it is associated with increased maternal serum AFP. Failure of closure of the caudal neuropore most often results in separation of the posterior lamina of the lumbosacral spine, with a dorsally protruding leptomeningeal sac containing cerebrospinal fluid (CSF; meningocele) and neural tissue (myelomeningocele). It is associated with mental retardation, incontinence, and motor impairment.

Another important parameter of the CNS assessment is the size of the lateral ventricles. Ventriculomegaly (>10 mm in the coronal plane) is associated with hydrocephalus, the most common CNS abnormality. Hydrocephalus ("water head") is called obstructive when there is a blockage of normal flow of CSF from the choroid plexus in the lateral and third ventricles, through the cerebral aqueduct, into the fourth ventricle, and out through the foramina of Magendie and Luschka into the subarachnoid space over the brain and spinal cord (**Fig. 7–33**). Myelomeningocele is a common cause of blockage, as is congenital aqueductal stenosis. A less common nonobstructive

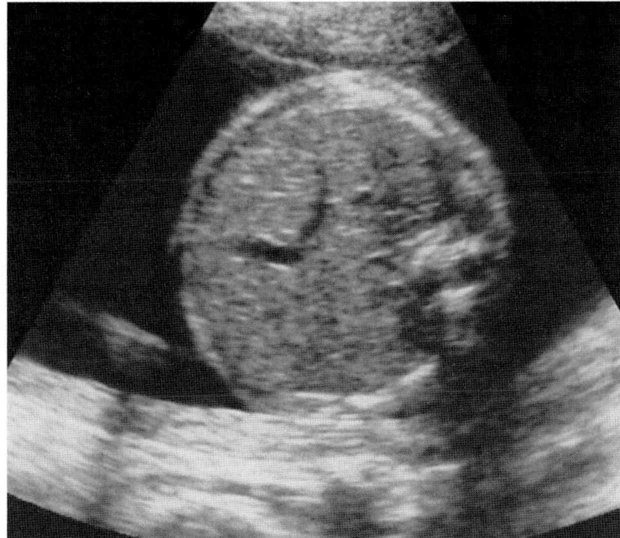

Figure 7–31 This transverse sonogram through the fetal abdomen demonstrates the absence of typical amniotic fluid in the stomach, the so-called stomach bubble. The exam was also remarkable for polyhydramnios. At birth, the baby was found to have esophageal atresia. (Reprinted with permission from Bluth, et al, eds. Bluth-Ultrasound: A Practical Approach to Clinical Problems. New York: Thieme; 2000:315, fig. 27–7.)

cause is prenatal hemorrhage, in which intraventricular blood degradation products may interfere with the absorption of CSF by the arachnoid granulations in the region of the superior sagittal sinus. It is important to bear in mind that ventriculomegaly is not the same entity as hydrocephalus, because cerebral atrophy secondary to in utero vascular insult or infection (particularly TORCH [*to*xoplasmosis, *r*ubella, *c*ytomegalovirus, and *h*erpes simplex] infections) may result in ex vacuo dilatation of the ventricles.

In practical terms, the triad of a normal cavum septum pellucidum, normal-sized lateral ventricular atria (<10 mm), and a normal-sized cisterna magna (2–11 mm) virtually excludes a CNS anomaly.

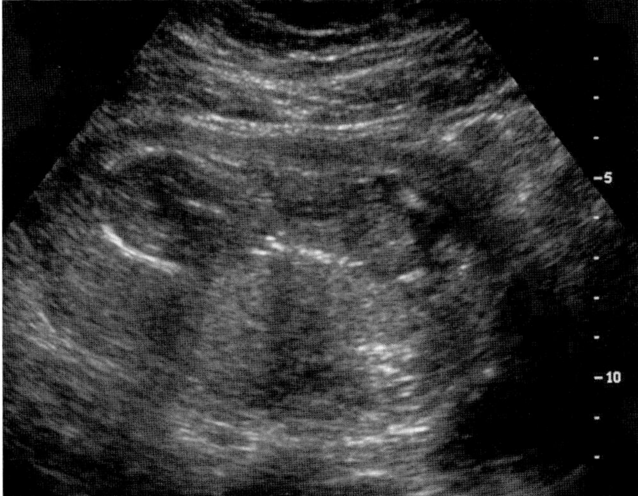

Figure 7–32 An obstetrical ultrasound image demonstrates the severest degree of oligohydramnios, with no fluid separating the longitudinally oriented fetus from the placenta and surrounding uterine walls.

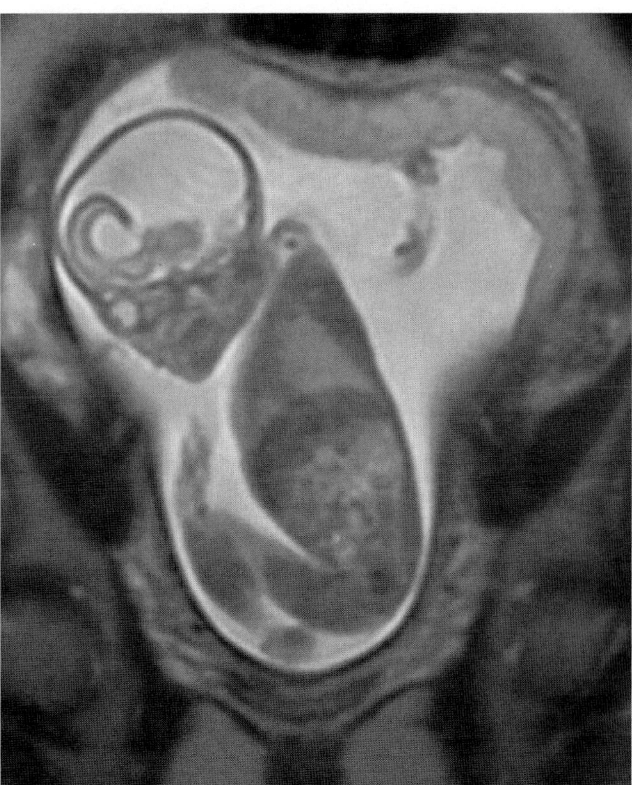

Figure 7–33 This fetal MR image demonstrates cerebrospinal fluid filling most of the fetal cranium, which raises suspicion for obstructive hydrocephalus. In this case, however, the primary anomaly lay with the development of the brain itself in this patient with alobar holoprosencephaly.

◇ Thorax

Evaluation of the fetal thorax includes primarily the heart and lungs. The prenatal detection of congenital heart disease is difficult due to the small size and rapid beating of the heart. Abnormalities visible on the four-chamber view include endocardial cushion defects, commonly seen in Down syndrome, and hypoplastic left heart syndrome, which manifests as absence of the left ventricle, with mitral and aortic atresia. The tetralogy of Fallot, the most salient feature of which is pulmonary stenosis, manifests as a large aorta and a small pulmonary artery on views of the outflow tracts. Important thoracic disorders that may be detected include congenital diaphragmatic hernia, with bowel present in the thorax; cystic adenomatoid malformation, characterized by a solid or cystic pulmonary mass; and masses in the mediastinum, including cystic hygromas (lymphangiomas) and neurogenic tumors.

◇ Abdomen

Assessment of the fetal abdomen includes the search for normal anatomic structures. Failure to visualize the stomach suggests such disorders as oligohydramnios (a paucity of fluid available to fill the gastric lumen), esophageal

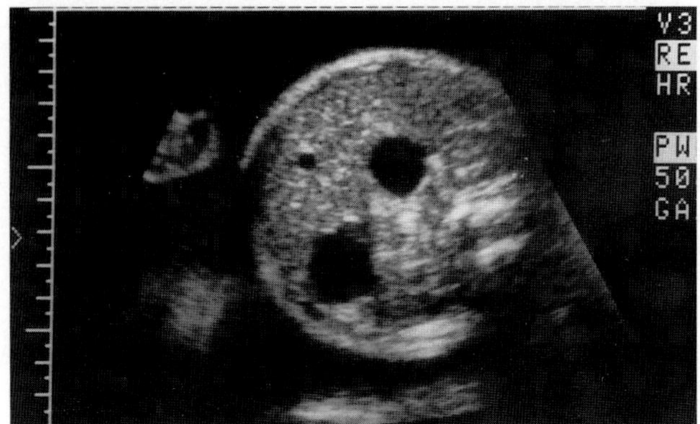

Figure 7–34 A transverse sonographic image of the fetal abdomen demonstrates the so-called double bubble sign of duodenal atresia, representing amniotic fluid–filled dilated stomach and proximal duodenum. (Reprinted with permission from Bluth, et al, eds. Bluth-Ultrasound: A Practical Approach to Clinical Problems. New York: Thieme; 2000:341, fig. 29–21.)

atresia, and a CNS defect with impaired swallowing (the latter two associated with polyhydramnios). Duodenal atresia classically presents with a combination of polyhydramnios and a "double bubble" sign, representing the dilated, fluid-filled gastric and proximal duodenal lumens (**Fig. 7–34**). Abnormalities of the abdominal wall include gastroschisis and omphalocele. Gastroschisis ("split stomach") involves a defect in all three layers of the wall, with herniation of abdominal contents through a small paraumbilical defect (**Fig. 7–35**). It is invariably associated with abnormalities of bowel rotation. Omphalocele (from the Greek *omphalos,* "navel," and *kele,* "hernia") involves a midline abdominal defect covered by peritoneum, with the umbilical cord inserting centrally into the hernia sac. Although gastroschisis is the more serious defect, omphalocele carries a graver prognosis, due to a 70% association with other malformations. One of the most important abnormalities of the urinary tract is obstruction, most prevalent at the level of the ureteropelvic junction. Multicystic dysplastic kidney is the most common renal mass and appears as a mass in the renal bed containing numerous cysts.

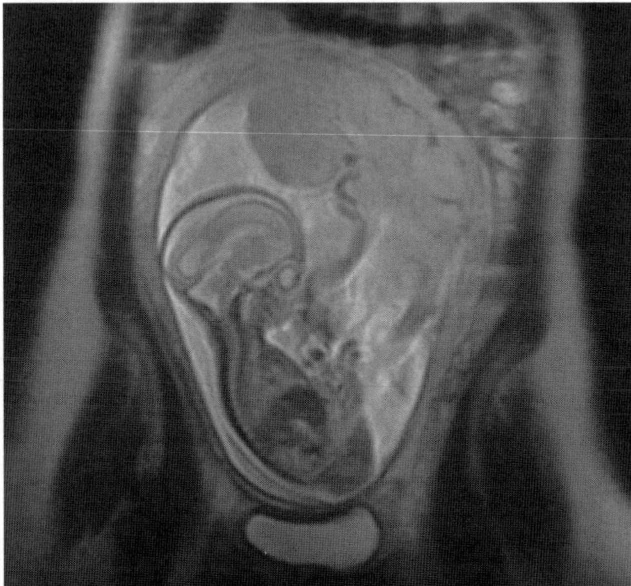

Figure 7–35 This fetal MR image demonstrates a sagittal view of the placenta, umbilical cord, and fetus. Note that there is bowel floating in the amniotic fluid anterior to the fetal abdomen, consistent with gastroschisis.

◇ Gestational Age

Gestational age can be assessed using a combination of biparietal diameter and femur length. Fetal growth is assessed primarily by measurement of abdominal circumference, which is especially important in detecting intrauterine growth retardation. IUGR is best diagnosed around the 34th week of gestation. The most important cause is uteroplacental insufficiency, most commonly of maternal etiology. Other causes include malnutrition, hypertension, and alcohol or tobacco use. IUGR is associated with a 5- to 10-fold increase in the risk of prenatal or neonatal death (**Fig. 7–36**). Macrosomia is associated with

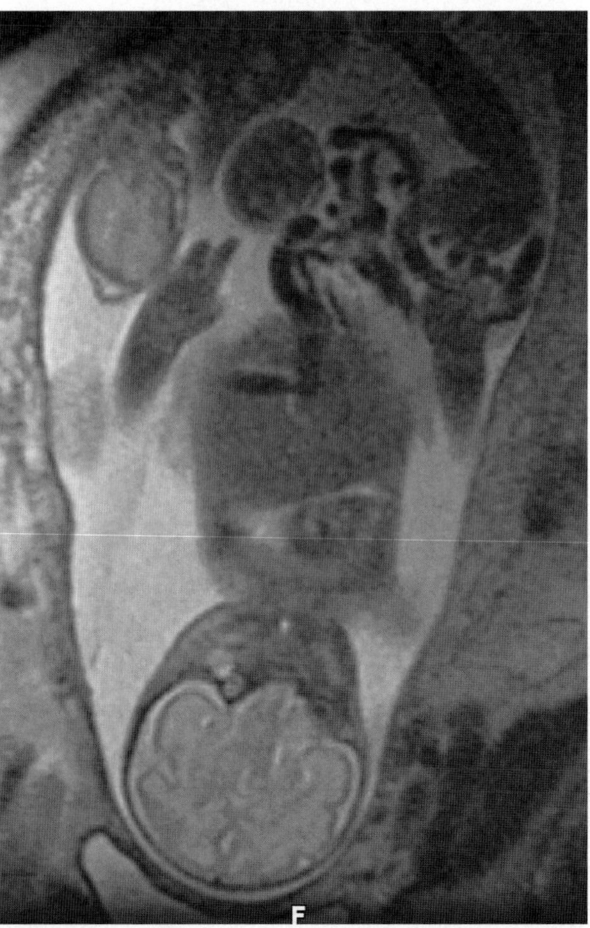

Figure 7–36 This patient's recent ultrasound examinations had shown growth retardation of one of her twin fetuses. The fetal MR image demonstrates a dramatic difference in size between the two fetuses, whose brains are clearly visualized. The larger, more caudally positioned fetus is normal in size, but the more cranial of the two demonstrates severe growth retardation. The latter eventually died due to twin–twin transfusion syndrome.

maternal diabetes and increases the risk of prolonged labor and meconium aspiration.

◆ Male Reproductive System

Anatomy and Physiology

The male gonads are suspended extra-abdominally within the scrotum, into which the testes (from the Greek for "witness," perhaps because a man testifying in court was required to place one hand on his scrotum) descend in the seventh month of intrauterine life (**Fig. 7–37**). Spermatogenesis takes place beginning at puberty within the seminiferous tubules, which account for 80% of the testicular mass. These highly coiled tubules measure ~250 m long and contain both the sperm-producing spermatogonia and the supporting Sertoli's cells. The seminiferous tubules converge on the rete (from the Latin for "net") testis, which empties into the epididymis (from the Greek for "upon" and "testicle"). The epididymis is another highly coiled tube that measures 6 m long and is located along the posterosuperior aspect of the testis. The epididymis empties into the vas deferens, which conveys sperm into the abdominal cavity and becomes the ejaculatory ducts at the base of the bladder. The secondary sex glands, the seminal vesicles and prostate gland, empty their secretions into the ejaculatory ducts. The ejaculatory ducts empty into the urethra, at which point the reproductive and urinary systems share a common pathway in the male. The penis contains cylinders of erectile tissue, the paired corpora cavernosa and the single corpora spongiosum, with the urethra traveling in the latter.

As in the female, the gonads perform the functions of gametogenesis and sex hormone production. In contrast to the female, the male hypothalamic gonadotropin-releasing hormone occurs in bursts every few hours, but otherwise does not exhibit the wide cycles that characterize female reproductive structure and function. The Leydig's cells, located within the testicular interstitium between the seminiferous tubules, produce testosterone. Testosterone is necessary for the normal in utero differentiation of the male reproductive tract and is also responsible for male secondary sexual characteristics such as growth of the beard, deepening of the voice, and broadening of the shoulders. A healthy young man produces several hundred million sperm per day, which are contained at ejaculation in ~3 mL of ejaculated semen. Produced by the accessory sex glands, the semen (from the Latin for "seed") contains fructose, an energy source for sperm; prostaglandins, which stimulate the smooth muscle of the female reproductive tract to aid in sperm transit; and alkaline secretions, which help to neutralize vaginal acidity.

Pathology

Scrotum

The most important scrotal pathologies may be divided into several categories, including tumors, inflammation, fluid collections, and vascular insult. In each case, the first and often only imaging study to be performed is ultrasound, because the scrotum and its contents are superficial structures containing no air or bone and are therefore readily accessible sonographically. Moreover, ultrasound does not subject the gonads to ionizing radiation.

Scrotal ultrasound embodies a key radiologic principle, namely, the use of the normal side for comparison. The bilateral symmetry of the vertebrate body plan constitutes one of nature's greatest boons to clinical imaging. Whether comparing testes, breasts, lungs, or hemispheres of the brain, the radiologist's eyes move back and forth from side to side, looking for asymmetries. In the case of the testes, key points of

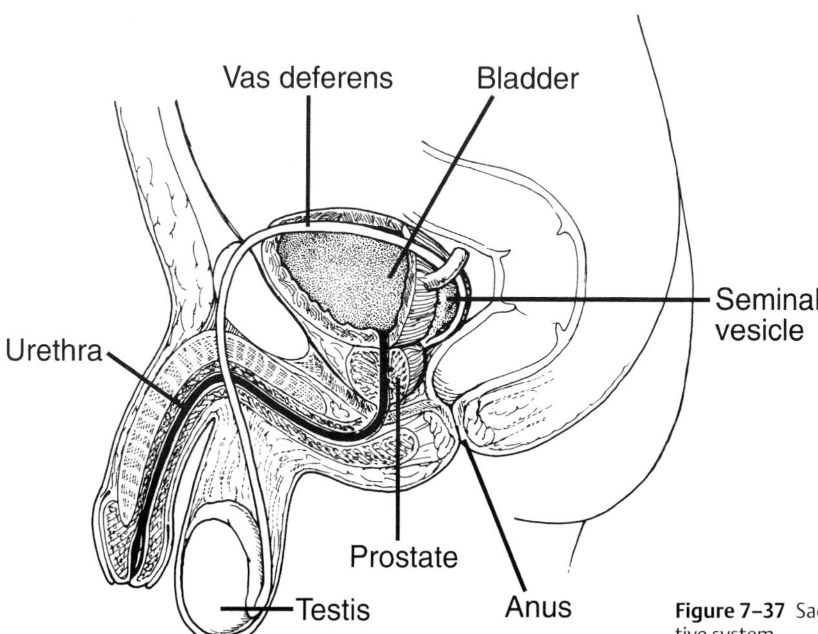

Figure 7–37 Sagittal view of the major structures of the male reproductive system.

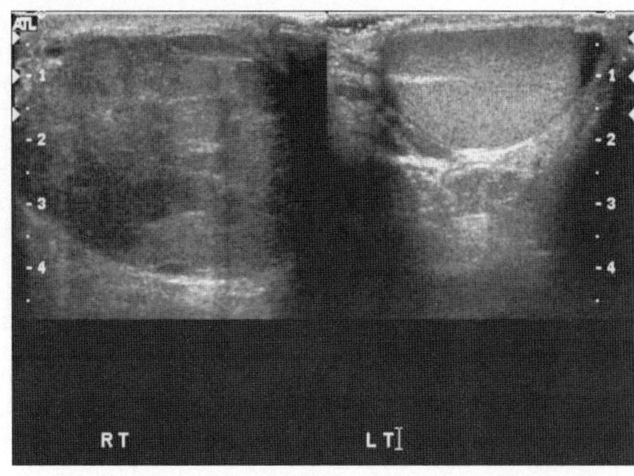

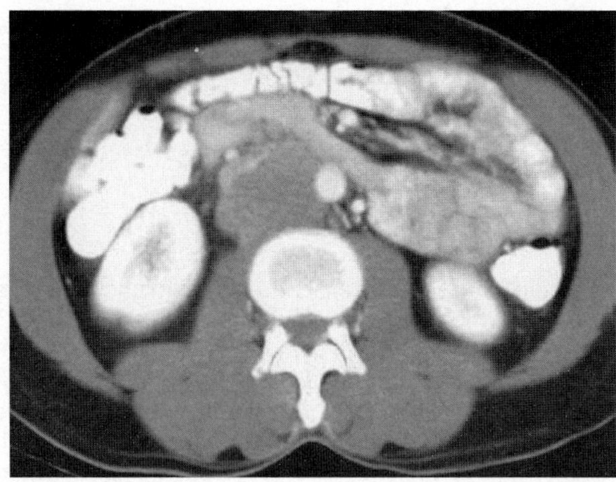

Figure 7–38 **(A)** Sonographic images of both testes demonstrate a normal left testis, but an enlarged and markedly heterogeneous right testis. **(B)** A staging CT exam reveals bulky periaortic adenopathy. Orchiectomy led to a diagnosis of metastatic testicular seminoma, proving that the imaging appearance is not always histologically diagnostic.

comparison include size, echotexture, and blood flow. When performing scrotal ultrasound, it is advisable to begin with the unaffected side. Not only is the unaffected side less tender, thereby enabling the examiner to put the patient somewhat at ease, but it provides a baseline against which to assess possible abnormalities on the symptomatic side.

◇ Tumors

Primary testicular neoplasms constitute 1% of all male malignancies, most commonly occurring in the 25-to-35-year age group. Ninety percent are germ cell neoplasms, with mixed tumors being the most common histologic type, followed by pure seminomas. Useful clinical adjuncts in diagnosis include the serum AFP and HCG. Both are typically negative in seminomas; however, the AFP will be elevated in a tumor with a yolk sac cell component, and the HCG will be elevated in choriocarcinoma (the tumor with the worst prognosis). Testicular neoplasms often present as painless masses.

Perhaps because the testis contains innumerable seminiferous tubules, each representing an acoustic interface, the normal testis is a relatively echogenic structure; therefore, tumors tend to demonstrate a relatively hypoechoic appearance. Seminomas exhibit well-defined margins and homogeneous hypoechogenicity, whereas nonseminomas tend to appear less well defined with a more heterogeneous echotexture (**Fig. 7–38**). Determining the cell type of a testicular neoplasm radiologically is not necessary, because the probability of malignancy in an intratesticular mass is high, and orchiectomy with definitive histologic diagnosis constitutes typical management.

The tunica albuginea, a tough membrane covering the testis, usually prevents local extension of neoplasms. Hence lymphatic and hematogenous routes of spread are most frequent, and it is not uncommon for a patient with testicular malignancy to present with massive retroperitoneal adenopathy. Overall, the prognosis is good, with stage I or II disease (confined to the scrotum or extension into the retroperitoneal lymph nodes, respectively) enjoying a better than 95% 5-year survival. Even stage III disease, which involves metastases beyond the retroperitoneum (especially the lungs) carries a 5-year survival rate of better than 70%. The most common metastatic malignancies to involve the testes are lymphoma and leukemia, which are only very rarely diagnosed on the basis of testicular involvement.

◇ Epididymitis

The two most common testicular pathologies to present acutely are epididymitis and torsion. Epididymitis typically involves the spread of lower urinary tract pathogens into the epididymis via the vas deferens. The most important pathogens in young men are the expected venereal organisms *Chlamydia* and gonococci. In about one quarter of cases, there is associated orchitis, or inflammation of the testis itself. Viral orchitis is associated with mumps. Findings on ultrasound examination include an enlarged, hypoechoic epididymis, which appears hyperemic as compared with the unaffected side on Doppler examination (**Fig. 7–39**).

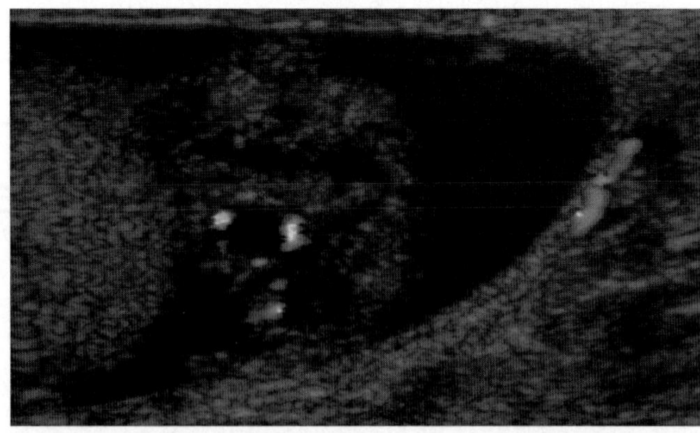

Figure 7–39 This scrotal ultrasound image in a patient with acute scrotal pain and swelling demonstrates a portion of the normal testis on the left side of the image with a swollen, heterogeneous epididymis on the right. The epididymis shows increased color Doppler flow compared with the testis. There is anechoic fluid around the testes and epididymis, a reactive hydrocele. These findings are consistent with epididymitis.

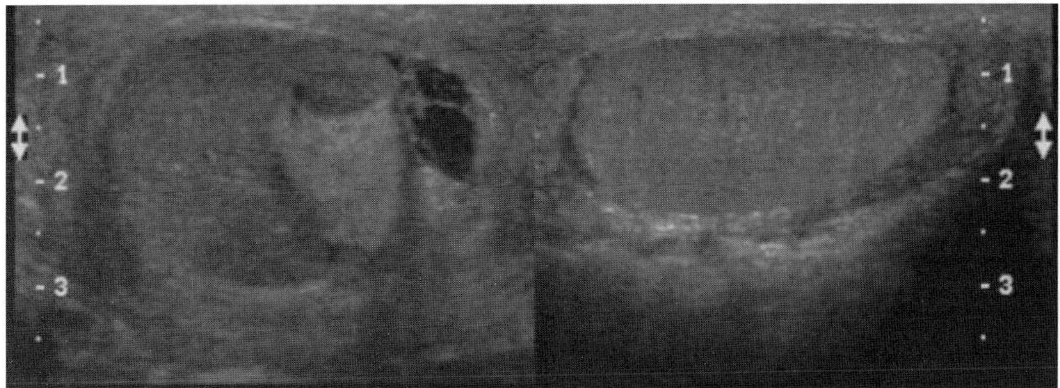

Figure 7–40 This teenage boy presented with acute scrotal pain and swelling for 3 days. Side-by-side sonographic images show the right testis to be larger and more heterogeneous in echogenicity than the left testis. Color flow and arterial Doppler waveforms could be visualized on the left but not on the right. Scrotal exploration demonstrated a hemorrhagic infarction of the right testis.

◇ Testicular Torsion

The key differential consideration in the acutely painful and swollen testis is epididymitis versus torsion, and the determination of whether torsion is present must be made immediately. The rate of salvage of torsed testes drops precipitously after the patient has been symptomatic for more than 6 hours, with a worse than 20% salvage rate after 12 hours. Torsion occurs secondary to trauma, sexual activity, or physical exertion, when the spermatic cord twists around its axis, impairing both venous drainage via the pampiniform plexus and arterial inflow via the testicular, deferential, and external spermatic arteries. Patients present with torsion most frequently in the newborn and teenage years. Certain individuals are predisposed to torsion because at least one of their testes is completely enveloped by the peritoneal membrane called the tunica vaginalis, which prevents secure anchoring of the testis to the scrotal sac. More than one half of patients exhibit this abnormality bilaterally, rendering bilateral orchiopexy standard surgical therapy when the affected testis is salvageable.

The key sonographic findings in testicular torsion can be visualized on color Doppler imaging. In complete torsion, the affected testis will demonstrate absence of flow, whereas an incomplete torsion may demonstrate markedly diminished flow. Additional findings of torsion on gray-scale imaging may include increased size and decreased echogenicity of the testis, as compared with the normal side (**Fig. 7–40**). Nuclear medicine imaging is less frequently employed today, but it remains a useful substitute when sonography is not available. After peripheral injection of technetium- (Tc-) 99m pertechnetate, a "cold" or photopenic area will be seen in the region of the affected testis, manifesting its lack of perfusion.

◇ Varicocele

A common fluid collection within the testis is a varicocele, a dilated and serpiginous pampiniform venous plexus (**Fig. 7–41**). This condition is clinically important because it may be associated with infertility, and varicoceles in fact constitute the most frequent correctable cause of infertility in the male. At least 95% of varicoceles are left-sided and probably result from incompetence of the valves in the internal spermatic vein. One hypothesis regarding the left-sided predominance of varicoceles is that the left-sided gonadal vein drains into the renal vein, and the right gonadal vein drains directly into the inferior vena cava. The finding of a new varicocele in a patient over age 40 is of special significance, because it may herald the development of a neoplasm causing obstruction of the gonadal or renal vein (most often a renal cell carcinoma).

Prostate

◇ Epidemiology

Approximately 200,000 cases of prostate cancer are diagnosed each year in the United States. This number has been increasing rapidly, primarily due to the aging of the population. Another factor in this increase is the detection of

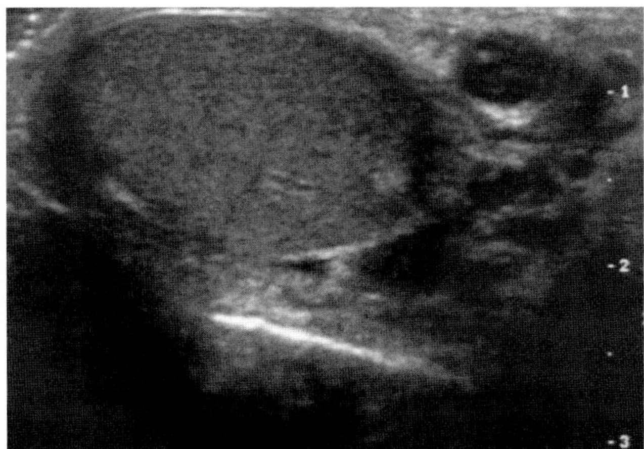

Figure 7–41 This middle-aged man presented with a scrotal mass that had been enlarging for several months. A longitudinal scrotal ultrasound image demonstrates serpiginous structures inferior and lateral to the testes. These showed increased signal on color Doppler imaging. Surgery confirmed a scrotal varicocele.

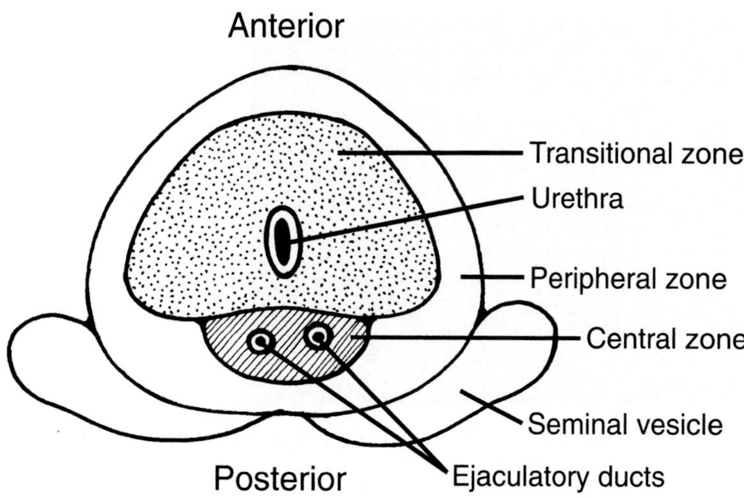

Figure 7–42 The key zones of the prostate gland seen on imaging studies such as ultrasound and magnetic resonance imaging.

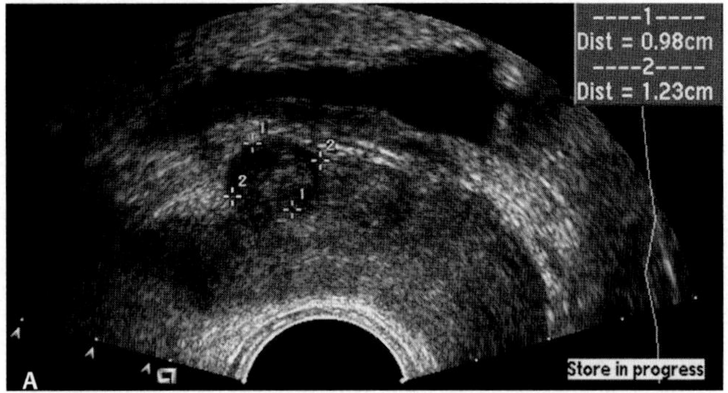

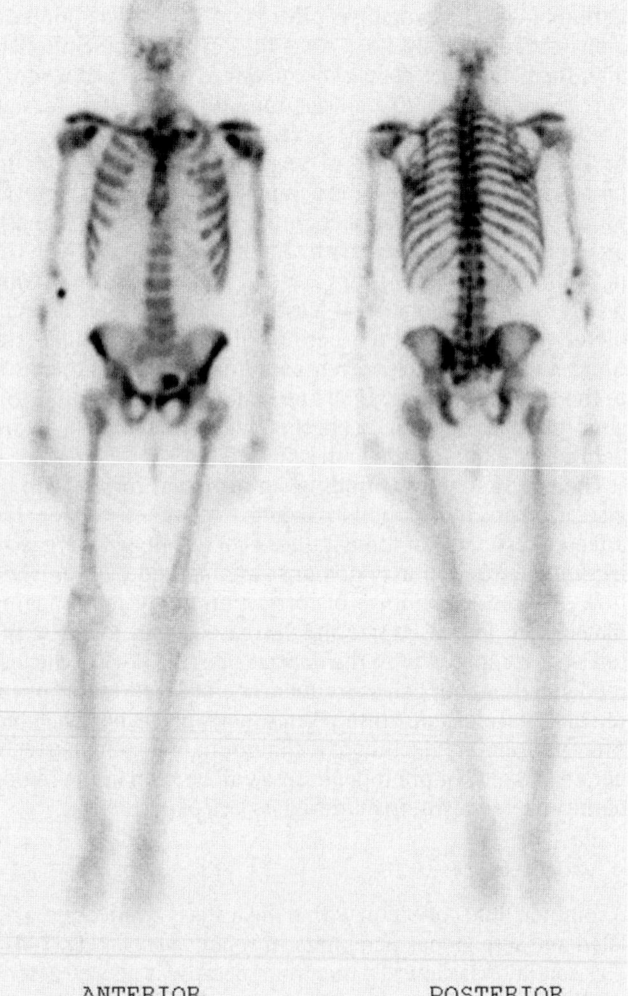

Figure 7–43 This middle-aged man's prostate-specific antigen (PSA) had been rising, although a digital rectal exam was normal. **(A)** Transrectal sonography reveals a 1 cm hypoechoic mass in the left lobe of the prostate gland. Biopsy demonstrated carcinoma. **(B)** A whole-body nuclear medicine bone scan in another patient with advanced prostate cancer demonstrates a so-called super-scan, with diffusely increased radiotracer activity throughout the axial skeleton as well as abnormal foci in the pelvis and the extremities. Note also that there is little renal activity, due to the avid bone uptake. This indicates diffuse skeletal metastatic disease.

clinically occult disease through screening programs. Prostate cancer is the second leading cause of cancer death in men, resulting in ~43,000 deaths per year, second only to lung cancer; however, the toll of prostate cancer in years of life lost is much less than that of breast cancer, due to the fact that it typically kills at a much later age; in the United States, breast cancer is responsible for over 100 years of life lost per 100,000 people under the age of 65, whereas prostate cancer is responsible for less than 10.

◇ Pathophysiology

An understanding of the anatomy of the prostate gland is critical in interpreting imaging studies, because different pathologic processes tend to arise in different portions of the gland (**Fig. 7–42**). The prostate gland surrounds the urethra at the base of the bladder and contains the junction point between the urethra and ejaculatory ducts. Approximately three fourths of the gland is located in the peripheral zone, which surrounds the remainder of the gland posterolaterally. Most prostate cancers arise here, and 95% of these malignancies are adenocarcinomas. The transitional zone, which surrounds the urethra, constitutes only 5% of the gland, but represents the site of benign prostatic hyperplasia (BPH), and hence may enlarge markedly.

The workup of a newly diagnosed patient generally includes measurements of serum alkaline phosphatase and liver function tests, as well as chest radiographs, bone scan, and abdominal and pelvic CT. MRI or transrectal ultrasound is more accurate than CT in assessing local extension of the disease. In patients presenting with an elevated prostate-specific antigen (PSA), transrectal ultrasound is often employed to guide biopsy of the gland.

◇ Clinical Presentation

The clinical presentation of prostate cancer includes symptoms such as urinary frequency, nocturia, and urinary urgency. Unfortunately, these same symptoms are associated with BPH, which is seen to some degree in most men as they age. A distinguishing feature that tends to favor malignancy is a relatively abrupt change in symptoms. The two most widely employed screening methods are serum assays for PSA and digital rectal examination. Digital rectal examination, performed by inserting a gloved finger into the rectum and palpating the prostate gland along the anterior rectal wall, is relatively sensitive but nonspecific. Findings worrisome for malignancy include a firm, asymmetrical mass or an irregularly enlarged gland.

Benign processes in the differential diagnosis of prostate carcinoma include BPH, which involves the transitional zone, and prostatitis, which generally causes the entire gland to become boggy, swollen, and edematous. The most common organism is *Escherichia coli.*

It is not uncommon for patients to present with metastatic disease, which manifests with such symptoms as impotence (due to disruption of neurovascular structures), as well as back pain and bone pain (due to skeletal metastases). Approximately 80% of patients with metastatic disease exhibit only bone involvement, but other sites include lymph nodes, liver, and lung.

◇ Imaging

Imaging findings that support the diagnosis of prostate carcinoma depend on the modality employed. Transrectal ultrasound findings include one or more hypoechoic nodules in the peripheral zone, mass effect on surrounding tissues, and asymmetric enlargement of the gland (**Fig. 7–43**). On T2-weighted MR images, cancers typically appear as hypointense (dark) lesions amid the relatively bright parenchyma of the peripheral zone. Ultimately, the diagnosis is established by biopsy, and ultrasound has the advantage that it readily guides biopsy of suspicious lesions via a transrectal route.

8

The Musculoskeletal System

◆ Anatomy and Physiology

Bone is living tissue, consisting of a combination of cells and an extracellular organic matrix laid down by those cells. The extracellular matrix (osteoid) consists of a combination of collagen fibers and a mucopolysaccharide-rich gel, referred to as ground substance. This ground substance or osteoid gives the bone a somewhat rubbery consistency that is responsible for its tensile strength. Precipitation of hydroxyapatite crystals (primarily calcium phosphate) within this matrix renders the bone hard, providing compressional strength. Cartilage is similar to bone, although it is unmineralized. The parts of a long bone include the epiphysis, the physis or growth plate, the metaphysis, and the diaphysis (**Fig. 8–1**).

Bone growth is growth hormone mediated. Bones grow in length through the addition of new chondrocytes at the epiphyseal end of the growth plate. These cartilage cells have no blood vessels and receive nutrients by diffusion through the ground substance. As the cartilage cells become mineralized toward the metaphyseal end, their tenuous blood supply is interrupted, and they die. Osteoclasts move in to clear out the dead chondrocytes, and osteoblasts move in to lay down bone in the remnants of the cartilage. Osteoblasts are literally bone formers, whereas osteoclasts are literally bone destroyers, which secrete acids that dissolve the hydroxyapatite crystals and enzymes that break down the organic matrix. Although the osteoblasts become entrapped in bone, and are then called osteocytes, they do not die due to the network of nutrient-conveying canaliculi to which they are connected. Long bones grow in diameter through the action of osteoblasts within the periosteum, the connective tissue sheath that covers the outer surface of the bone. Osteoclasts simultaneously dissolve away the inner cortex of the bone, allowing the marrow cavity to expand apace.

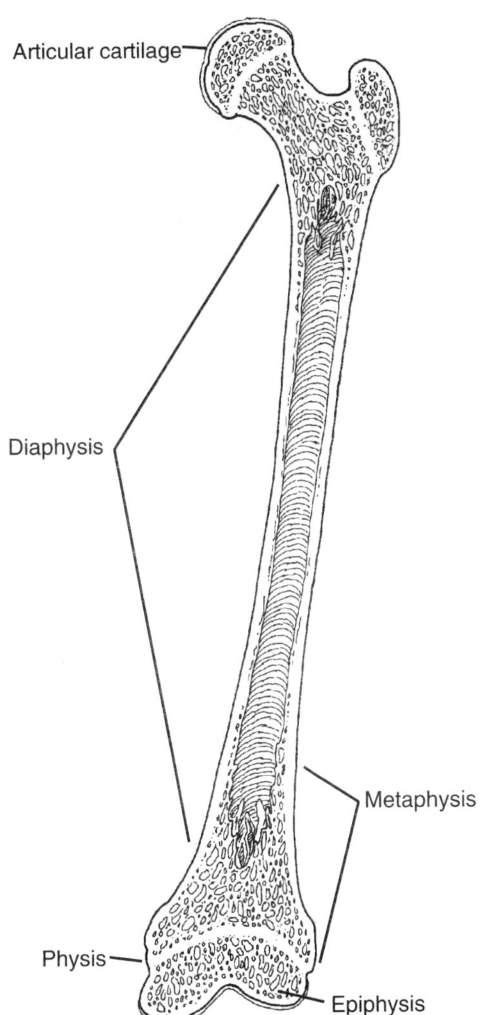

Figure 8–1 The principal parts of a long bone, in this case the femur.

The skeleton performs several functions. First, it provides the mechanical scaffolding necessary to support the body and allow for movement through the lever action of skeletal muscles. Second, it protects vital internal organs such as the brain, spinal cord, heart, and lungs. Third, blood cells are manufactured in the bone marrow. Fourth, the skeleton serves as a storage reservoir for calcium and phosphate; 99% of the calcium in the body is found in the bones. The key regulator of serum calcium levels is parathyroid hormone (PTH), produced by the four parathyroid glands found posterior to the thyroid gland in the neck. Absence of PTH is incompatible with life, and a patient without it typically dies within several days when hypocalcemia-induced respiratory muscle spasm results in asphyxiation.

To understand the myriad pathologic processes to which bone is subject, it is first necessary to understand normal bone anatomy and physiology. Consider the following example. It is often observed that patients with severe neurologic impairment that confines them to bed develop articular deformities, involving such joints as the hip and knee joints. Why? Part of the answer lies in the normal physiology of articular cartilage. The cartilage of the hip and knee joints receives its nutrients not from blood vessels, but from the synovial fluid within the joint space itself. The cartilage and synovial fluid function rather like a sponge and water, respectively. When we place weight on the joint, the cartilage is compressed, and some of the synovial fluid is squeezed out. When mechanical force is removed, the cartilage expands slightly and draws in fresh fluid, from which it extracts nutrients. Hence the maintenance of normal joint morphology is dependent on regular joint function, a principle that applies more broadly to the whole of the skeleton.

The structure of bone is of a more dynamic nature than the structure of any other adult organ. Bone undergoes continual remodeling throughout life. Both the mass of bone and the three-dimensional orientation of bone elements respond to the functional demands placed on the skeleton, a principle that applies in both health and disease; therefore, individuals who exercise regularly tend to have stronger bones than those who do not.

The observation that exercise increases bone mass is especially notable in light of the fact that maximum bone mass is attained early in the third decade of life. To avoid the ravages of osteoporosis, exercise during young adult life is therefore critical, as bone mass usually increases no further after that time. A person's bone mass at that age constitutes the point of departure for a subsequent inexorable decline after age 40, which becomes more rapid in women after menopause. An example of the rapidity with which bone loss may occur is seen in astronauts, who tend to undergo very rapid loss of bone mass due to the lack of mechanical stress in a weightless environment. Early astronauts lost 20% of their bone mass during only a short time in orbit, and resistance exercises are now a routine part of life in space. The adage "Use it or lose it" is an especially apt description of bone physiology.

Osteoporosis does not represent the death of bone or a decline in bone function; in fact, truly dead or devascularized bone cannot become osteoporotic in the first place, because it lacks not only osteoblastic but also osteoclastic activity. Rather, osteoporosis represents a change in the balance of osteoblastic and osteoclastic activity. Living bone is anything but a static structure. The term *osteoporosis,* which refers to decreased density of bone, should be distinguished from the more general term *osteopenia* (from "bone" and "poor"), which simply means an increased radiolucency of bone. Aside from osteoporosis, another cause of osteopenia is osteomalacia, which results from abnormal bone mineralization.

Another graphic example of the dynamic nature of bone is seen in the bone's response to osseous lesions. If the lesion grows slowly enough to give the bone a chance to react, it will tend to have sclerotic (dense) margins, representing in part an attempt by the remaining intact bone to compensate for the lack of mechanical support provided by the abnormal bone. So, too, in cases of traumatic fracture, the formation of callus can be regarded as a process of physiologic casting, with the callus temporarily assuming the burden of weight bearing while the underlying bone heals. Highly aggressive bone malignancies, on the other hand, tend to destroy surrounding bone at such a rapid pace that no osseous response can be mounted, and thus tend to manifest a lytic appearance (**Fig. 8–2**). The stress fractures that occur in individuals who undertake rigorous exercise programs likewise reflect the fact that the bone must first become weaker before it can be made stronger; the attempt to remodel the bone for greater strength entails an initial loss of osteoid and mineral.

Although many factors are involved, the primary players in the dynamic remodeling of bone are the osteoblasts and osteoclasts. Osteoblastic activity is stimulated by compressive forces on the bone, by the thyroid hormone calcitonin, and by low local pO_2, or passive hyperemia. Osteoclastic activity is stimulated by tensile forces on the bone, by parahormone, and by high local pO_2, or active hyperemia. Because the osteoclasts are more efficient than the osteoblasts—a single osteoclast working at maximum capacity would require over 100 osteoblasts to counterbalance it—negative bone balance is an ever-present propensity.

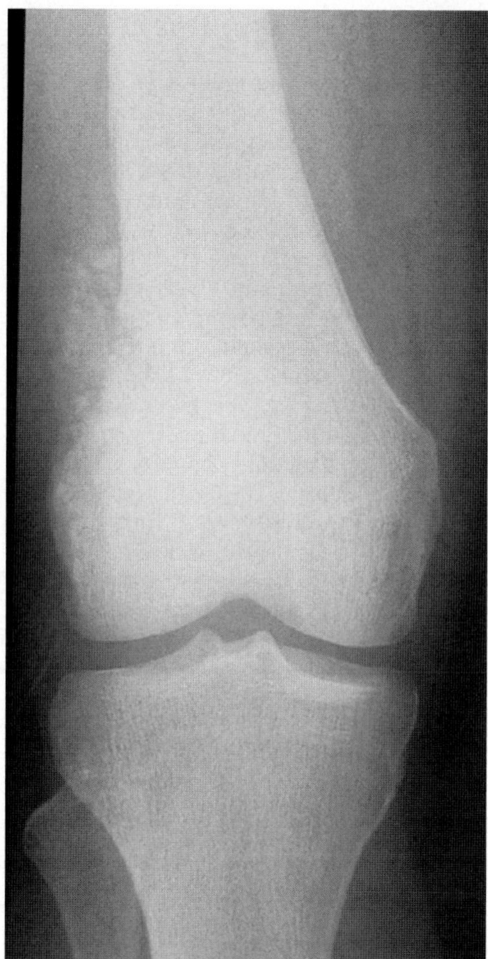

Figure 8–2 A frontal radiograph of the right knee demonstrates a combination of erosive change in the lateral aspect of the femoral metaphysis as well as cloudlike extraosseous osteoid formation. This is typical behavior of an osteogenic osteosarcoma.

◆ Imaging Modalities

The modalities employed in musculoskeletal imaging include magnetic resonance imaging, computed tomography, nuclear medicine, ultrasound, and plain radiography. MRI plays an increasing role in the evaluation of joints, soft tissues, and the spine because of its unique strengths in assessing tissue composition, imaging lesions in multiple planes, and accurately delineating geographic relationships. CT provides accurate assessment of osseous lesions and is especially useful in evaluating calcification, although its capabilities in evaluating the soft tissues are considerably inferior to MRI. Multidetector CT can provide multidimensional imaging that rivals that of MRI. Radionuclide bone scans provide physiologic information on cell turnover and generally constitutes the best means of screening for lesions throughout the skeleton, although limited MRI sequences of the entire skeleton can also play the role. Ultrasound has played a more limited role in the assessment of joint effusions, blood flow, and the presence of foreign bodies within the soft tissues, although it is being used increasingly to assess soft tissue structures such as tendons. Despite the important contributions of other modalities, plain radiography stands out as the single most useful skeletal diagnostic study in most situations.

◆ Pathology

Congenital

Congenital or developmental dysplasias exert their effects at the physis (growth plate), impacting such processes as cartilage cell proliferation (achondroplasia), cartilage matrix production (mucopolysaccharidoses), or the mineralization of cartilage matrix with calcium hydroxyapatite (rickets).

Rickets, which usually represents an acquired metabolic disorder, is discussed in Chapter 10. A variety of noxious agents, including infections such as syphilis and toxins such as alcohol, may also interfere with this process.

Achondroplasia

Achondroplasia is the most common nonlethal skeletal dysplasia and the most prevalent form of short-limbed dwarfism. It is characterized by rhizomelic (proximal segment) limb shortening and is inherited in an autosomal dominant fashion, although most cases are sporadic. The fundamental abnormality is a defect in enchondral bone formation. Characteristic findings on clinical examination include short, stubby fingers, extremities that are disproportionately short in relation to the trunk, and a prominent calvarium with frontal bossing.

Radiographic findings include a small foramen magnum and narrowing interpediculate distances as one moves from cephalad to caudad down the spine. As a result, patients are predisposed to spinal stenosis, with neurologic complaints secondary to compression of the spinal cord and nerve roots.

Thanatophoric Dysplasia

This is the most common skeletal dysplasia that is lethal in the neonatal period. Its name is derived from the Greek for "death-bringing." It is associated with severe limb shortening, thoracic narrowing, macrocephaly, and normal trunk length. Infants usually die of respiratory insufficiency or brainstem compression (**Fig. 8–3**).

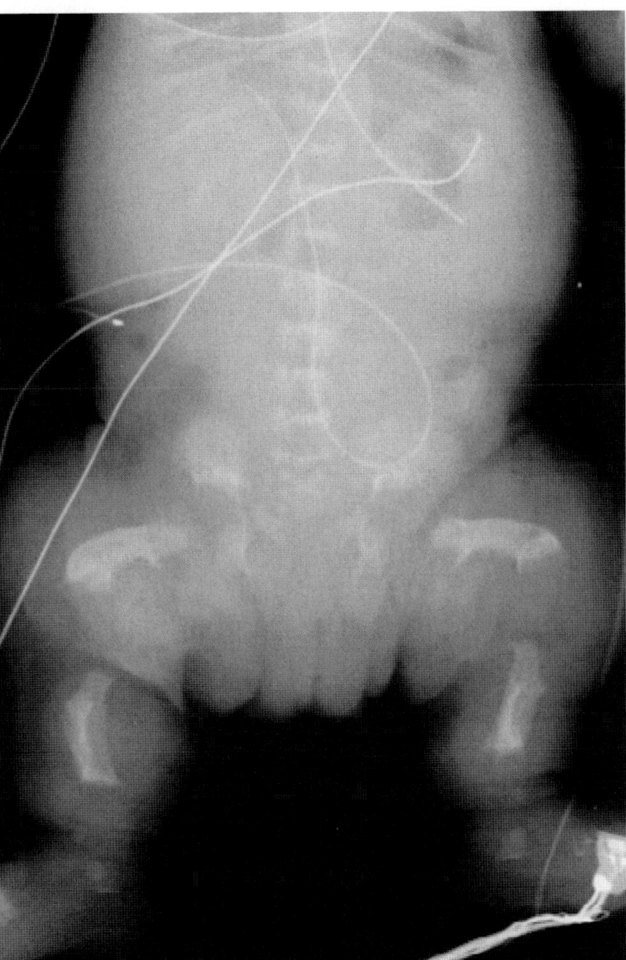

Figure 8–3 This radiograph of the abdomen of a neonate demonstrates classic findings of thanatophoric dysplasia, including severe limb shortening, platyspondyly (flattening of the vertebral bodies), narrowing of the chest from short ribs, and "telephone receiver–shaped" femurs.

Osteopetrosis

Osteopetrosis is a rare but edifying disease that illustrates some of the essential principles of bone pathophysiology. It is transmitted in both autosomal recessive (fatal) and autosomal dominant forms and is caused by an enzymatic abnormality that results in impaired osteoclastic function. As a result, bone remodeling, which is critical in both bone's growth and its response to mechanical stress, occurs abnormally. Patients with the nonlethal form of this disease present with frequent fractures and anemia, among other problems. The fractures stem from the fact that bone cannot adapt to mechanical stresses by remodeling normally. The anemia results from a lack of normal bone tubulation, with diminution or even obliteration of the marrow space, and resultant decreased hematopoeisis.

Radiographic findings are predictable and include generalized osteosclerosis (dense bones), the so-called Erlenmeyer flask deformity of the distal femur (due to abnormal remodeling of the metaphysis with growth), and frequently, pathologic fractures (**Fig. 8–4**).

Infectious

Osteomyelitis

◇ Epidemiology

Osteomyelitis typically refers to pyogenic infection of the medullary canal of bone. It results from two principal routes of infection: hematogenous spread and local extension from soft tissues. Hematogenous spread is the most frequent, often from a source in the urinary tract, lungs, or skin. Hematogenous osteomyelitis tends to occur in the young and old, generally sparing patients between 20 and 50 years of age. Local spread may occur at any age and tends to occur in patients with circulatory or immune disorders, such as diabetic patients, who often suffer infected skin ulcers.

Pathogens can often be predicted according to the clinical circumstances. After the newborn period, *Staphylococcus aureus* is the most likely organism. *Salmonella* is relatively more common in sickle-cell disease patients, and *Pseudomonas* deserves special consideration in intravenous drug abusers and patients with a history of a puncture wound to the foot, especially through a shoe. Polymicrobial infection is common in situations such as diabetic foot ulcers. Numerous other etiologies, including tuberculosis, are also possible.

◇ Pathophysiology

The damage to bone in osteomyelitis results from a vicious cycle of infection and host response. Initially, an inoculum of bacteria is deposited hematogenously, which then begins to

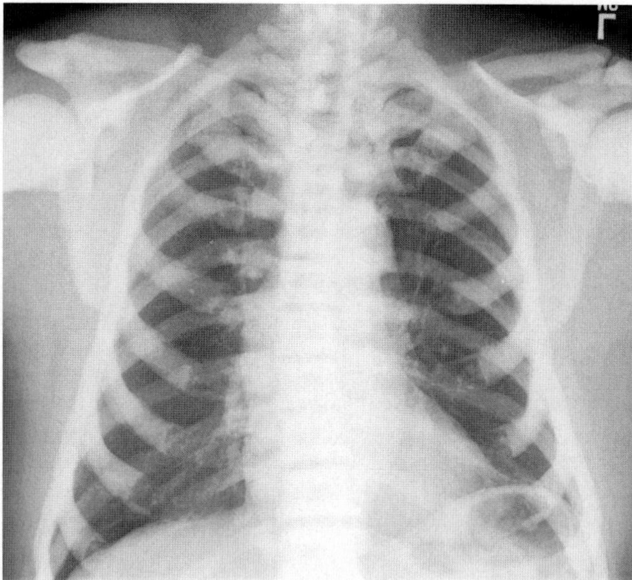

Figure 8–4 This child presented with chest pain. A frontal chest radiograph demonstrates markedly increased density of all the bones, which have an ivory or rocklike appearance. This is a typical appearance of osteopetrosis. Note that there is also thoracic dextroscoliosis, a rightward curve to the spine. The patient had suffered multiple fractures of the extremities in the past.

colonize the perivascular space. The host inflammatory response produces local inflammation and edema, which often extends into the surrounding soft tissues (**Fig. 8–5**). The associated increase in local tissue pressure, related to both hemostatic and oncotic factors, has four potential consequences. First, there is wider dissemination of the infection, as cells are forced out into the lower pressure trabecular spaces surrounding the infectious focus. Next, there results a reduction in the blood supply to the region, which both impairs the delivery of immune cells (and antibiotics) and eventually produces a rim of infarction. Thereafter, an abscess forms in an effort to contain the infection, which unfortunately renders eradication of the infectious focus more difficult. Eventually, there results a sequestrum, an area of osseous infection completely cut off from the rest of the bone.

Two forces produce the characteristic bone destruction seen both pathologically and radiographically. The first is a hyperemically stimulated increase in osteoclastic activity surrounding the focus of infection. The second is frank marrow necrosis.

The distribution of the focus of infection within long bones varies according to the age of the patient. Infectious organisms tend to deposit in the regions of most sluggish blood flow, the most distal arterioles and capillaries. In patients younger than 1 to 2 years of age, in whom arteries coming from the metaphyseal side of the physis cross over into the epiphysis, infections often involve the epiphysis.

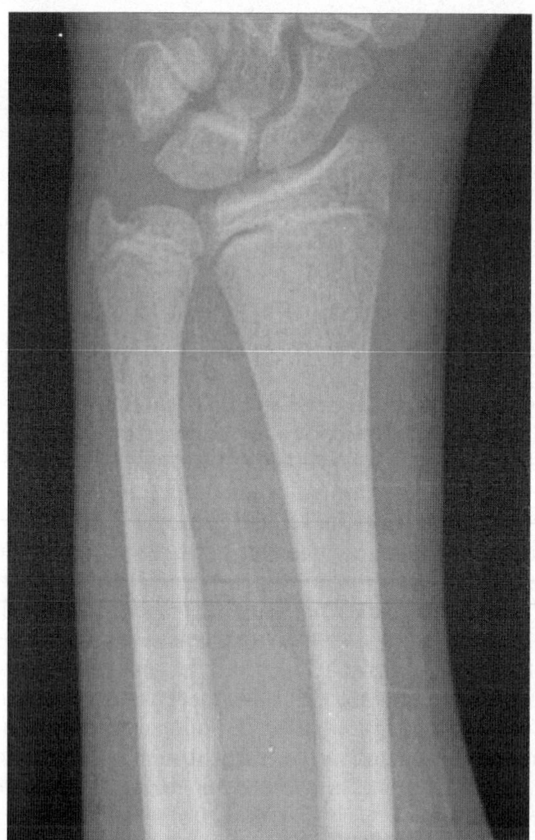

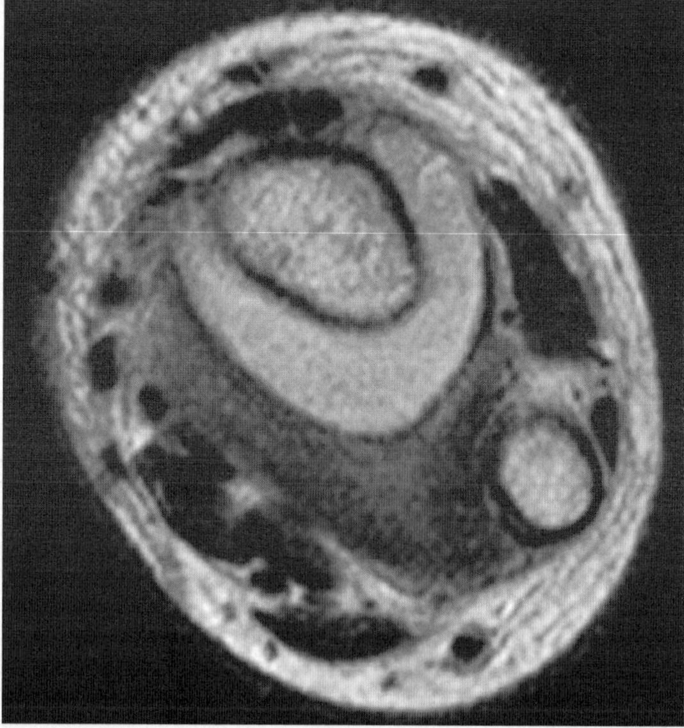

Figure 8–5 This 14-year-old boy presented with pain and swelling of the left forearm. **(A)** A radiograph of the wrist demonstrates no osseous abnormality, which is commonly the case early in osteomyelitis. **(B)** However, an axial T2-weighted MR image demonstrates a large subperiosteal fluid collection around the distal radial cortex. This represented early *Staphylococcus* osteomyelitis.

After ~2 years of age, the transphyseal supply is eliminated, and most infections occur in the metaphysis. In the adult, closure of the growth plate again allows metaphyseal vessels to reach the epiphysis, which again becomes a prime site of inoculation. In the adult, the most frequently involved sites are the tibia, femur, and humerus, as well as the vertebrae.

◇ Clinical Presentation

Patients of any age tend to present with an increased white blood cell (WBC) count, fever, and other systemic evidence of infection, which may be accompanied by local symptoms such as pain and swelling. However, neonatal osteomyelitis, typically secondary to group B *Streptococcus, Escherichia coli,* or staphylococcal infection, often presents with little symptomatology. In older pediatric age groups, there is often a history of refusal to bear weight or to use the affected limb. Additional pediatric signs include fever, irritability, and lethargy. Many adults will complain of vague extremity or back pain. At every age of presentation, physical examination may disclose point tenderness, muscle spasm, or even a draining sinus (the so-called cloaca, which may be thought of as nature's way of draining an abscess). A common but nonspecific laboratory finding is an elevated erythrocyte sedimentation rate.

◇ Imaging

Blood cultures should be obtained in every patient in whom osteomyelitis is a consideration, because they identify an organism in ~50% of cases, and antimicrobial therapy can be tailored accordingly. One reason that osteomyelitis requires weeks of antibiotic therapy is that the conduits of local antibiotic delivery, the capillaries, are compromised, and only with time can adequate antibiotic concentrations in the focus of infection be attained.

Plain radiography is not as sensitive as bone scan or MRI, but is routinely obtained. In the first week of infection, there is likely to be little or no discernible change. The first sign of infection is swelling of the surrounding soft tissues, a nonspecific finding that can be seen in cellulitis or deep soft tissue infection. The first finding in the bone is osteoporosis, which results from the local active hyperemia produced by the inflammatory response (**Fig. 8–6**). At ~2 weeks, periosteal reaction may be seen. Eventually, signs such as sequestrum and cloaca formation may be seen, although today it is rare for osteomyelitis to progress to these points.

A more sensitive study, likely to be positive within the first 2 days of infection, is a radionuclide bone scan utilizing technetium- (Tc-) 99m methylene diphosphonate (MDP), which will usually demonstrate increased uptake at the site of infection (**Fig. 8–7**). Even more sensitive and specific are radionuclide-labeled WBC scans, utilizing indium 111 or Tc 99m, which demonstrate the site of acute infection after 24 hours. MRI is also quite sensitive for acute infection, demonstrating low signal in the marrow on T1-weighted images and high signal on T2-weighted images, secondary to the increased edema associated with infection. Adjacent soft tissues also become hyperintense on T2-weighted images early in the infection (**Fig. 8–7**).

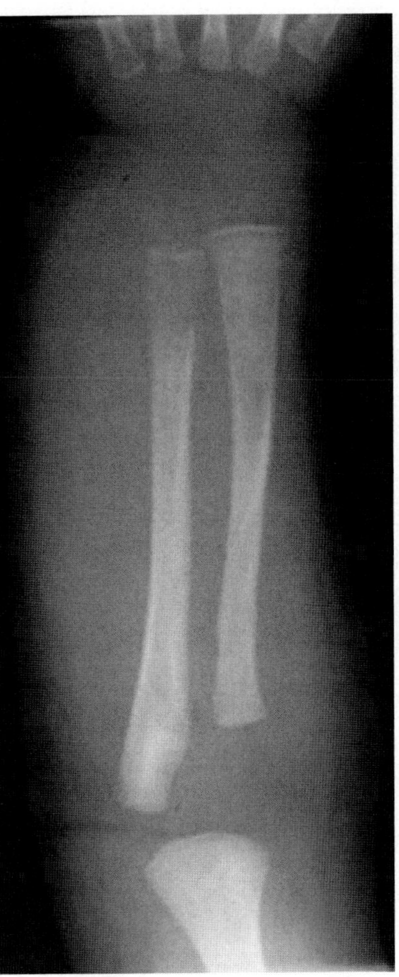

Figure 8–6 This infant presented with a swollen and tender wrist. A radiograph demonstrates marked soft tissue swelling along the ulnar aspect of the wrist, as well as lytic changes (increased lucency) in the distal ulnar metaphysis. The diagnosis was bacterial osteomyelitis.

Septic Arthritis

◇ Epidemiology

Septic arthritis is often associated with osteomyelitis, but it frequently occurs alone. From the Greek *sepsis,* meaning "putrefaction," *arthron,* meaning "joint" (related to *art*iculation), and *-itis,* meaning "inflammation," septic arthritis is a rapidly progressive pyogenic infection of the joint space, which, if untreated, results in loss of joint function (**Fig. 8–8**). Patients at increased risk include those with preexisting arthritis, diabetes, alcoholism, and immunocompromising disorders. Septic arthritis with osteomyelitis most often results from trauma, such as animal or human bites, puncture wounds, and surgery. The most common organism is *S. aureus,* although *Neisseria gonorrhoeae* is more prevalent in the sexually active young population. Intravenous drug abusers and diabetic patients are at increased risk for gram-negative organisms.

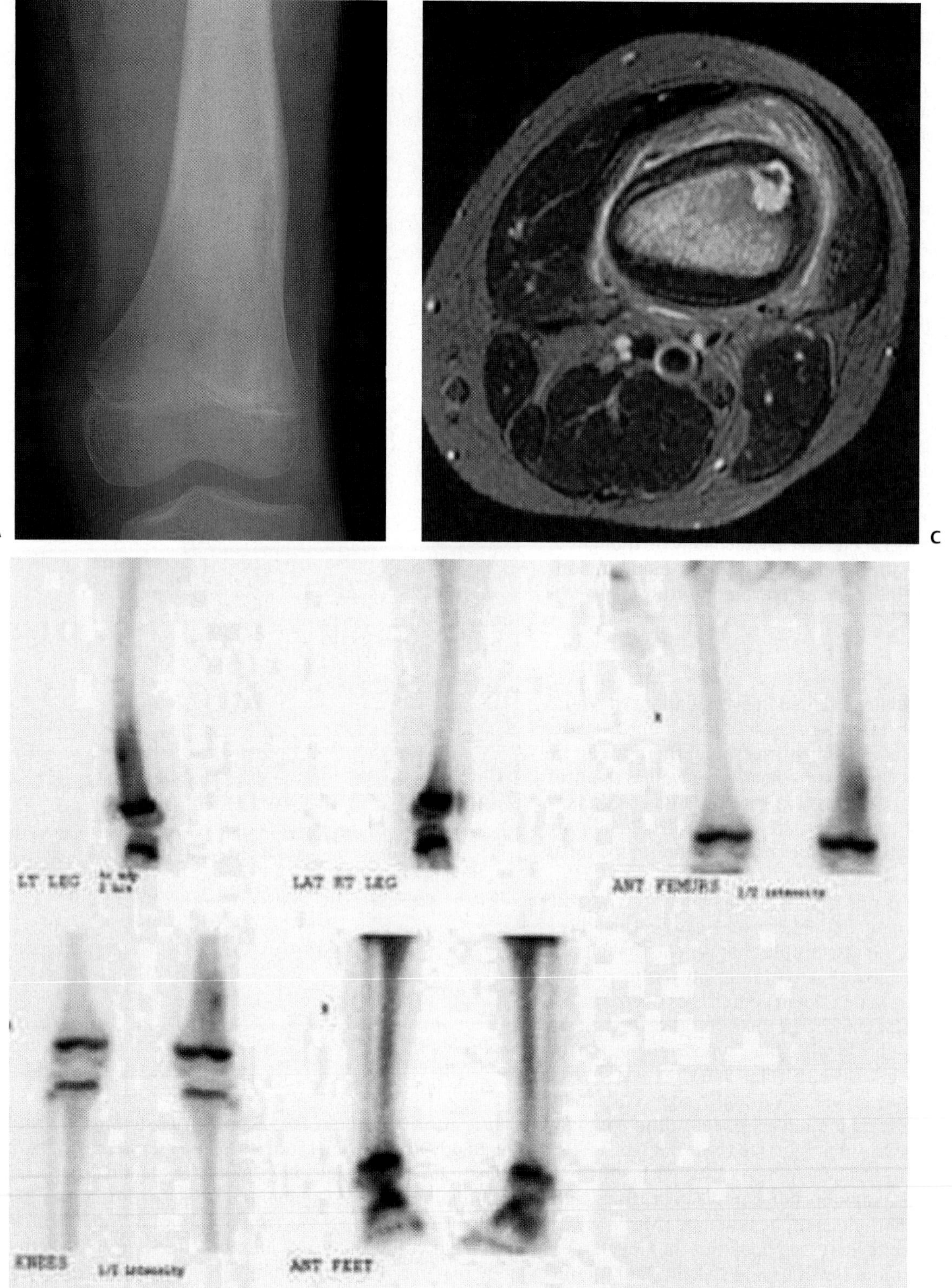

Figure 8–7 This 10-year-old girl presented with left leg pain and fever. **(A)** A frontal radiograph demonstrates cortical and periosteal thickening of the lateral metaphysis of the left femur. There is some endosteal erosion. **(B)** Delayed images from a nuclear medicine bone scan with technetium- (Tc-) 99m methylene diphosphonate (MDP) demonstrate increased radiotracer activity (a "hot" area) in the anterolateral femur. **(C)** An axial STIR MR image demonstrates bone marrow edema, edema surrounding the cortex, and a subcortical fluid collection consistent with a Brodie's abscess, a form of subacute osteomyelitis.

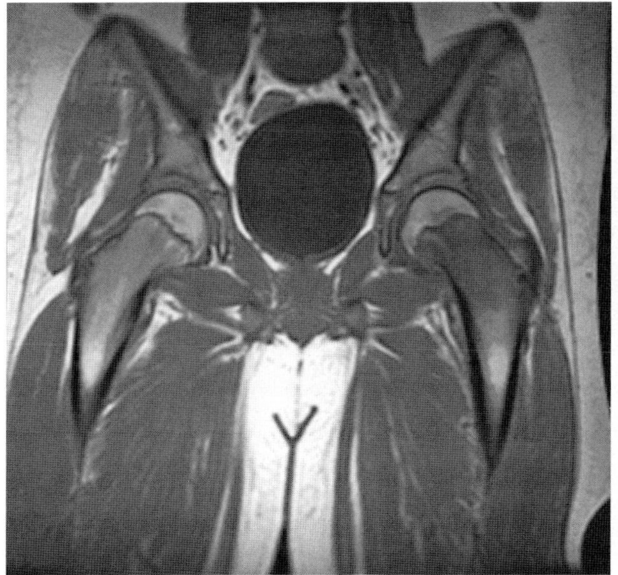

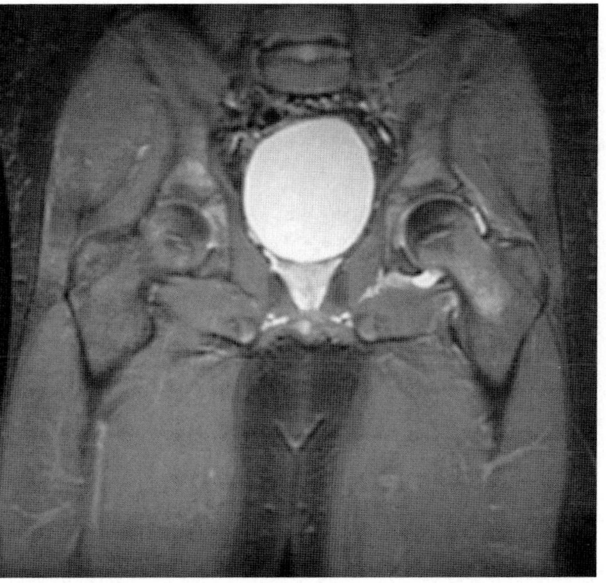

Figure 8–8 This 13-year-old boy presented with fever, leukocytosis, and severe left hip pain. Blood cultures subsequently grew out *Staphylococcus aureus.* **(A)** A T1-weighted coronal MR image of the pelvis demonstrates decreased signal in the bone marrow of the left femoral neck. **(B)** A T2-weighted image demonstrates a left hip joint effusion and increased signal (edema) within the left femoral neck. This represented a combination of septic arthritis and osteomyelitis. Note the urine in the urinary bladder, which (like water) is dark on T1 and bright on T2.

◇ Pathophysiology

The pathophysiology of septic arthritis includes synovial hyperemia with exudation of fluid. Because of this fluid's high fibrin content and the rapid consumption of nutrients in the synovial fluid due to bacterial proliferation, cartilage nutrition is inhibited. Once cartilage cells are lost, they cannot be replaced. The release of cytotoxic enzymes by inflammatory cells also produces tissue destruction. Septic arthritis is treated similarly to osteomyelitis, with intravenous antibiotics over a period of weeks, as well as, in some cases, repeated joint aspirations and immobilization.

◇ Clinical Presentation

Patients present with the classic signs of local inflammation: rubor, tumor, calor, and dolor (redness, swelling, warmth, and pain) and with systemic signs of infection, including fever and leukocytosis.

◇ Imaging

Septic arthritis is not a radiographic diagnosis. By the time radiographic signs of infection appear, irreversible joint damage has already occurred. The key to diagnosis is joint aspiration, which in some cases may require ultrasonographic or fluoroscopic guidance. Joint fluid is opaque, demonstrates a low glucose, and has a WBC count greater than 100,000. Radiographic findings include soft tissue swelling extending to the joint, joint space loss, and periarticular osteopenia, as well as the findings of periosteal reaction and cortical destruction associated with osteomyelitis (**Fig. 8–9**).

Tumorous

Bone tumors can be classified based on many criteria, including benign versus malignant and primary versus metastatic. Let us begin by considering the distinction between primary and metastatic lesions.

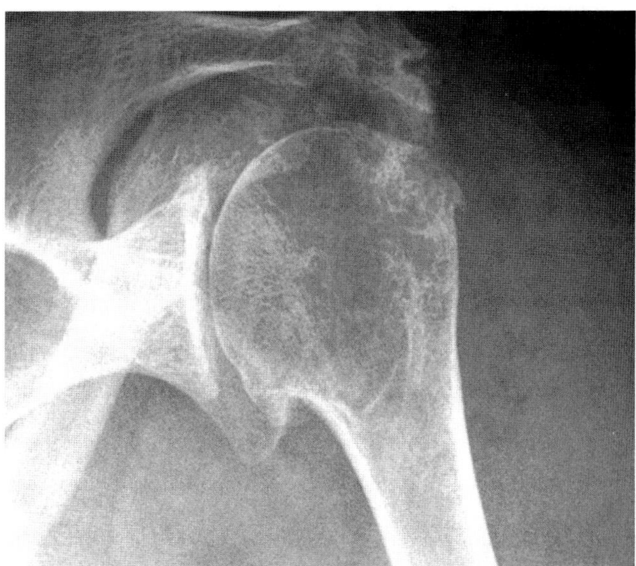

Figure 8–9 This elderly man presented with left shoulder pain and fever. A frontal radiograph of the shoulder demonstrates advanced osteoarthritis with glenohumeral joint space narrowing and osteophytosis. More importantly, there are multiple lucent gas collections deep to the deltoid muscle. Aspiration of the joint yielded pus, indicating septic arthritis. The gas collections represented associated gas gangrene.

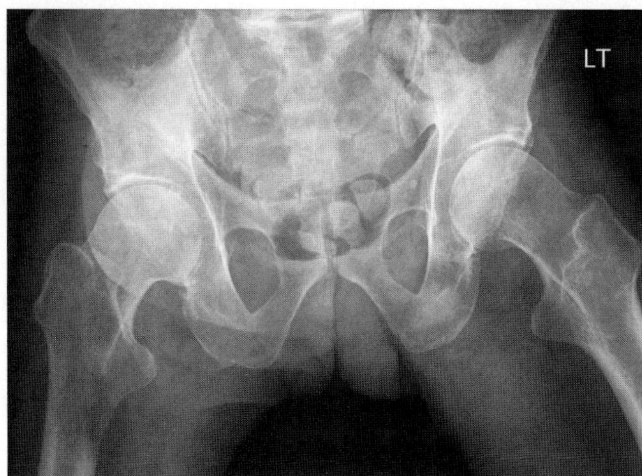

Figure 8–10 This elderly man with a history of lung cancer presented with right hip pain. A frontal radiograph of the pelvis demonstrates a large lytic lesion in the proximal right femoral diaphysis. This was a metastasis from the patient's lung cancer. The lesion is large enough and involves a sufficient amount of the cortex to increase the risk of pathologic fracture.

Metastases

◇ Epidemiology

Bone metastases are ~50 to 100 times more frequent than primary bone malignancies. The finding of even a single skeletal metastatic lesion is of immense clinical significance, because it indicates that the primary tumor cannot be surgically resected for cure.

◇ Pathophysiology

Hematogenous dissemination is the most frequent route by which metastatic cells reach the skeleton. Most metastatic lesions appear in multiples, because multiple cells from the primary tumor tend to gain access to the bloodstream. A truly solitary bone lesion has only a 1 in 10 chance of representing a metastatic process (**Fig. 8–10**).

What percentage of cancer patients develop bone metastases? The lung and the liver, and not the skeleton, are in fact the two most common sites of metastatic spread. Yet the rich blood supply of the skeleton's hematopoietic tissues explains why approximately one third of all cancer patients eventually develop bone metastases. The rich sinusoidal bed of the marrow capillaries, with its large gaps between endothelial cells, presents a very hospitable environment for wayward tumor cells. This explains why metastatic lesions are much more common in bone than in, for example, the soft tissues surrounding the bone, such as muscle, tendons, ligaments, and fat.

Of all skeletal metastases in adults, more than 80% can be traced to one of five primary malignant sources: prostate, breast, lung, kidney, and thyroid. Prostate carcinoma accounts for more than one half of all skeletal metastases in men, as does breast carcinoma in women. Of these, prostate carcinoma has a special anatomic propensity to metastasize to bone. Its venous drainage through Batson's plexus renders the lumbar spine, pelvis, and proximal femur the first capillary beds reached by blood-borne tumor cells (**Fig. 8–11**).

Although the most frequent carcinomas may metastasize to virtually any location, certain sites tend to suggest particular types of primary lesions. When metastatic lesions are found in the distal extremities, particularly the hands and feet, bronchogenic carcinoma is the most likely culprit. The most common tumors to affect the skull are multiple myeloma and carcinomas of the lung and breast. Breast cancer is also the most likely culprit when metastatic lesions are found in the axial skeleton, and accounts for approximately three quarters of spine metastases.

◇ Clinical Presentation

Clinically speaking, bone metastases may represent the first indication of a malignancy, although the vast majority of patients in whom metastatic skeletal lesions are found have known primary tumors. Clinical signs of skeletal metastases include hypercalcemia and the syndrome known as hypertrophic pulmonary osteoarthropathy (HPO). HPO consists of clubbing of the digits, periosteal reaction, and pain. Approximately 1 in 20 patients with bronchogenic carcinoma develops the syndrome (**Fig. 8–12**).

Bone metastases typically present in one of two ways. Pain is the most common presentation, seen in most patients, and the other is pathologic fracture. Although from one point of view all fractures are by definition "pathologic," the term refers to fractures that take place through preexisting bone lesions, which weaken the bone and predispose it to mechanical disruption. Obviously, the bone lesions most likely to develop pathologic fractures are those in the weight-bearing skeleton, and the most prevalent sites are the spine and the femur. Approximately 5 to 10% of all patients with skeletal metastases eventually develop a pathologic fracture. One key role of the radiologist, once metastatic lesions have been detected, is to determine which lesions are at significant risk for fracture, so that prophylactic measures can be instituted, such as radiating the lesion or decreasing the mechanical load on the bone.

◇ Imaging

Radiologic indicators of an increased risk of pathologic fracture include destruction of more than 50% of bone cortex (with a 60–70% risk of fracture), lesions of 3 cm or greater in the proximal femur, and an appropriately positioned lesion that continues to cause pain even after radiotherapy. Lesions that involve substantially less than 50% of the cortex produce pathologic fractures in less than 20% of cases. Although every metastatic lesion would, in theory, eventually become large enough to cause a fracture, most patients with metastatic disease will die of other consequences of their malignancy before this occurs.

Lytic versus Blastic Although metastases can have virtually any appearance, certain metastatic lesions tend to exhibit characteristic radiographic patterns. For example, breast and prostate carcinoma should be at the top of any differential for blastic (sclerotic) lesions, whereas renal cell and thyroid carcinoma characteristically exhibit a lytic appearance. Another

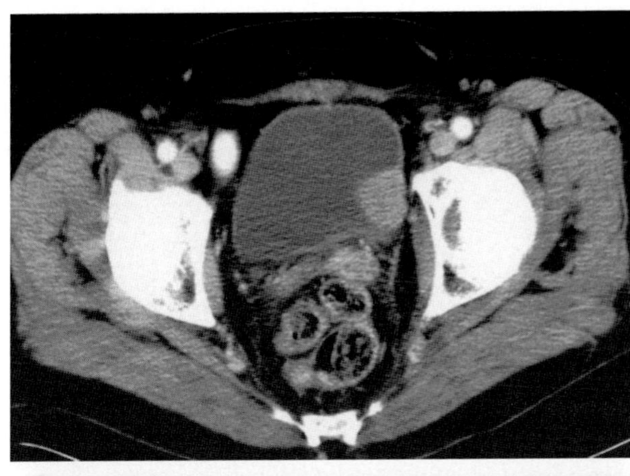

A

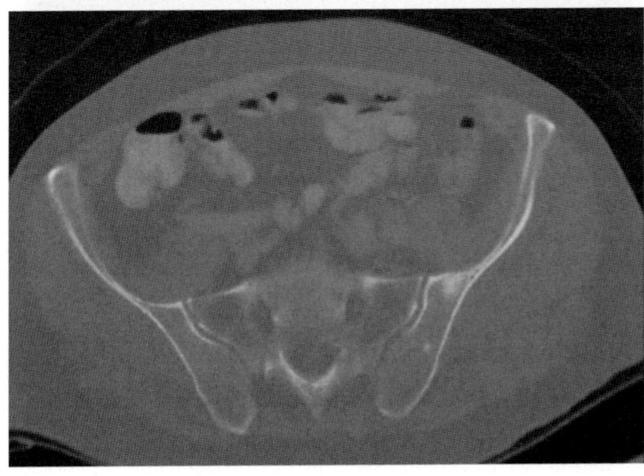

B

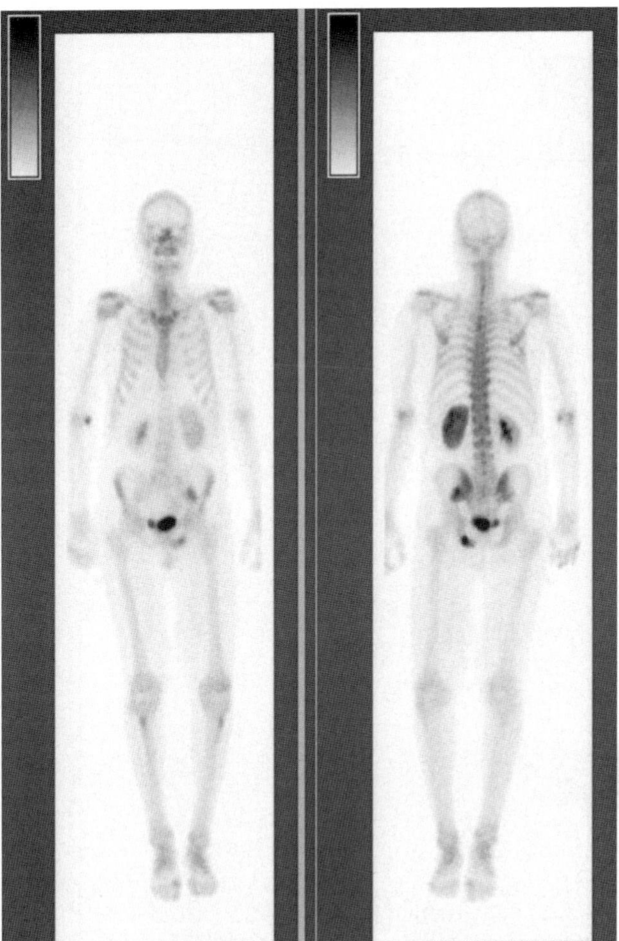

C

Figure 8–11 This 52-year-old man has prostate cancer. **(A)** An axial CT scan of the pelvis at soft tissue settings shows a portion of the primary tumor, indenting the left side of the urinary bladder at the point where the left ureter drains into the bladder lumen. **(B)** This bone-window axial CT image shows two osteoblastic lesions in the medial aspect of the left ilium. **(C)** These anterior and posterior whole-body bone scan images demonstrate delayed excretion of radiotracer from the left kidney due to hydroureteronephrosis, as well as multiple abnormal foci of activity in the left side of the pelvis, due to metastatic prostate carcinoma.

lesion that is typically lytic is multiple myeloma (**Fig. 8–13**). Breast, lung, and gastrointestinal metastases often exhibit a mixed lytic and blastic appearance.

Hidden in these figures is an important principle—less common presentations of common diseases are usually more common than common presentations of uncommon diseases. Most metastases from breast carcinoma are lytic (two thirds), and only 10% present with a blastic appearance. Why, then, should one think “breast” when a blastic lesion is encountered in a woman? The answer is that breast carcinoma is the single most prevalent source of skeletal metastases, and even its less common presentations will be seen more often than the typical presentations of much less common malignancies, such as thyroid carcinoma.

It should be noted again that a lytic appearance generally suggests an aggressive lesion, whereas a blastic appearance indicates a more indolent process. The latter implies that the surrounding bone has had sufficient time to mount an osteoblastic response. The typically lytic appearance of renal cell carcinoma and thyroid carcinoma can be explained on the basis of the extreme hypervascularity of these tumors, with associated hyperemia and increased osteoclastic activity.

Aside from pathologic fracture and the presence of a lytic or blastic lesion, other radiographic indicators of metastatic disease include destruction of a vertebral pedicle, the presence of a soft tissue mass, periosteal reaction, compression fracture of a vertebral body (another type of pathologic fracture), and an “ivory” or unusually dense (and hence white) vertebra. When an ivory vertebra is seen, metastatic disease is a strong possibility, although two other processes are more likely culprits—Paget’s disease and Hodgkin’s lymphoma (**Fig. 8–14**).

Bone Scan In a patient with a primary malignancy in whom skeletal metastases need to be ruled out, the optimal study is generally the nuclear medicine bone scan, which efficiently and relatively inexpensively screens the entire skeleton. The bone scan employs Tc-99m–labeled diphosphonate compounds. Tc-99m is an excellent radiolabel, due to its ready availability, low cost, 140 kilo-electron-volt (keV) principal photon (meaning that it is easily detected by conventional

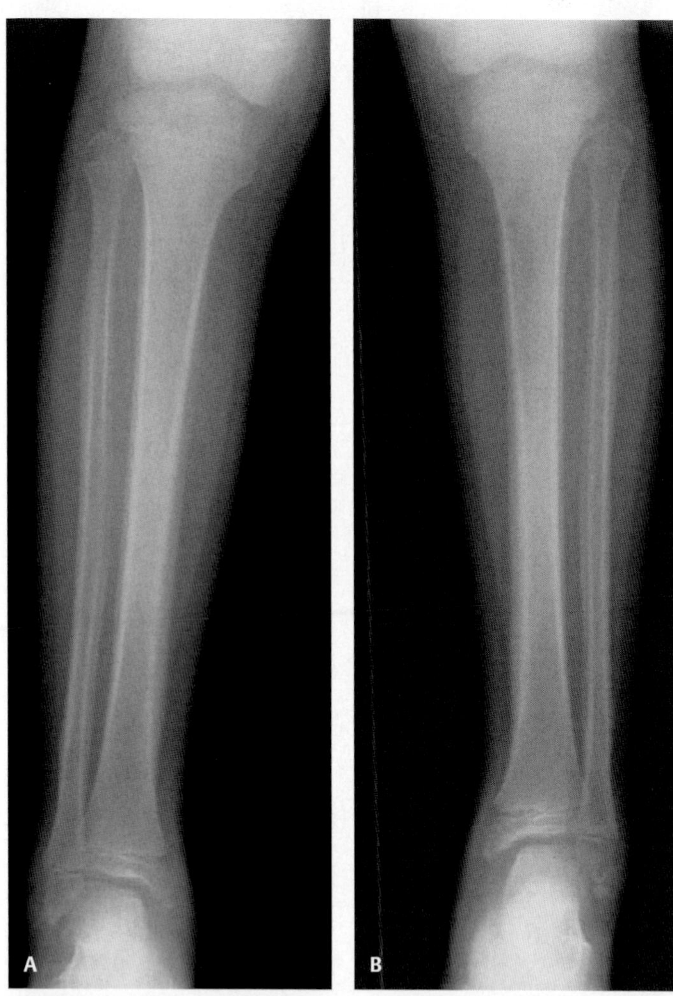

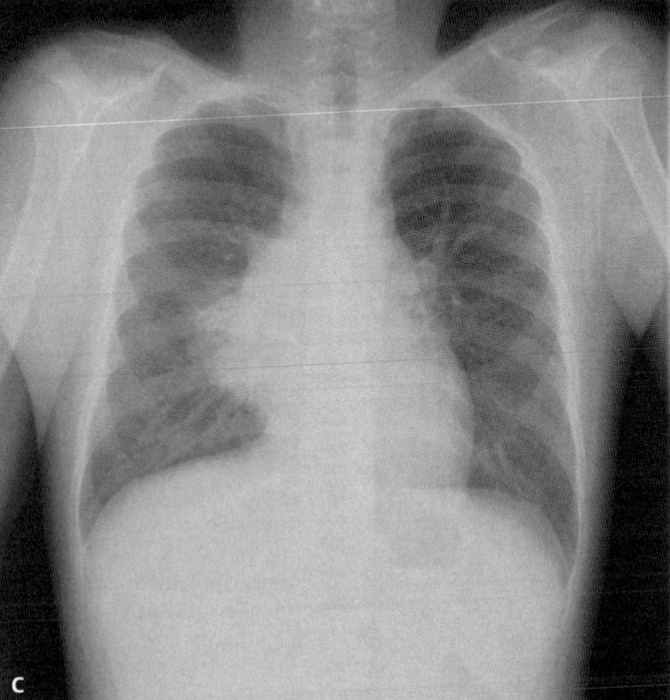

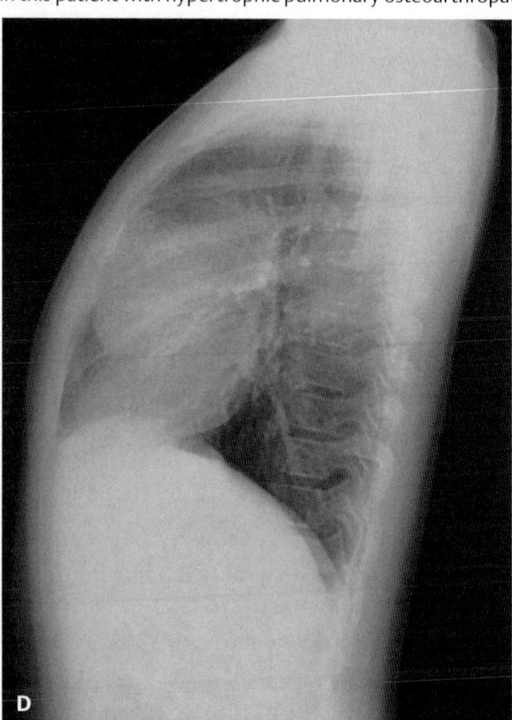

Figure 8–12 This teenage boy presented with bilateral lower leg pain. Frontal radiographs of the right **(A)** and left **(B)** lower legs demonstrate bilaterally symmetrical tibial and fibular periosteal reaction. Frontal **(C)** and lateral **(D)** chest radiographs demonstrate an anterior mediastinal mass, subsequently proven to be a lymphoma in this patient with hypertrophic pulmonary osteoarthropathy.

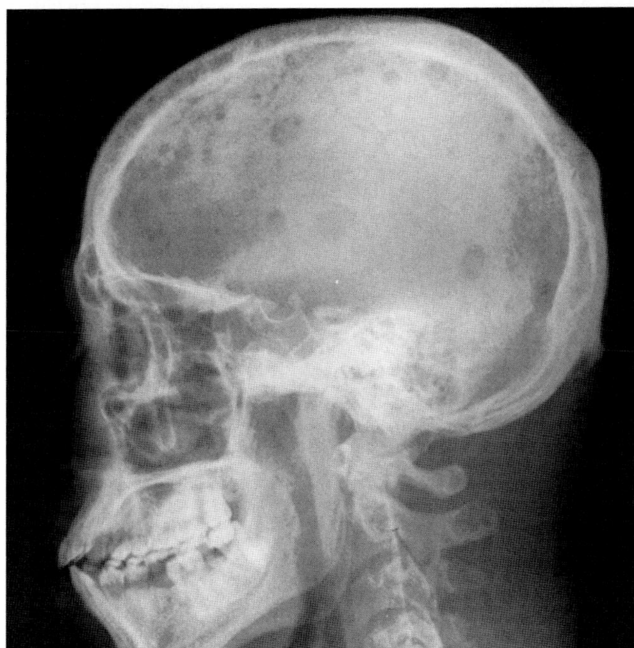

Figure 8–13 A lateral skull radiograph demonstrates innumerable variably sized lytic lesions throughout the skull. This appearance is typical for advanced multiple myeloma, which was this patient's diagnosis.

scintigraphic detectors), and 6 hour half-life, which limits the patient's absorbed radiation dose.

Perfusion and Osteoblastic Activity The distribution of radiotracer within bone is dependent on two factors: regional blood flow and osteoblastic activity. A change in either can cause an abnormal pattern of activity on bone scan. In the case of blood flow, an increase in perfusion will tend to cause increased radiotracer activity, whereas oligemia will tend to cause decreased activity. Similarly, an increase in osteoblastic activity results in the incorporation of more of the diphosphonate molecule into the mineral matrix of bone, causing it to appear "hot" or "dark"; absence of osteoblastic activity produces a "cold" or photopenic ("photon poor") area, due to decreased radiotracer localization and photon emission. Examples of photopenic lesions on bone scan include bone infarcts (no blood flow) and bone destruction (no osteoblasts); lesions that appear hot on bone scan include healing fractures and osteoblastic tumors, such as osteogenic sarcoma (**Fig. 8–15**).

Technique The bone scan is probably the most frequently performed nuclear medicine study in the United States. Hence some familiarity with its technique is desirable. Because Tc 99m is excreted via the kidneys, the urinary bladder represents the critical organ; that is, the bladder is the organ that typically receives the highest radiation dose. A typical bladder dose for the study would be ~3 rads. In an effort to minimize absorbed dose, patients are kept well hydrated and encouraged to void frequently after the procedure, which lasts ~3 hours (by which time 50% of the injected dose will have been taken up by bone). Images are obtained using whole-body scintillation detectors, in both anterior and posterior projections.

Even when clinical concern is focused only on a particular region, whole-body images are obtained. Why? The answer lies in the fact that, once the radiotracer is injected, the whole body has been "dosed," and therefore it makes sense to obtain at least survey views of the entire skeleton. Of course, in the case of a search for bone metastases, such whole-body views are the purpose of the study. When an abnormality is detected on whole-body views or a specific region is of particular clinical concern, spot views are obtained, which provide significantly better resolution of the area in question.

Findings Multiple areas of increased activity can be predicted in the normal patient. In children and adolescents, whose growth plates have not yet closed, increased activity will be seen in these regions. The "hottest" areas are those undergoing the most rapid growth, including the distal femur, the proximal tibia, and the proximal humerus. In the adult, greater activity is seen in the axial skeleton than in the appendicular skeleton (i.e., the spine and pelvis are hotter than the limbs), and the kidneys are routinely visualized.

Greater than normal activity in the kidneys is most commonly due to urinary tract obstruction, and bilaterally decreased activity most often reflects renal failure. An important exception to the latter is the absence of renal activity in the so-called superscan, in which diffuse skeletal uptake is so avid that renal uptake is undercut. A common condition producing a superscan is diffusely metastatic prostate carcinoma (**Fig. 8–16**).

When bone scanning is employed in the search for skeletal metastatic disease, the likely skeletal sites of metastasis should be noted. Because the vast majority of bone metastases are deposited hematogenously, metastatic disease is most frequently found in bones that receive the greatest blood supply. By far the most richly perfused bone is that which contains red (hematopoietic) marrow, which in adults is found in the axial skeleton (spine and pelvis), as well as the cranium and the proximal humeri and femurs.

Sensitivity and Specificity Bone scan is much more sensitive than plain radiography in the detection of metastatic lesions, because the latter requires at least a 30 to 50% alteration in bone density before a lesion becomes detectable, whereas the former can detect much smaller alterations in local bone metabolism. These alterations result from the bone remodeling stimulated by tumor growth. The amount of osteoblastic remodeling may not be enough to produce a blastic appearance on plain radiography, but it will generally be more than sufficient to cause increased radiotracer uptake on bone scan.

The site of increased activity is not the tumor per se, but the interface between the tumor and the remodeling bone; thus, many larger lesions will manifest as a central "cold" area (representing "pure" tumor) surrounded by a rim of tumor–bone interface, where remodeling is taking place. MRI is actually superior to bone scanning in detecting the earliest lesions, due to its ability to display alterations in marrow signal accompanying tumor invasion. Moreover, both MRI and

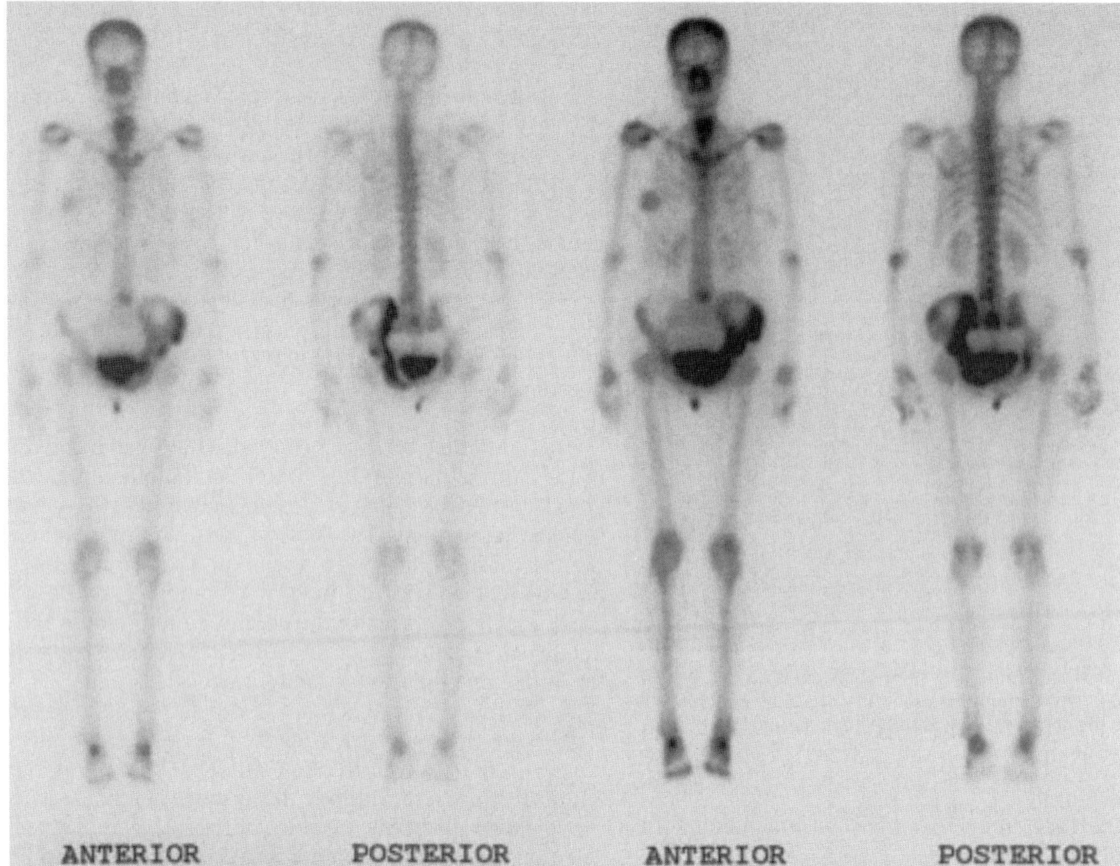

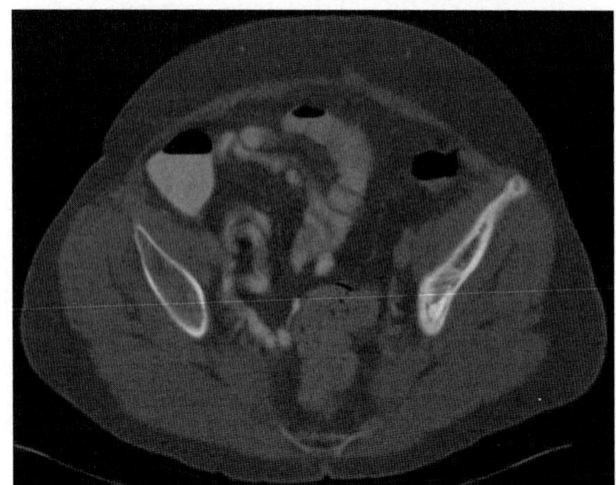

Figure 8–14 This elderly woman was recently diagnosed with breast cancer. A whole-body bone scan was performed for staging. **(A)** These images demonstrate increased activity in the right breast (site of the primary tumor) as well as in the fourth lumbar vertebra and the left hemipelvis. **(B)** A bone-window CT image demonstrates marked sclerosis of the left ilium. This pattern is much more typical of Paget's disease than breast cancer metastases, and the former proved to be the correct diagnosis.

plain films are much more effective at characterizing individual lesions; however, despite these advantages, to screen the entire skeleton by radiography proves relatively time-consuming and costly, and the bone scan is often the study of choice. The most important exception to this general rule is multiple myeloma, the lesions of which typically do not exhibit increased radiotracer accumulation, and thus may be missed. In the case of multiple myeloma, the plain film skeletal survey, including both the axial and appendicular skeleton, is often more sensitive, and an MRI survey of the skeleton using T2-weighted imaging is even better. Similar principles can also apply to leukemia and lymphoma in the skeleton.

The bone scan is a highly sensitive but nonspecific study, as many processes other than metastatic disease may produce multiple foci of radiotracer accumulation. One process that may produce multiple "hot" areas is osteoarthritis (OA); however, the appearance is not typical of metastatic disease because the abnormalities tend to be bilaterally symmetrical and found in locations very unusual for metastases, such as the knees and ankles. When suspicious hot spots are seen in the spine or involving such joints as the hips or shoulders, it may

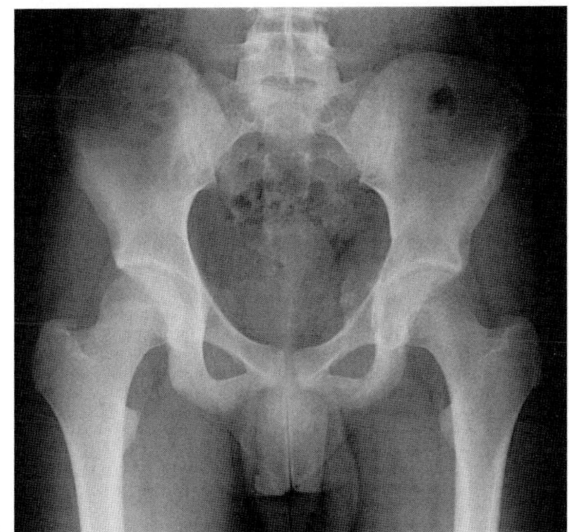

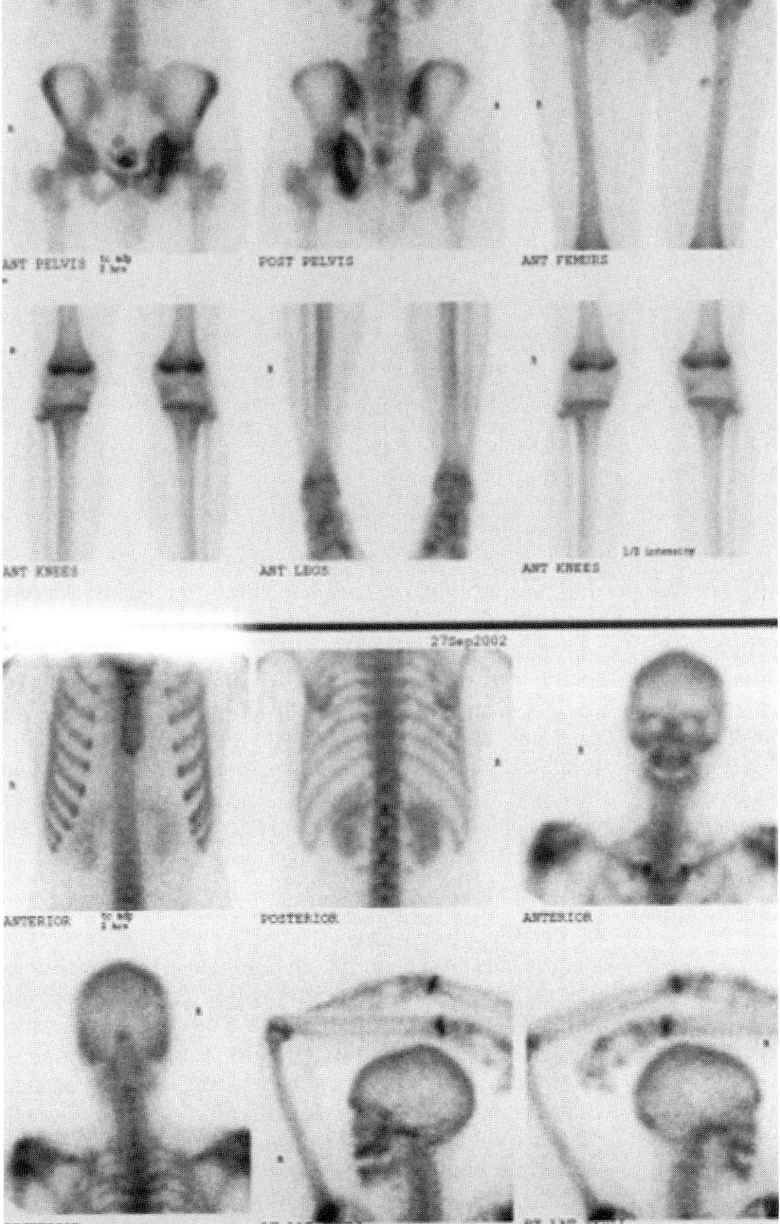

Figure 8–15 This 16-year-old boy presented with left hip pain. **(A)** A frontal pelvis radiograph demonstrates a calcified soft tissue mass along the medial aspect of the left ischium. **(B)** These images from a whole-body bone scan show increased radiotracer activity at his location. No distant metastases are seen. This represented an osteogenic osteosarcoma, a classically "blastic" lesion.

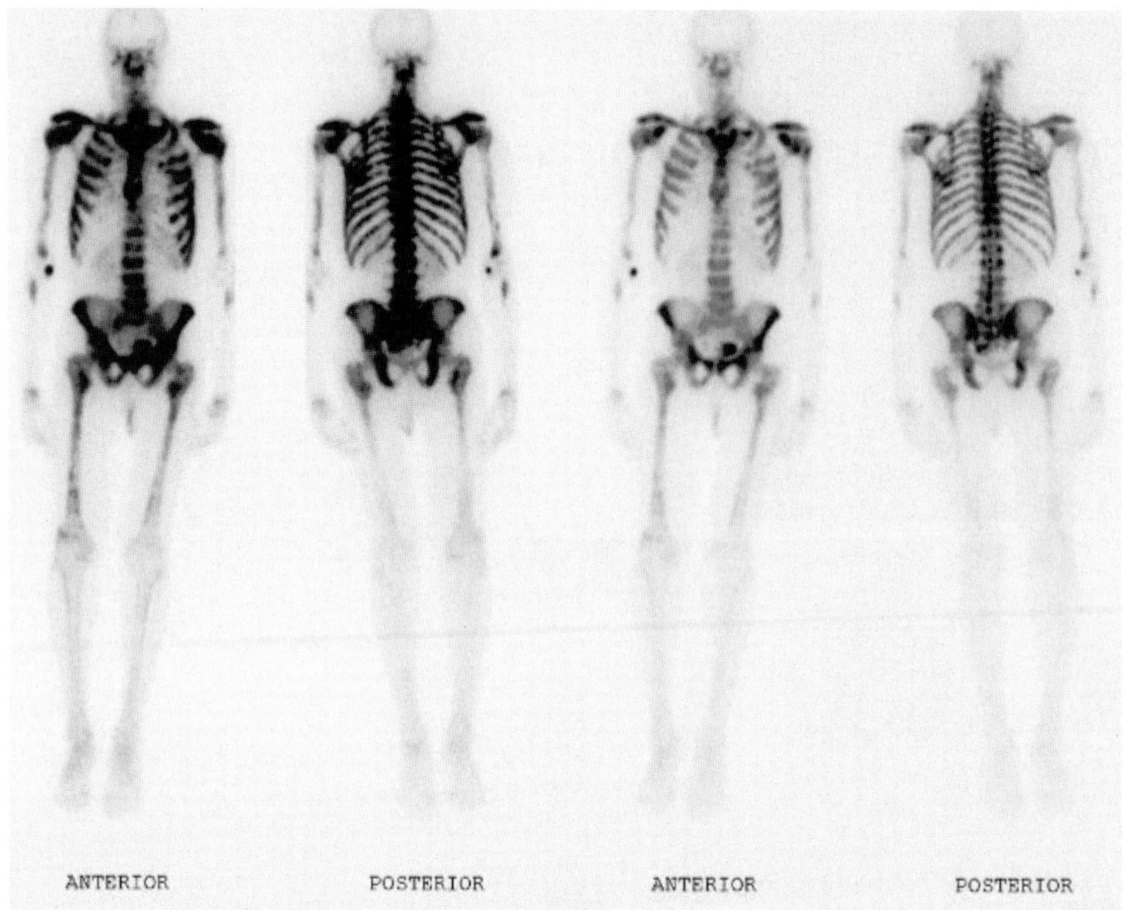

Figure 8–16 This elderly man underwent a staging whole-body bone scan after being diagnosed with prostate cancer. The anterior and posterior images demonstrate diffusely increased activity in the axial skeleton with little activity in the appendicular skeleton or kidneys. This "superscan" indicates diffuse metastatic disease in the axial skeleton. There is actually also increased uptake in the right femur and both humeri, indicating involvement of the appendicular skeleton as well.

be necessary to obtain plain films or MRI for further evaluation. Another prevalent cause of multiple hot spots is trauma, which tends not to be bilaterally symmetrical. Trauma often enters the differential diagnosis in the ribs, and obtaining a good history from the patient often proves critical in sorting out whether metastatic disease or trauma is responsible.

In the setting of a known primary tumor with a tendency to metastasize to bone, however, multiple abnormal areas of increased radiotracer activity are virtually diagnostic of metastatic disease. Of course, the ultimate means of discriminating between benign and malignant etiologies of increased bone agent uptake is tissue biopsy, for which imaging guidance is often used.

Primary Bone Tumors

◇ Epidemiology

Depending on how one defines a primary malignant bone tumor, the incidence of these lesions is relatively low, with only ~3000 new cases diagnosed each year in the United States (not counting multiple myetoma). In decreasing order of frequency, the most important primary malignant lesions of bone include multiple myeloma, osteogenic sarcoma, chondrosarcoma, lymphoma, and Ewing's sarcoma (**Fig. 8–17**). Benign primary tumors are much more common; for example, it is estimated that as many as 40% of children harbor at least one benign fibrous cortical defect or nonossifying fibroma somewhere in their skeletons. At the opposite end of the lifecycle, evidence of Paget's disease can be found in 4% of persons older than age 50 and 10% of persons older than 80.

◇ Pathophysiology

Predictably, primary bone tumors tend to occur in certain locations in the skeleton, with the highest incidence of both benign and malignant tumors in the regions of the most rapid and prolonged bone growth. These include the metaphyseal regions of the distal femur and the proximal tibia. When in doubt about the most frequent site of any particular primary bone tumor, the distal femur, the site of greatest growth, represents the best guess.

Primary bone tumors are classified according to the pattern of their cellular differentiation, meaning the cell type

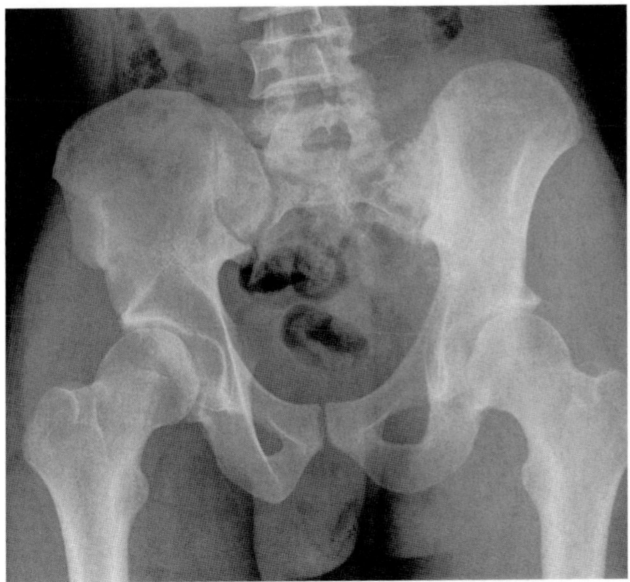
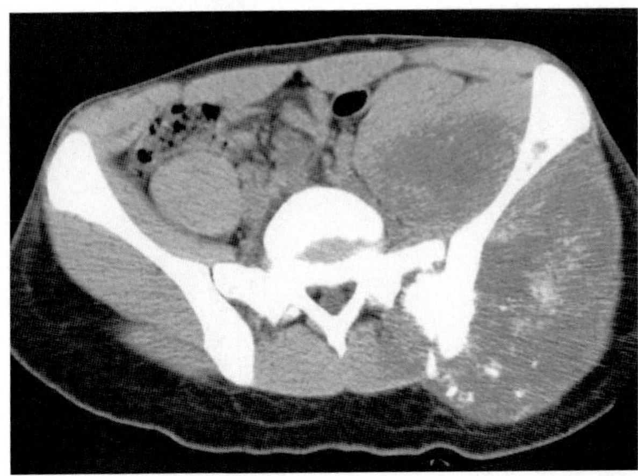

Figure 8–17 This young man presented with left hip pain. **(A)** Plain radiograph of the pelvis demonstrates abnormal lucency of the left side of the sacrum with a soft tissue mass containing a calcific matrix. **(B)** A soft tissue window CT of the pelvis demonstrates a large soft tissue mass involving the left ilium and sacrum, which contains multiple areas of calcification. This was a chondrosarcoma.

of which they most remind the pathologist. Among the principal cell types are bone cells (as in osteogenic sarcoma), cartilage cells (chondrosarcoma), primitive mesenchymal cells (Ewing's sarcoma), lipid cells (liposarcoma), neural cells (neurofibroma), and fibroblasts (fibrosarcoma). A variety of hematopoietic cell types may be seen, the most prominent of which is the plasmacytoma, the isolated harbinger of multiple myeloma. Tumor grading, which tends to correlate directly with the aggressiveness of the lesion and inversely with prognosis, is based on the degree of cellular anaplasia or dedifferentiation.

◇ Clinical Presentation

Many bone tumors are identified incidentally on radiologic studies undertaken for other purposes, but others are evaluated on the basis of their clinical presentation. The principal presenting symptoms include mass, pain, and impairment of function.

◇ Imaging

A key distinction to be made in the evaluation of bone tumors, whether benign or malignant, is between single and multiple lesions. As we have seen, myeloma and metastases are the malignant lesions by far most likely to be multiple at the time of diagnosis. The most prevalent benign polyostotic lesions include Paget's disease (most likely due to a chronic paramyxovirus infection of bone), fibrous dysplasia, and eosinophilic granuloma. In the remainder of this discussion, we will concern ourselves primarily with the radiographic evaluation of isolated lesions.

One of the most difficult tasks of the radiologist is simply to detect lesions, which may exhibit a quite subtle appearance. In some cases, lesions on radiographs are detected only in retrospect, after they have undergone additional growth and development. Once a solitary bone lesion is identified, a variety of factors go into its analysis.

Age Even if one knows little about the particular radiologic characteristics of bone tumors, the correct diagnosis can often be predicted merely on the basis of the incidence of different tumors at various ages. In the case of malignant tumors, most tumors in the first 2 decades will be either Ewing's sarcoma or osteosarcoma, with the former tending to occur earlier than the latter. After age 40, solitary metastases, multiple myeloma, and chondrosarcoma are the most likely diagnoses. If the patient has a known primary tumor that generally metastasizes to bone, metastasis will usually become the primary suspect at any age.

Lesion Margins How does the radiologist determine if the lesion is likely to be malignant? The single most useful criterion is the radiographic appearance of the lesion's margins, which more than any other characteristic reflects its biologic behavior (**Fig. 8–18**). Lesions with narrow, well-defined zones of transition with adjacent normal bone tend to be benign, whereas lesions with wide, ill-defined zones of transition tend to be malignant. Radiologists often describe the margins of bone lesions as geographic, implying a clear demarcation between the normal and abnormal regions due to a slow rate of growth, usually indicating benignity; moth-eaten, implying a less well-defined margin with a wider zone of transition and indicating a more rapid rate of growth; or permeative, denoting a very rapidly growing lesion that merges imperceptibly with normal bone. Certain processes, such as simple bone cyst, characteristically exhibit geographic borders; others, such as Ewing's sarcoma and metastatic neuroblastoma, have characteristically permeative

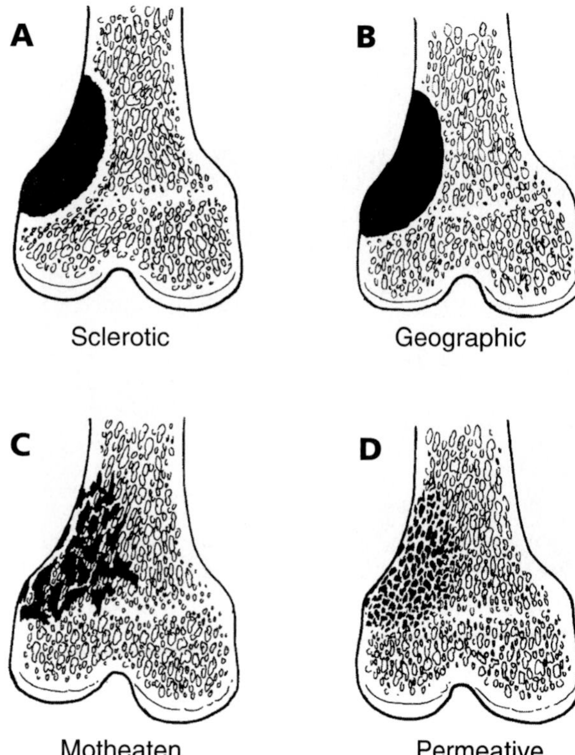

Figure 8–18 The radiographic terms used to describe the degree of definition of a lesion's margins, varying from **(A)** extremely well-defined, sclerotic margins in sclerotic lesions, to **(B)** well-defined but nonsclerotic margins in geographic lesions, to **(C)** poorly defined margins in motheaten lesions, to **(D)** margins that merge imperceptibly with normal bone in permeative lesions.

borders. Still other processes, such as infection and metastases, may exhibit any type of border (**Fig. 8–19**).

Periosteal Reaction The response of the periosteum to a contiguous lesion may also supply important information about the lesion's biologic behavior. Generally speaking, a slow-growing, benign process will give the periosteum time to lay down dense, uniform, or solid new bone, whereas a fast-growing, malignant tumor process will not allow the periosteum a chance to complete its work, and the pattern of periosteal reaction will be interrupted, with a lamellated ("onion skin"), sunburst, or amorphous appearance (**Fig. 8–20**). Another type of aggressive periosteal reaction is the so-called Codman's triangle, in which the periosteum is lifted progressively farther from the bone as one moves toward the center of the lesion. Again, benign lesions such as infection, eosinophilic granuloma, and osteoid osteoma may produce aggressive periosteal reaction; however, when a benign pattern of periosteal reaction is seen, the probability of malignancy is very low.

Osseous Distribution A final characteristic of note in any solitary osseous lesion is its location within the bone (**Fig. 8–21**). This location should be described in both longitudinal and axial dimensions, with different tumors tending to occur in characteristic locations (**Fig. 8–22**). In the axial plane, the central medullary cavity of bone is a characteristic location for enchondroma and simple bone cysts; osteosarcoma tends to occur in an eccentric medullary position, and benign fibrous cortical defects and osteoid osteomas are characteristically cortical. In the longitudinal plane, chondroblastoma (a benign lesion of children and young adults) and giant cell tumor are epiphyseal lesions, osteogenic sarcoma and chondrosarcoma are characteristically metaphyseal in location, and Ewing's sarcoma and fibrous dysplasia are typically diaphyseal (**Fig. 8–23**).

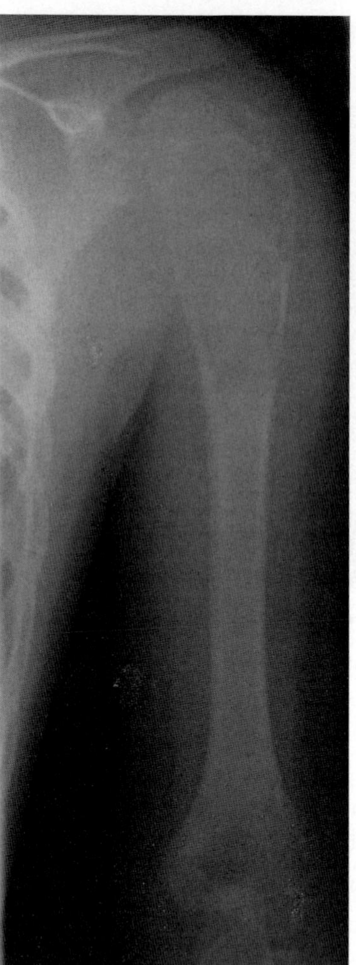

Figure 8–19 This young boy presented with shoulder pain. A frontal radiograph demonstrates an expansile lytic lesion of the proximal humeral metaphysis. It has sharply demarcated, geographic borders. This is a classic location and appearance for a benign unicameral bone cyst.

The role of the bone scan is typically less in the workup of primary bone malignancies than in metastatic disease. In the case of a primary bone tumor, the orthopedic surgeon needs to assess the extent of the lesion within bone and surrounding soft tissues, neither of which is well evaluated by the scintigram. Bone scanning, however, does play a role in the evaluation of tumors that often produce distant metastases, such as osteogenic sarcoma. In the case of an osteogenic sarcoma, increased tracer activity may be detected not only in bone metastases, but in pulmonary and soft tissue metastases as well, due to the tendency of metastatic deposits to form bone matrix. Even tumors that do not produce an osteoblastic response may be detected on bone scintigraphy, due to the regional hyperemia they produce.

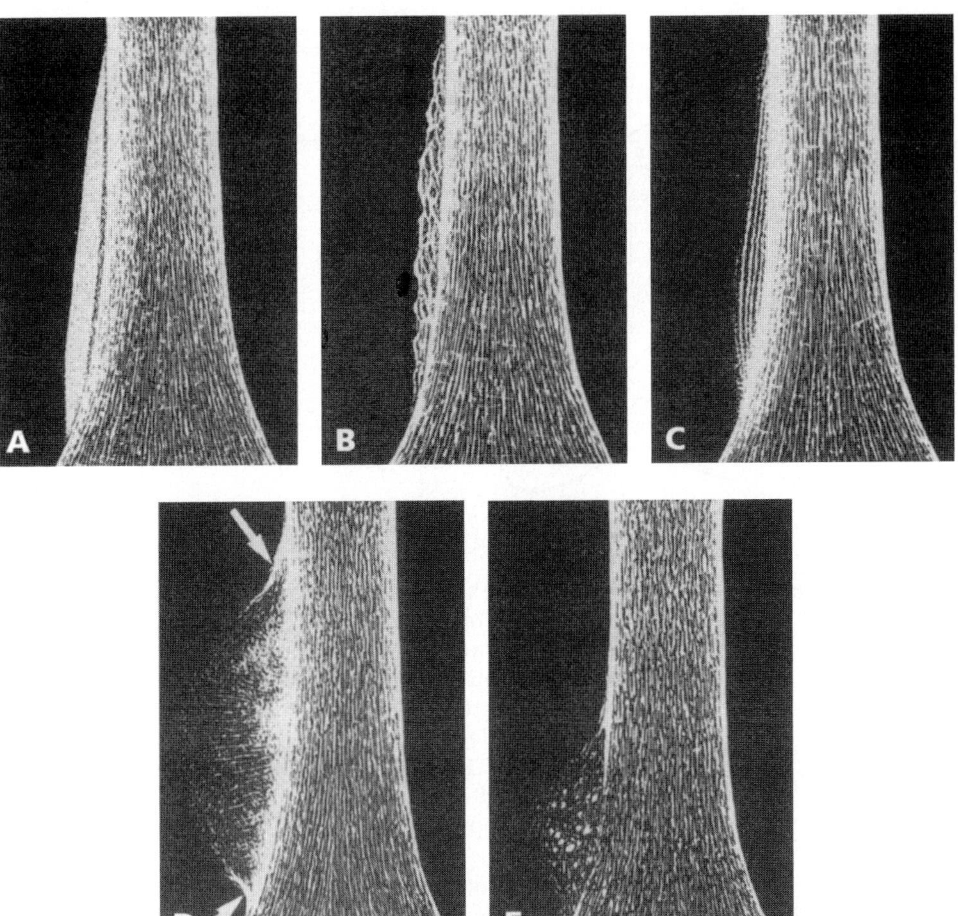

Figure 8–20 The various types of periosteal reaction. Types A and B are benign in appearance, and may be described as **(A)** thick and **(B)** undulating. Types C through E are more aggressive and more likely malignant and may be described as **(C)** laminated or "onion skin," **(D)** perpendicular or "sunburst," and **(E)** amorphous. Although not a perfect indicator, the pattern of periosteal reaction is one visual manifestation of a lesion's biological behavior.

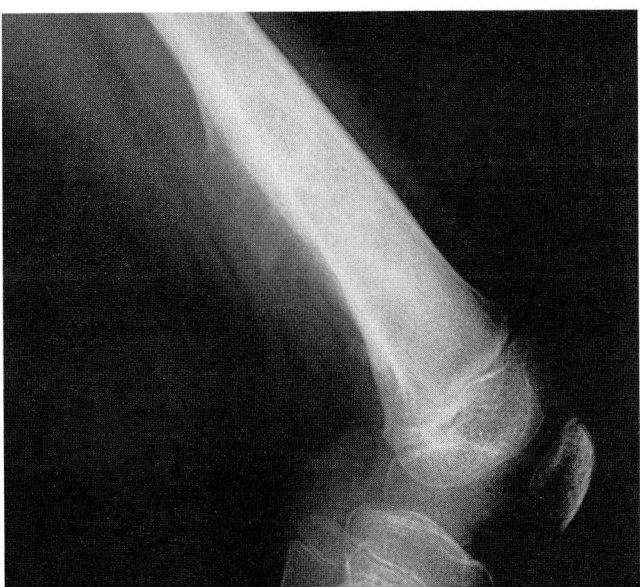

Figure 8–21 This 9-year-old girl presented with leg pain. A lateral radiograph of the knee demonstrates a sclerotic lesion in the distal femur with poorly defined borders that exhibits aggressive periosteal reaction, including a Codman's triangle. This represented an osteogenic osteosarcoma.

Multiple myeloma, a malignant tumor of B lymphocytes, arises in the hematopoietic marrow in the skull, axial skeleton, pelvis, and proximal portions of the humeri and femurs. It is associated with monoclonal protein spikes, Bence Jones proteinuria, and other signs of a bone marrow malignancy, such as anemia, infection, increased alkaline phosphatase, and hypercalcemia. Characteristic features of multiple myeloma on plain radiography include a punched-out appearance with endosteal scalloping (implying a site of origin within the central, marrow-containing portion of the bone) and a bubbly appearance that may be associated with a soft tissue mass.

Inflammatory

The suffix *-itis* is used to denote an inflammatory condition. In the case of OA, the inflammatory suffix is probably something of a misnomer, because the true pathophysiology of the condition likely consists instead of repeated episodes of microtrauma, with secondary inflammatory reaction; however, rheumatoid arthritis (RA), the other major form of joint pathology, is undoubtedly inflammatory in nature, and because the two represent the most important joint pathologies,

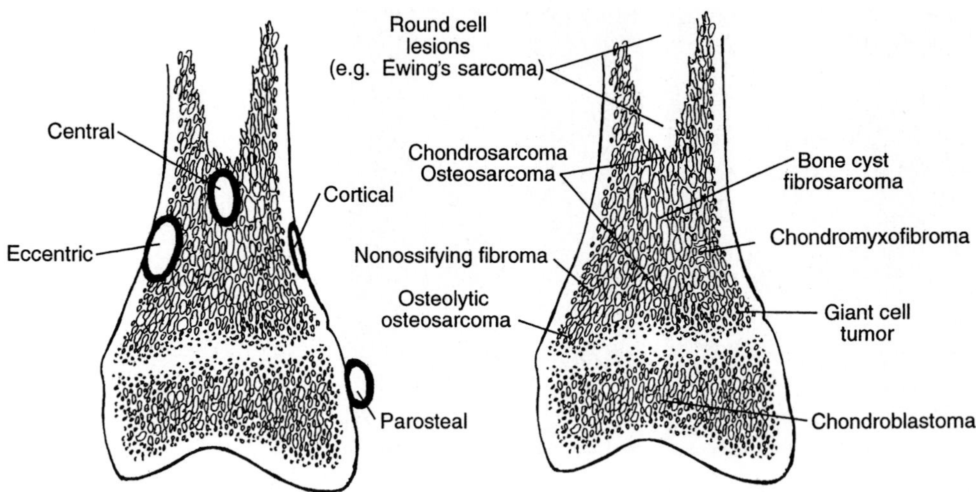

Figure 8–22 The typical location within long bones of various bone lesions, which can be very helpful in formulating a differential diagnosis.

both OA and RA are considered under the heading of inflammatory disease.

Osteoarthritis

◇ Epidemiology

The most common joint disease of human beings, OA, also commonly referred to as degenerative joint disease, clinically afflicts more than one half of persons older than 65 years of age. It is one of the leading causes of disability in this age group. It is estimated that at least 80% of persons harbor at least radiographic evidence of OA by the time they reach 50 years of age. Although hereditary factors have been implicated in the development of OA, most cases are idiopathic, and mechanical factors are usually invoked. For example, ballet dancers suffer a higher incidence of ankle and toe OA than the general population.

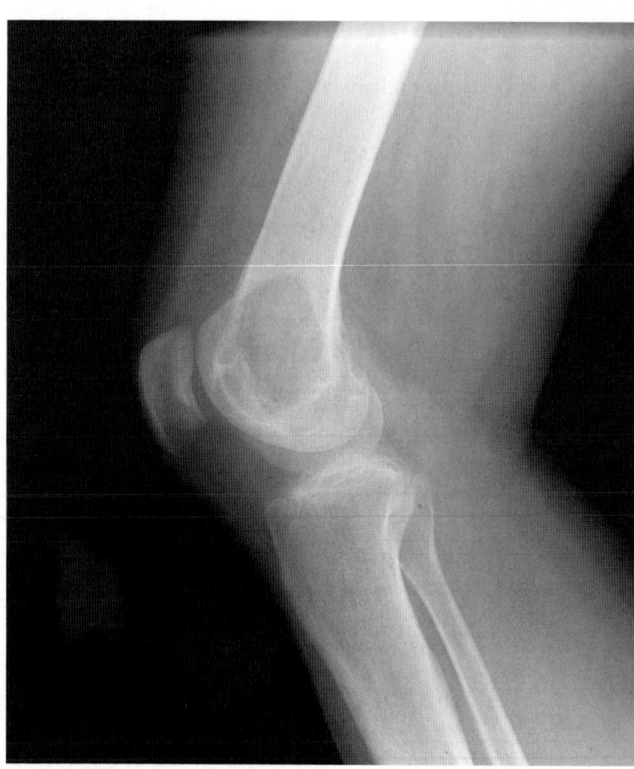

Figure 8–23 This 48-year-old woman presented with knee pain. A lateral knee radiograph demonstrates a large, well-circumscribed lytic lesion arising in the distal femoral epiphyseal region and extending into the metaphyseal region. This is the classic appearance of a giant cell tumor.

◇ Pathophysiology

OA is often categorized into primary and secondary forms. Primary OA results from abnormal mechanical forces on a normal underlying joint and is age-related. Secondary OA results from normal forces on an abnormal joint and is seen in conditions such as calcium dihydrate pyrophosphate deposition disease (CPPD), rheumatoid arthritis (discussed later), trauma, and septic joint.

Strictly speaking, OA afflicts only the synovial joints. Important mechanical characteristics of synovial joints include stability during motion, joint lubrication, and uniform load distribution. The articular cartilage is vital in providing a smooth and relatively frictionless surface for joint motion and in helping to dissipate loading forces as one bone mechanically compresses another. Articular cartilage itself contains only one cell type, the chondrocyte, and an extracellular matrix. It contains no nerves or blood vessels. As noted earlier in this chapter, chondrocytes depend for their metabolism on the diffusion of nutrients and metabolites through the cartilage matrix. Despite their relatively precarious nutritional state, they maintain a level of metabolic activity similar to that of some cells in vascularized tissues.

The cyclic loading and unloading of cartilage stimulates matrix synthesis, whereas prolonged stable loading or the absence of loading and motion (as in prolonged immobilization) causes degradation of the matrix and eventually leads to joint degeneration. In addition to prolonged immobilization, another disorder that predisposes to OA is a septic joint, in which bacteria compete with chondrocytes for glucose and other nutrients in the synovial fluid.

OA is not primarily an inflammatory process. Instead, it consists of a retrogressive sequence of cell and matrix changes that result in loss of articular cartilage structure and function, accompanied by attempted cartilage repair and bone remodeling. Three phases can be discerned: cartilage damage, chondrocyte response, and over time, a gradual diminution in chondrocyte response.

The first sign of OA pathologically is softening and loss of articular cartilage. As OA progresses, cartilage thins and becomes fibrillated, with eventual uncovering of underlying bone. This causes eburnation (sclerosis), microfractures with cyst formation, and osteophyte formation. Why does the bone form osteophytes? The proliferation of these outgrowths of bone around joint surfaces may be regarded as an attempt by bone to increase the surface area of the joint and thereby distribute mechanical forces more widely. With loss of the shock-absorbing properties of articular cartilage, fragments of cartilage or bone may break off from the articular surface and become loose intra-articular bodies, interfering with joint motion and causing sudden "locking."

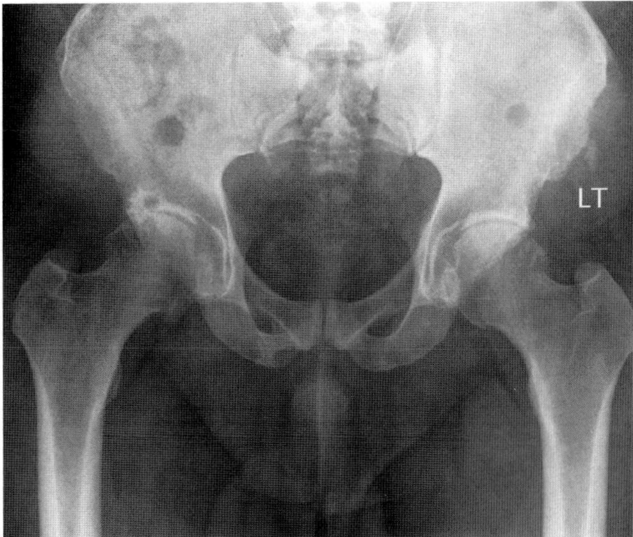

Figure 8–24 This obese middle-aged man presented with bilateral hip pain. A frontal radiograph of the pelvis demonstrates classic findings of osteoarthritis in a weight-bearing joint, involving both hips, but more severe on the right. These include superior joint space narrowing, subchondral cysts, and osteophytosis.

◇ Clinical Presentation

OA usually presents with mono- or pauciarticular involvement. Patients complain of an aching pain that is aggravated by use and alleviated by rest. The pain originates not within the cartilage, which is uninnervated, but within the periosteum and subchondral bone, secondary to structural distortion and microfractures. Physical examination discloses swelling and tenderness around the involved joint, crepitus (from bone rubbing on bone), and effusion. The warmth and swelling are less than that seen in RA. Moreover, in contrast to the hour or more of morning stiffness associated with RA, that experienced by OA patients usually lasts only a period of 10 to 20 minutes.

◇ Imaging

The radiographic hallmarks of OA, in contrast to RA, include normal mineralization, productive changes (osteophyte and subchondral bone formation), and nonuniform joint space loss (**Fig. 8–24**). In the hand, the joints most often involved by OA include the distal interphalangeal joints (producing Heberden's nodes) and the proximal interphalangeal joints (Bouchard's nodes). The metacarpophalangeal joints are characteristically spared, whereas they are generally involved by RA. Other prominent sites of involvement by OA include the base of the thumb, the hip, the knee, and the spine.

A strong indication that OA is a mechanical disorder is the fact that the risk of OA is increased in obese patients, patients with congenitally dislocated hips, and those who have suffered prior trauma associated with cartilage disruption. In the hip, there is nonuniform loss of joint space and superolateral migration of the femoral head (**Fig. 8–25**). In the knee, joint space loss is likewise nonuniform and more often involves the medial than lateral femoral-tibial compartment. Strictly speaking, OA of the spine refers only to degeneration of the apophyseal joints; *spondylosis* is the term for degenerative disk disease. The osteophyte production associated with OA of the spine often encroaches on the neural foramina, resulting in spinal nerve root compression (see the discussion of back pain in Chapter 9).

Initial treatment of OA is primarily symptomatic, employing aspirin or acetaminophen. As the disease progresses, preservation of mobility and function become increasingly important concerns, and improvement of joint mechanics and physical therapy often prove helpful. In patients who are refractory to medical therapy, orthopedic surgery is often performed to repair or replace the damaged joint. Approximately 250,000 joint replacements are performed each year in the United States, the majority of which involve the hip and the knee. Hemiarthroplasties involve replacement of only one side of a joint, whereas total arthroplasties involve prosthetic components in both sides. Prosthetic components are attached to bone with cement (methylmethacrylate) that has been made radiopaque by the addition of barium; press fitting, so that there is direct contact between the prosthesis and the bone cortex; or biologic methods, in which fenestrations are created in the prosthesis, into which new bone can grow. Another common reason for joint replacement is trauma, particularly femoral neck fracture.

Radiography is one of the most important tools available to the orthopedic surgeon in assessing joint prostheses. In the immediate postoperative period, radiographs are taken to ascertain component position and to detect intraoperative fractures or dislocation (**Fig. 8–26**). The most common delayed complications, which should be suspected in patients with recurrent or persistent pain, are loosening and infection. Unfortunately, the two can be difficult to differentiate radiographically. Signs especially suspicious for infection include irregular periostitis, poorly marginated lucencies, and sinus tracts. The presence of infection can be verified by needle aspiration. Signs of loosening include migration of the components (hence the importance of comparison with previous

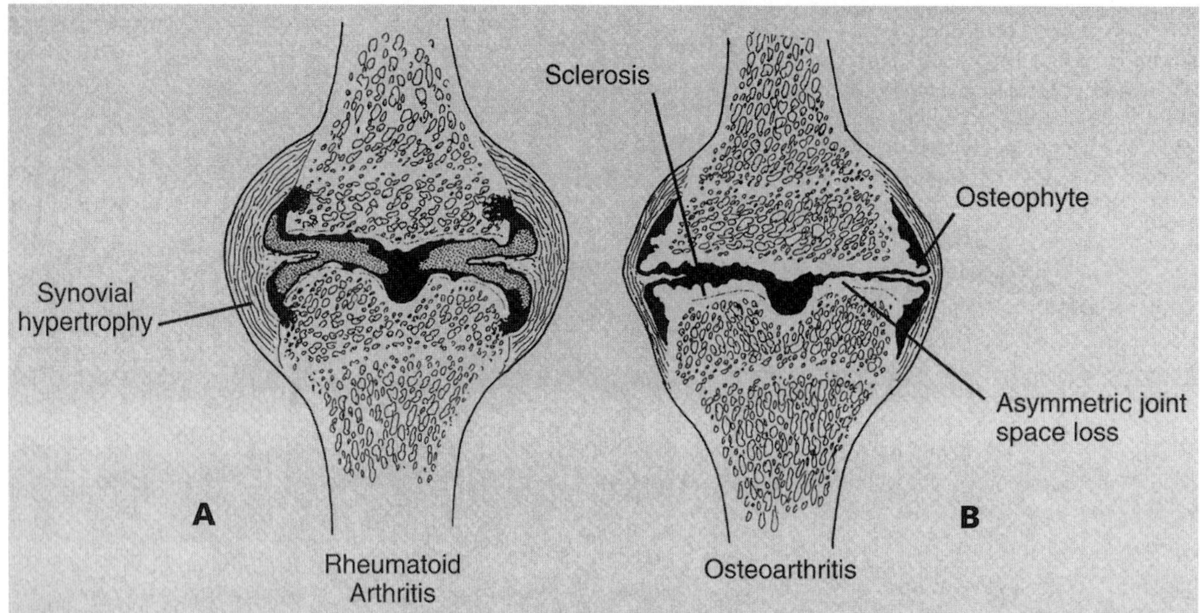

Figure 8–25 The important morphologic differences between **(A)** rheumatoid arthritis (RA) and **(B)** osteoarthritis (OA). Note that OA involves little or no loss of mineralization, osteophyte formation, and nonuniform loss of joint space. RA, in contrast, involves juxta-articular osteoporosis, periarticular erosions, and an absence of productive changes (osteophytes).

radiographs), fracture of the cement or prosthesis, and widening of the prosthesis–cement interface. Additional complications include profuse heterotopic bone formation, dislocation, and stress fractures.

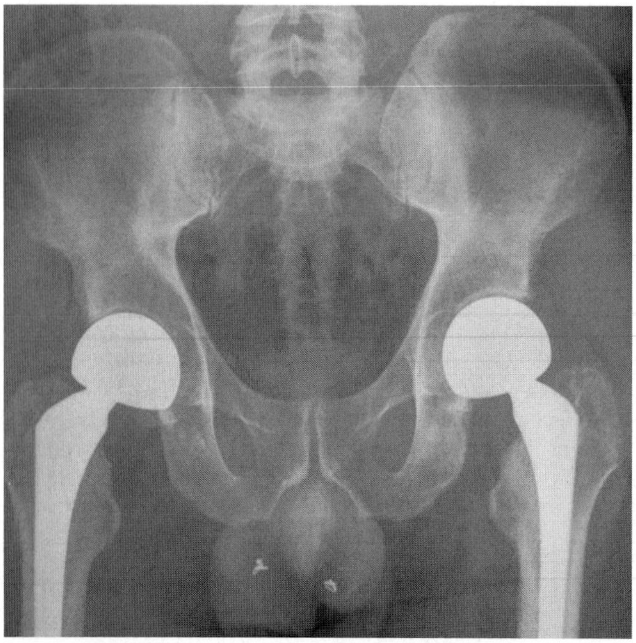

Figure 8–26 This 33-year-old man with a long history of vasculitis resulting in bilateral avascular necrosis of the hips underwent placement of bilateral hip prostheses, which have a normal appearance.

Rheumatoid Arthritis

◇ Epidemiology

Afflicting ~1% of the population, RA is a major source of disability in the United States. Women are afflicted approximately 3 times as often as men, and in 80% of cases the onset of symptoms occurs between the ages of 35 and 50. Although genetic susceptibility is a definite factor, environmental factors appear also to play a role. Some patients develop only mild symptoms that spontaneously and completely remit, whereas others suffer profound systemic sequelae and marked joint deformities. Most patients experience a course somewhere between these two extremes. If RA persists for more than a decade, more than four of five patients will have some degree of joint deformity.

◇ Pathophysiology

The pathophysiology of RA is the subject of debate. Immune phenomena are clearly implicated. More than two thirds of adult RA patients exhibit circulating rheumatoid factor, which consists of autoantibodies reactive with the Fc portion of immunoglobulin G (IgG). It has been hypothesized that complexes of circulating rheumatoid factor and IgG may be the inciting factors in synovial inflammation. However, rheumatoid factor may also be present in systemic lupus erythematosus (SLE), sarcoidosis, and infectious mononucleosis, among other disorders. Early inflammatory changes of RA include synovial hypervascularity, edema, and cellular infiltration (**Fig. 8–27**). Synovial inflammation and associated hyperemia induce osteoclastic activity, resulting in bone "washout" around joints seen on radiographs as juxta-articular osteoporosis. With time, the synovium hypertrophies, a process called pannus formation. This synovial proliferation

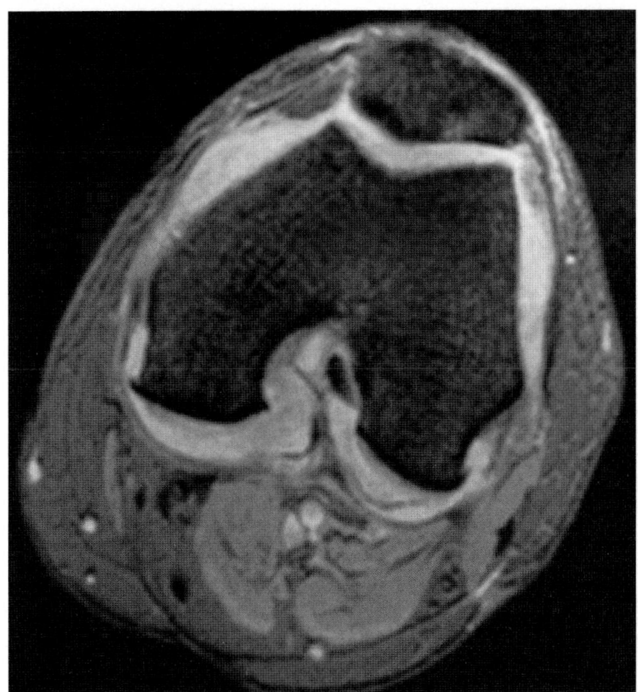

Figure 8–27 This 45-year-old woman presented with left knee pain. An axial STIR MR image of the knee demonstrates marked synovial proliferation, manifest as a thick rim of high signal around the distal femoral cortex. This is a characteristic finding in early rheumatoid arthritis.

produces erosion of subchondral bone and ligamentous laxity, which may be followed by subluxation and ankylosis.

◇ Clinical Presentation

The onset of RA is usually insidious, with constitutional symptoms such as fatigue, anorexia, and weakness, although several patients will also note vague musculoskeletal symptoms. Over a period of months, more specific musculoskeletal symptoms appear, with pain, swelling, tenderness, and limitation of motion symmetrically involving the hands, wrists, knees, and/or feet. Prolonged morning stiffness (>1 hour) helps to distinguish a truly inflammatory arthritis such as RA from noninflammatory arthritides such as OA. Because the joint capsule is richly innervated with pain fibers, swelling secondary to hyperemia, edema, and accumulation of synovial fluid, with distension of the joint capsule, can produce severe pain. As a result, patients often hold the joint in a flexed position, to maximize joint volume and minimize pressure.

The extra-articular manifestations of RA are legion. These include rheumatoid nodules, which develop in one quarter of patients and vary in size and consistency but are usually found in periarticular locations, on extensor surfaces, or in areas subject to mechanical pressure. Pleural and pericardial manifestations include effusions and inflammation. Pulmonary fibrosis may result. Other manifestations include vasculitis, scleritis, osteoporosis, and Felty's syndrome, which consists of RA, splenomegaly, neutropenia, and anemia.

◇ Imaging

Although RA is a systemic disease, it nearly always presents with inflammation in the synovial lining of the joints. As one would expect, these inflammatory changes and the associated hypervascularity cause hyperemia-induced juxta-articular osteoporosis, which, along with soft tissue swelling, are the first radiographic signs of the disease. The later hallmarks of RA include articular erosions, bilaterally symmetrical involvement, and absence of bone production (osteophyte formation).

The hands are the most commonly involved region where, following symmetrical soft tissue swelling and juxta-articular osteoporosis, RA produces characteristic erosions in the "bare areas" of the joints, where bone is directly exposed to the synovium because it is not protected by articular cartilage. Characteristic locations include the entire carpal compartment, as well as the metacarpophalangeal and proximal interphalangeal joints, with sparing of the distal interphalangeal joints.

Characteristic deformities are seen clinically and radiographically in RA (**Fig. 8–28**). These include the swan-neck deformity, with hyperextension of the proximal interphalangeal joints and flexion of the distal interphalangeal joints; boutonniere deformity, with flexion deformity of the proximal interphalangeal joints and extension of the distal interphalangeal joints; and "Z" deformity, with radial deviation of the wrist and ulnar deviation of the digits (if ulnar deviation is seen without erosions, one should think of SLE) (**Fig. 8–29**). These can be traced to destruction or weakening of ligaments, tendons, and cartilage; muscle imbalance; and altered physical forces produced by the use of affected joints.

Other characteristic areas include the feet, hips (with axial migration of the femoral head and protrusio acetabuli deformity), knees (with tricompartment joint space narrowing, including the medial and lateral femoral-tibial compartments and the patellofemoral joint), and shoulder (with chronic rotator cuff tear and erosion of the distal clavicle). Nearly 50% of RA patients have involvement of the cervical spine, while the thoracic and lumbar spines are generally not involved. One of the most important findings is atlantoaxial subluxation, which is best detected on flexion views.

Seronegative Spondyloarthropathies

The seronegative spondyloarthropathies are an important class of joint diseases that are distinguished from RA in part by the fact that the rheumatoid factor is negative. These include disorders such as ankylosing spondylitis and psoriatic arthritis. Ankylosing spondylitis is far more common in men than women, and 95% of patients are human leukocyte antigen (HLA)–B27 positive. Around age 20, patients begin to note the insidious onset of back stiffness and pain. Radiographically, the initial site of involvement is the sacroiliac joint, but the process gradually progresses to involve the entire spine. The sacroiliac joints eventually ankylose (fuse), as do the vertebral bodies. The characteristic intervertebral fusion produces the so-called bamboo spine (**Fig. 8–30**). Psoriasis usually manifests first with skin changes, and only 10 to 20% of patients develop psoriatic arthropathy. In contrast to ankylosing spondylitis, psoriatic arthritis tends to involve the peripheral joints as well as the axial skeleton and often produces asymmetric involvement in the spine and sacroiliac joints. Characteristic findings include a combination of erosive and proliferative changes (in contrast to RA, which is only erosive), soft tissue swelling of the digits producing a so-called sausage digit, and the presence of periosteal reaction.

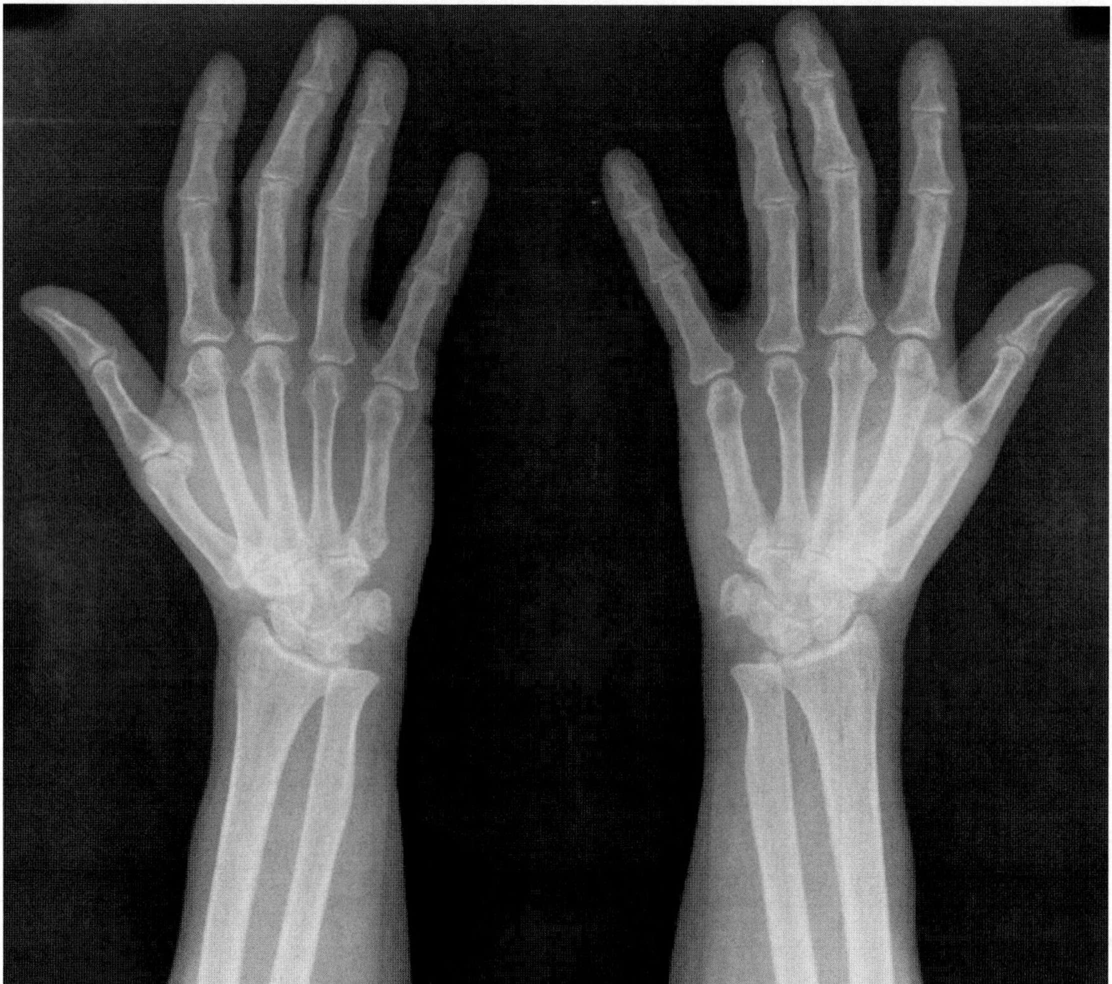

Figure 8–28 A so-called ball catcher's view of both hands demonstrates bilateral subarticular erosions of the carpal bones and osteopenia of the wrists. There is no osteophyte formation, and the process is bilaterally symmetrical. This is a typical location and appearance for rheumatoid arthritis.

Metabolic

Acromegaly

Acromegaly is a classic metabolic bone disorder that usually stems from autonomous hypersecretion of pituitary somatotropin by a functional microadenoma. The excess growth hormone results in overstimulation of cartilage growth. When this occurs prior to growth plate closure, it results in gigantism. After closure of the growth plate, it results in acromegaly. The effects of acromegaly are most dramatically seen in structures with the greatest number of cartilage end plates, such as the hands, feet, skull (where sutures remain open until age 45), and face. Hence the inclusion of hat, glove, and shoe sizes in the endocrinologic history, as well as the value of old photographs to assess for coarsening of the facial features.

Radiographic features include widened joint spaces due to cartilage growth, which is associated with secondary osteoarthritic changes. The osteoarthritic changes are presumed to result from impaired diffusion of nutrients from synovial fluid through the thickened cartilage. Other findings include prognathism (protrusion of the jaw), frontal bossing due to overgrowth of the frontal sinuses, and in some cases, enlargement of the sella turcica. As discussed in Chapter 9, MRI is often used to localize the pituitary lesion.

Chronic Renal Failure

◇ Epidemiology

One of the most prominent metabolic disorders of bone stems from renal dysfunction. Chronic renal failure is a relatively common condition in the United States, representing the final common pathway of several prevalent diseases. The most important is diabetes, which is responsible for 28% of cases and is associated pathologically with the Kimmelstiel-Wilson lesion (nodular glomerulosclerosis). The second most common is prolonged hypertension, the cause of 24% of cases, which is associated pathologically with nephrosclerosis. Other major causes include glomerulonephritis and polycystic kidney disease.

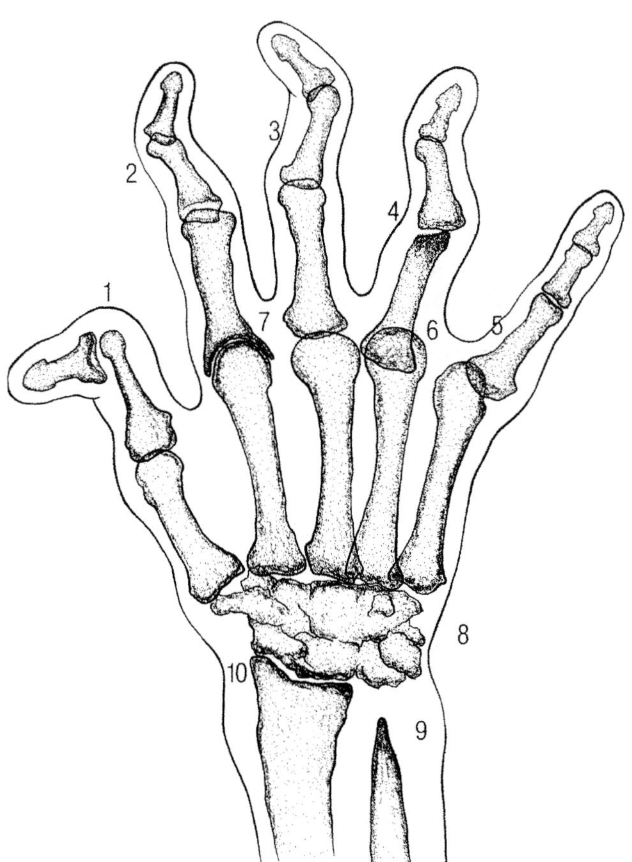

Figure 8–29 Many of the characteristic hand deformities seen in rheumatoid arthritis. 1, hyperextension and subluxation of the distal phalanx of the thumb; 2, flexion at the proximal and extension at the distal interphalangeal joint (boutonniere deformity); 3, extension at the proximal and flexion at the distal interphalangeal joint (swan-neck deformity); 4, destruction of bone ends; 5, ulnar deviation at the metacarpophalangeal joints with subluxation; 6, dislocation of the metacarpophalangeal joints ("main en lorgnette" or "telescoping"); 7, erosion and compression of the metacarpophalangeal joints ("ball in socket"); 8, erosion, sclerosis, and partial fusion of the carpal joints; 9, tapering of the distal ulna; 10, sclerosis, narrowing, or ankylosis of joints.

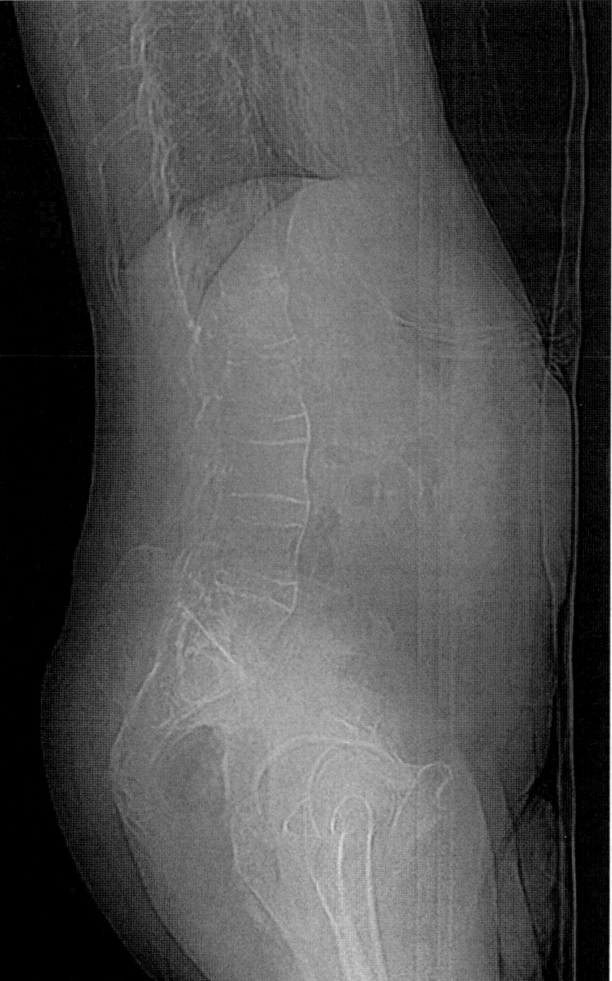

Figure 8–30 This 49-year-old man presented with low back pain. A lateral "scout" view for a CT scan demonstrates characteristic fusion of the lumbar vertebral bodies, producing the "bamboo spine" of ankylosing spondylitis.

◇ Pathophysiology

The term *chronic renal failure* encompasses decreased glomerular filtration, renal tubular dysfunction, and decreased enzymatic activity, particularly the conversion of 25-OH-vitamin D to 1,25-$(OH)_2$-vitamin D. Secondary hyper-parathyroidism results from the kidney's inability to normally excrete phosphate, resulting in hyperphosphatemia, consequent hypocalcemia, and increased secretion of PTH. The hypocalcemia is exacerbated by loss of renal 1-hydroxylase activity, with a deficiency of the active form of vitamin D. Renal osteodystrophy refers to the production of bone that is deficient in mineral content, with increased liability to fractures.

Secondary hyperparathyroidism is distinguished from both primary and tertiary hyperparathyroidism. Primary hyperparathyroidism, which is especially common in middle-aged and elderly women, results in at least 80% of cases from a benign, autonomous adenoma, which causes suppression of the three remaining parathyroid glands. Other causes of primary hyperparathyroidism include hyperplasia (seen most often in the multiple endocrine neoplasia syndromes) and carcinoma. Tertiary hyperparathyroidism refers to autonomous gland function following long-standing renal failure.

Therapies employed in chronic renal failure include chronic hemodialysis, peritoneal dialysis, and renal transplantation. Transplantation now enjoys a 1-year survival rate in most centers of greater than 90%.

◇ Clinical Presentation

Nearly all patients with end-stage renal disease will eventually develop secondary hyperparathyroidism. The clinical manifestations of secondary hyperparathyroidism include bone pain, proximal muscle weakness, pruritis, and eventually, diffuse soft tissue calcification. The latter finding is more likely when the product of the serum calcium and phosphate exceeds 50 mg/dL.

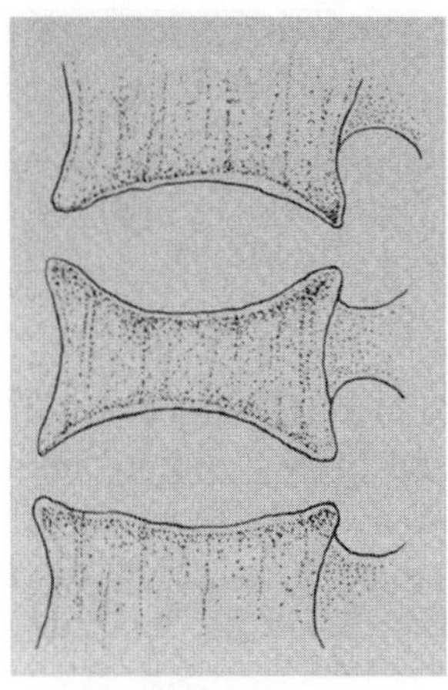

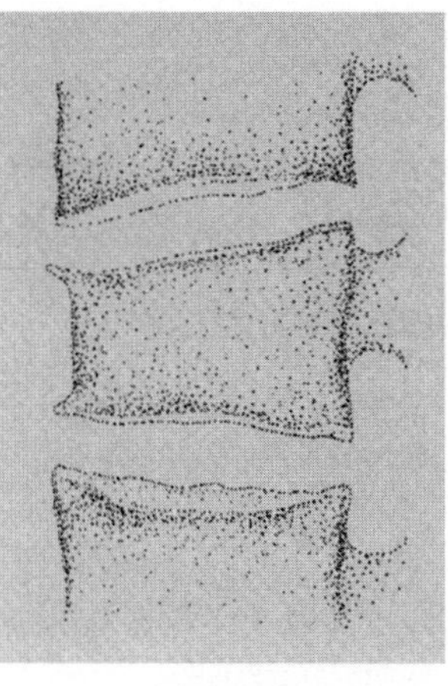
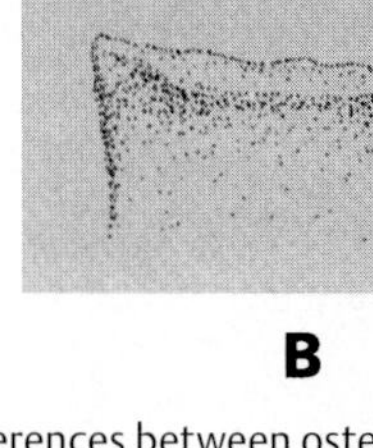

C

Figure 8–31 The characteristic differences between osteoporosis, osteomalacia, and hyperparathyroidism in the spine. **(A)** Osteoporosis manifests as a biconcave vertebral body with prominent vertical trabeculae. **(B)** Osteomalacia manifests as uniform deossification with a loss of trabecular detail and anterior wedge-shaped compression fractures. **(C)** The "rugger jersey" spine of secondary hyperparathyroidism manifests as increased density adjacent to the vertebral end plates.

◇ Imaging

Numerous radiographic findings are possible. Osteosclerosis, the cause of which is unknown, refers to an apparent increased bone density in certain areas, especially the "rugger jersey" spine (**Fig. 8–31**). Bone resorption is seen in up to 70% of long-standing cases. Subperiosteal resorption is pathognomonic and characteristically involves the radial aspects of the middle phalanges. Endosteal resorption causes a classic "salt and pepper" appearance of the calvarium. Subchondral resorption is often seen in the hands and may simulate the erosions of inflammatory arthritis. Brown tumors are localized areas in which bone is replaced by fibrous tissue and appear as well-defined, lytic lesions, which may cause osseous expansion. Another finding is soft tissue and vascular calcifications (**Fig. 8–32**).

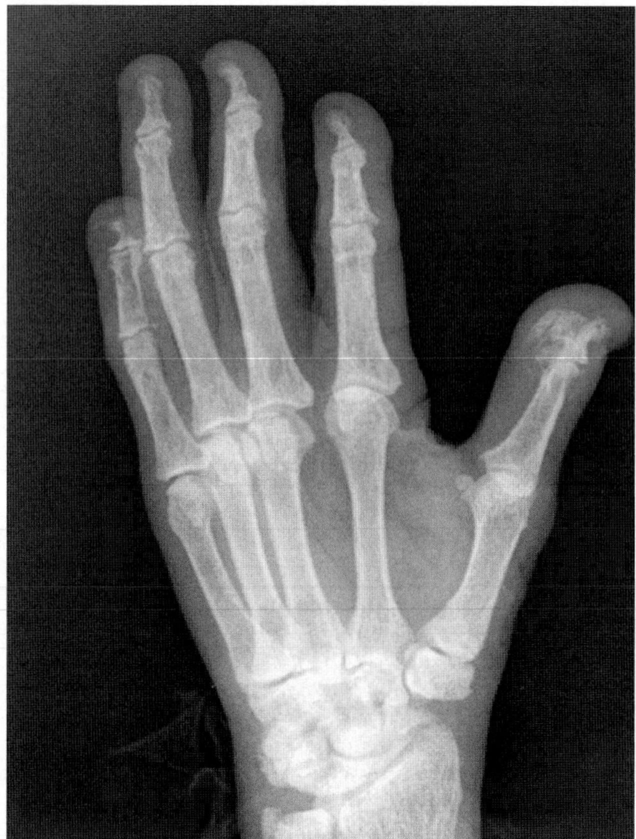

Figure 8–32 This patient with long-standing renal failure exhibits classic findings of renal osteodystrophy involving the hand, including subperiosteal resorption of metacarpophalangeal joints and soft tissue calcifications, most prominent in the distal thumb.

Crystalopathies: Gout

◇ Epidemiology

A disease of middle-aged and elderly men and postmenopausal women, gout afflicts ~3 of every 1000 people in the United States, although it is found in up to 5% of patients with clinical arthritis.

◇ Pathophysiology

The risk of suffering an attack of gout is directly proportional to the plasma level of uric acid; a person with a uric acid level of greater than 10 mg/dL has a greater than 90% probability of suffering an attack. The attack is thought to occur when uric acid crystals begin to precipitate in the synovial fluid and cartilage, with phagocytosis of the crystals by leukocytes, which are subsequently damaged by the "indigestible" crystals and release the toxic contents of their phagolysosomes into the joint, causing inflammation. When aspirated joint fluid is inspected microscopically, monosodium urate crystals appear as needle-like refractile bodies, which are strongly negatively birefringent (yellow when aligned parallel to the compensatory axis).

Gout is divided into primary and secondary forms, depending on the underlying etiology of the increased uric acid levels. Primary gout is seen in patients with an underlying disorder of purine metabolism, which is heritable and predominantly afflicts males, or in patients who undersecrete uric acid. Most patients with idiopathic gout fall into the latter category. Secondary gout is seen in patients with some other primary disorder that increases uric acid levels. Secondary gout may be further divided into disorders associated with increased uric acid production, such as leukemia and cytotoxic chemotherapy, and disorders associated with decreased uric acid excretion, such as renal failure. Risk factors for gout include alcoholism, which both increases uric acid production and decreases excretion, and salicylate use, which decreases excretion. Treatment of gout is directed at the acute manifestation, synovitis, as well as the underlying etiology, the increased uric acid level.

◇ Clinical Presentation

Only ~5% of hyperuricemic patients develop gout. The typical attack of acute gouty arthritis is that of an exquisitely painful monoarthritis, most often the first metatarsophalangeal (MTP) joint (podagra). The patient with podagra finds weight bearing impossible, and the joint often appears red and swollen. The attack generally subsides within days to weeks, and the patient becomes asymptomatic until the next attack. Eventually, the patient may develop tophi and chronic gouty arthritis, with nodular deposits of monosodium urate involving the external ears and the ulnar surface of the forearms.

◇ Imaging

Radiographic changes of gout are seen in up to 50% of patients. The most commonly involved joint is the first MTP joint, which is the initial finding in 60% of patients. After the first MTP joint, other common sites of gouty arthritis include other toes, ankles, hands, and the olecranon bursa, typically with sparing of the hips and shoulders. Bone mineralization is initially normal. Findings include soft tissue tophi (containing birefringent monosodium urate crystals), punched-out erosions with sclerotic borders and overhanging edges, and preservation of the joint space (**Fig. 8–33**). As the disease progresses and more uric acid crystals deposit in the articular cartilage, the cartilage itself is eroded away, and secondary arthritis with joint space narrowing ensues.

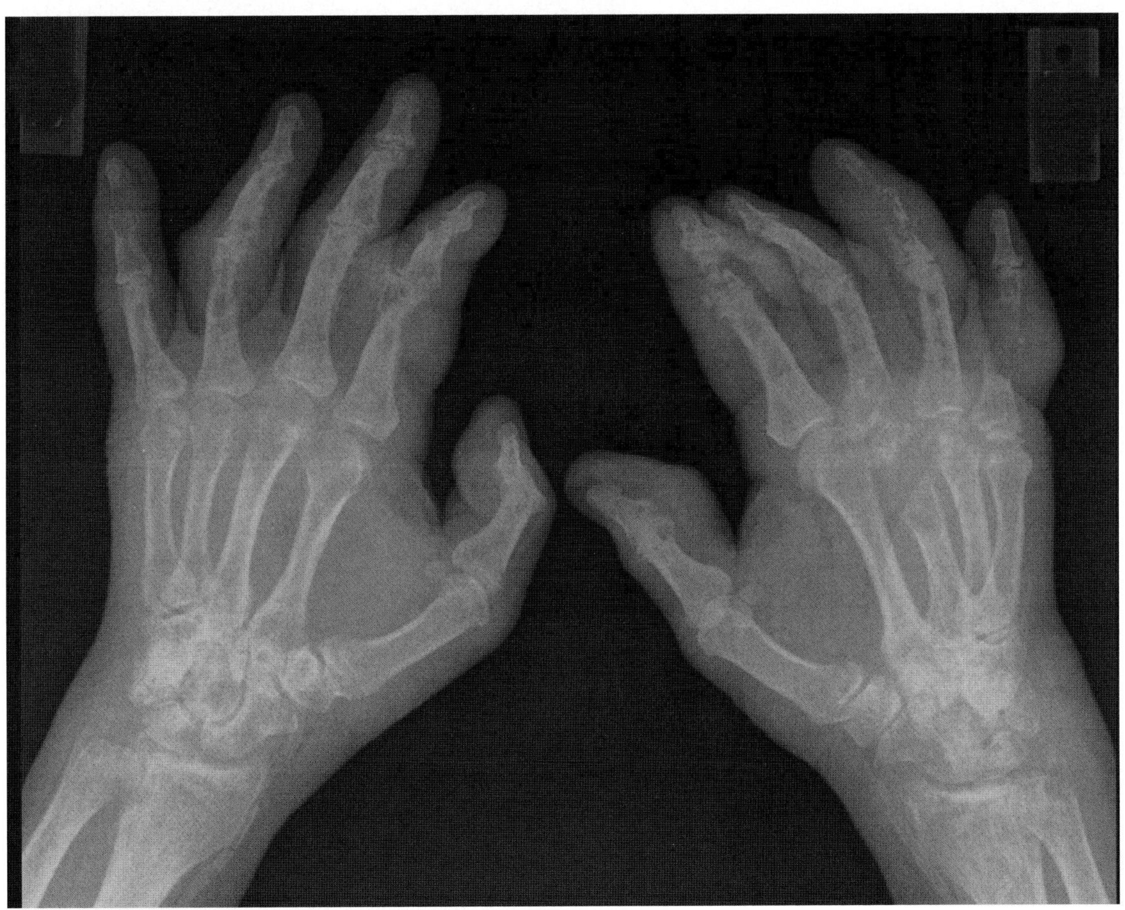

Figure 8–33 This man with long-standing gout exhibits classic radiographic findings in the hands, including asymmetric polyarticular punched-out lesions and overhanging erosions in many joints.

Crystalopathies: Pseudogout

◇ **Epidemiology**

Pseudogout, better termed *calcium pyrophosphate dihydrate deposition disease*, afflicts predominantly elderly patients and is found in up to 5% of the general population, rendering it much more common than gout. It is seen with increased frequency in patients with hyperparathyroidism, gout, and hemochromatosis.

◇ **Pathophysiology**

CPPD is defined as calcification in the hyaline cartilage of articular surfaces and is seen as a thin rim of calcification outlining the surface of the joint. It most often involves the knees (especially the patellofemoral joint), the pubic symphysis, and the hands and wrist (especially the radial-carpal and carpal-lunate joints). These calcium deposits interfere with normal cartilage structure and function, and predispose to secondary OA.

◇ **Clinical Presentation**

Only ~25% of patients with CPPD present with an acute pseudogout attack, most frequently involving the knee. The involved joint is red, swollen, warm, and painful. A minority of patients experience attacks involving multiple joints, which can be confused with RA.

◇ **Imaging**

Because articular cartilage is radiolucent, the rim of surface calcification associated with CPPD appears to be "floating in space" above the end of the bone (**Fig. 8–34**). It should be suspected when OA-like changes are seen in unusual joints, such as the elbow, shoulder, and the metacarpal-phalangeal joints of the hand, or when joints commonly involved with OA demonstrate an unusual appearance, such as a hip with uniform joint space loss. The definitive diagnosis rests on the finding of calcium pyrophosphate crystals in synovial cells, which appear blunt and rectangular, and demonstrate slight positive birefringence, thus appearing blue.

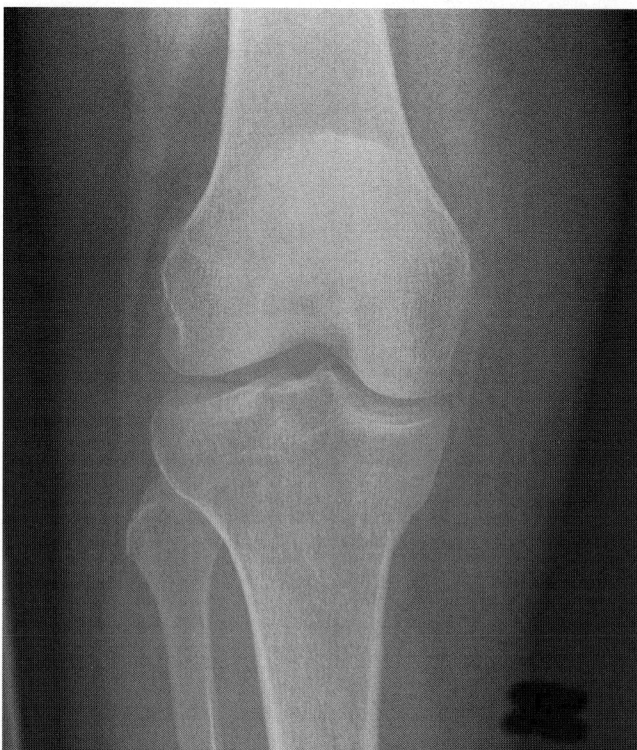

Figure 8–34 This 89-year-old man complained of knee pain. A frontal radiograph of the right knee demonstrates calcification of the articular cartilage, typical of calcium dihydrate pyrophosphate deposition disease (CPPD).

Hydroxyapatite Deposition Disease

While calcium pyrophosphate deposits in articular cartilage, the form of calcium that deposits in tendons, ligaments, and bursae is calcium hydroxyapatite. This type of soft tissue calcification is seen on a secondary basis in several conditions, including collagen vascular diseases such as scleroderma, dermatomyositis, and lupus, as well as hyperparathyroidism and hypervitaminosis D. Hydroxyapatite deposition may also occur on an idiopathic basis, especially in the shoulder and the wrist (**Fig. 8–35**).

Traumatic

Joint Injury

Displacement of a bone relative to another bone at a joint may be described as a dislocation, a subluxation, or a diastasis. A dislocation is diagnosed when there is complete loss of continuity of the bones at a joint surface. A subluxation, by contrast, occurs when the bones are less severely displaced and some degree of continuity at the joint surface remains (**Fig. 8–36**). A diastasis occurs with displacement at a slightly moveable joint, such as the sacroiliac joint, and is often associated with a fracture elsewhere.

Fracture: Extremity Trauma

◇ **Epidemiology**

The first clinical use of the x-ray in the United States took place just 5 weeks after Roentgen's announcement of its discovery. On February 3, 1896, at Dartmouth University, astronomy professor Edwin Frost radiographed a young man's fractured forearm. Fracture remains one of the most common emergency room diagnoses in the United States, and nearly every patient with a suspected fracture undergoes plain film radiography.

◇ **Pathophysiology**

Newton's laws of motion supply the physical principles vital to understanding musculoskeletal trauma. Newton's second law states that energy is neither created nor destroyed, but only changes form. This law provides the theoretical framework for understanding the events that transpire when the human body and another object collide. Suppose, for

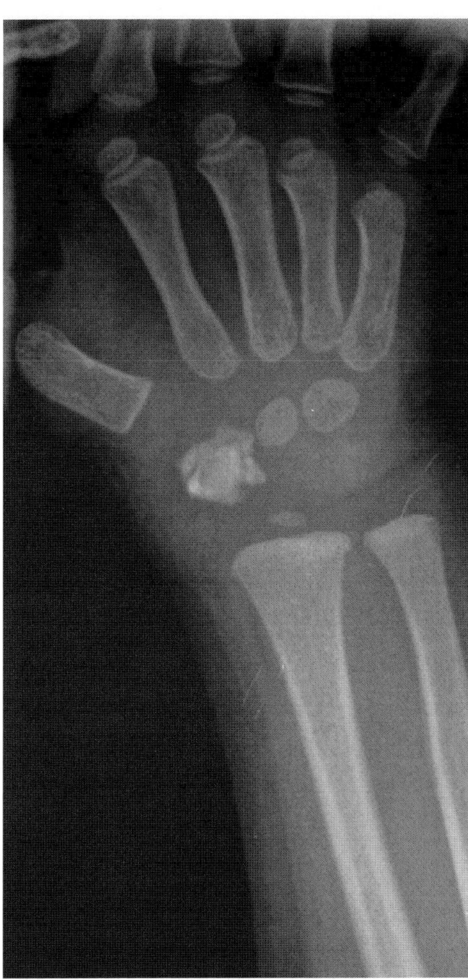

Figure 8–35 This toddler fell and injured her wrist several months ago, and now complains of wrist pain. A plain radiograph demonstrates bulky mineral deposition in the radial aspect of the wrist, representing hydroxyapatite deposition.

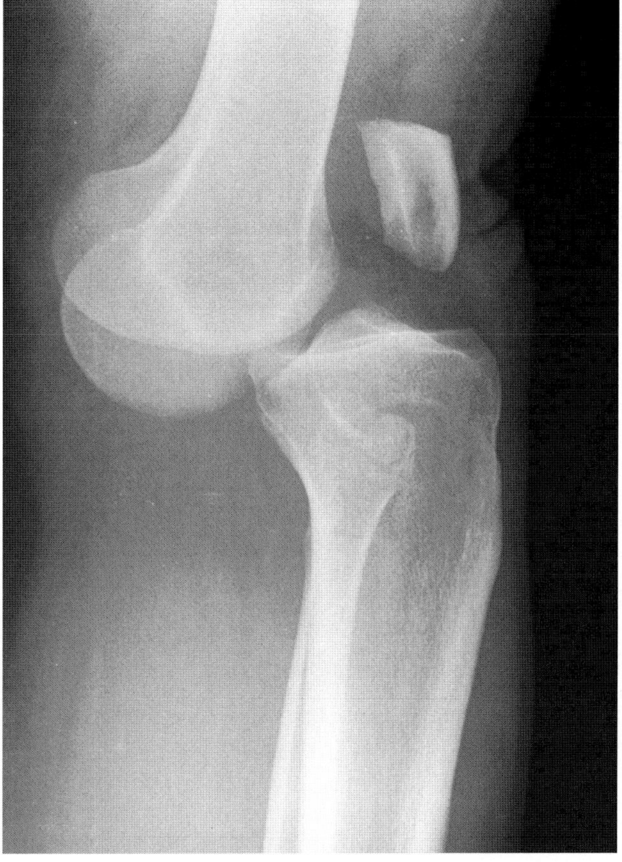

Figure 8–36 This lateral view of the knee demonstrates nearly complete posterior subluxation of the femur relative to the tibia.

example, that in a motor vehicle accident an unrestrained passenger is thrown against the dashboard. The car is decelerated from a speed of 30 miles per hour to 0 mile per hour, as is the passenger within. In order for an object to come to a complete stop, its kinetic energy must be absorbed. In the case of the automobile, energy is absorbed by the front end of the car, as the sheet metal and frame in this region buckle. The biological analogy of the automobile's sheet metal and frame is the passenger's soft tissues and skeleton.

Two additional principles vital to understanding the physics of trauma are kinetic energy and force. In assessing the kinetic energy of an object, it is important to recall the equation

$$KE = 1/2\ mv^2,$$

where *KE* is kinetic energy, *m* is mass, and *v* is velocity. This relationship implies that velocity is relatively more important than mass in determining an object's kinetic energy. Doubling an object's velocity does not merely double, but in fact quadruples, its kinetic energy; hence, 4 times as much energy must be absorbed in the impact. Force introduces the additional element of time, the rate at which the object's velocity reaches 0. Force is equal to the product of mass and acceleration (the rate of change in velocity). A common unit of acceleration is the "G," equivalent to the acceleration due to gravity. A high-speed motor vehicle accident might produce a deceleration equivalent to 30 G, indicating that both the dashboard and the 150-lb passenger who strikes it would feel a force at impact of ~4500 lb (**Fig. 8–37**).

Bone provides a lightweight yet strong scaffold for the soft tissues, and as such can support considerable loads with merely elastic deformation, not suffering any permanent deformity. Despite the fact that the 206 bones of the human skeleton support the entire weight of the body, the skeleton itself accounts for only ~18% of that weight. A general principle underlying all fractures is that of the load-deformation curve, which describes the strain that occurs with increasing stresses. The differing concentrations of calcific extracellular matrix in the bones of adults and children accounts for the different patterns of fracture seen in the two groups. The bones of children have a relatively long plastic deformation phase, during which the bone will bend without fracturing

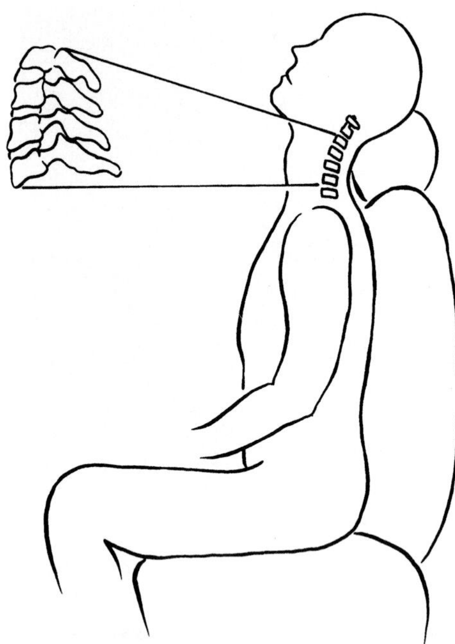

Figure 8–37 A rear-impact collision pushes forward all components of the body that are in contact with the seat. If the head restraint is not high enough to contact the posterior skull, severe angulation of the neck occurs.

completely, because it contains relatively little rigid extracellular matrix. The bones of adults, however, contain more mineral, and are therefore stronger but more brittle.

Fractures may be classified according to the health of the underlying bone and the nature of the stresses placed upon them. The most common type of fracture is that which occurs from a single episode of major trauma to a normal bone, and these are the sorts of fractures seen many times every day in a busy hospital emergency room. A second type of fracture is the so-called fatigue fracture, which results from the application of lower magnitude, repetitive stresses to normal bone, as in military recruits subjected to a program of markedly increased physical activity, such as marching and running (**Fig. 8–38**). Insufficiency fractures are seen in osteopenic individuals, most notably elderly patients, in whom normal stresses surpass the weakened bone's mechanical capacity. Pathologic fractures occur in tumor-containing bone and are usually associated with normal stresses.

◇ Clinical Presentation

Most cases of trauma present no great challenge to the clinician, consisting of isolated extremity fractures and the like. They present with point tenderness, deformity, and loss of normal function, and the patient may report having felt or even heard the bone break.

◇ Imaging

The subject of extremity trauma is vast. What follows are brief descriptions of some of the most common and illustrative osseous injuries.

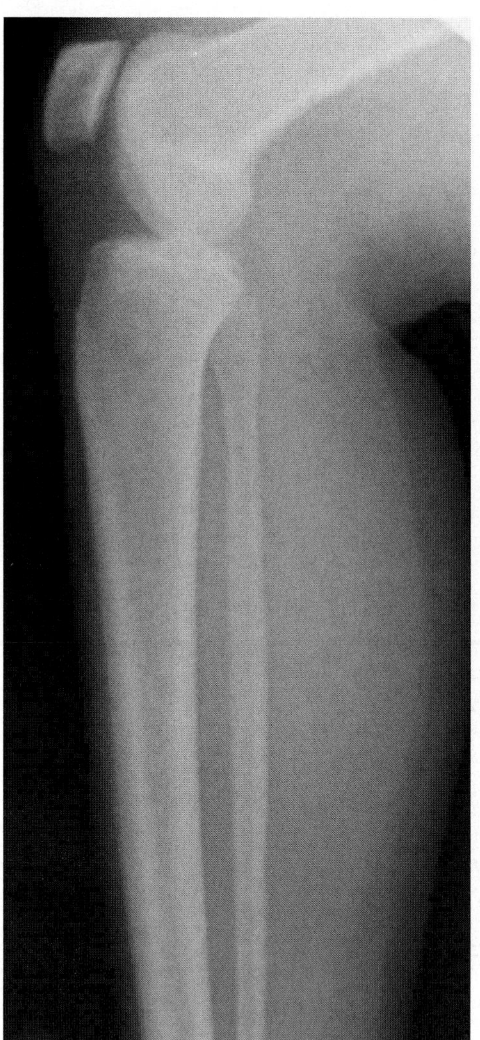

Figure 8–38 This young woman recently took up jogging but had to stop due to severe knee pain. A lateral radiograph demonstrates anterior cortical thickening and a subtle horizontal lucency of the tibia, consistent with a stress fracture, likely of the fatigue variety.

Elbow A key radiographic principle in the diagnosis of trauma about the elbow is the so-called fat-pad sign. An anterior fat pad, detected as a subtle luceny anterior to the distal humerus on the lateral view, is seen normally; however, if this fat pad is elevated from the bone, assuming a sail-like configuration, it is abnormal. There is also a posterior fat pad behind the humerus, but it cannot normally be visualized; however, in the case of an elbow joint effusion in a trauma patient, visualization of either the posterior fat pad or an elevated anterior fat pad constitutes presumptive evidence of a fracture within the elbow joint capsule. In a child, the most common type of fracture is a supracondylar fracture of the humerus. In an adult, a radial head fracture is most common.

Wrist and Hand There are 27 bones in the human hand, including the carpals, the metacarpals, and the phalanges. Fully 90% of carpal bone fractures involve the scaphoid. Most of these are transverse fractures across the scaphoid waist, which may not be visible on initial films and should be followed up 7 to 10 days later, if clinically indicated based on pain and point tenderness in the snuffbox. These fractures exhibit a high rate of nonunion and avascular necrosis, due to the fact that the blood supply to the proximal pole comes from the more distal portion of the bone. This means that a fracture through the waist, especially proximally, is likely to compromise the proximal pole's blood supply (**Fig. 8–39**). The next most often seen fracture is an avulsion from the triquetrum, which is seen as a dorsal bone fragment on lateral views.

Common fractures of the metacarpals include the boxer's fracture, which typically occurs when delivering a punch with a closed fist. These are most often seen in the fourth and fifth metacarpals, with the expected volar (palmar) angulation of the distal fragment. Whenever a boxer fracture is seen, vigilance is warranted regarding a possible septic arthritis, due to inoculation of the puncher's metacarpophalangeal joint with oral flora from the victim's teeth. Infections associated with human bites are among the most difficult to eradicate with antibiotics. Fractures in the phalanges include avulsion injuries, which may involve either the flexor or extensor tendons. An extensor tendon injury is known as a "baseball" (mallet) finger, and the flexor tendon avulsion is described as a "volar plate" injury (**Fig. 8–40**).

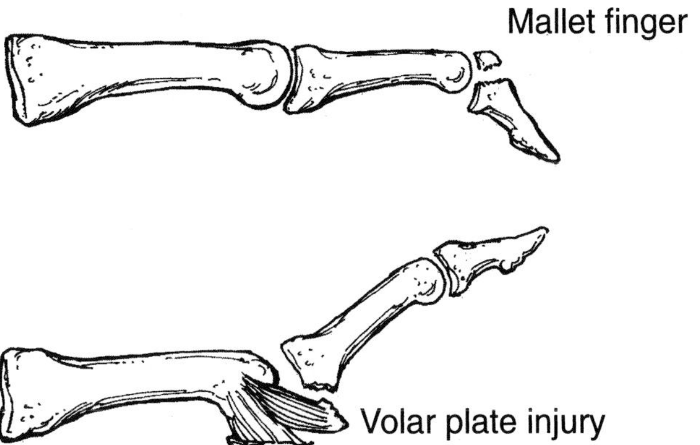

Figure 8–40 The characteristic appearances of mallet finger and volar plate injuries. The mallet finger results from a hyperflexion injury, and the volar plate injury results from excessive extension.

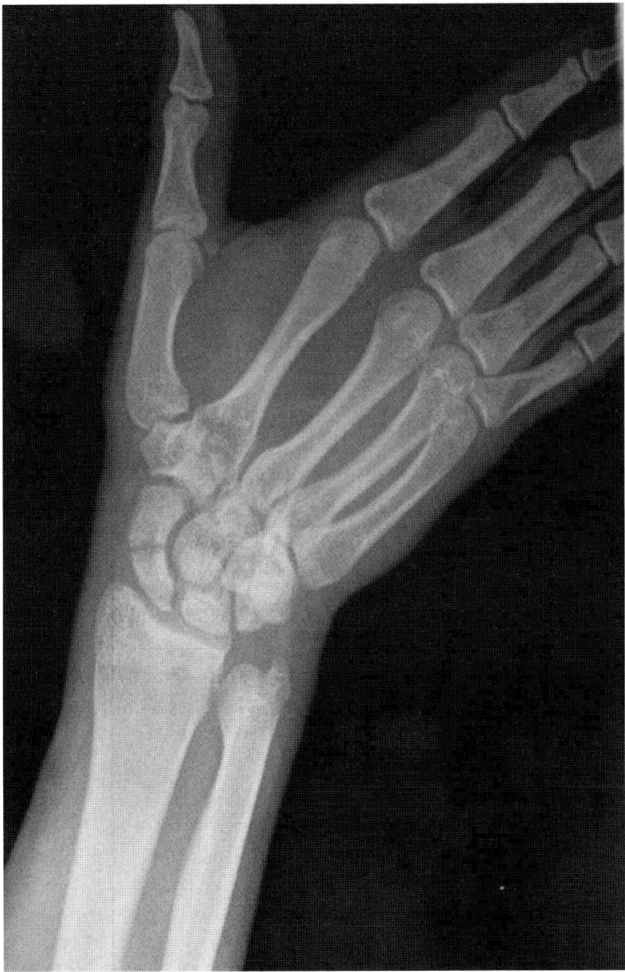

Figure 8–39 This man suffered from persistent wrist pain 2 days after trauma. Initial plain radiographs (not shown) were interpreted as normal. With pain still persisting 2 weeks later, a dedicated scaphoid view was obtained, which demonstrates a transverse fracture across the midscaphoid. Many fractures that are initially occult become more apparent with time due to hyperemia at the fracture site, with bone resorption.

Hip More than 250,000 subcapital ("below the head") femoral fractures occur each year in the United States, the vast majority of which are secondary to osteoporosis (**Fig. 8–41**). They represent the single greatest source of morbidity and mortality associated with osteoporosis, with a nearly 10% mortality rate secondary to the immobilization that tends to accompany such fractures in elderly patients (with cardiac deconditioning, risk of deep venous

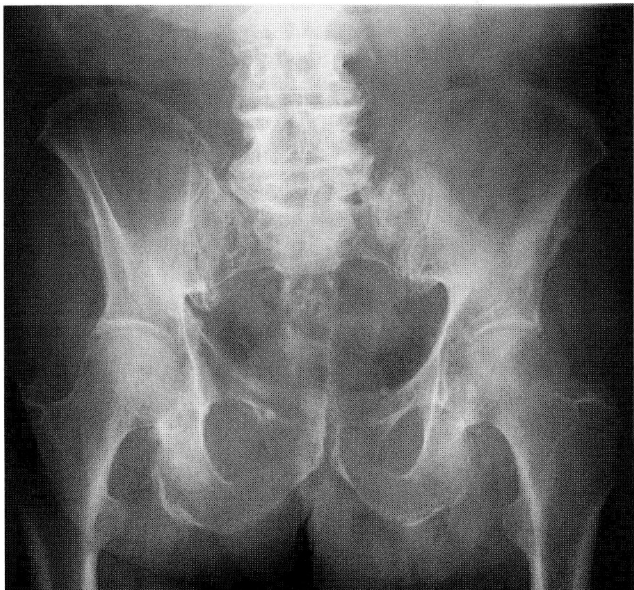

Figure 8–41 This 94-year-old man complained of left hip pain after a fall. A frontal pelvis radiograph demonstrates slight shortening of the left femoral neck compared with the right, with a subtle transverse band of sclerosis in the subcapital area, a subcapital femur fracture.

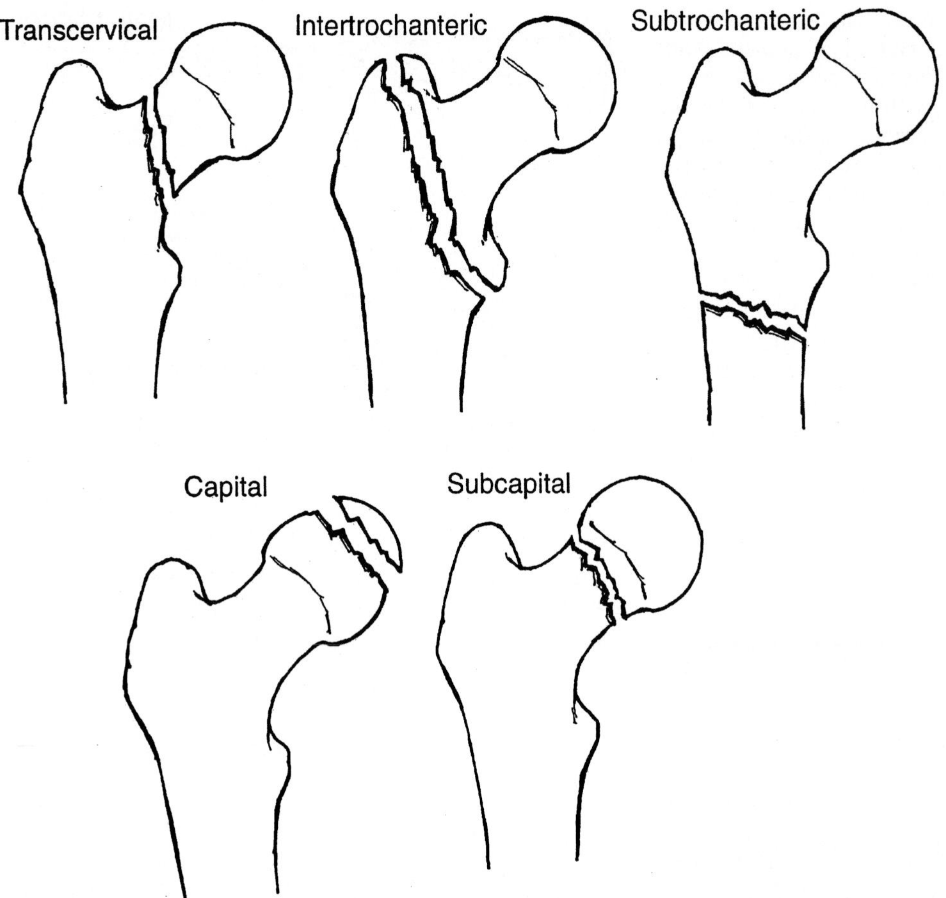

Figure 8–42 The anatomic classification of femoral fractures. The inter- and subtrochanteric fractures are outside the joint capsule, whereas the others are within the hip joint capsule. Subcapital fractures are common and carry a 25% risk of avascular necrosis.

thrombosis, etc.). By the age of 80, 20% of white women and 10% of white men will sustain a hip fracture.

Intracapsular fractures (above the trochanters) are associated with a high risk of avascular necrosis, because the blood supply enters the femoral neck and head from distal to proximal (**Fig. 8–42**). Such fractures are usually apparent on plain radiographs, but if clinical suspicion of fracture is high and the diagnosis cannot be established radiographically, MRI is extremely sensitive. Fractures are seen on T1-weighted images as a transverse band of low-intensity marrow replacement, with surrounding edema (high signal) on T2-weighted images. Fatigue fractures are seen in the medial femoral neck in young patients, while insufficiency fractures may also involve the acetabulum or pubic rami in the elderly.

Knee No joint in the body is more commonly imaged by MRI than the knee. MRI offers several important advantages over other imaging modalities, including noninvasiveness, ability to evaluate soft tissue structures such as tendons, ligaments, menisci, and cartilage, and its multiplanar capabilities. The complex anatomy of the knee as revealed by MRI makes it especially important that a systematic approach be used in every case. T1-type coronal sequences should be evaluated for marrow signal of the femur, tibia, and fibula, as well as osteophyte formation. Sagittal T2-type sequences are best for inspecting the anterior and posterior cruciate ligaments for the presence of tears, as well as for detecting the presence of joint effusions (**Fig. 8–43**). Proton density-weighted sagittals provide optimal assessment of the menisci. Coronal images are employed to evaluate the medial and lateral collateral ligaments. Plain films are useful in acute fracture detection and the evaluation of secondary OA, and occasionally reveal abnormalities of the soft tissues.

Foot The 26 bones of the foot include the tarsals, the metatarsals, and the phalanges. One of the most common injuries is fracture of the calcaneus. Although approximately one quarter of such injuries are avulsions; the remaining three quarters are secondary to axial loading, as when someone leaps out of a second-story window to escape a fire (**Fig. 8–44**). One of the most serious injuries of the midfoot is the Lisfranc's tarsometatarsal dislocation, named after the surgeon in Napoleon's army who used to perform foot amputations at that joint. It is detected as a lack of continuity along the medial aspects of the second cuneiform and the second metatarsal. One of the most prevalent forefoot fractures is the

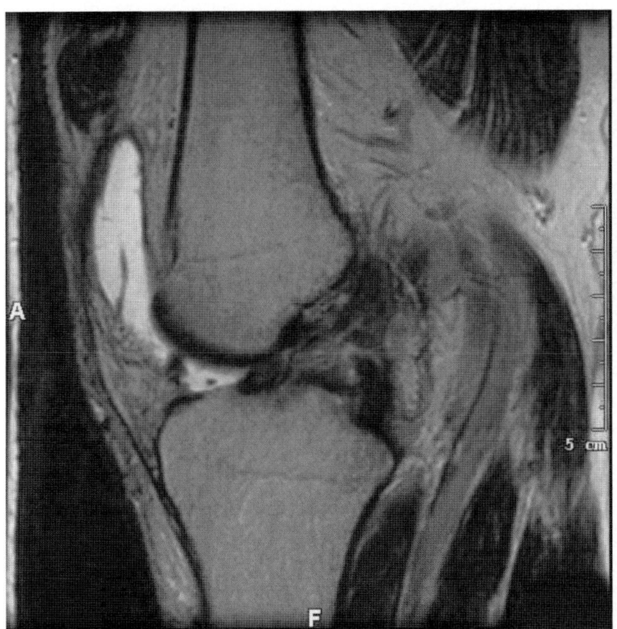

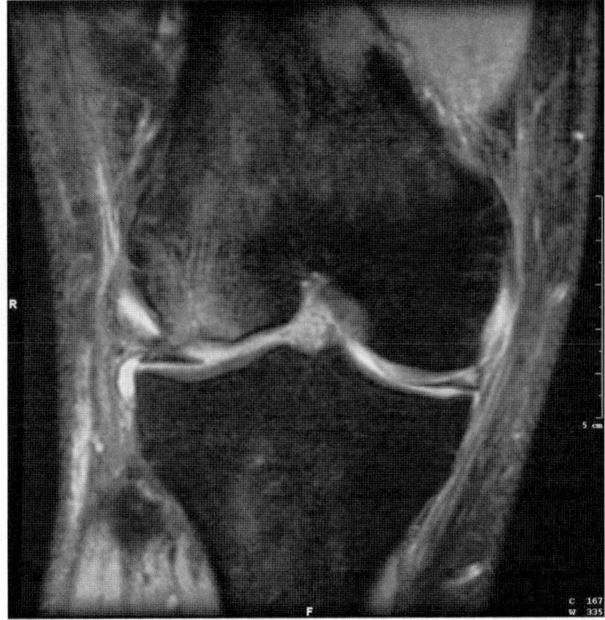

A B

Figure 8–43 (A) This sagittal T2-type image of the knee demonstrates a large knee joint effusion and disruption of the anterior cruciate ligament. **(B)** A coronal view demonstrates sprains of both the medial and lateral collateral ligament complexes, as well as a contusion of the lateral femoral condyle.

Jones fracture of the base of the fifth metatarsal, named after the physician who diagnosed his own Jones fracture after a dancing injury. It most often stems from repetitive stress.

Nondisplaced fractures may require no treatment, or if the bone is subject to continued use, may be splinted or casted to ensure immobility at the fracture. Even many displaced fractures will heal well without reduction; however, such outcomes as lower limb length discrepancy, significant rotation, and displacement of articular surfaces (with subsequent secondary OA) must be avoided. Many displaced fractures do require reduction, which may be either closed (nonsurgical) or open (surgical). Aside from assessing the adequacy of reduction, follow-up radiographs are employed to rule out complications (e.g., fracture and dislocation) and to verify healing. Signs of healing include periosteal reaction, bony callus bridging the fracture, and indistinctness of the fracture line itself.

Fracture: Cervical Spine

◇ Epidemiology

The initial imaging study in the multiply traumatized patient typically consists of portable cervical spine radiography. Spinal injuries are a major source of disability and mortality, and rapid evaluation and treatment are critical in preserving spinal cord function.

◇ Pathophysiology

The most common mechanisms of cervical spine fractures are flexion (e.g., sudden deceleration in a forward-moving vehicle) and axial loading (e.g., diving head first into a shallow swimming pool). The levels between C5 and C7 are most commonly involved (**Fig. 8–45**). A critical distinction is that between stable and unstable fractures. In unstable fractures, the spinal canal is no longer protected by its ligamentous and osseous supports, meaning that any movement of the neck could result in damage to the cord.

Examples of unstable fractures include a flexion teardrop fracture (with ligamentous instability secondary to avulsion) and a "hangman's" fracture (with fracture of the pars interarticularis of C2 and anterolisthesis of C2 on C3), an extension injury (**Fig. 8–46**). Fractures that may or may not be stable (possibly unstable), depending on the extent of injury, include a Jefferson fracture (a "burst" fracture of C1 secondary to axial loading, with fractures of the anterior and posterior arches on at least one side), and a unilateral facet lock, seen on the lateral view as a slight anterolisthesis and rotation of one vertebral body on the other (**Fig. 8–47**). Stable injuries (assuming they are isolated) include a fracture of the posterior arch of C1 and the so-called clay-shoveler's fracture, caused by avulsion by the supraspinatus ligament.

◇ Clinical Presentation

In the case of the multiply traumatized patient, acute management decisions may determine whether the patient lives or dies, as well as the level of residual disability. Before any radiologic study is ordered, the presence of life-threatening injuries must be assessed, and the patient must be stabilized. The five steps of acute management consist of the well-known A-B-C-D-E mnemonic: airway management, breathing, circulation (with control of bleeding), disability

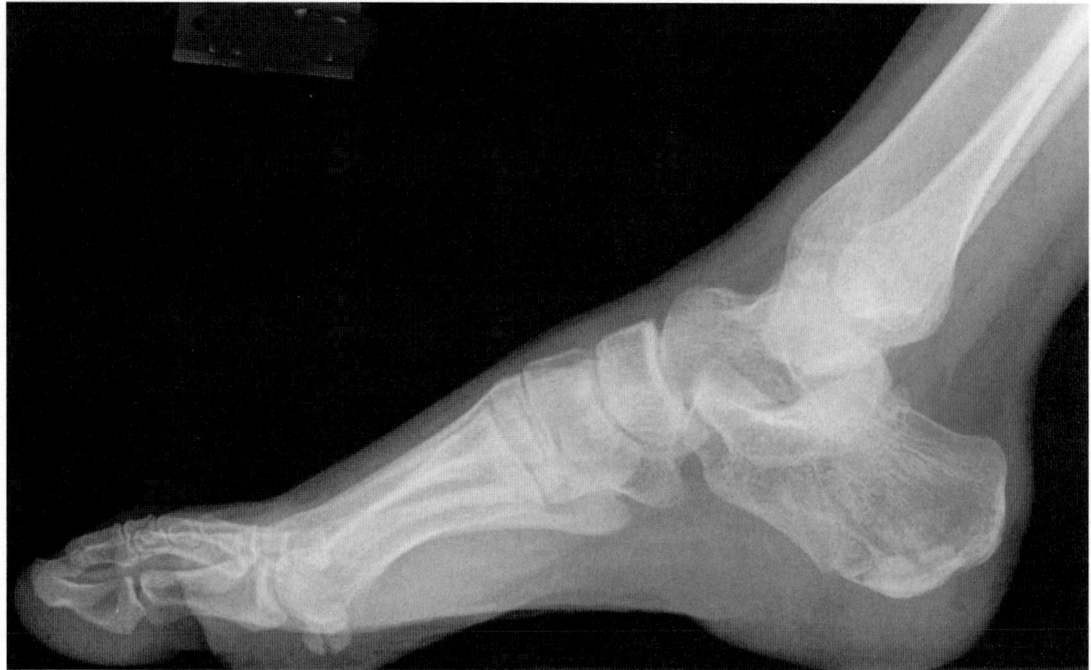

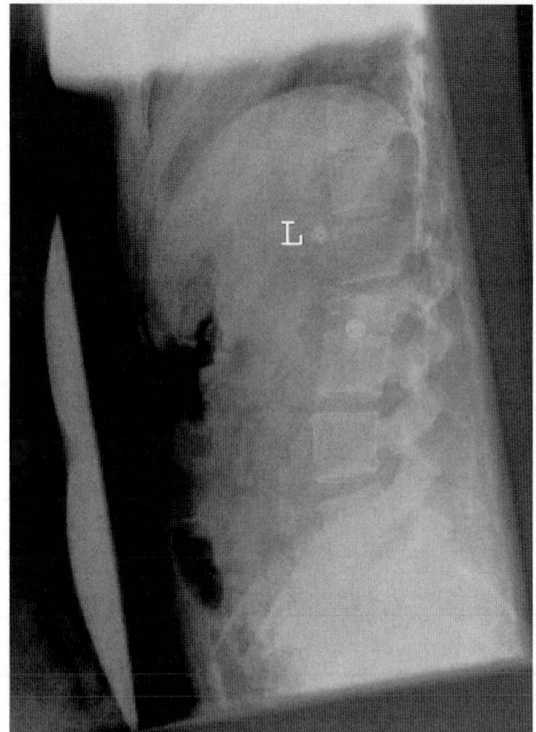

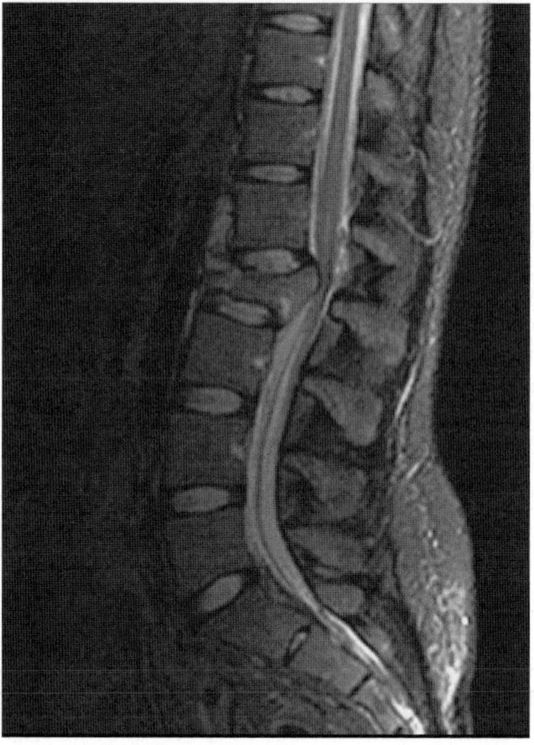

Figure 8–44 This young woman jumped out a second-story window and now complains of heel and low back pain. **(A)** A lateral view of the right foot demonstrates a comminuted fracture of the base of the calcaneous. **(B)** A lateral radiograph of the lumbar spine demonstrates a compression fracture of the second lumbar vertebral body. **(C)** This T2-weighted sagittal MR image demonstrates compression of the distal spinal cord by the retropulsed vertebral body fragments.

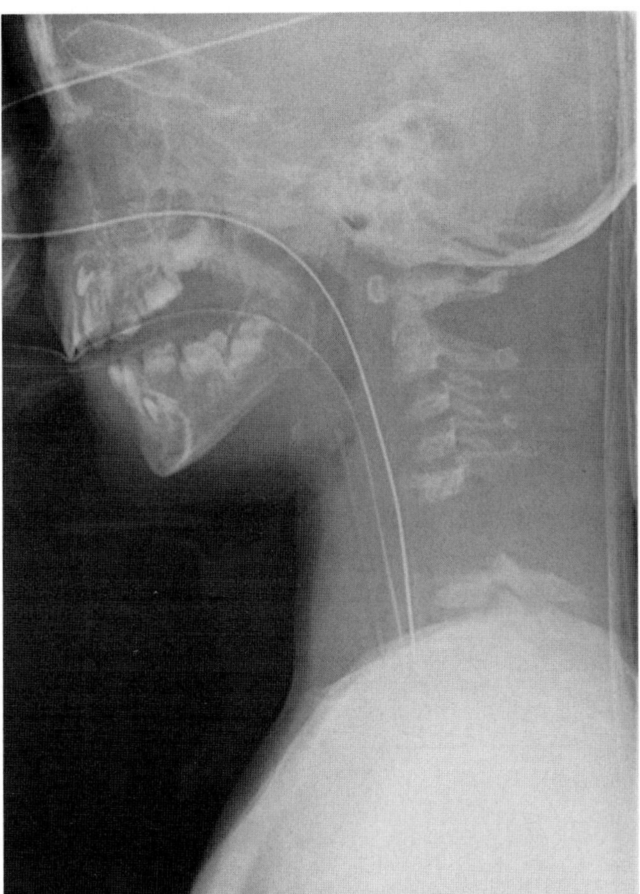

Figure 8–45 This child was improperly restrained at the time of a motor vehicle collision. A lateral C-spine radiograph demonstrates nasogastric tube and endotracheal tubes, as well as a catastrophic distraction injury between the fifth and sixth cervical vertebrae. This is obviously an extremely unstable injury.

(neurologic assessment), and exposure (cutting off clothing). A helpful mnemonic in neurologic assessment of deep tendon reflexes is that sacral level 1–2 is responsible for the Achilles' tendon reflex, lumbar level 3–4 is responsible for the patellar tendon reflex, cervical level 5–6 is responsible for the biceps tendon reflex, and cervical level 7–8 is responsible for the triceps tendon reflex.

Even once the patient is stabilized, the clinician must continue to balance the need for definitive diagnostic information against the need to monitor and manage the patient. Moving the patient from the emergency room to the radiology suite typically compromises access to the patient by personnel and equipment that would be vital if acute resuscitation becomes necessary. Simply put, the radiology department is not the ideal environment in which to manage a cardiac arrest or a disoriented and combative patient. Despite these caveats, however, diagnostic imaging constitutes a vital ingredient in the acute care of the vast majority of multiply traumatized patients.

Imaging evaluation of the cervical spine is indicated in patients whose mental status is altered (compromising history taking and neurologic evaluation), who complain of neck pain, who are tender to palpation of the cervical spine, whose neurologic examination is abnormal, who are at high risk due to the mechanism of injury (fall from a height greater than 10 feet or high-speed motor vehicle accident), or who suffer severe pain at another site that may distract them from neck pain. Depending on the clinical setting, evaluation of the thoracic and lumbar spine may also warrant consideration.

To properly care for the patient in whom spinal trauma is being assessed, it is essential that the patient be handled as though serious injury were present. The patient with an unstable spinal injury may suffer further serious injury if mishandled, and the possibility of inducing quadriplegia is

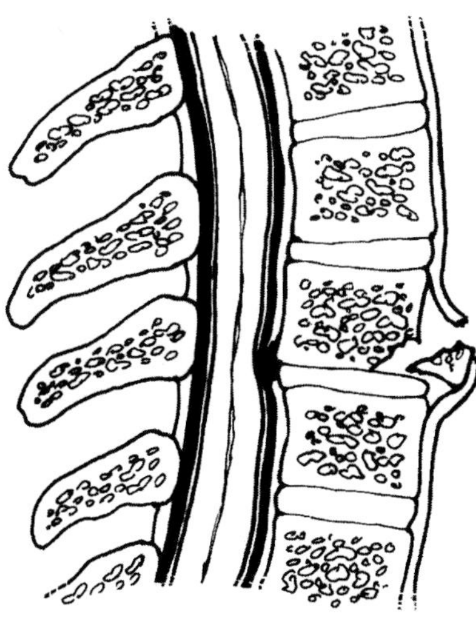

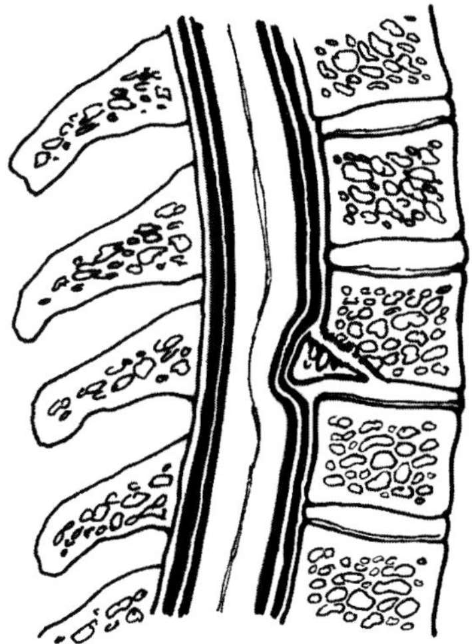

Figure 8–46 Typical appearances of unstable fractures of the cervical spine. (A) A flexion teardrop fracture is seen, with a fragment avulsed off the anteroinferior portion of a vertebral body and disruption of the supporting ligaments. (B) A fragment of a vertebral body has been retropulsed into the vertebral canal, where it exerts mass effect on the spinal cord.

sufficient justification for always erring on the side of overprotection. The patient should be transported with a cervical collar in place, and immobilized on a long spine board, and the patient and the board are moved as a unit until serious injury is radiographically ruled out.

◇ Imaging

The initial view obtained is generally a cross-table lateral, with the patient lying supine in a cervical collar. Once the cervical spine has been "cleared" by a combination of this view and clinical findings, additional radiographs are necessary to fully exclude injury. These include an additional lateral view, an anteroposterior view, an open-mouth odontoid view, and two supine obliques, making a total of five films in a complete cervical spine series. In some cases, CT examination of the cervical spine may be indicated. Many trauma patients will undergo CT scanning of the head to rule out intracranial injury in any case, and it is simple to add on axial images of the cervical spine. This may be especially helpful in patients in whom standard views are unsatisfactory, as when superimposition of shoulder structures compromises views of the lower cervical spine. Moreover, CT is helpful in better delineating equivocal findings on plain films and in further evaluating the extent of definite injuries detected by plain radiography.

The key to evaluating the cervical spine is to approach the radiograph systematically. Many systems are possible, and the following is but one example. Here is a seven-step checklist to employ in evaluating the cross-table lateral view. Although this list is by no means complete, it suffices to rule out most serious injuries in the acute setting.

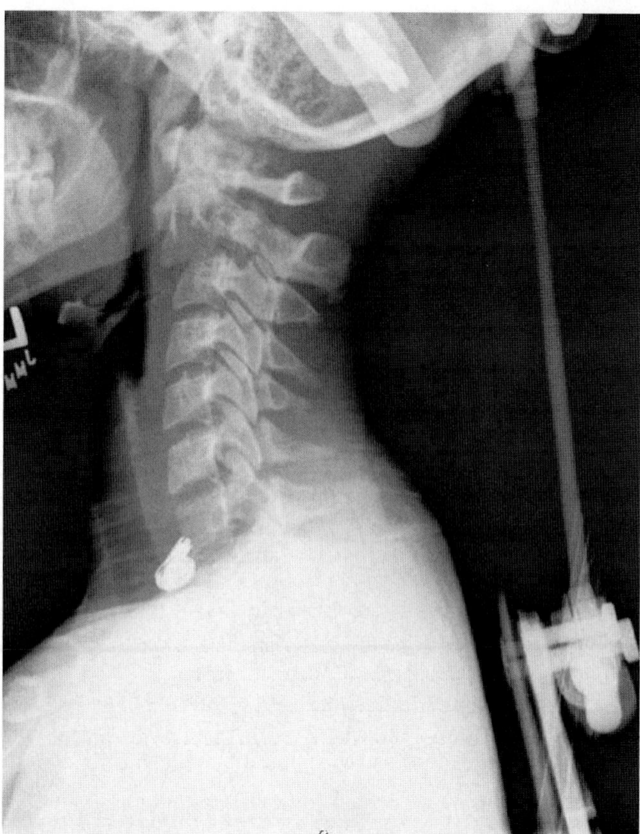

Figure 8–47 This lateral C-spine radiograph demonstrates anterolisthesis of C2 on C3, a classic finding in a "hangman's" fracture.

1. Count the number of vertebrae. A good cross-table lateral view should display all seven cervical vertebrae, as well as the upper portion of the T1 vertebral body. Often the shoulder obscures the lower cervical spine, and a "swimmer's view" must be obtained (the arm closest to the film is extended cranially, as though the patient were reaching to retrieve an object from a high shelf). Just as one would not "clear" a patient's chest after listening to only one lung, one must not "clear" the cervical spine unless the whole cervical spine has been adequately visualized. Although C2 is the single most commonly fractured vertebra in the cervical spine, approximately three fourths of cervical spine fractures involve the lower levels, and adequate visualization is essential in ruling these out. To assess adequate visualization, begin counting below the base of the skull at C1, then count downward.
2. Assess the curvature of the spine. The normal cervical spine is slightly lordotic (convex anteriorly). If this lordosis is exaggerated or lost, it may indicate ligamentous injury, although poor positioning or muscle spasm occurs more commonly.
3. Assess vertebral alignment. Four lines drawn along the axis of the cervical spine should demonstrate smooth, gentle curves (**Fig. 8–48**). These include the anterior vertebral line, the posterior vertebral line, the spinolaminal line, and the posterior spinal line. Any irregularity in any of these lines should raise suspicion for a fracture or dislocation. Because the spinal cord is housed between the posterior vertebral line and the spinolaminal line, an

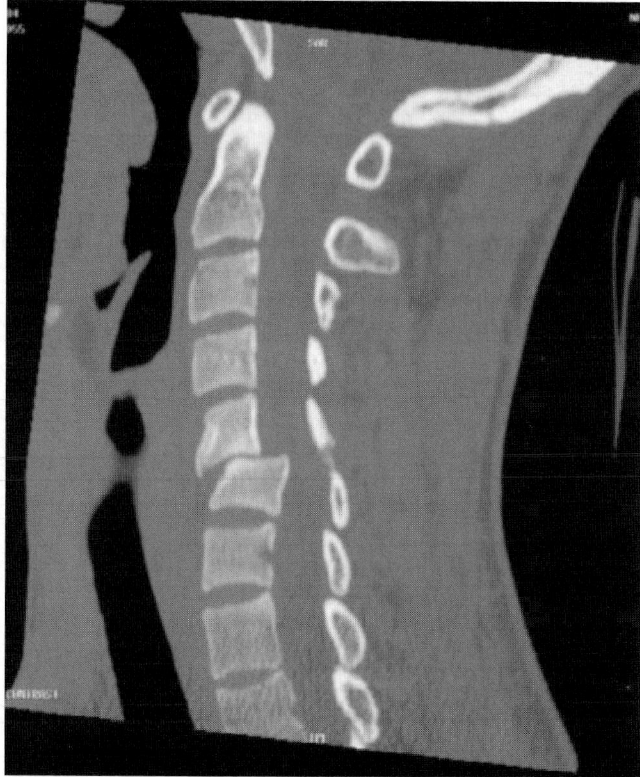

Figure 8–48 This sagittal reformat of axially acquired CT data demonstrates anterolisthesis of the fifth cervical vertebra on the sixth vertebra, which was associated with locking of the facet joint.

irregularity in either of these carries the greatest probability of cord injury (**Fig. 8–49**).

4. Assess bone integrity. Different types of vertebral deformity imply different mechanisms of injury. A hyperflexion injury, as in a head-on collision, tends to produce compression of the anterior portions of the vertebral bodies, with tearing of the intraspinous ligaments. Hyperextension injuries, however, tend to fracture the posterior elements and disrupt the anterior longitudinal ligament. So-called burst fractures result from a force directed along the axis of the spine, as when someone dives head first into a shallow pool. These fractures tend to spare the ligamentous components, but fracture fragments may be directed into the vertebral canal, damaging the cord.
5. Assess the intervertebral disk spaces. The space separating the inferior end plate of one vertebral body from the superior end plate of another should be similar at each level. If a single disk space is narrowed, and there are no other signs of long-standing pathology, such as advanced OA of the spine, one must suspect that the disk space narrowing resulted from trauma. This may be associated with ligamentous injury, and there may also be extrusion of disk material into the vertebral canal, compromising the spinal cord. This could be directly imaged by MRI.
6. Assess the cranium and the first two cervical vertebrae. To ensure that there is no dissociation of the cranium from the spine, make sure that a line drawn along the clivus intersects the odontoid process of C2 at the junction of its anterior and middle thirds, and that the distance between the anterior arch of C1 and the odontoid does not exceed 3 mm (in adults). In children, this measurement may be as great as 5 mm, due to their greater ligamentous laxity.
7. Assess the prevertebral soft tissues. Widening of these tissues may reflect edema or hemorrhage, indirect signs of cervical spine trauma. As a general rule, the soft tissues in front of C2 should not measure more than 4 mm, or measure more than three fourths of a vertebral body diameter in the lower cervical spine. Prevertebral gas is suspicious for abscess.

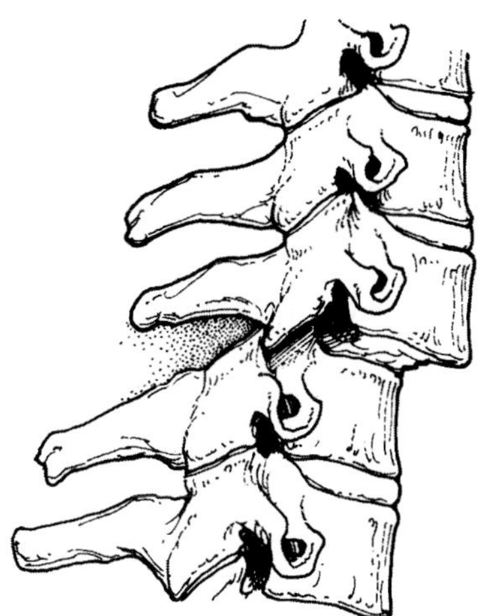

Figure 8–49 A 50% anterolisthesis of one vertebral body on another, with the inferior articular facets of the upper vertebra locked in front of the superior articular facets of the lower vertebra. Naturally, this anterolisthesis tends to compromise the vertebral canal and threatens the cord.

Vascular

Circulatory disorders can be divided into two categories, based on whether they involve increased or decreased flow. Increased flow is seen in many conditions discussed previously. The effects of active hyperemia are readily manifest in bone adjacent to fracture lines, which undergoes an initial loss of osteoid and mineral in response to the associated inflammatory response of healing.

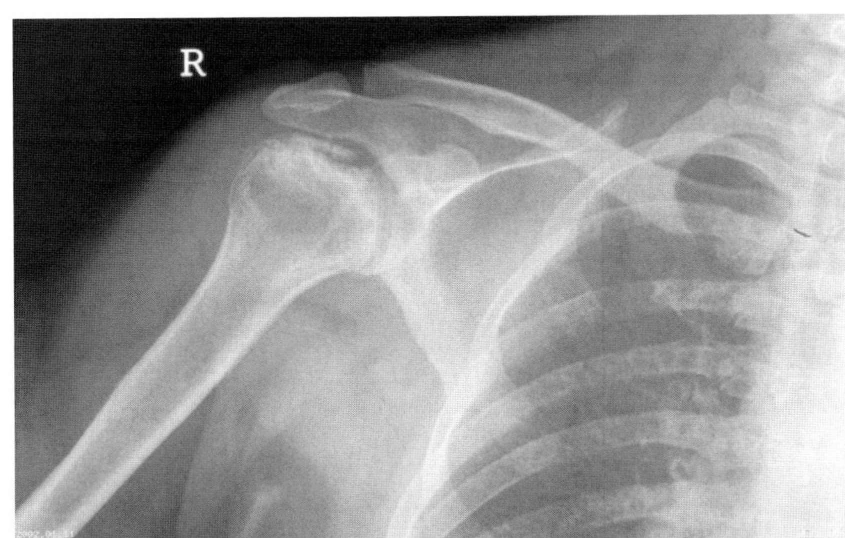

Figure 8–50 This patient on corticosteroids complained of long-standing right shoulder pain. A frontal radiograph of the right shoulder demonstrates irregularity and fragmentation of the humeral head, consistent with advanced avascular necrosis.

Examples of bone disease due to impaired blood flow include avascular necrosis and bone infarct. The classic location of avascular necrosis is the femoral head, and patients at increased risk for this form of osteonecrosis include alcoholics and patients receiving high-dose steroid therapy. Why? Recent experimental evidence suggests that both conditions promote an increase in the amount of marrow fat, which compromises the capillary bed of the femoral head. Other predisposing conditions include sickle-cell anemia, trauma, and collagen vascular diseases.

One of the earliest plain radiographic signs of avascular necrosis is mixed areas of sclerotic and lytic change (**Fig. 8–50**). Although it is tempting to suppose that the lytic areas represent the infarcted tissue, in fact it is the sclerotic areas that have suffered the ischemic insult. These "sclerotic" areas actually represent normally mineralized bone that has died, and which therefore cannot undergo osteoclastic activity. The lytic areas represent inflammation-associated osteoclastic activity in adjacent viable areas of bone. Eventually, the femoral head may collapse, which invariably results in secondary osteoarthritic changes in the hip joint. MRI is far more sensitive than plain film in detecting the early changes of avascular necrosis (**Fig. 8–51**).

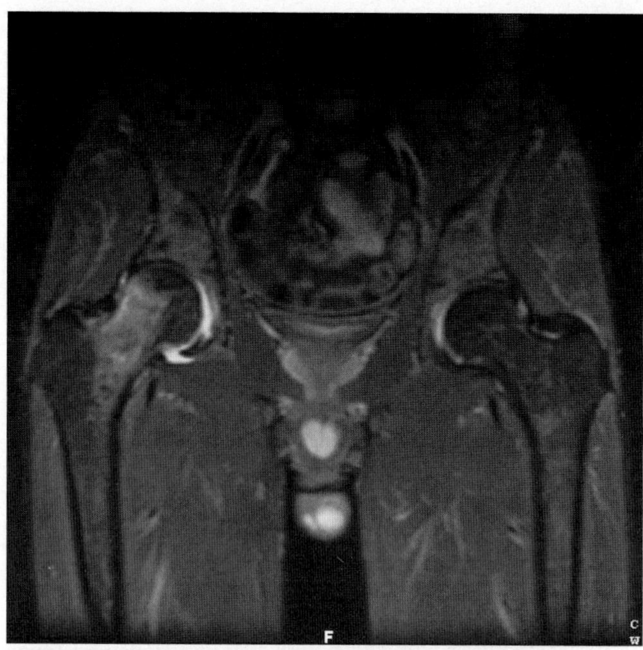

Figure 8–51 This coronal STIR-weighted MR image of the pelvis demonstrates a right hip effusion and abnormally increased signal in the right femoral neck and head, consistent with avascular necrosis.

9

Neuroimaging

◆ Anatomy and Physiology

The central nervous system (CNS), consisting of the brain and spinal cord, is connected to the peripheral nervous system by afferent (Latin for "to bear toward") and efferent ("to bear away from") neurons. Efferent neurons outnumber afferent neurons by a ratio of 10:1, while interneurons, which function in integration, make up ~99% of the 100 billion neurons in the CNS. However, neurons themselves make up only ~10% of the cells in the CNS, the rest consisting of glial cells (from the Greek, *gloios*, "glue"). Glial cells guide the growth of neurons during development, support them both structurally and metabolically, and induce changes in blood vessels that are responsible for the blood–brain barrier. Under normal circumstances, adult neurons do not divide, and the primary neoplasms of the CNS arise from other cell types, such as glial cells (which give rise to gliomas).

The brain itself may be divided into the brainstem, the cerebellum, and the forebrain (**Fig. 9–1**). The brainstem, the oldest region of the brain, functions primarily in a variety of vegetative functions, such as the control of heartbeat, respiration, and digestion. The cerebellum functions in the coordination of motor activity. The forebrain consists of both the diencephalon (the thalamus and hypothalamus) and the cerebrum, which is most highly developed in human beings, where it constitutes ~80% of brain volume. The thalamus is a critical relay station for all synaptic input, and the hypothalamus functions primarily in homeostasis. The cerebrum is divided into the right and left hemispheres, each of which may be divided into an outer shell of gray matter and an inner core of white matter; however, there are numerous gray matter nuclei within the inner portions of the hemispheres. Gray matter consists of densely packed neurons and glial cells, and white matter is made up of myelinated fiber tracts connecting parts of the CNS. Because white matter contains more lipid than gray matter, it appears relatively dark compared with gray matter on CT images (the increased lipid in the form of myelin makes it less dense), and relatively bright compared with gray matter on T1-weighted MR images.

The cerebrum may be divided into four lobes. Broadly speaking, the occipital lobes are responsible for visual processing. The temporal lobes play important roles in hearing, motivation and emotion, and memory. The parietal lobes function in somatosensory and proprioceptive roles, and contain the somatosensory cortex, located immediately posterior to the central sulcus (which divides the frontal and parietal lobes). The frontal lobes contain the motor cortex (immediately anterior to the central sulcus), as well as regions responsible for speech and abstract thought. In addition, there is some division of labor between the two hemispheres, with the right excelling in spatial, artistic, and musical functions, and the left in language and analytical tasks. Hence, a unilateral stroke that leaves a patient mute more likely affects the left hemisphere. Because both sensory and motor tracts generally cross to the contralateral side between the brain and the spinal cord, the left half of the brain is connected to the right half of the body, and vice versa.

The brain and spinal cord have several special protective structures. The brain is encased in the rigid cranium, and the spinal cord by the vertebral column. Although the cranium protects the relatively soft brain from mechanical trauma, it also poses special problems when intracranial pressure rises from hydrocephalus, diffuse edema, or neoplasm, because the brain has no safe means of decompressing itself. The meninges lie beneath the cranium and vertebral column and consist of the outer dura mater (Latin for "tough mother"), beneath which is the subdural space; the arachnoid (Latin for "spider," because it resembles a cobweb), beneath which is the subarachnoid space, which is accessed during a spinal tap; and the pia mater ("soft mother"), which is attached to the brain and dips down into

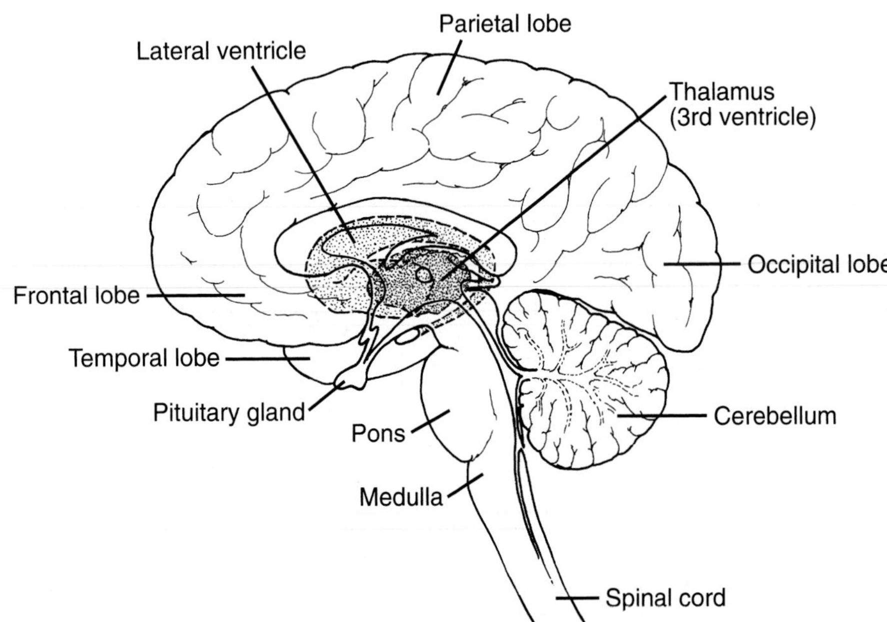

Figure 9–1 The basic anatomy of the brain as seen on a sagittal view of the midline.

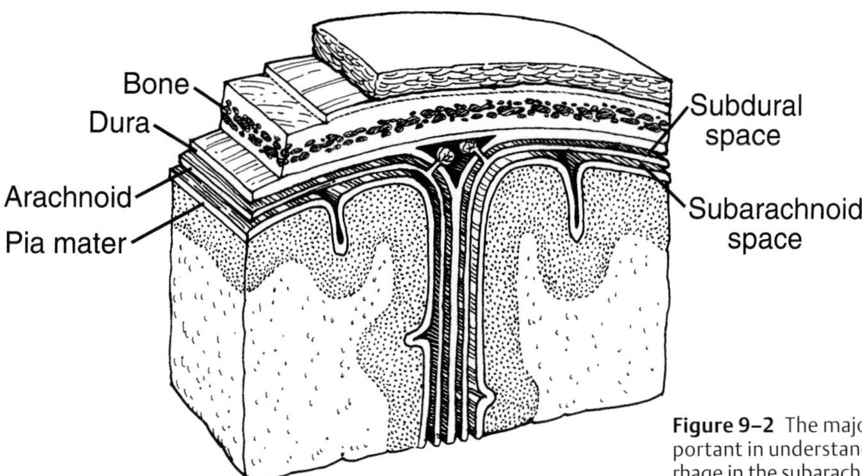

Figure 9–2 The major protective coverings of the brain, which are important in understanding the appearance of processes such as hemorrhage in the subarachnoid, subdural, and epidural spaces.

sulci (**Fig. 9–2**). A subarachnoid hemorrhage will extend down into cerebral sulci, while a subdural hematoma will not.

The brain is cushioned both internally and externally by the cerebrospinal fluid (CSF), which is produced by the choroid plexus of the lateral, third, and fourth ventricles, and is absorbed by the arachnoid granulations in the region of the superior sagittal sinus. The normal CSF production and absorption rate is ~30 mL per hour. The normal circulation and drainage of CSF can be impeded at several critical points, including the foramen of Monro (connecting the lateral ventricles with the third ventricle), the aqueduct of Sylvius (connecting the third and fourth ventricles), and the foramen of Magendie and Luschka, where CSF leaves the ventricular system and circulates in the subarachnoid space around the brain and cord (**Fig. 9–3**). Obstruction to either flow or resorption may result in hydrocephalus.

The brain's other protective structure is the microscopic blood–brain barrier, which prevents most blood-borne substances from leaving the CNS capillaries and entering surrounding tissues. The blood–brain barrier is made up of glial cell foot processes and tight junctions between capillary endothelial cells. Only simple sugars, oxygen, carbon dioxide, amino acids, and lipid-soluble substances such as anesthetic

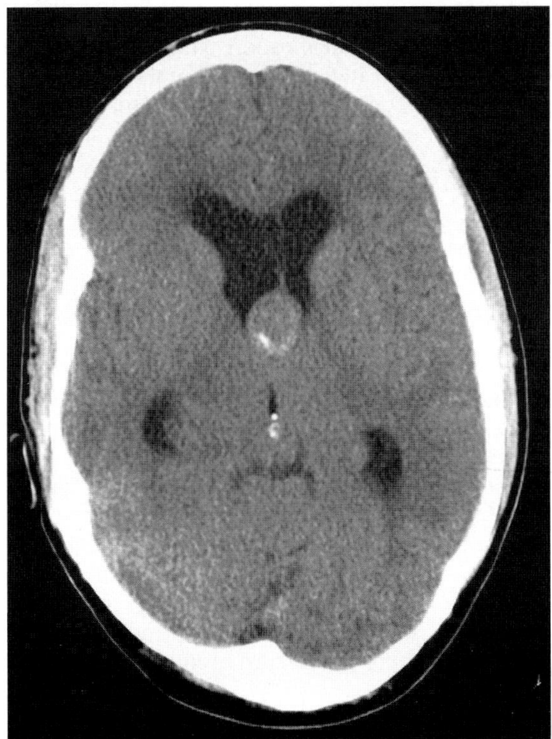

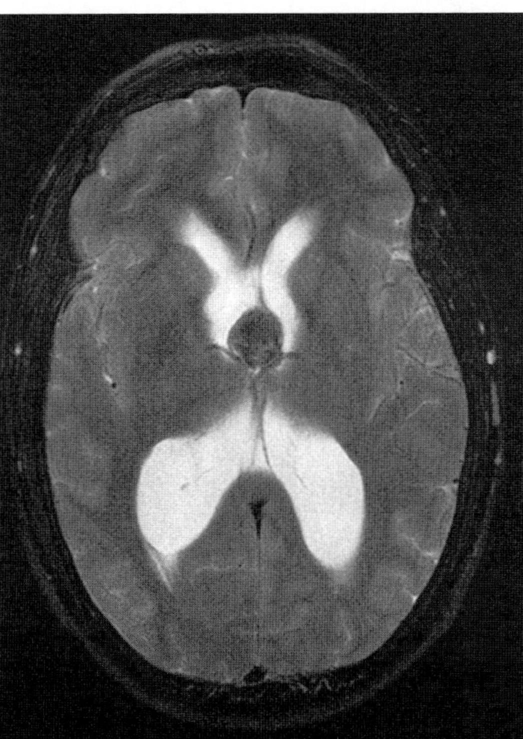

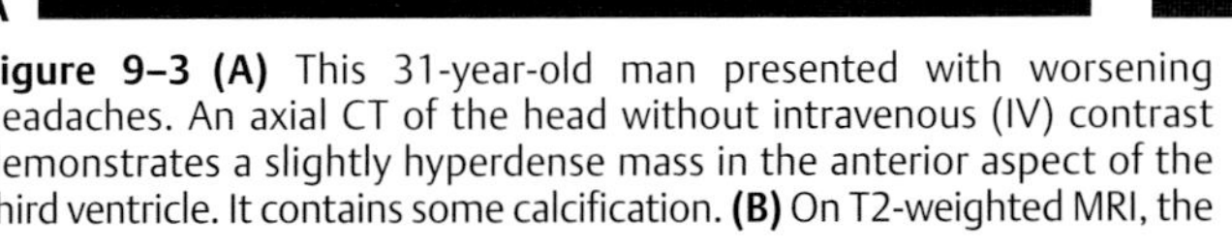

Figure 9–3 (A) This 31-year-old man presented with worsening headaches. An axial CT of the head without intravenous (IV) contrast demonstrates a slightly hyperdense mass in the anterior aspect of the third ventricle. It contains some calcification. **(B)** On T2-weighted MRI, the mass is hypodense to brain. There is enlargement of the lateral ventricles with transependymal flow of cerebrospinal fluid (CSF) into the adjacent brain parenchyma. These imaging findings are typical of a colloid cyst, in this case obstructing the foramen of Monro and causing hydrocephalus.

gases can pass through it. Even alterations in serum potassium ion concentration produce little change in its concentration in CSF. This prevents circulating hormones that can also act as neurotransmitters from wreaking havoc in the brain, and also screens out a variety of foreign chemicals and microorganisms. Unfortunately, the human immunodeficiency virus (HIV) is able to circumvent this defense, probably entering the CNS in macrophages. Moreover, the blood–brain barrier can prove an obstacle in eradicating certain neoplasms, such as lymphoma, from the brain, and chemotherapeutic agents often must be administered directly into the CSF. Leakiness in the blood–brain barrier, which may accompany processes such as tumor and infection, is responsible for contrast enhancement, as discussed later.

The brain is critically dependent on a constant blood supply. It receives ~15% of resting cardiac output and consumes 20% of the body's oxygen supply. Because it is incapable of anaerobic metabolism, it requires oxygen to produce adenosine triphosphate (ATP). Moreover, the brain has no glucose stores. Thus, an interruption in the brain's oxygen supply for more than 5 minutes or its glucose supply for more than 15 minutes results in irreparable brain damage. The availability of oxygen can be reduced due to hypoxia (as in asphyxiation) or ischemia (as in hypotension or vessel occlusion). The blood supply of the brain arrives by four principal arteries: the paired internal carotid arteries and the paired vertebral arteries (**Fig. 9–4**). The internal carotid arteries arise at the carotid bifurcation in the neck and represent the primary supply of the anterior and middle cerebral arteries; the vertebral arteries represent the first branches of the subclavian arteries and constitute the primary supply of the posterior circulation. The circle of Willis provides a built-in backup system in the event that one of these vessels should be compromised, with connections between the internal carotid arteries and the posterior circulation via the posterior communicating arteries (**Fig. 9–5**); however, the circle is complete in only 25% of patients. The venous drainage of the brain is directed toward the occiput, eventually emptying into the internal jugular veins.

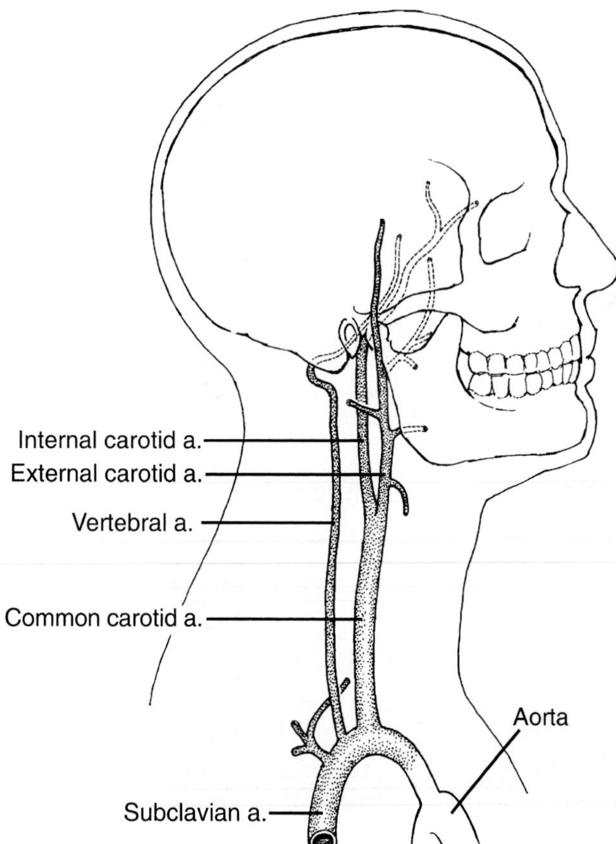

Figure 9–4 The course of the carotid and vertebral arteries in a lateral projection as they course toward the brain.

◆ Imaging

Choice of Modality

Plain radiography plays essentially no role in evaluation of the CNS, although it can be very useful in evaluating bony lesions of the skull and spine, such as bone tumors and fractures. In adults, ultrasound is used to assess the carotid arteries, and angiography is used as a secondary study to assess for vascular stenoses, aneurysms, and the like. In the acute setting, however, the choice is between CT and MRI (**Fig. 9–6**). The widespread clinical application of CT antedated that of MRI by ~15 years, and, although MRI has supplanted CT in many clinical settings, CT remains the modality of choice in several important situations. In general, the advantages of CT over MRI include speed (examinations lasting minutes rather than tens of minutes or even hours), cost, and wide availability. CT is more sensitive than MRI for the detection of small amounts of calcification, which can be helpful in diagnosing tumors that frequently contain calcifications. Moreover, even if all other factors were equal, noncontrast CT would be the preferred modality in most acute settings because of its superior ability to detect acute hemorrhage, and because the CT scanner is a much more hospitable environment for the seriously ill patient, whose presence in the radiology department often requires a retinue of monitoring and life support equipment and personnel. Examples of settings where a noncontrast CT generally remains the examination of choice include acute trauma, acute stroke, severe acute headache, and acute coma.

There are, however, acute situations in which MRI is clearly superior to CT, for example, to evaluate suspected spinal cord compression. Like the brain, the spinal cord does not respond well to lesions exerting mass effect upon it, as in trauma or neoplasms involving the spine or its contents. In the case of a patient presenting with the acute onset of neurologic deficits such as lower extremity weakness, paresthesias, or the loss of bowel or bladder control, MRI is the study of choice to rule out cord compression and should be performed urgently, before sustained pressure on the cord produces an irreversible neurologic deficit.

In the vast majority of nonacute clinical settings, MRI is superior to CT. Although CT is generally confined to imaging in the axial plane (coronal scanning is often used in imaging osseous structures and the paranasal sinuses), MRI is capable of multiplanar imaging (axial, coronal, sagittal, and obliques),

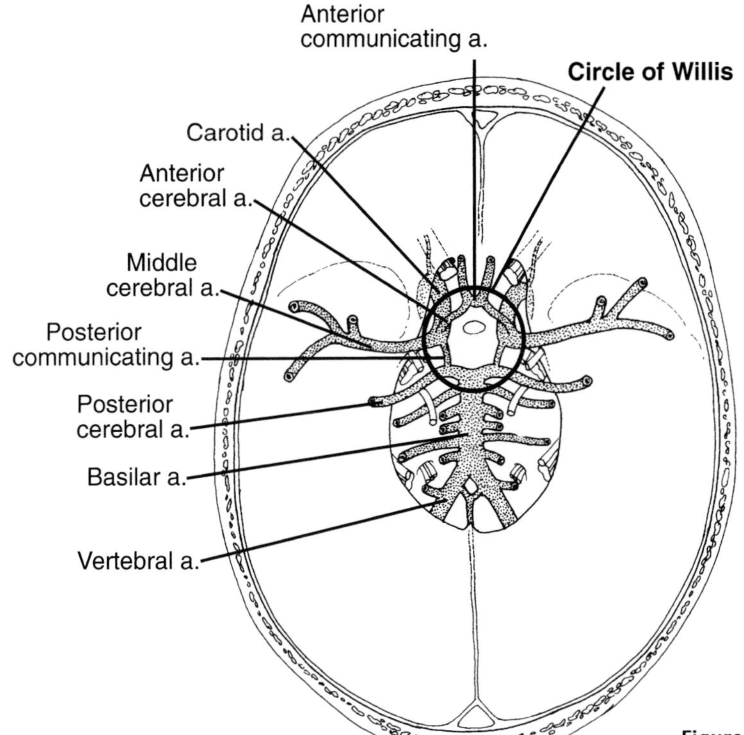

Figure 9–5 The major vessels of the intracranial circulation, including the circle of Willis.

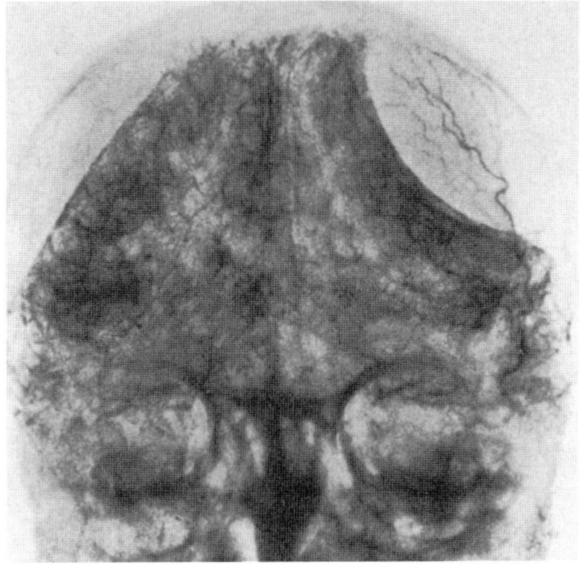

Figure 9–6 This frontal image from a bilateral internal carotid artery angiogram provides some indication of how far neuroimaging has progressed since the 1970s. This patient suffered from chronic bilateral subdural hematomas, which can be seen displacing the enhancing vessels of the cerebral parenchyma inferiomedially, away from the inner table of the skull. Prior to the advent of computed tomography, angiography represented a primary modality in the diagnosis of such lesions, the presence of which could be inferred by the displacement of normal vessels. Today, however, the diagnosis of a subdural hematoma can be rendered much more rapidly, inexpensively, and with less risk via a CT scan (or MRI).

and these multiplanar capabilities can be further customized to answer specific questions about the extent of lesions and their impact on adjacent structures (**Fig. 9–7**).

MRI provides greater differentiation of gray and white matter structures, is more sensitive for the detection of subacute and chronic bleeds, and generally provides a more detailed and precise view of anatomic structures. MRI can be used to determine the structure and patency of vascular structures with greater sensitivity than CT, and even without the use of intravascular contrast agents. CT is relatively poor at visualizing soft tissue structures surrounded by or adjacent to large amounts of bone, such as the inferior temporal lobes, which produce so-called streak artifact, whereas MRI is immune to this problem. Situations in which MRI generally represents the study of choice include suspected tumor or infection, nonacute trauma, seizures, chronic headache, and dementia.

When faced with the decision of which neuroimaging study to order, the physician should consider consulting a radiologist; however, in the vast majority of cases, the following guidelines should hold. If the process in question began less than 48 hours prior to imaging, noncontrast CT is a logical starting point. If the findings suggest a tumor or abscess, consider contrast infusion, which will increase the sensitivity due to the differential enhancement patterns of normal and abnormal tissues. If concern for vascular pathology such as stroke is high, contrast should probably be withheld, because extravasated iodinated contrast may increase edema in the vicinity of the lesion, exacerbating mass effect on surrounding normal parenchyma. If the process is older than 48 hours,

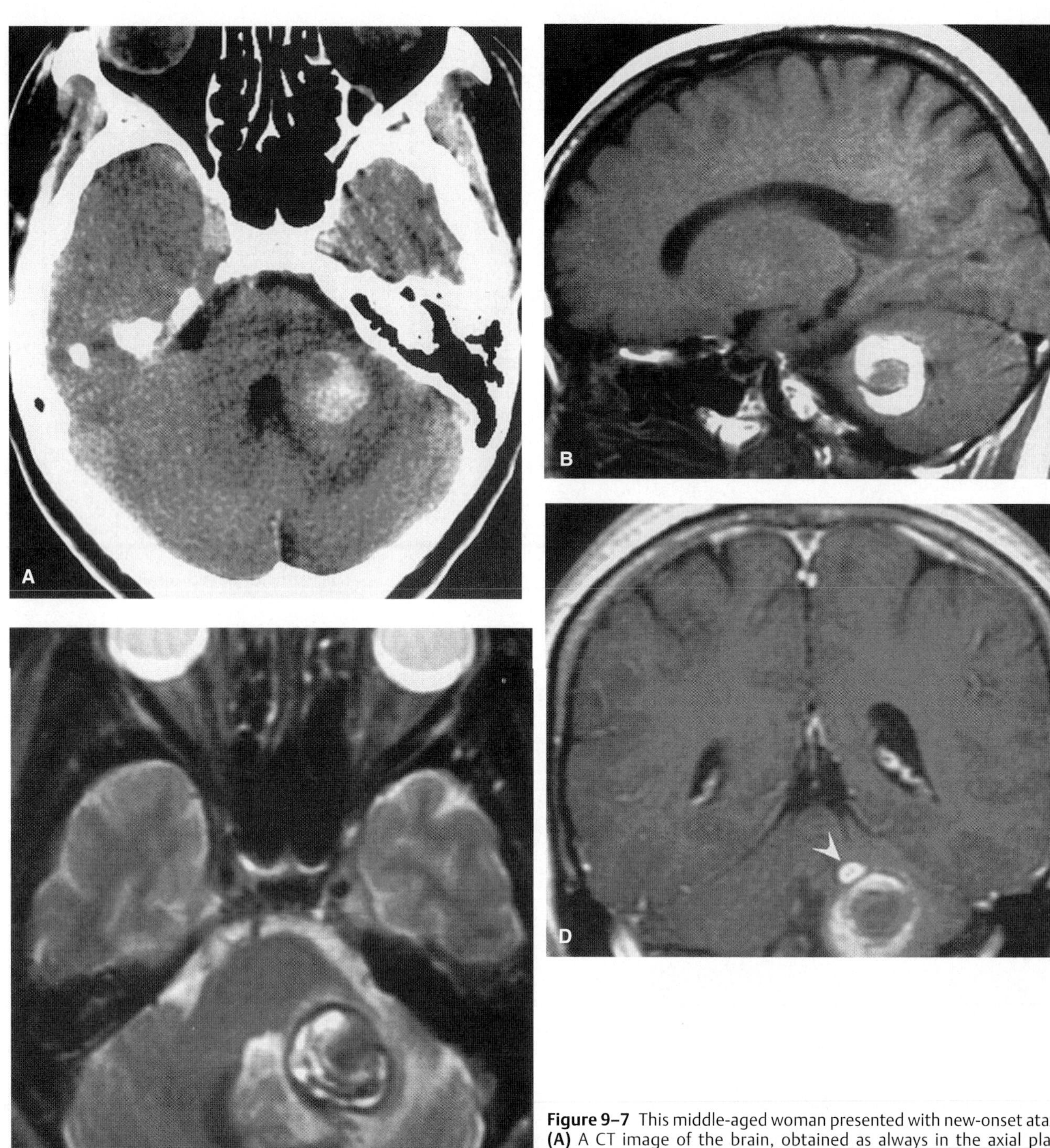

Figure 9–7 This middle-aged woman presented with new-onset ataxia. **(A)** A CT image of the brain, obtained as always in the axial plane, demonstrates a dense lesion in the left cerebellar peduncle, likely representing acute hemorrhage. Sagittal TI **(B)**, axial T2 **(C)**, and coronal T1 postcontrast. **(D)** MR images better demonstrate the mass's location and relationship to adjacent structures. The mass was a cavernous malformation that had bled acutely. (Reprinted with permission from Fischbein, Dillon, Barkovich, eds. Teaching Atlas of Brain Imaging. New York: Thieme; 2000:272,273, figs. A–D.)

begin where possible with MRI. Gadolinium should be given if a primary or metastatic neoplasm is a strong consideration, if the patient suffers seizures, or if the patient has localizing neurologic symptoms. Particularly in the case of MRI, which can be performed in many different planes with many different pulse sequences, good clinical history is imperative in enabling the radiologist to tailor the examination to the clinical situation. There are exceptions to the 48-hour rule. For example, it is important to recognize herpes encephalitis as early as possible, and MRI is much superior to CT in demonstrating characteristic inflammatory changes in the frontal and temporal lobes.

Comparison of T1- and T2-Weighted MRI

MRI of the brain generally includes T1- and T2-like sequences. T1-weighted images usually provide the greatest anatomic detail, whereas T2-weighted images are preferred for evaluating pathologic lesions. Why? Most processes that involve inflammation or neoplasia are accompanied by some disturbance of the blood–brain barrier, rendering the capillary endothelium in the region "leakier." This leakiness permits the extravasation of proteins and solutes into the surrounding tissue, with a resultant increase in interstitial osmolality, which draws water to the area. This increase in water is represented on T2-weighted images as increased brightness. Hence, abnormally "bright" or high-signal regions on T2-weighted images should be regarded with suspicion (**Fig. 9–8**). In addition to signal abnormality (which, as we will see, involves more than just abnormal water content), another category of abnormality to look for on MRI is mass effect, the displacement of normal structures from their usual positions by a pathologic lesion.

How does one determine whether an MR image of the CNS is T1- or T2-weighted? First, it is important to note that not all images are either T1- or T2-weighted. For example, so-called proton density images rely on a technique that minimizes the effects of the T1 and T2 characteristics of tissues and highlights the differences in their proton density. One way to determine if an image is T1- or T2-weighted is to determine the time of repetition (TR) and time to echo (TE) settings utilized in the scan, by looking at the scan data. TR is a measure of the time protons are given between radiofrequency pulses to align with the main magnetic field, and TE is a measure of the time allowed for the energy absorbed from the radiofrequency pulse to be released. T1-weighted images have a short TR (<800 msec) and short TE (<30 msec). T2-weighted images have a long TR (>2000 msec) and long TE (>60 msec). Proton density images, in contrast, have a long TR and a short TE. Diffusion-weighted imaging, a sequence that relies on a different physical property, can be useful for the detection of processes such as acute stroke, which appear as regions of increased signal intensity.

Even if the scan parameters are not known, however, T1- and T2-weighted images can be differentiated based on the fact that water (including CSF) appears dark (or low signal) on T1 and bright (or high signal) on T2. Fat, by contrast, appears bright on T1 and dark (compared with water) on T2. Hence, the CSF in the ventricles will appear dark on T1-weighted images and bright on T2-weighted images,

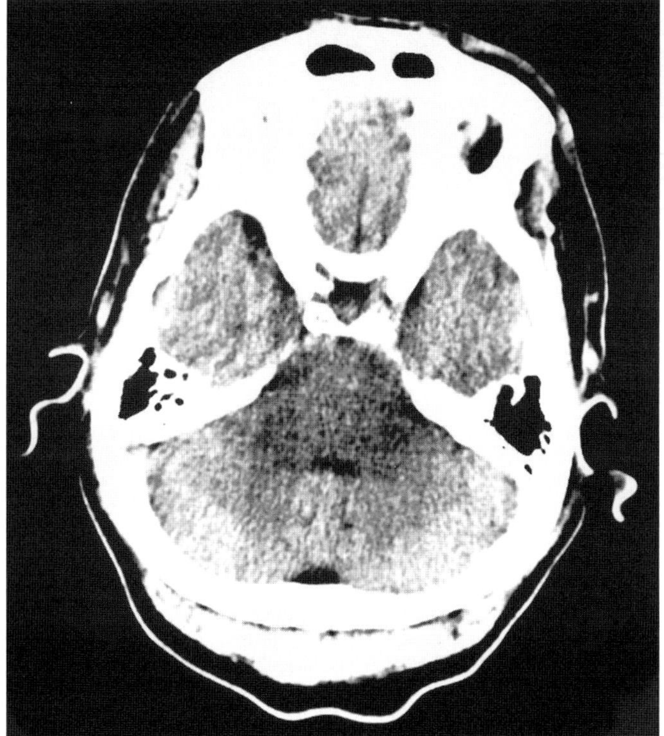

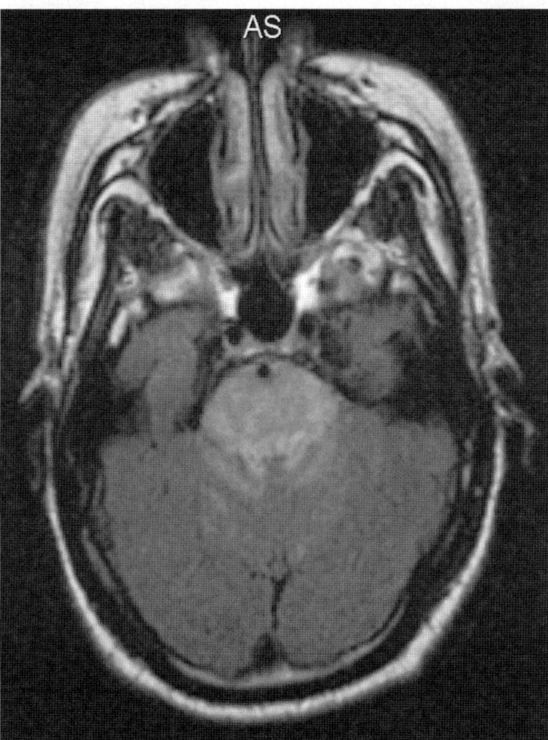

Figure 9–8 (A) This axial CT image demonstrates the obscuration of brain parenchyma that can result from close proximity to a large osseous structure, such as at the skull base. There is a suggestion of general hypodensity in the midbrain and pons, but might this merely reflect streak artifact? **(B)** This T2-weighted axial MR image clearly shows that there is abnormal increased signal in this region. The hypodensity (darkness) on CT and hyperintensity (brightness) on T2 MRI both reflect increased water content in this patient with a diffuse brainstem glioma.

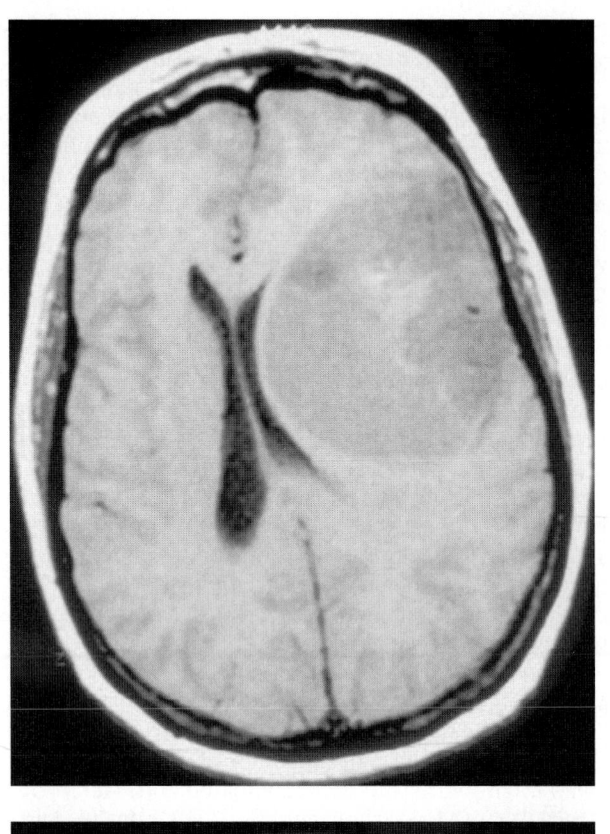

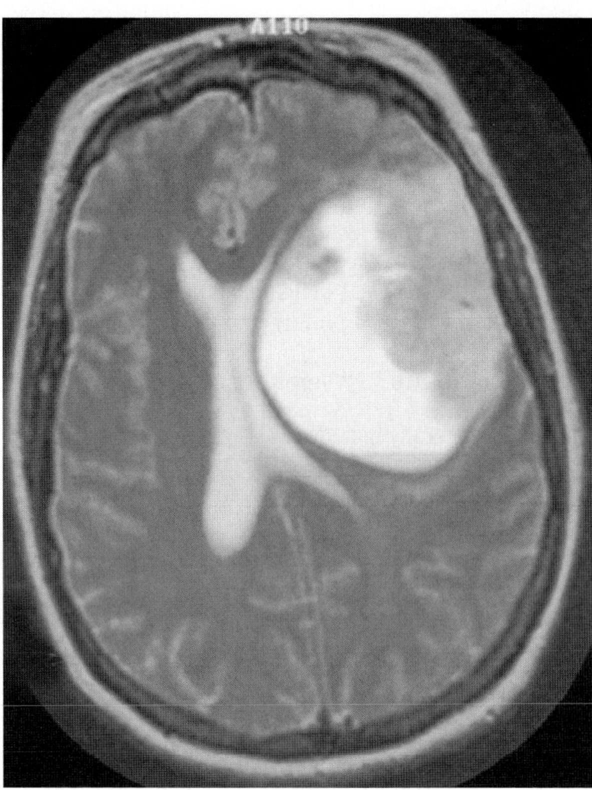

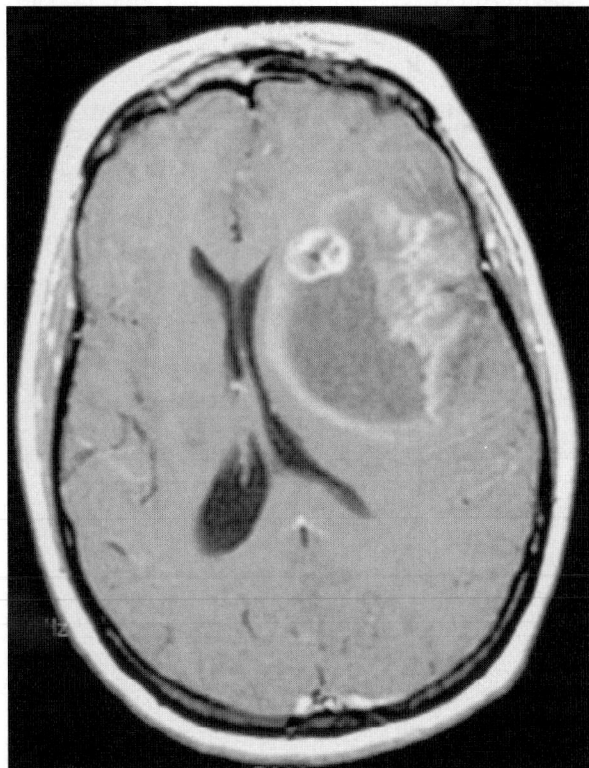

Figure 9–9 **(A)** This T1-weighted axial MR image demonstrates a large mass in the left frontal lobe. Note that the CSF in the lateral ventricles is dark on T1, and the subcutaneous fat of the scalp is bright. **(B)** On the T2-weighted image, the CSF is now bright, and the subcutaneous fat is relatively dark. **(C)** On this image, the CSF is dark, but peripheral portions of the lesion appear bright. Why? This is a postcontrast T1-weighted image, and the bright rim reflects peripheral enhancement in this largely necrotic glioblastoma multiforme.

and the lipid-rich myelin of the white matter will appear brighter than the gray matter on T1-weighted images and darker than the gray matter on T2-weighted images (**Fig. 9–9**).

Contrast Enhancement in CT and MRI

To interpret examinations in which intravenous contrast material was administered, it is important to understand the mechanisms of contrast enhancement in both CT and MRI. As previously noted, "enhancement" occurs when an anatomic structure or lesion becomes more conspicuous after the administration of intravascular contrast. CT enhancement occurs on the basis of the increased attenuation of the x-ray beam by iodine-containing molecules. MRI enhancement relies on the T1-shortening effect of gadolinium-containing molecules. From a diagnostic point of view, the fact that a structure or lesion does not enhance may be just as important as the fact that it does.

In interpreting an examination, how does one determine whether contrast material was utilized? One means of doing so is to inspect the scan data accompanying the images, looking for such telltale indications as "C+," "postinfusion," or the brand name of the contrast agent, all of which suggest that contrast material was used; however, a superior method of detecting contrast infusion is to look for increased "brightness" in structures that should normally enhance. In CT, this means inspecting the most highly vascular structures of the head, such as the cerebral vessels and the dura mater. In MRI, the best place to look is the richly vascular erectile tissues of the nasal mucosa, as well as the pituitary gland and the dura mater of the cavernous sinus.

Having said that the cerebral vessels enhance with contrast infusion on CT, why is contrast enhancement of the vessels not visible when contrast is administered in MRI? On standard T1- and T2-weighted imaging, the flow of blood within the cerebral arteries and veins is rapid enough that vascular structures are seen as so-called flow voids. The reason is that protons in the flowing blood move out of the plane of imaging in the time that elapses between the absorption of the energy of the radio wave pulse and the detection of its release, meaning that rapidly flowing blood produces no signal. The "flow void" phenomenon occurs both in blood and in any imaged structure moving at sufficient velocity relative to the imaging apparatus. If the patient's head were moving at sufficient speed, the entire head, too, would not be visible. Under normal conditions, however, the blood is the only substance moving with sufficient velocity to produce the flow void phenomenon. The nasal mucosa does enhance because the blood in it is moving very slowly. This principle can be of immense clinical value. For example, a thrombus, which is stationary, appears as a intravascular soft tissue signal where a flow void would have been expected (**Fig. 9–10**).

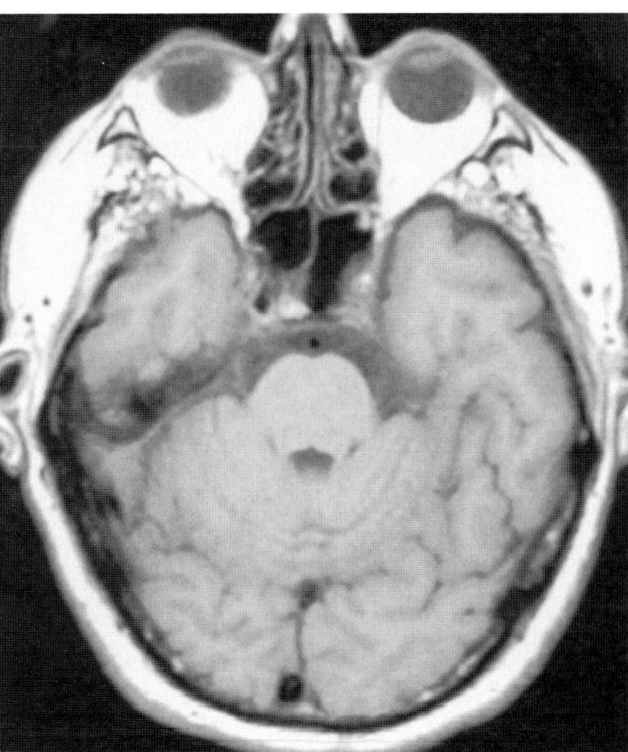

Figure 9–10 This T2-weighted MR image demonstrates a normal flow void in the right internal carotid artery, but absence of the expected flow void on the left. This patient presented with a left-sided stroke, due to thrombotic occlusion of the left internal carotid artery.

With respect to CNS imaging, contrast enhancement may be divided into two phases. The first is the intravascular phase, which lasts so long as a sufficient concentration of contrast agent is present within the vascular lumen, whether that of arteries, veins, or capillaries. This is essentially the only phase of enhancement seen on conventional angiography and is also clearly visible on CT (which is why we can inspect the cerebral vasculature to determine if the examination was performed with contrast infusion). The gray matter is several times as vascular as the white matter (because it contains cells that are 3 to 4 times more active metabolically); hence, the parenchyma of the gray matter will tend to enhance more than the white matter in the intravascular phase. However, intravascular enhancement does not occur on routine T1- and T2-weighted MR images, where a flow void is seen instead. Other MR sequences, such as time-of-flight angiography, can make flowing blood appear bright, even without the use of contrast material.

The second phase, the interstitial phase, is seen with both CT and MRI contrast infusion. To understand how the interstitial phase of contrast enhancement occurs, it is necessary to briefly discuss the blood–brain barrier. The blood–brain barrier is found in 99% of the brain's volume, and, as previously discussed, represents the seal formed by the tight junctions between closely abutting capillary endothelial cells. In addition, there is relatively little pinocytosis across the capillary cells of the brain, with the exception of metabolic substrates as glucose. Of course, certain areas of the brain are notable for the absence of a blood–brain barrier, such as the pituitary gland, chemoreceptors in areas of the brain connected to the brainstem vomiting center, and the dura, and these areas normally exhibit contrast enhancement. The pituitary gland and the vomiting center do not have a blood–brain barrier, because to perform their functions (regulating the serum concentrations of various hormones and ridding the body of potential poisons, respectively), access of brain cells to the chemical contents of the blood must be preserved (**Fig. 9–11**). As a result of the blood–brain barrier, the relatively high molecular weight, nonlipophilic contrast agents used in CT and MRI cannot cross normal brain capillaries into the interstitium of the brain.

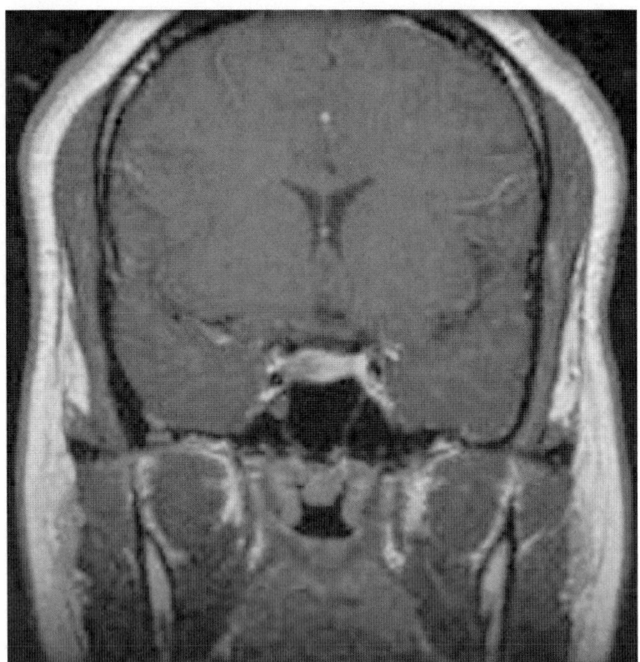

Figure 9–11 This coronal T1-weighted MR image at the sellar region was obtained after gadolinium–pentetic acid (DTPA) infusion. It demonstrates a hypointense mass in the right lobe of the pituitary gland. This is a pituitary microadenoma. Why is it less intensely enhanced (darker) than the normal left lobe? Because the normal pituitary gland lacks a blood–brain barrier and enhances more intensely than the tumor.

If contrast agents cannot cross the blood–brain barrier, of what use are they in diagnostic imaging? The answer is that, although they cannot cross the blood–brain barrier when it is intact, they can cross it when it is disrupted. Generally speaking, the blood–brain barrier is disrupted by acute inflammation (as in demyelinating diseases such as multiple sclerosis, where chemical mediators increase capillary permeability), neoplasm (where the capillaries formed in conjunction with the growing tumor possess an abnormal endothelium), infection (which produces inflammation), and ischemia (which damages the endothelial cells of capillaries along with the parenchymal cells). In these cases, contrast leaks out of defective vessels into the interstitium, and the surrounding parenchyma demonstrates enhancement (**Fig. 9–12**).

Different pathologic processes tend to produce characteristic patterns of enhancement.

Search Pattern in MRI

To ensure that common and important abnormalities are not missed, it is helpful to develop an ordered approach to the brain. In MRI, images are usually obtained in sagittal, axial, and coronal dimensions. Beginning with the midline sagittal view, examine the corpus callosum (the major connection between the two cerebral hemispheres, subject to partial or complete agenesis in several conditions), the aqueduct of Sylvius (connecting the third and fourth ventricles, and associated with hydrocephalus in aqueductal

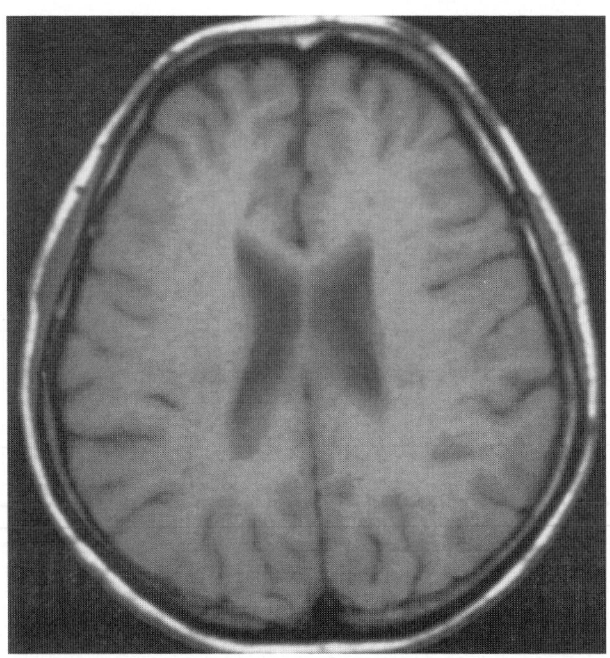

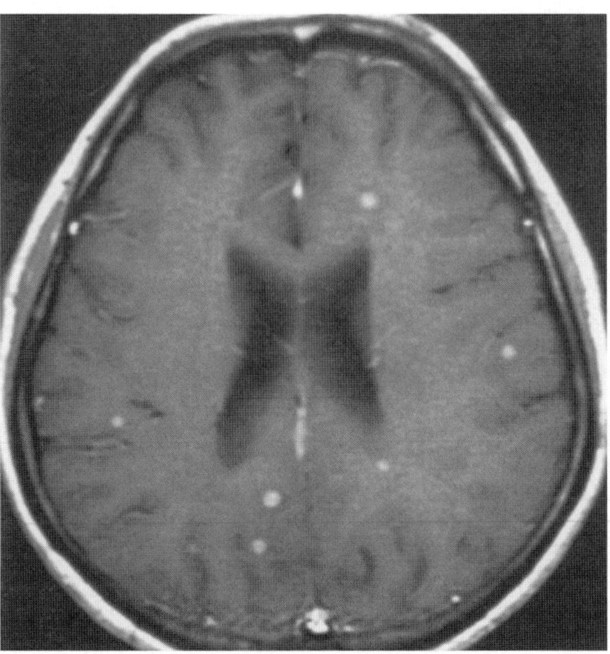

Figure 9–12 **(A)** This 5-year-old boy presented with new-onset seizure, having complained for several days of headache and low-grade fever. His axial T1-weighted MR image appears unremarkable. **(B)** After administration of IV contrast, however, multiple nodular areas of abnormal enhancement are visible at gray-white matter junctions. The diagnosis is miliary tuberculosis. Different pathologic processes tend to produce characteristic patterns of enhancement. (Reprinted with permission from Fischbein, Dillon, Barkovich, eds. Teaching Atlas of Brain Imaging. New York: Thieme, TK:165, figs. B,C.)

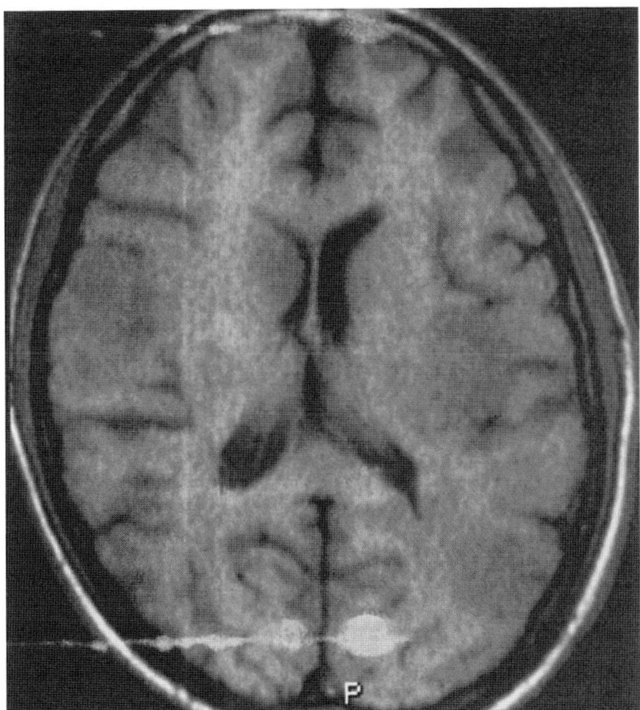

FIGURE 9–13 This human immunodeficiency virus (HIV)–positive patient presented with seizure. An axial T1-weighted MR image shows several areas of abnormal signal, but note the mass effect on the frontal horn of the right lateral ventricle, making it appear slitlike compared with the left. The mass in the right caudate nucleus represented a central nervous system (CNS) lymphoma. (Reprinted with permission from Fischbein, Dillon, Barkovich, eds. Teaching Atlas of Brain Imaging. New York: Thieme, TK:32, fig. A.)

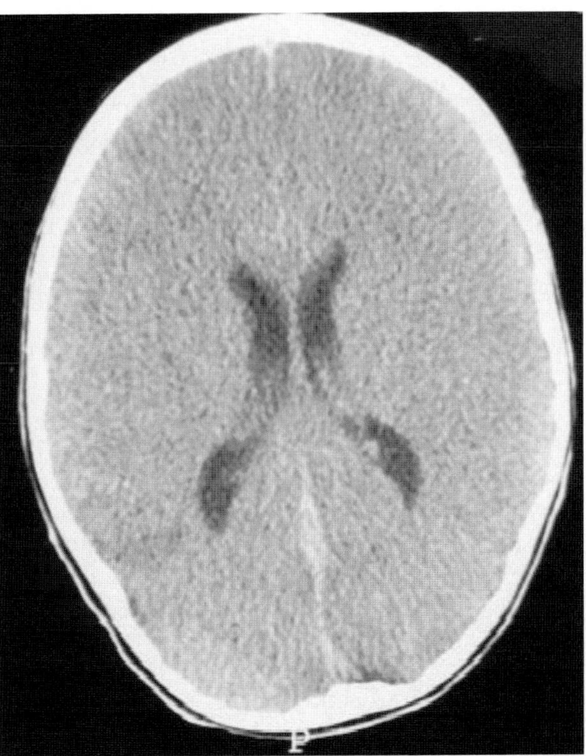

Figure 9–14 An axial CT image demonstrates a diffuse decrease in the density of the brain parenchyma with loss of the normal density difference between gray matter and white matter. This patient suffered prolonged hypoglycemia, with severe acute brain injury.

stenosis), and the optic chiasm and pituitary gland (pituitary tumors may compress the optic chiasm from below, producing bitemporal hemianopsia). Posterior fossa structures to be evaluated include the brainstem, the fourth ventricle, and the position of the cerebellar tonsils, which are inferiorly displaced in an Arnold-Chiari malformation.

On axial images, key structures to assess include the orbits and sinuses, the brainstem, thalamus, basal ganglia, cerebellum, and the frontal, parietal, temporal, and occipital lobes of the brain. Key features to evaluate include the symmetry of the intracranial structures, with special attention to the presence of asymmetric signal abnormalities (as in hemorrhage or tumor); masses or mass effect (displacement of adjacent structures, such as ventricles) (**Fig. 9–13**); midline shift (e.g., subfalcine herniation); extra-axial fluid collections (subdural and epidural hematomas); effacement of ventricles and sulci (as in increased intracranial pressure); and loss of the normally clear demarcation between gray and white matter (diffuse anoxia with edema) (**Fig. 9–14**). When an abnormal space-occupying lesion is detected, determining its location is critical.

◆ Pathology

Congenital

Congenital disorders of the CNS are also discussed in Chapter 7's section on obstetrical sonography. There are numerous types of congenital CNS lesions, but three of the most important are neural tube closure defects, migrational anomalies, and the phakomatoses. One of the most common neural tube closure defects is a Chiari type II malformation (Arnold-Chiari malformation), which is related to the presence of a smaller than normal posterior fossa. The cramped posterior fossa results in herniation of the cerebellar tonsils and vermis through the foramen magnum and compression of the fourth ventricle, with resultant hydrocephalus that may be amenable to surgical decompression (**Fig. 9–15**).

Migrational abnormalities result from the arrested migration of neurons from the subependymal regions outward toward the cortical surface, with gray matter cells ending up where they do not belong. One such migrational abnormality is schizencephaly, in which a cleft of gray matter extends from the cortical surface down to one of the ventricles. Such migrational abnormalities, which are usually associated with abnormal cerebral electrical activity, must be borne in mind when imaging a child who presents with seizures.

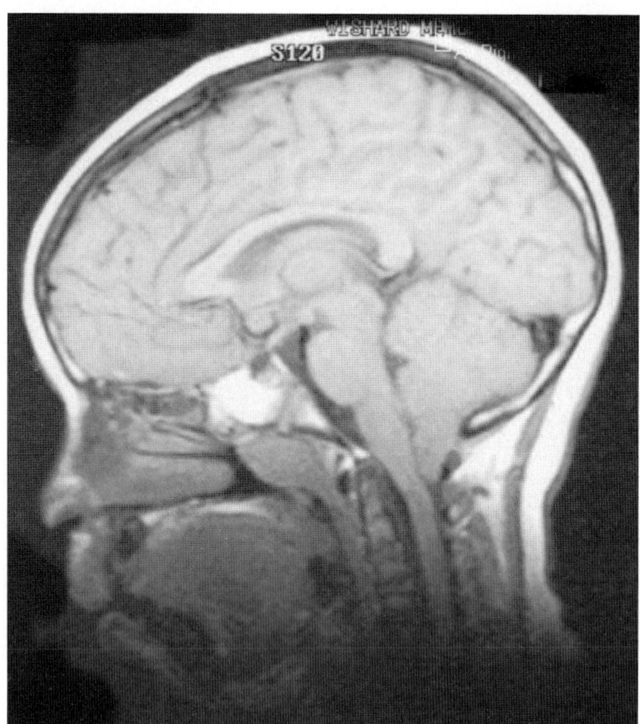

Figure 9–15 This sagittal T1-weighted MR image demonstrates extension of the cerebellar tonsils down through the foramen magnum, diagnostic of a Chiari I malformation. Similar displacement can be seen in the more complex Chiari II malformation, which is almost always associated with a myelomeningocele.

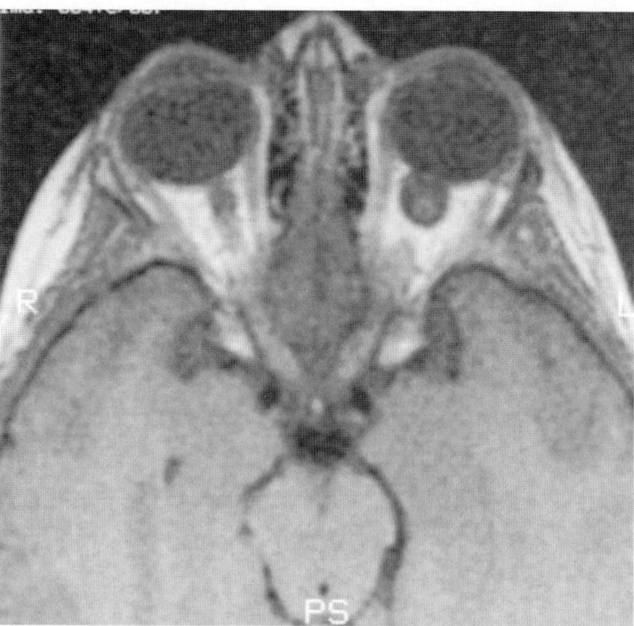

Figure 9–16 This T1-weighted axial MR image of the orbits demonstrates a left optic nerve glioma and dilation of the nerve sheath in a patient with neurofibromatosis type I. Note that there is also a smaller lesion on the right.

Phakomatoses

The phakomatoses are neuroectodermal disorders characterized by coexistent skin and CNS hamartomas and neoplasms. Among the most common are neurofibromatosis types I and II, tuberous sclerosis, von Hippel-Lindau disease, and Sturge-Weber syndrome. Neurofibromatosis type I (NF-I) is the most common phakomatosis, found in 1 in 3000 persons, half of whom represent spontaneous mutations and half of whom inherited the disorder via an autosomal dominant route. It is associated with abnormalities of chromosome 17. It is associated clinically with cutaneous café au lait spots and axillary or inguinal freckling, among other findings. Neuroimaging findings include optic nerve gliomas and spinal neurofibromas (**Fig. 9–16**).

Skeletal findings in NF-I related to the presence of neurofibromas include a sharply angled kyphosis of the spine, twisted ribs, and pseudoarthroses (due to improper healing of a tibial bowing fracture). NF-II is considerably less common, seen in 1 in 50,000 persons, and is associated with chromosome 22 defects. Imaging findings include bilateral eighth cranial nerve schwannomas, as well as meningiomas (**Fig. 9–17**).

Tuberous sclerosis is characterized by the clinical triad of mental retardation, seizures, and "adenoma sebaceum," and is inherited in an autosomal dominant fashion in up to 50% of cases. Imaging findings include multiple CNS tubers (hamartomas), angiomyolipomas in the kidneys, and spontaneous pneumothorax in up to 50% of patients (**Fig. 9–18**).

Von Hippel-Lindau disease, incidence 1 in 40,000, is inherited in autosomal dominant fashion and represents the most life-threatening of the phakomatoses discussed here. It is associated with cerebellar hemangioblastomas and/or renal cell carcinomas in 40% of patients, as well as pheochromocytomas and retinal angiomas and pancreatic cysts (**Fig. 9–19**).

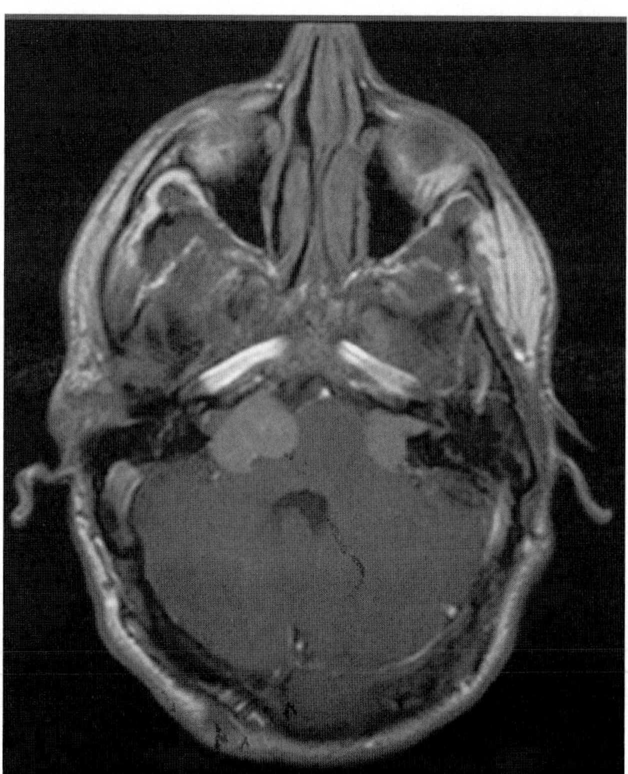

FIGURE 9–17 A post-contrast T1-weighted axial MR image of the brain demonstrates bilateral cerebellopontine angle masses involving both internal auditory canals. These are vestibular schwannomas in a patient with neurofibromatosis type II.

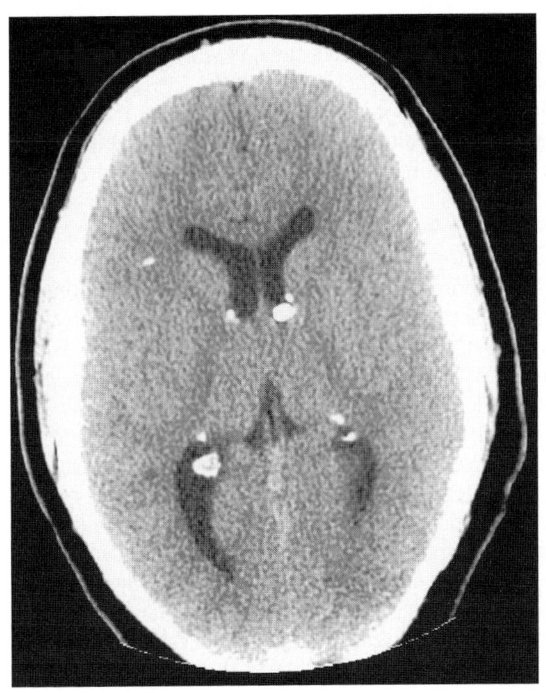

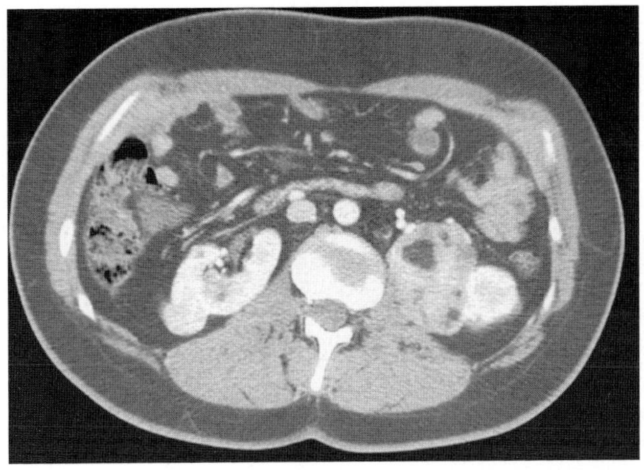

Figure 9–18 (A) This noncontrast head CT image demonstrates bilateral calcific nodules, most in a periventricular location. **(B)** An axial CT image of the abdomen after IV contrast demonstrates bilateral renal masses. Note that the left-sided mass clearly contains fat. This patient has tuberous sclerosis, with cerebral tubers and renal angiomyolipomas.

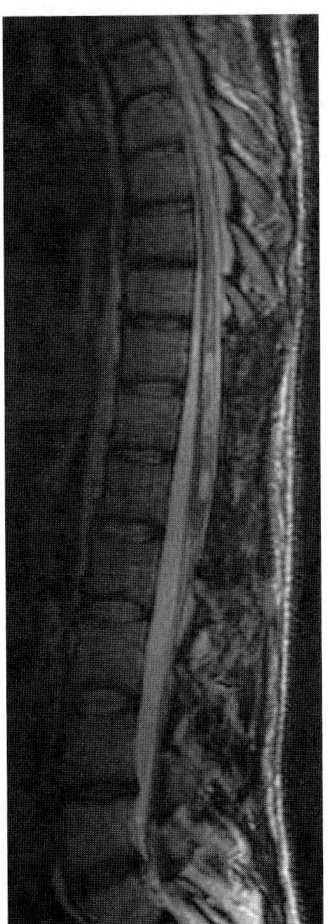

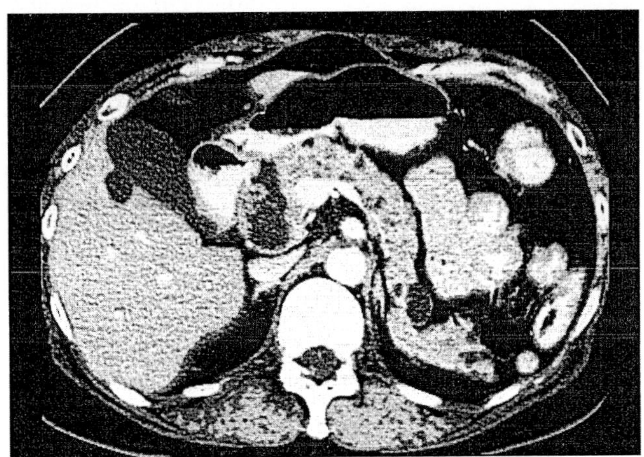

Figure 9–19 (A) This sagittal T2-weighted image demonstrates multiple high-intensity lesions in the spinal cord, representing spinal hemangioblastomas. **(B)** The axial CT image after IV and oral contrast shows multiple pancreatic cysts and a single liver cyst. The patient had von Hippel-Lindau disease.

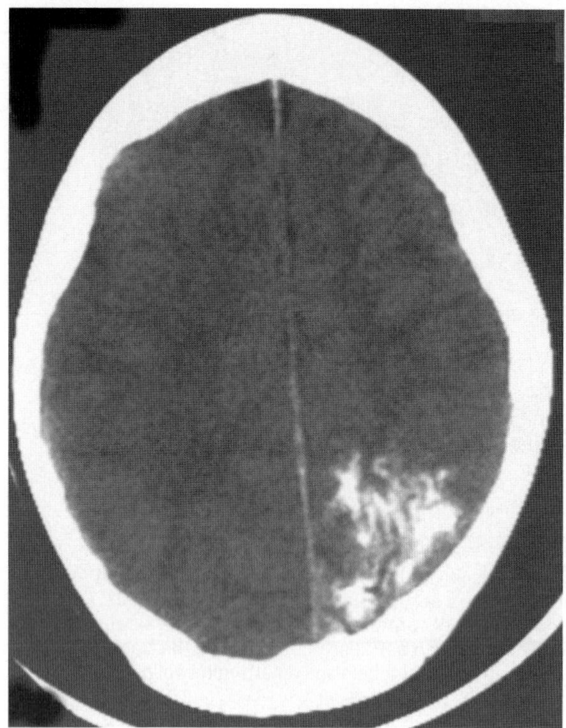

Figure 9–20 An axial CT image demonstrates left-hemispheric atrophy and gyriform calcification in the posterior aspect of the left cerebral hemisphere in this patient with Sturge-Weber syndrome.

Sturge-Weber syndrome involves ipsilateral capillary angiomas of the face (port-wine nevus of the first division of the trigeminal nerve) and the cerebral hemisphere. Imaging findings include a highly characteristic pattern of unilateral curvilinear calcification that follows the convolutions of the brain, better detected on CT than MRI (**Fig. 9–20**).

Inflammatory

Multiple Sclerosis

◇ Epidemiology

Multiple sclerosis (MS) is a relatively common disorder, afflicting ~350,000 Americans, two thirds of whom are women. Each year, ~10,000 new cases are diagnosed, most frequently in patients between the ages of 20 and 40 years. Curiously, MS is virtually unknown in arctic and tropical climates, and is most common in the temperate regions of Europe and the United States, although the risk profile of adults depends not on where they live now, but where they spend their first 15 years. Unfortunately, a significant percentage of patients, approximately one third, eventually develop severe disability, including the loss of ambulation, and two thirds of patients eventually lose their jobs due to the disease; however, it is not associated with a large increase in mortality, and the average patient lives with the disease for 40 years.

◇ Pathophysiology

Multiple sclerosis belongs to a major class of neurologic diseases, the demyelinating diseases. In contrast to the dysmyelinating diseases, such as adrenoleukodystrophy, in which the myelin that is produced is abnormal, the demyelinating disorders are associated with the subsequent destruction of initially normal myelin. Normally, the axons of the CNS are enveloped along their course by spiraled layers of the myelin sheath, which are produced by oligodendrogliocytes (while myelin in the peripheral nervous system is the product of Schwann's cells). Myelin sheaths with intervening nodes of Ranvier permit saltatory conduction of axonal impulses, which renders conduction through myelinated fibers ~50 times faster than that through nonmyelinated ones. Myelin also allows conservation of energy, by permitting sodium–potassium pump action to be largely restricted to the nodes of Ranvier.

At least half of the weight of the white matter of the CNS is made up of myelin, which helps to explain why demyelinating diseases are seen to affect predominantly the white matter. In multiple sclerosis, immune-mediated destruction of myelin occurs anywhere in the CNS, producing a protean array of symptoms. The etiology of this attack is unknown, although genetics appears to play a role, as monozygotic twins have an ~25% rate of concordance. The disease is defined clinically as multiple CNS lesions separated in time and space; this correlates pathologically with the presence of multiple separate sclerotic plaques demonstrating loss of oligodendrogliocytes and myelin, with an accumulation of antibody-producing plasma cells.

◇ Clinical Presentation

Symptoms are correlated with the function of the affected white matter. Common sites of involvement include the optic nerves, the periventricular cerebral white matter, and the cervical spinal cord. Optic nerve lesions are associated with blurred vision and blindness. On physical examination, patients demonstrate upper motor neuron signs such as hyperreflexia, as well as other long-track signs such as a positive Babinski's sign. The clinical course is characterized by alternating periods of remission and relapse, which may or may not eventuate in residual symptoms. Diagnostic tests other than imaging include examination of CSF for so-called oligoclonal bands of immunoglobulin G (IgG), the use of electrophysiologic evoked potentials to measure the delayed conduction velocities associated with demyelination, and blood tests to rule out multiple sclerosis mimics.

◇ Imaging

MRI has revolutionized the diagnosis of multiple sclerosis. In clinically confirmed cases, MRI demonstrates lesions over 90% of the time, whereas CT is positive in the minority of cases, and evoked potentials and oligoclonal bands are positive in fewer than 70%. The most sensitive images are heavily T2-weighted MR sequences, in which plaques typically appear as round or oval lesions of increased signal intensity, especially in the periventricular and deep white matter regions (**Fig. 9–21**).

Often, lesions will be seen to radiate out perpendicularly from the lateral ventricles. Such an appearance is not specific to multiple sclerosis, however, and can be seen in other demyelinating disorders such as Lyme disease. As the disease progresses, global cerebral atrophy, atrophy of the corpus callosum, and increased iron deposition are seen.

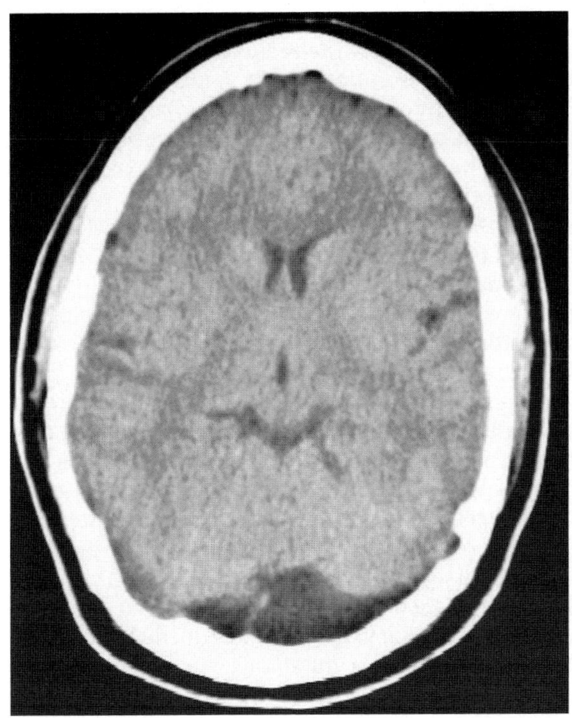

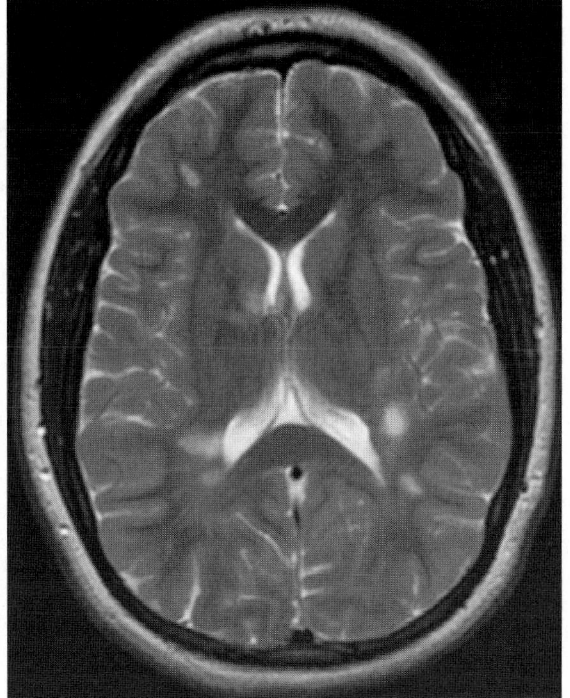

Figure 9–21 **(A)** This noncontrast axial CT image demonstrates mild atrophy but no clearly definable focal lesions. Note that the patient happens to have a posterior fossa arachnoid cyst. **(B)** On T2-weighted MRI, however, there are multiple bilateral predominantly periventricular foci of increased signal intensity, representing white matter plaques in this patient with multiple sclerosis.

Contrast administration does not increase the sensitivity of MRI in lesion detection, but the presence of enhancement within plaques (indicating breakdown of the blood–brain barrier) is thought to indicate active demyelination, which is correlated with clinical activity. Therefore, the finding of new areas of enhancement is correlated with a worsening clinical picture. As newer therapies continue to emerge, MRI is likely to play an increasing role in monitoring treatment response.

Tumorous

◇ Epidemiology

CNS neoplasms are diagnosed in ~17,000 patients per year in the United States and account for ~1% of all hospital admissions. Included in these figures are both primary and metastatic lesions.

◇ Pathophysiology

Given the fact that metastatic lesions are far more common than primary malignancies in organs such as lung, liver, and bone, one would predict that intracranial metastases are a more prevalent form of intracranial neoplasm than primary lesions. In fact, however, metastases from extracranial sources constitute only approximately one third of intracranial malignancies, with the remaining two thirds representing primary lesions. The most common tumors to metastasize intracranially in adults include lung and breast carcinomas and malignant melanoma (**Fig. 9–22**).

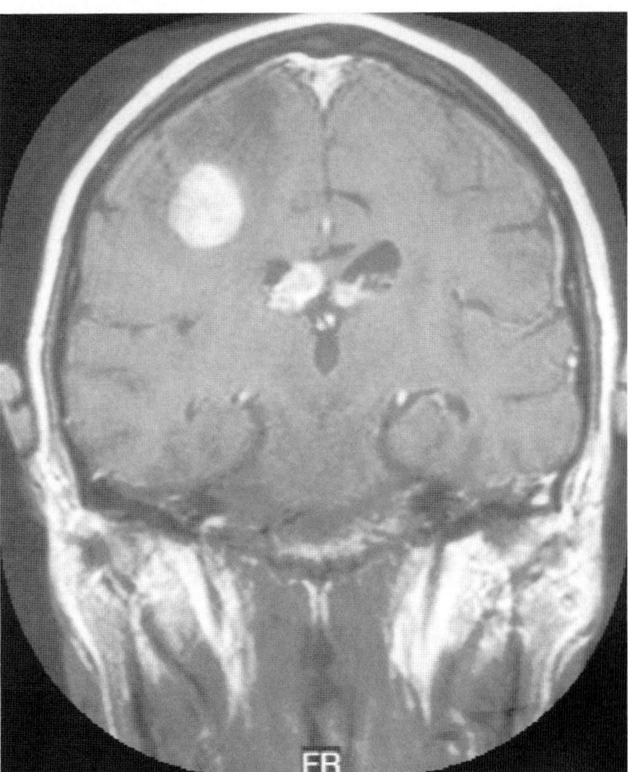

Figure 9–22 A coronal T1-weighted MR image demonstrates high-signal masses in the choroid plexus and right cerebral hemisphere in a patient with hemorrhagic metastases. Likely primary lesions would include malignant melanoma and renal cell carcinoma, among other possibilities.

In children, metastases to the brain are comparatively rare, but skull metastases are not uncommonly seen in neuroblastoma and leukemias. Tumors such as breast and lung cancer may also metastasize to the meninges, where they produce focal or diffuse pial enhancement that may resemble meningitis.

Tumors of the CNS differ from tumors elsewhere in the body in interesting ways. Histologic features are less reliable in predicting benign versus malignant behavior, a "benign" tumor is much more likely to prove life threatening due to mass effect within the skull, surgery to remove tumors is much riskier due to damage to surrounding normal tissue, and tumors are very unlikely to metastasize outside the CNS. Primary brain neoplasms are defined as tumors that arise from the brain or its linings, but typically included in this category are lesions such as craniopharyngiomas and chordomas, which are intracranial and may cause CNS symptoms.

◇ Clinical Presentation

Numerous neurologic symptoms may result from intracranial neoplasms, including alterations in consciousness and behavior, cranial nerve palsies, endocrinologic abnormalities, and seizures. Obviously, the location of the tumor is manifest by its clinical presentation, with monocular blindness an indication of a retinal or optic nerve tumor, while headaches could indicate a tumor obstructing CSF flow.

◇ Imaging

In both CT and MRI, contrast administration is vital to reliably identify and characterize intracranial neoplasms, although precontrast imaging should be performed first to determine the presence of hemorrhage. The radiologist attempts to answer three questions: (1) Is a mass present, as manifest by mass effect on adjacent structures? (2) Is the mass intra-axial or extra-axial in origin? An intra-axial lesion originates in the brain or spinal cord, whereas an extra-axial lesion originates external to them (and by convention, includes the ventricles). (3) What are the mass's intrinsic imaging characteristics, such as signal intensities on T1- and T2-weighted images, presence or absence of calcification, and contrast enhancement characteristics?

One of the most crucial determinations the radiologist can make regarding an intracranial neoplasm is whether it is intra-axial or extra-axial in location, because the differential diagnosis of intra- and extra-axial lesions is completely different. For example, astrocytomas are not extra-axial tumors, and meningiomas are not intra-axial tumors. Some characteristics of intra-axial masses include limited contact with the dura, acute angles between the mass and the dura, white matter expansion, absence of a "dural tail," and absence of bone destruction. Extra-axial masses, however, usually exhibit such characteristics as a broad base of contact with the dura, an obtuse angle of dural contact, white matter buckling, medial or central displacement of vessels, a dural tail, and bone destruction (**Fig. 9–23**). As one would expect, if a mass is extra-axial in origin, a rim of CSF is often interposed between the mass and underlying brain. Because a lesion with an apparently indeterminate point of origin in one plane of imaging may demonstrate a clear origin when imaged in another plane, MRI represents a major advance in brain tumor imaging due to its multiplanar capabilities, not to mention its superior contrast resolution.

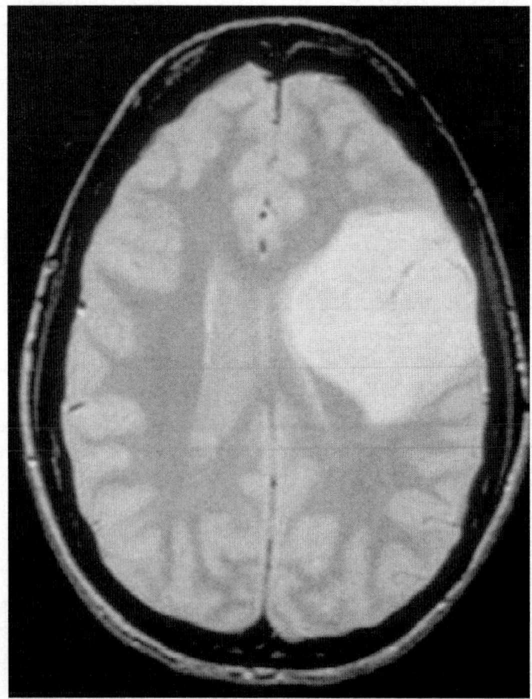

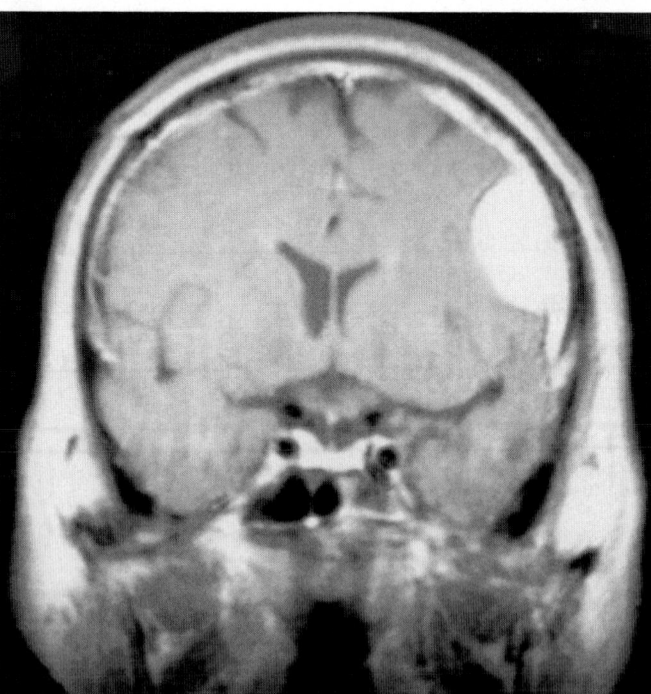

Figure 9–23 **(A)** This axial proton density-weighted image of a patient with a large left hemisphere oligodendroglioma demonstrates typical features of an intra-axial mass. The mass appears to arise from within the brain, demonstrating white matter expansion, and has acute angles where it touches the dura. **(B)** The coronal postcontrast T1-weighted image of the brain in a patient with meningioma demonstrates classic signs of an extra-axial mass. Note the highly vascular mass appears to arise from outside the brain and press down into it. Note also the large dural tail and its obtuse margins with the skull.

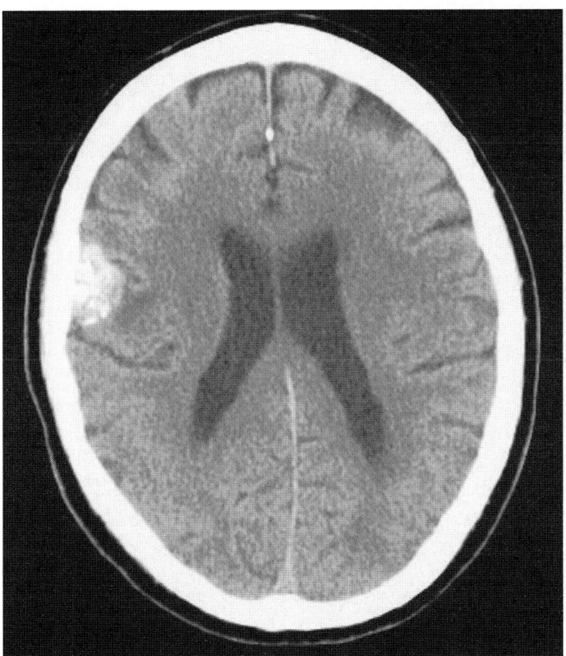

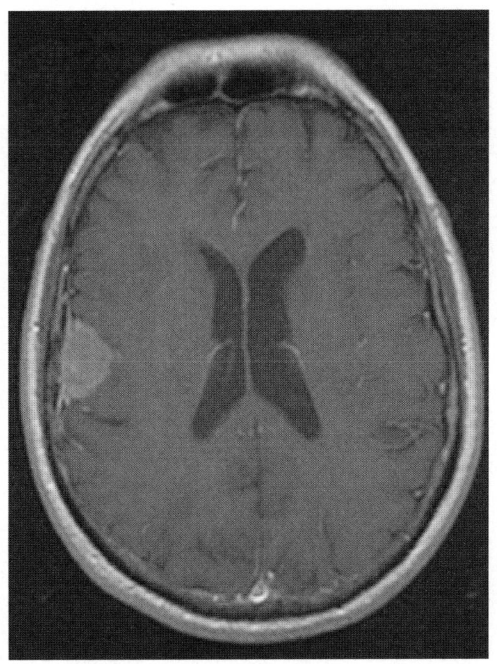

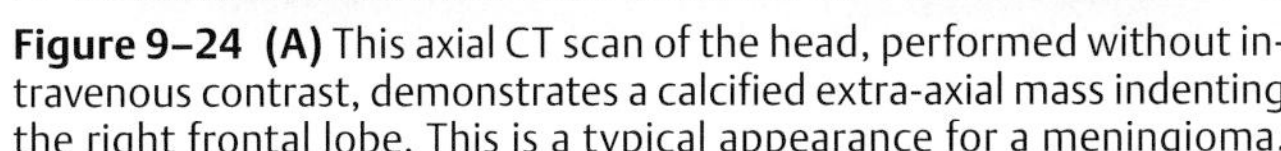

Figure 9–24 **(A)** This axial CT scan of the head, performed without intravenous contrast, demonstrates a calcified extra-axial mass indenting the right frontal lobe. This is a typical appearance for a meningioma. **(B)** Note its bright enhancement on this axial T1-weighted MR image, obtained after gadolinium infusion.

Extra-axial Neoplasms

Two of the most common extra-axial neoplasms are meningiomas and schwannomas. Meningiomas constitute 20% of all adult brain tumors, occurring mainly in middle and old age, and are more common in women than in men (3:2). They are histologically benign tumors that grow slowly and produce symptoms secondary to compression of adjacent brain. Because of their slow growth and lack of irritation of brain parenchyma, they may be large at the time of diagnosis.

Meningiomas are multiple in up to 10% of cases. Typical locations include the frontal and parietal convexities and the parasagittal region. Approximately one quarter of meningiomas demonstrate calcification (**Fig. 9–24**). Another characteristic finding in meningioma, related to its location next to the overlying skull, is hyperostosis. Meningiomas typically demonstrate intense and homogeneous contrast enhancement on both CT and MRI.

The schwannoma is a tumor of the Schwann's cells that produce myelin around peripheral nervous system axons—in the case of intracranial tumors, around the axons of the cranial nerves. The acoustic schwannoma is the most common type of intracranial schwannoma. Arising from the vestibular portion of the eighth cranial nerve, it is the most common mass in the cerebellopontine angle, the angle between the cerebellum and the pons. It can be differentiated from a meningioma in this location by the fact that it typically extends into and expands the internal auditory canal. These benign tumors produce symptoms secondary to their size and location, which may result in compression of the cochlear and vestibular nerves, with progressive neurosensory hearing loss and tinnitus.

Intra-axial Neoplasms

Intra-axial primary neoplasms exhibit different profiles in adults and children. In children, two thirds of lesions are infratentorial; that is, they are located below the tentorium cerebelli, which separates the anterior and middle cranial fossae from the posterior fossa (**Fig. 9–25**).

Most intra-axial primary neoplasms in adults are gliomas, tumors that arise from the glial cells, including astrocytomas, oligodendrogliomas, and ependymomas. Gliomas are graded histologically, based on criteria such as the number of mitoses, the presence of necrosis, and nuclear pleomorphism. Eighty percent of adult primary brain tumors are astrocytomas. Grade I astrocytoma is the least aggressive, and grade IV represents the highly malignant glioblastoma multiforme. Recent genetic studies have suggested that these various grades in fact represent stages in the evolution of a single tumor, which tends to progress over time toward higher and more malignant forms. Imaging characteristics on MRI include low signal on T1-weighted images, high signal on T2-weighted images, and enhancement that may be solid or ringlike.

Associated findings include surrounding edema and mass effect, which can cause more extensive symptoms than would be predicted based on the size of the tumor alone. Glioblastoma multiforme may exhibit considerable necrosis and hemorrhage (**Fig. 9–26**). Glioblastoma and lymphoma are the only two tumors that can cross the corpus callosum into the opposite hemisphere (**Fig. 9–27**).

Primary lymphoma of the brain is a non-Hodgkin's lymphoma that occurs without evidence of involvement outside the CNS. It is the most common CNS neoplasm in immunocompromised patients, such as those with acquired immunodeficiency syndrome (AIDS). The tumors are highly cellular and proliferate

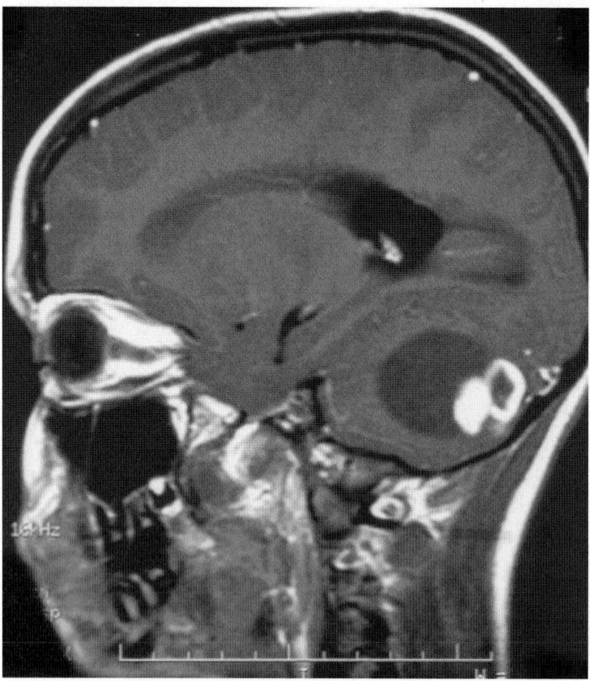

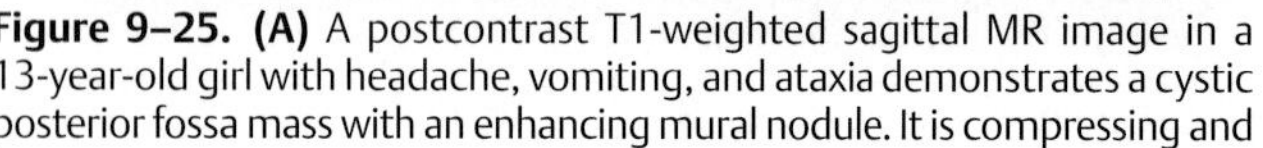

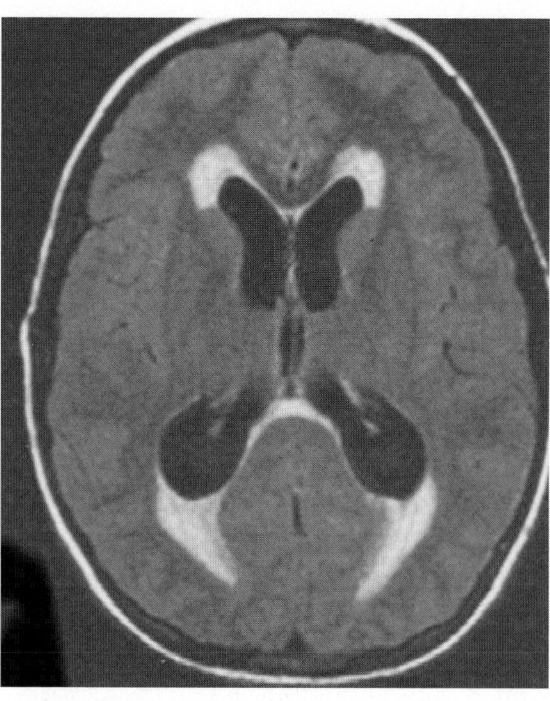

Figure 9–25. (A) A postcontrast T1-weighted sagittal MR image in a 13-year-old girl with headache, vomiting, and ataxia demonstrates a cystic posterior fossa mass with an enhancing mural nodule. It is compressing and obstructing the fourth ventricle. This is a typical appearance of a juvenile pilocytic astrocytoma. **(B)** This axial proton density-weighted MR image demonstrates the hydrocephalus as well as transependymal flow of CSF.

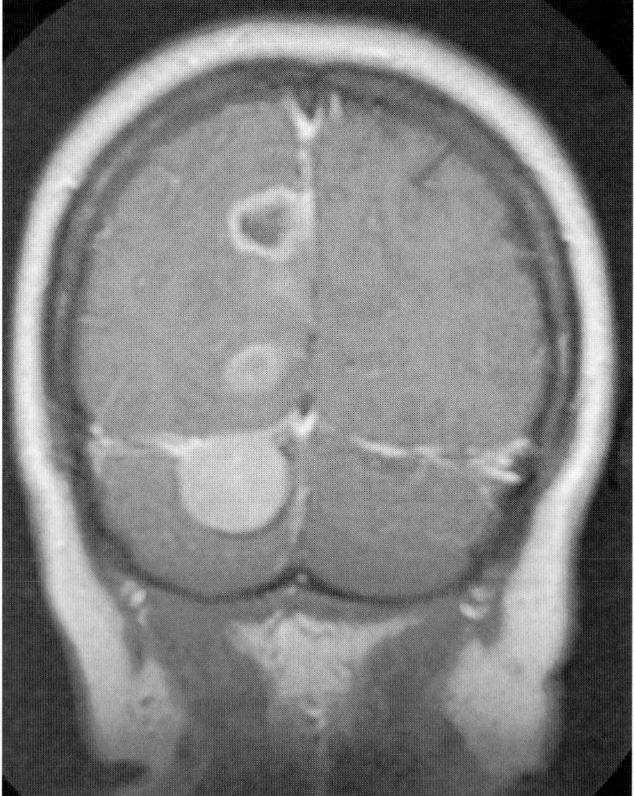

Figure 9–26 This postcontrast coronal MR image demonstrates two masses. The more inferior of the two demonstrates a solid pattern of enhancement and arises from the tentorium. It represented a meningioma. The superior mass demonstrates central necrosis and ring enhancement. On other images, it is connected to the more inferior enhancing lesion in the right cerebral hemisphere. It was a glioblastoma multiforme.

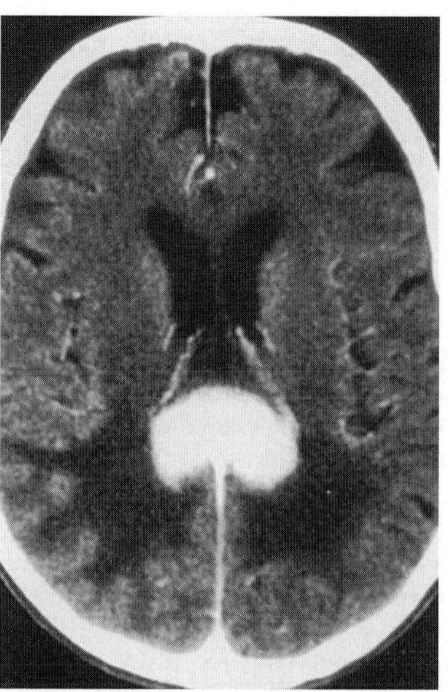

Figure 9–27 A postcontrast CT scan demonstrates an enhancing lesion in the splenium of the corpus collosum, with surrounding edema in both cerebral hemispheres. This represented a primary CNS lymphoma. (Reprinted with permission from Fischbein, Dillon, Barkovich, eds. Teaching Atlas of Brain Imaging. New York: Thieme, 2000:31, fig. E.)

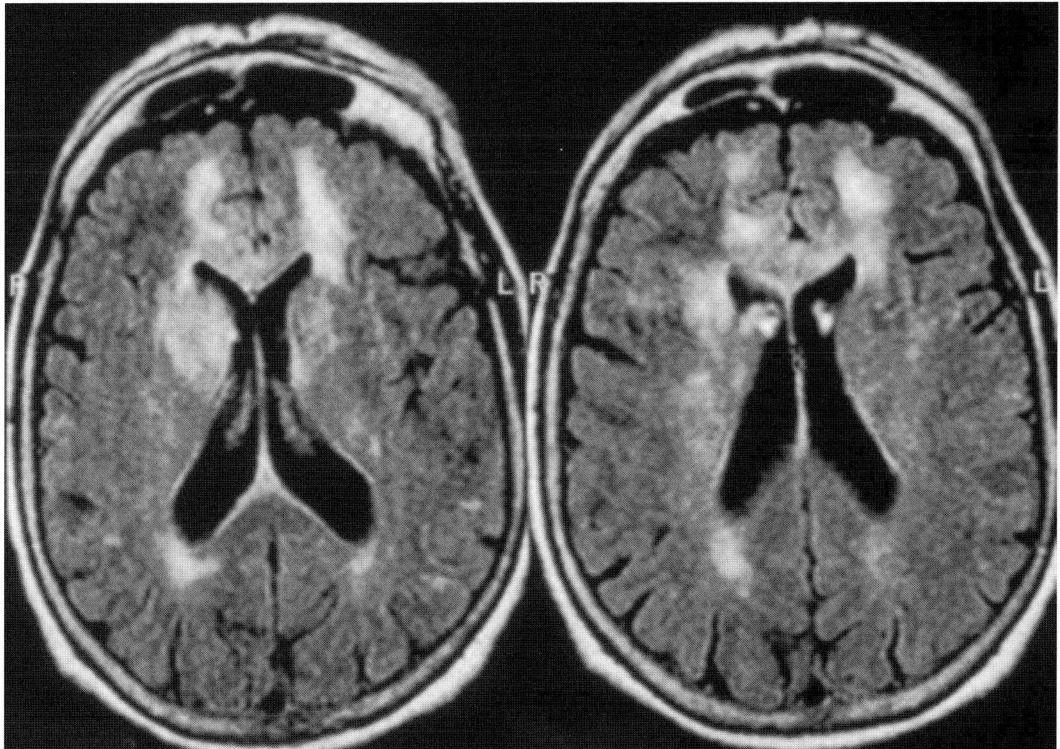

Figure 9–28 These axial FLAIR MR images demonstrate multiple bilateral areas of signal abnormality in this 73-year-old man with CNS lymphoma.

rapidly; thus, they tend to exhibit a good response to radiation and steroids, though their behavior is modified for the worse in AIDS patients. Distinguishing imaging characteristics include multiplicity, lack of necrosis, a tendency to cross the midline, mild edema, and a relative lack of mass effect. Multiple lesions are present in as many as one half of patients (**Fig. 9–28**).

Epilepsy

One of the most classic presenting complaints in adult intracranial neoplasms is new-onset seizure. In aggregate, ~150,000 new cases of epilepsy, or chronic seizure disorder, are diagnosed each year, and there are ~2 million patients with epilepsy in the United States. The lifetime risk of developing a seizure disorder is ~3%. Numerous causes other than tumor, such as congenital anomalies, trauma, infection, and metabolic disorders, may be responsible. In patients without an underlying neoplasm, medical therapy is effective in controlling seizures two thirds of the time. Of the remaining one third, ~5000 surgical candidates are identified each year.

Whenever a previously healthy adult develops a seizure disorder, CNS imaging is warranted to rule out the presence of a neoplasm. Because fewer than 5% of strokes present with seizure, one should think twice before attributing a seizure disorder to stroke (**Fig. 9–29**). Even imaging findings typical for stroke should not eliminate suspicion for an underlying neoplasm. One clue to the presence of an underlying neoplasm is a substantial amount of vasogenic edema, which is typically seen in neoplasm or abscess.

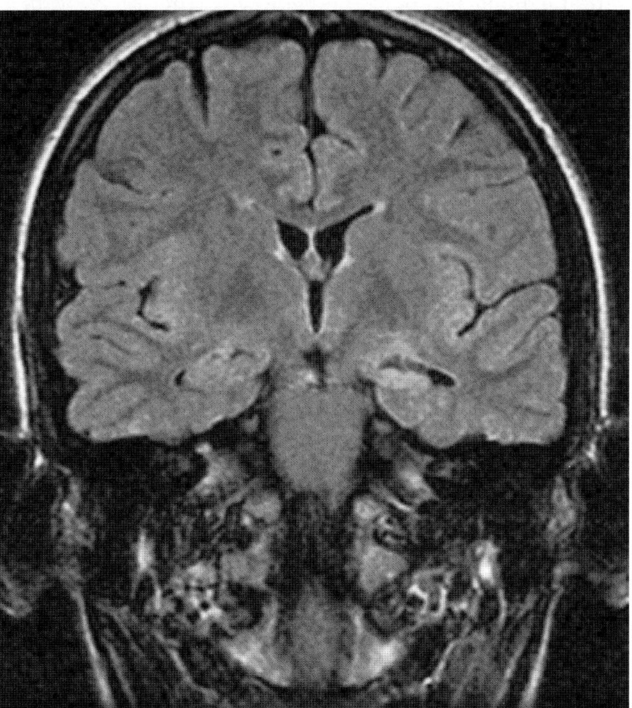

Figure 9–29 This patient presented with complex partial seizures refractory to medical therapy. A coronal FLAIR MR image demonstrates atrophy and increased signal in the left hippocampus, typical of mesial temporal sclerosis, a lesion associated with seizure disorders.

Vasogenic edema occurs with disruption of the normal blood–brain barrier, with movement of water into the intercellular space, whereas cytotoxic edema implies increased intracellular water due to cell injury, as might occur in ischemia. Although the surgical objective in many tumor cases is to debulk the lesion, surgery for epilepsy aims for complete removal of the epileptogenic lesion, as even a small lesion residual may result in continued or recurrent seizures.

Infectious

Meningitis

◇ Epidemiology

Infectious meningitis accounts for ~1 in every 1000 hospital admissions. It is the most common form of CNS infection, and can be divided into three clinical and pathologic categories: acute superative meningitis, usually due to bacterial infection; lymphocytic (aseptic) meningitis, which is usually viral; and chronic meningitis, as seen in tuberculosis and coccidiodomycosis, although any infectious agent can be responsible. This discussion focuses on acute meningitis.

◇ Pathophysiology

Organisms usually reach the meninges via one of three routes: hematogenously in septic patients, direct invasion in postsurgical or post-traumatic settings, or contiguous spread from the sinuses or middle ear. The infection is spread via the CSF, which circulates between the pia mater and arachnoid layers of the meninges. The infection may disseminate to involve the full extent of the meningeal membranes. Hydrocephalus may be precipitated by a combination of congestion of venous sinuses and postinflammatory fibrosis.

The pneumococcus, meningococcus, and *Haemophilus influenzae* (or *H. flu*) are the principal etiologic organisms. Pneumococcal meningitis is the most common form in adults and was uniformly fatal before the introduction of antibiotics. Currently, mortality may range as high as 30%, and many survivors are left with neurologic residua such as seizure disorders and deafness. Meningococcal meningitis may be associated with a characteristic skin rash. *H. flu* was the most common in children, although this is changing with immunization against more common strains of the organism, a practice that is also affecting the epidemiology of epiglottitis.

◇ Clinical Presentation

The patient with meningitis classically presents with severe headache, stiff neck, and fever. The most striking physical examination finding is nuchal rigidity, reflecting the underlying inflammation of the pia and arachnoid membranes, which are stretched when the neck is flexed.

◇ Imaging

Bacterial meningitis is not an imaging diagnosis. The diagnosis can only be made with confidence through examination of the CSF, usually obtained via lumbar puncture, which is typically performed at or below the L2–L3 level, because the spinal cord typically terminates at approximately the level of L1. A spinal tap reveals cloudy CSF under increased pressure, an increased neutrophil count and protein level, and decreased glucose, secondary to bacterial glycolysis.

Imaging is often obtained to rule out the presence of other conditions that may mimic meningitis, such as a mass lesion, and to detect the presence of increased intracranial pressure, which might preclude lumbar puncture due to the danger of transtentorial herniation.

Increased intracranial pressure is defined as a pressure above 200 mm water in a supine patient. Signs suggestive of meningitis on CT include cerebral edema, manifested as a loss of the usually sharp demarcation between gray and white matter, and the presence of communicating hydrocephalus, which appears as enlargement of the ventricles and effacement of the basilar cisterns. Although post-contrast MRI is not routinely obtained, it may demonstrate enhancement of the meninges and ependymal lining of the ventricles (**Fig. 9–30**).

Abscess

Most abscesses result from the contiguous spread of infection from the paranasal sinuses, the mastoid air cells, or the middle ear, although dental and facial sources may also be involved. Some abscesses result from hematogenous

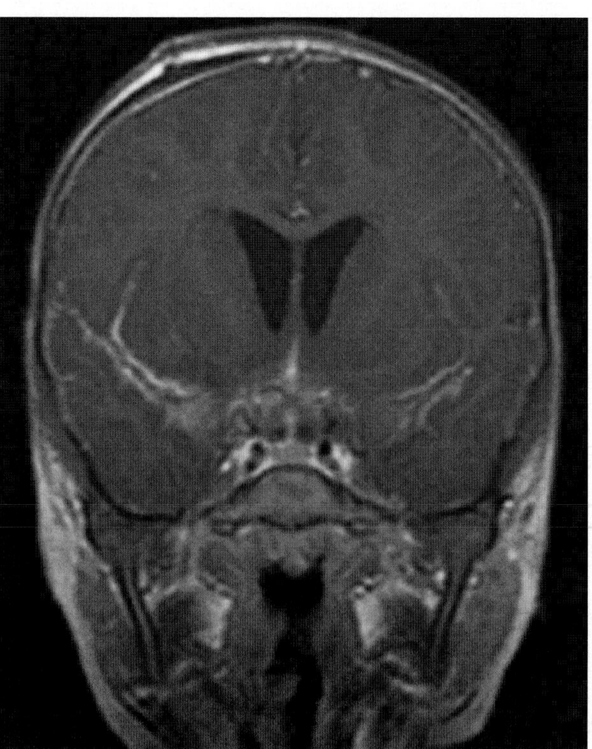

Figure 9–30 This 3-year-old patient presented with fever and obtundation. This coronal T1-weighted MR image after administration of gadolinium-DTPA demonstrates thickening and intense enhancement of the basal cisterns and sylvian fissures in this patient with tuberculous meningitis.

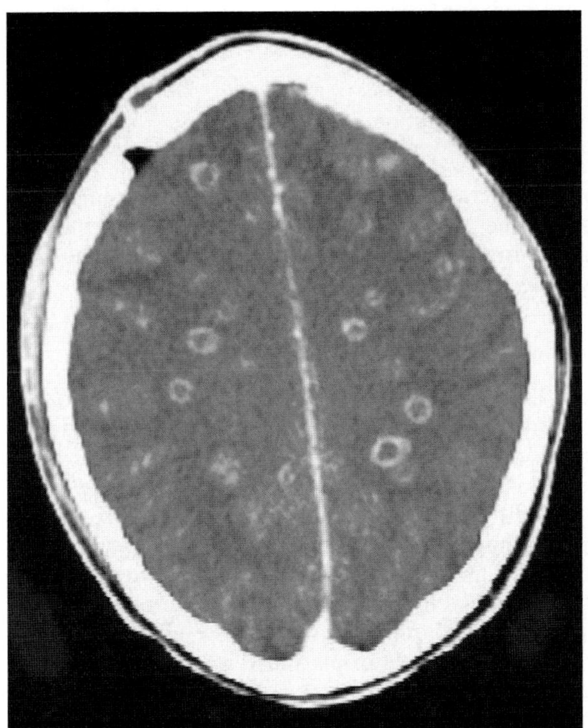

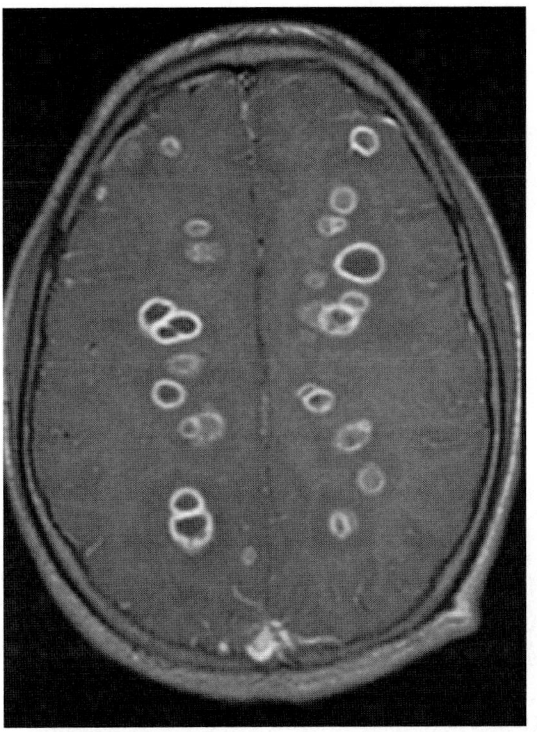

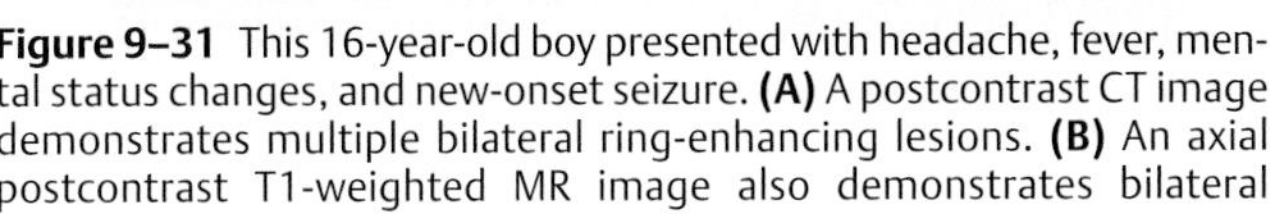

Figure 9–31 This 16-year-old boy presented with headache, fever, mental status changes, and new-onset seizure. **(A)** A postcontrast CT image demonstrates multiple bilateral ring-enhancing lesions. **(B)** An axial postcontrast T1-weighted MR image also demonstrates bilateral ring-enhancing lesions. These turned out to represent abscesses due to septic emboli containing group A streptococci. The patient improved rapidly on intravenous antibiotics.

spread, most commonly in endocarditis. In contrast to meningitis, lumbar puncture should demonstrate a normal glucose level. A brain abscess begins when a portion of the brain is inoculated with a pathogen, which leads to cerebritis. Direct microbial cytotoxicity and host inflammatory response are accompanied by vascular congestion and increased vascular permeability, with the development of edema. If severe enough, capillary perfusion pressure may be overcome by locally increased interstitial pressure, causing necrosis, which appears pathologically as softening and liquefaction. Within a period of days to weeks, the necrotic region becomes encapsulated by a rim of highly vascular granulation tissue, presumably in an attempt to isolate the infection and protect the surrounding tissue. CT findings include a ring-enhancing lesion, reflecting the increased vascularity of the capsule, with a low-density center of necrosis. MRI likewise demonstrates an enhancing rim, the differential for which can include neoplasm and resolving hematoma (**Fig. 9–31**).

Encephalitis

The most common and dangerous form of encephalitis is caused by the herpes simplex virus. It is almost always of the type I variety, except in neonates, who may acquire type II (genital) infection during vaginal delivery. The organism exhibits a distinct predilection for the inferior frontal and temporal lobes, producing predictable symptoms such as seizures, personality changes, and confusion, often preceded by a flulike prodrome of headache and fever. For antiviral therapy to be effective, it must be instituted within the first several days of the illness, placing a premium on early diagnosis. MRI is more sensitive than CT and demonstrates an increased signal on T2-weighted images, as well as gyral enhancement in the temporal lobes (**Fig. 9–32**). Immunofluorescent staining and viral cultures from CSF and/or brain biopsy can definitively establish the diagnosis, but often antiviral therapy must be instituted with only a presumptive diagnosis in hand, to prevent rapidly irreversible brain damage. Although the majority of patients survive the illness, many are left with permanent and devastating neurologic effects, including severe personality and behavioral changes.

Parasitic Infections

Although parasitic infections are less common in industrialized nations than in developing countries, they are seen often enough to warrant brief discussion. The most prevalent parasitic CNS infection in the United States may be toxoplasmosis, which is discussed later in connection with HIV disease. In immunocompetent patients, cysticercosis is the principal infection. It results from fecal-oral transmission of the eggs of the pork tapeworm *Taenia solium* and is most frequently encountered in Latin American immigrants. Organisms that reach the parenchyma of the CNS take up residence as viable cysts, often distributed along the gray matter–white matter junctions. When the organism dies, it incites a local

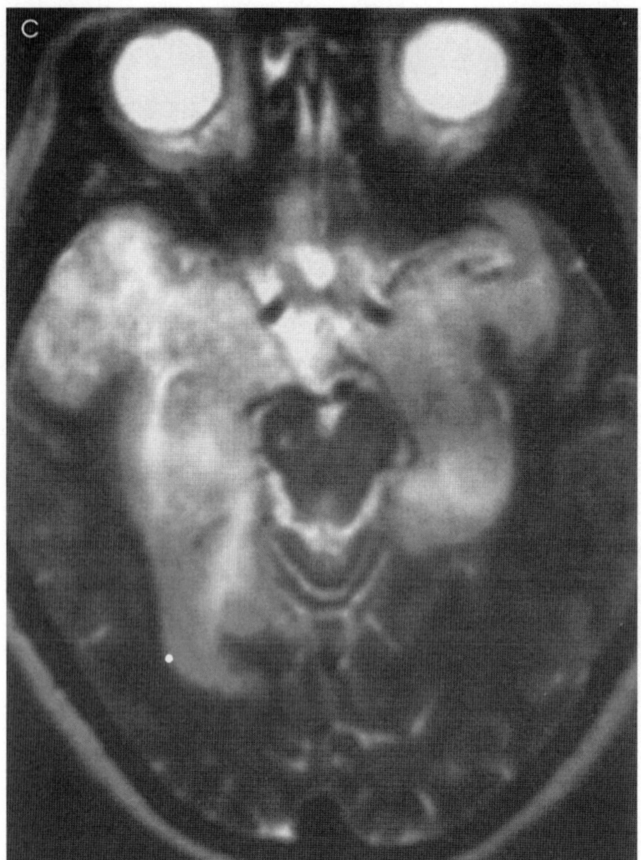

Figure 9–32 This elderly woman presented with confusion. An axial T2-weighted MR image demonstrates hyperintensity in the anterior and medial aspects of both temporal lobes, greater on the right than on the left. This is a typical pattern for herpes simplex type I encephalitis. (Reprinted with permission from Fischbein, Dillon, Barkovich, eds. Teaching Atlas of Brain Imaging. New York: Thieme, TK:158, fig. C.)

inflammatory reaction that causes clinical symptoms such as seizures and, on imaging studies, contrast enhancement (**Fig. 9–33**). The dense scolex of the organism may be visible within the lumen of the cyst.

Human Immunodeficiency Virus

◇ **Epidemiology**

As many as 60% of patients with AIDS eventually develop neurologic symptoms, and neurologic complaints represent the presenting symptom of HIV infection in approximately one tenth of patients. CNS involvement is found in 80% of AIDS patients at autopsy.

◇ **Pathophysiology**

The neurologic manifestations of HIV infection can be traced to one of three etiologies: opportunistic infections related to immunodeficiency, vascular insults, or direct HIV-mediated neurotoxicity. Toxoplasmosis is the principal HIV-related opportunistic infection. Seropositivity to this ubiquitous protozoan is found in up to 70% of the American population, and it causes disease in ~10% of AIDS patients, usually as a reactivation of latent infection.

◇ **Clinical Presentation**

The presentation of patients with HIV-associated CNS infection is generally nonspecific but will vary depending on whether the patient suffers from an opportunistic infection, a vascular insult, or primary HIV encephalopathy. The latter is associated with a progressive subcortical dementia.

◇ **Imaging**

The CNS lesions of toxoplasmosis are usually well localized, with an abscess-like appearance. A minority may be hemorrhagic. When a mass lesion is detected in an HIV-positive patient with new-onset neurologic symptoms, the most important differential diagnosis is that between toxoplasmosis and lymphoma. The incidence of primary CNS lymphoma in AIDS is as high as 6%. In contrast to toxoplasmosis, lymphoma often exhibits a hyperdense appearance on noncontrast CT scan. Moreover, lymphoma tends to occur in a periventricular location, whereas toxoplasmosis is often seen in the basal ganglia. Lesions of toxoplasmosis tend to be more numerous, whereas those of lymphoma tend to be larger. The key distinguishing feature, however, is prompt response to antibiotic therapy, only seen in toxoplasmosis (**Fig. 9–34**).

Traumatic

◇ **Epidemiology**

Trauma is the leading cause of death in the United States in persons younger than 44 years of age, and approximately one half of those deaths are the result of brain injury. Only 10% of CNS trauma is fatal, however, and each year, 100,000 patients who survive are left with permanent neurologic sequelae ranging in severity up to paralysis and persistent vegetative state. The suffering occasioned by CNS trauma is further heightened by the fact that it tends to strike individuals in the "prime of life," with nearly two thirds of cases occurring in men between the ages of 20 and 30 years.

◇ **Pathophysiology**

Head trauma is categorized in several important ways. Closed-head trauma refers to injuries in which the dura remains intact, whereas in open head trauma it is disrupted. Primary brain injury refers to damage occurring at the moment of impact, whether it be an object penetrating the head, a collision between the head and an external object, or a deceleration injury in which the head itself does not collide with any object, but differential inertial properties of gray and white matter result in shearing of tissues. Examples of primary traumatic injuries include contusions and hematomas, vascular injury, and so-called shearing injury, including diffuse axonal injury (**Fig. 9–35**).

Secondary injuries include infarction due to edema, herniation, embolism, and infection resulting from penetrating trauma.

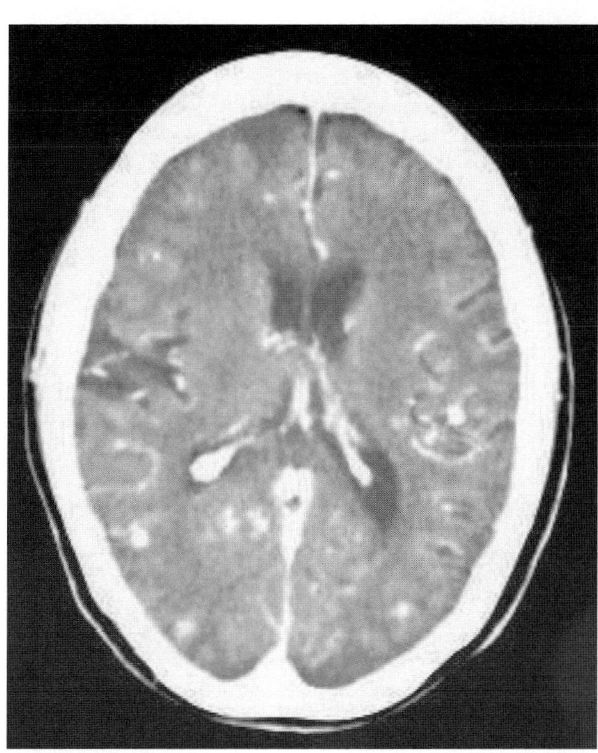
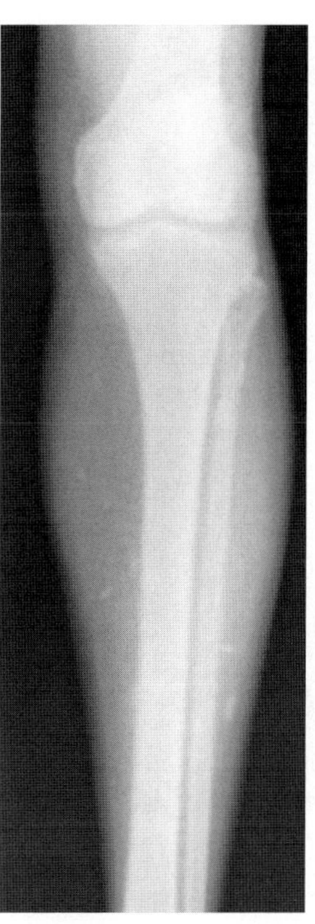

Figure 9–33 (A) This postcontrast axial CT image demonstrates numerous enhancing nodules in both cerebral hemispheres situated mainly at gray matter–white matter junctions. **(B)** A frontal radiograph of the tibia and fibula demonstrates many rice grain–shaped densities in the skeletal muscles, oriented parallel to the muscle planes. This 57-year-old patient was found to be suffering from cysticercosis.

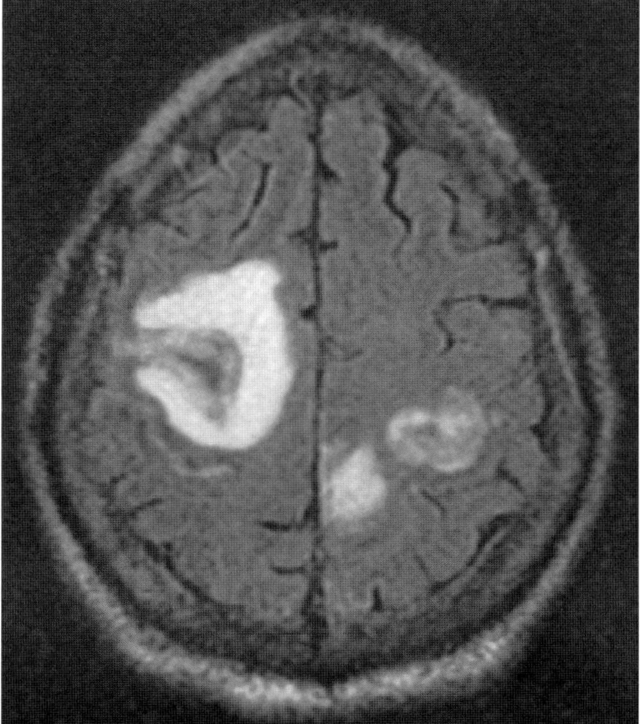

Figure 9–34 This 54-year-old HIV-positive man presented with headache, confusion, and fever. An axial FLAIR MR image demonstrates bilateral somewhat ringlike foci of increased signal, which represented toxoplasmosis. These resolved with appropriate medical therapy.

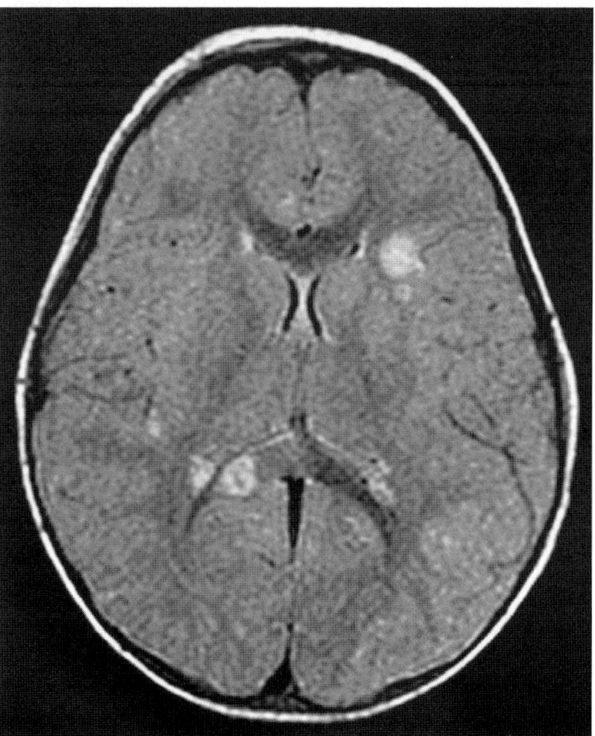

FIGURE 9–35 This axial FLAIR MR image in a patient unconscious after a high-speed motor vehicle accident demonstrates multiple bilateral foci of increased signal intensity in the corpus collosum and at gray matter–white matter junctions, indicating diffuse axonal injury.

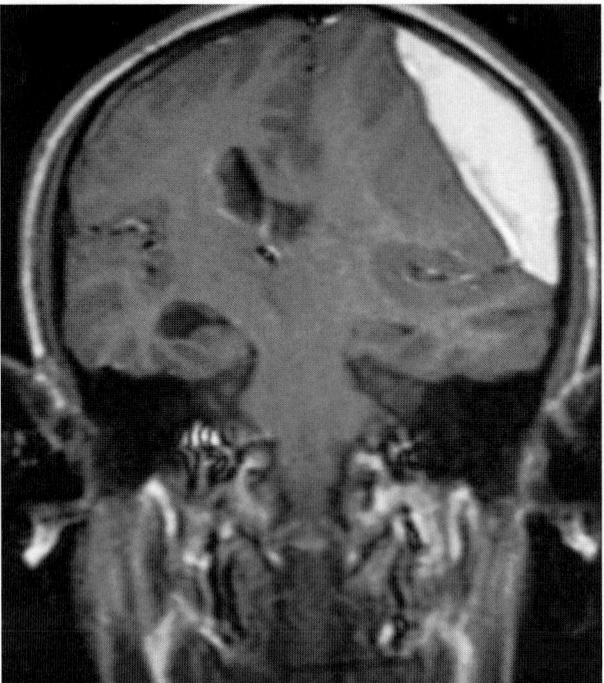

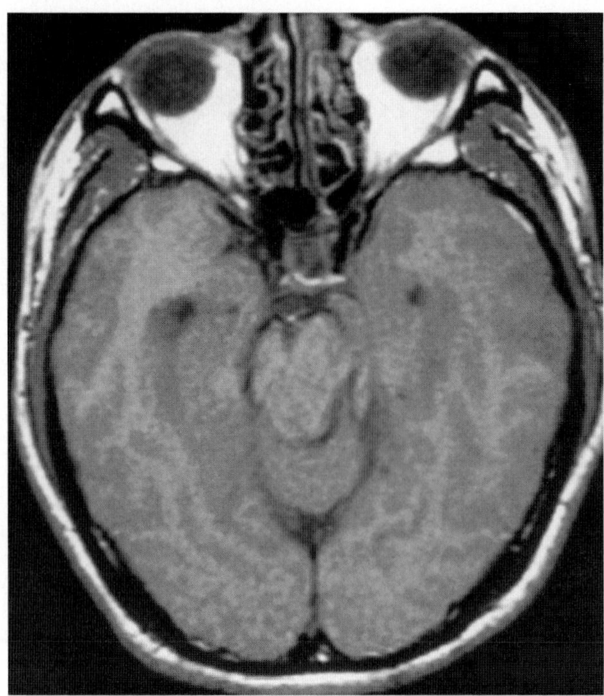

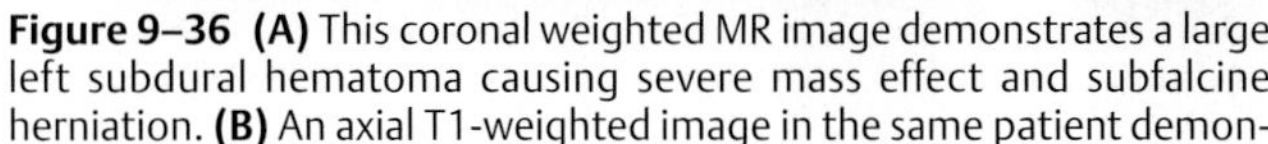

Figure 9–36 (A) This coronal weighted MR image demonstrates a large left subdural hematoma causing severe mass effect and subfalcine herniation. **(B)** An axial T1-weighted image in the same patient demonstrates uncal herniation, with compression of the midbrain by the downward displacement of the temporal lobe.

A key element in the pathophysiology of head trauma is the fact that the brain is a relatively noncompliant tissue within a closed, rigid space. Severe head trauma may initiate a vicious cycle, producing inexorably rising increased intracranial pressure. The inciting trauma causes tissue damage, with disruption of blood vessels, inflammation, and resultant edema and swelling. This results in an increase in interstitial pressure outside the capillaries, which has the effect of diminishing blood flow. If autoregulatory compensation is not effective, further tissue damage then results, with further swelling and edema, further increased intracranial pressure, and so on. Hence, one of the principal roles of surgery in head trauma is to reduce intracranial pressure, by decompressing the brain. For example, an acute hematoma may be evacuated through burr holes. Medical measures include mannitol infusion to increase intravascular osmotic pressure, thereby reducing transcapillary flow of fluid into the brain parenchyma, and hyperventilation, which normally results in hypocarbia and an autoregulatory decrease in cerebral perfusion (which may help to reduce hyperemic swelling).

Any force that increases intracranial pressure, whether it be diffuse cerebral swelling from hyperemia or edema, or more focal mass effect from a hematoma, tumor, or infarction, will press brain tissue into the path of least resistance. In a unilateral hematoma along one of the cerebral hemispheres, the brain will tend to shift toward the opposite side, effacing or obliterating the ipsilateral ventricle and causing subfalcine herniation (ipsilateral brain tissue crossing the midline under the falx cerebri into the opposite side). If supratentorial pressure is sufficient, uncal herniation may result, in which the uncus (the medial portion of the temporal lobe) moves medially and inferiorly, compressing the oculomotor nerve (with pupillary dilatation), the posterior cerebral artery, and the midbrain, which may result in death (**Fig. 9–36**).

◇ Clinical Presentation

Fully one half of cases of CNS trauma result from motor vehicle accidents. A large percentage of cases involve alcohol or drug use, which hampers clinical assessment of the acutely injured patient and renders neuroimaging even more important, because history and physical examination are not as useful in the intoxicated patient. When a history cannot be obtained, it is often impossible to be certain whether superficial injuries are the result of a primary traumatic event or if the "trauma" resulted from some other neurologic deficit, for example, a patient who suffered a stroke or a seizure, then fell over and struck his head. Again, neuroimaging is key in diagnosis.

◇ Imaging

The most important imaging modality in suspected or known acute head trauma is the noncontrast CT. CT is superior to MRI for the detection of acute blood and fractures, and is more readily available, quicker, and more accommodating to the patient requiring close clinical monitoring (**Fig. 9–37**). MRI is the most sensitive modality for the detection of more subtle regions of parenchymal injury, but these need not be demonstrated emergently, because their detection does not alter therapeutic management. The acute question is simply whether there is a treatable lesion. To answer this question, CT is the modality of choice.

The role of plain skull radiographs is highly limited, for the following reason. Suppose the clinician orders skull films, and a fracture is detected; a CT of the head is indicated to

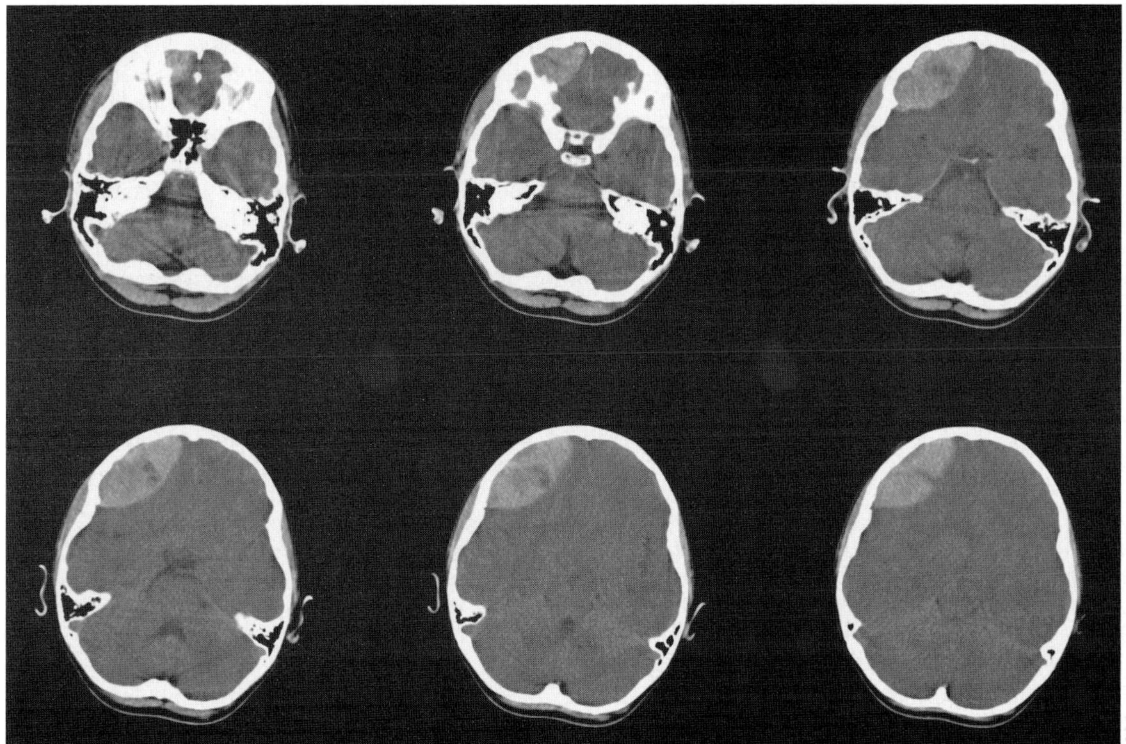

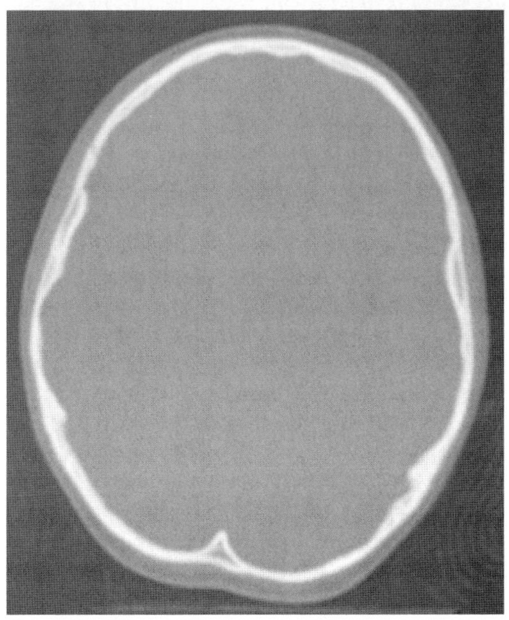

Figure 9–37 This 7-year-old boy fell and hit his head, and now presents with altered mental status. **(A)** These contiguous axial CT images at "blood" windows demonstrate a large acute right frontal epidural hematoma. The fact that the blood is denser (brighter) than brain indicates that it is acute. **(B)** A single bone-window image demonstrates a nondisplaced right frontal skull fracture. Note that such fractures are typically occult unless viewed on bone windows.

assess for the possibility of intracranial injury. Suppose the clinician orders skull radiographs, and no fracture is detected; if there is clinical suspicion of trauma of sufficient force to fracture the skull, a CT is also indicated to rule out intracranial injury, even if no fracture is seen. CT may, however, miss nondisplaced fractures parallel to the plane of imaging, and skull radiographs may still be warranted if the diagnosis of a nondepressed skull fracture would have important medicolegal implications, as in suspected child abuse.

The triage of head trauma may be divided into surgical and nonsurgical findings. Nonsurgical findings include contusion, infarction, and mild to moderate edema. Surgical findings, those warranting emergent surgical consultation, would include more severe edema threatening herniation, or subdural or epidural hematomas.

Which trauma patients should receive CNS imaging? The imaging yield will generally be quite low in patients who do not have a clinically apparent neurologic deficit, an obvious injury such as a depressed skull fracture or penetrating trauma, a history of loss of consciousness, or severe headaches or seizures. When the patient cannot give a history due to age or intoxication, the history is inconsistent or unreliable, or physical examination is deemed unreliable due to factors such as intoxication, seizure, or associated injuries, most clinicians will choose to scan the patient; however, before radiological evaluation takes place, the patient must be stabilized, and at least a single lateral view of the cervical spine should be obtained to rule out spinal instability or injury to the cord. The cervical spine may be further evaluated by CT at the same time the head is scanned. Following is a brief discussion of some of the most frequent and important imaging findings in acute head trauma.

Subdural Hematoma

Young patients typically develop subdural (below the dura) hematomas secondary to motor vehicle accidents, whereas those in older patients typically result from falls. The mortality rate associated with these injuries is high, at least 50%, and only one fifth of those who survive can expect to recover fully. Subdural hematomas may result from closed or open injury, with tearing of bridging veins and bleeding into the potential space between the dura mater and pia arachnoid membranes. Because this space is interrupted by the falx cerebri, these hematomas do not cross the midline, but they will cross sutures, to which only the overlying dura is adherent. Because they are not bounded by sutures, they tend to spread out over the underlying hemisphere, giving them an elongated, crescentic shape (**Fig. 9–38**).

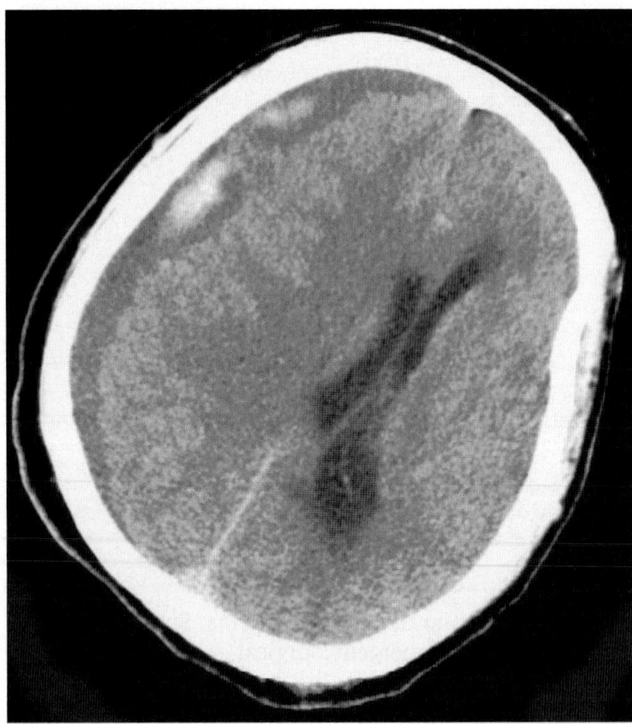

Figure 9–38 This elderly patient experienced mental status changes two days after head trauma. This non-contrast CT image demonstrates a large right crescent-shaped extra axial fluid collection extending along the right cerebral hemisphere. It contains both hypodense (dark) and hyperdense (bright) fluid, the former representing chronic blood and the latter acute blood. Note the severe mass effect, with leftward displacement of the midline and effacement of the right lateral ventricle. This was an acute chronic subdural hematoma.

Because acutely extravasated blood is usually high attenuation (bright) on CT, acute subdural hemorrhages are generally easily detected; however, some subdural hematomas may be isodense, and a careful search must be made for midline shift, ventricular distortion, and sulci that do not extend all the way to the apparent brain surface. What could make an acute subdural hematoma isodense? The density of acutely extravasated blood is related to the concentration of red blood cells. Hence, erythrocyte-poor blood (as in anemia) or dilution of blood (as with CSF if the arachnoid membrane is torn) may render the hematoma isodense.

Epidural Hematoma

Approximately 90% of epidural (above the dura) hematomas result from temporal bone fracture, with tearing of the middle meningeal artery or veins. The resultant blood collection strips the dural membranes from the inner table of the skull; hence the name *epidural*. As in subdural hematoma, patients may exhibit a so-called lucid interval after the injury before deteriorating, during which time intracranial pressure has not yet increased sufficiently to impair consciousness. Patients are usually younger than those suffering subdural hematomas, and because many of these bleeds are self-limited and the patients have a greater neurologic resiliency, the prognosis is not as poor. These hematomas cannot cross sutures (unless there is diastasis or "opening up" of the suture secondary to fracture), and for this reason the blood is more tightly contained and tends to assume a "biconvex" or "lens" shape, meaning that, in contrast to the subdural hematoma, the collection bulges inward toward the brain (**Fig. 9–39**).

Intracerebral Contusions and Hematomas

Both contusions and hematomas result from regions of parenchymal hemorrhage, with accumulation of blood. The term *hematoma* is used to describe a well-defined, homogeneous density collection of blood; *contusion* refers to a lesion of mixed density with less clearly defined margins. These lesions are most often found in the anterior frontal and temporal lobes, where the brain is accelerated against bone in a frontal impact (**Fig. 9–40**).

A clue to the presence of both is extracranial swelling, which indicates the site of impact. When the hemorrhage is on the same side of the brain as the impact, the lesion is called a *coup* (French for "blow") injury, whereas when it is opposite the impact, it is called a *contrecoup* ("opposite the blow") injury. With time, these lesions become isodense and then hypodense, and are eventually replaced by an area of encephalomalacia.

Diffuse Axonal Injury

Diffuse axonal injury is the principal cause of persistent coma immediately following trauma and is the primary lesion responsible for poor long-term outcome in head trauma patients. The injury results from disruption of axonal fibers by deceleration forces, typically at gray matter–white matter interfaces, because the gray matter is more gelatinous in

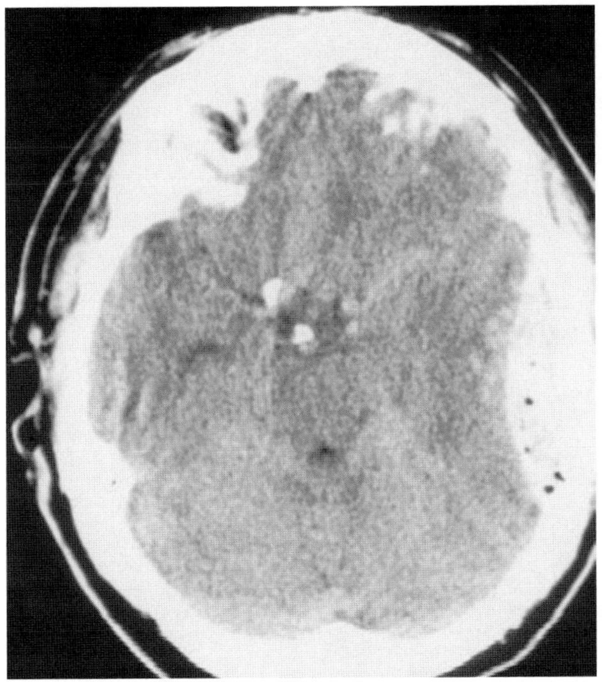

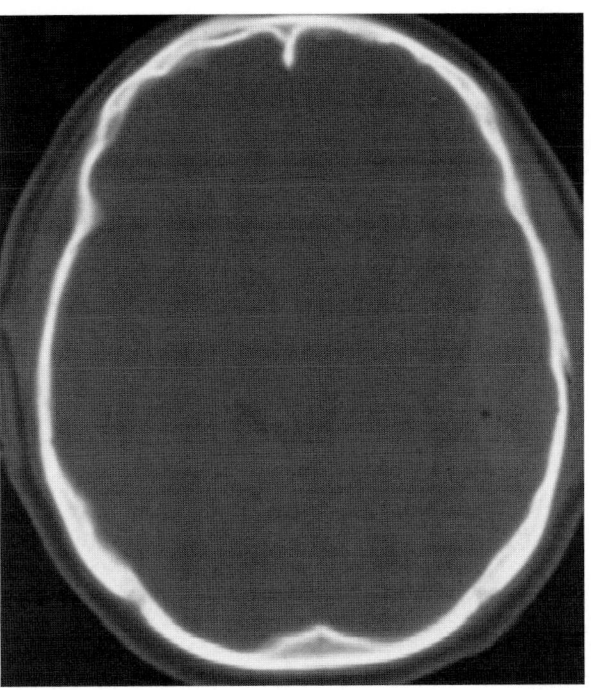

Figure 9–39 (A) A noncontrast axial CT image demonstrates a large, hyperdense left extra-axial fluid collection, causing significant mass effect. Its biconvex shape indicates that it represents an epidural hematoma, and its hyperdensity indicates that it is acute. **(B)** This bone-window image demonstrates a step-off in the overlying portion of the skull, diagnostic of a minimally displaced fracture.

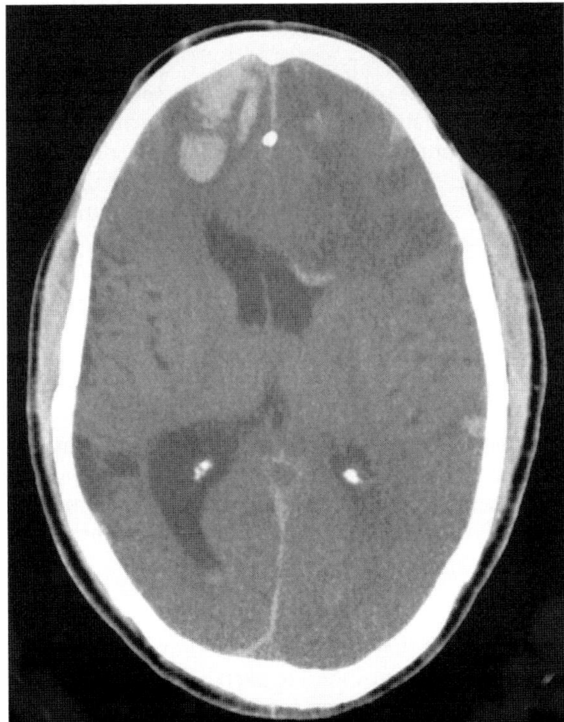

Figure 9–40 This noncontrast axial CT image demonstrates bilateral frontal lobe contusions with surrounding edema. Note the mass effect on the lateral ventricles, especially on the left. There is also both subarachnoid and intraventricular blood. Because the extravasated blood is bright, we can be confident that this represents acute hemorrhage.

consistency than the firmer white matter. Eventually, wallerian degeneration results, with loss of axons in distal white matter tracts. Although CT may detect associated hemorrhage, only MRI can detect nonhemorrhagic lesions, which appear bright on T2-weighted images and are associated with a poorer prognosis.

Vascular

Stroke

◇ Epidemiology

Stroke refers to an abrupt neurologic deficit stemming from a vascular insult. Although the incidence of stroke in the United States has steadily declined over the past few decades, it remains the third leading cause of death in the United States. More than 750,000 Americans still suffer strokes each year, resulting in over 160,000 deaths. Perhaps even costlier is the heavy toll it exacts among survivors, many of whom are left with severe neurologic impairment. Stroke is the number one hospital discharge diagnosis for patients entering long-term care facilities. The principal risk factor is hypertension, which afflicts one third of adult Americans, and increases the risk of stroke 6 times.

◇ Pathophysiology

The two principal types of ischemic injury are global (due to decreased cerebral perfusion as from cardiac arrest or shock) and focal (due to thrombosis or embolism). Because neurons

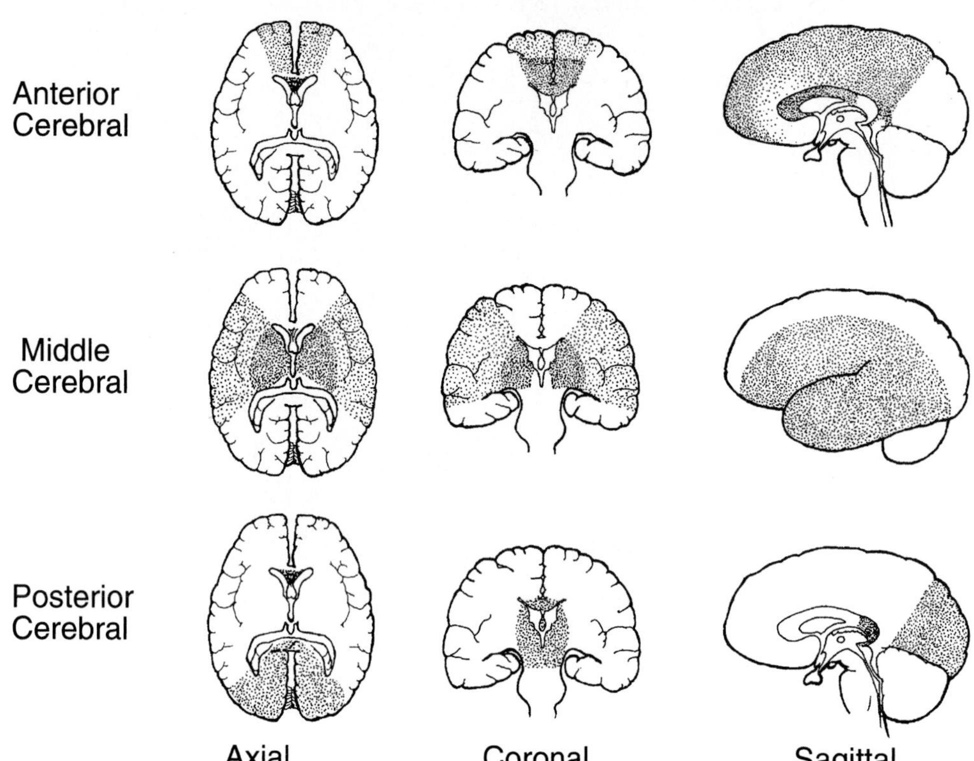

Figure 9–41 The arterial territories of the brain, as visualized on axial, coronal, and sagittal views.

in the adult generally do not divide, the damage caused by a stroke is irreversible; however, strokes are sometimes preceded clinically by so-called transient ischemic attacks (TIAs), neurologic deficits that completely resolve within 24 hours, and many other strokes pursue a stuttering course; therefore, although completed strokes are not amenable to therapy (except rehabilitation), preventive measures such as carotid endarterectomy and anticoagulation may be indicated in patients who have suffered a TIA, and therapeutic maneuvers such as heparinization and even thrombolysis may be warranted in some patients whose stroke is not completed.

Clinically, the site of stroke can often be discerned on the basis of the patient's neurologic deficit. The most common location of stroke is in the middle cerebral artery (MCA) distribution, which supplies the bulk of the frontal, temporal, and parietal lobes (**Fig. 9–41**). Patients with MCA strokes may present with contralateral hemiplegia and hemianesthesia, and when the dominant hemisphere (usually the left) is involved, aphasia. The anterior cerebral artery (ACA) supplies portions of the frontal and parietal lobes, especially along the midline. ACA occlusion may cause contralateral foot and leg weakness. The posterior cerebral artery (PCA), or vertebrobasilar system, supplies the cerebellum, the occipital lobes, the thalamus, and the upper midbrain, through which most of the brain's input and output pass. Even a small infarction in some portions of the PCA territory may produce catastrophic consequences, including apnea, coma, cranial nerve deficits, and major motor and sensory deficits.

◇ Imaging

Stroke versus Another Process Imaging has several critical roles in stroke, all related to its pathophysiology and therapy. One often underappreciated role of imaging is to determine whether the patient's neurologic deficit may stem from some process other than stroke. It is not uncommon for patients to be referred for head CT scans with the history of "Stroke—rule out hemorrhage," who turn out to be suffering from non-vaso-occlusive processes, such as a subdural hematoma, tumor, or encephalitis. Although this occurs in only a minority of patients, all patients with suspected stroke deserve imaging to rule out such mimics, some of which can be highly treatable. Other unusual disease processes that may "mimic" conventional stroke are vasculitis, coagulopathies, and venous occlusion; these are called mimics because, even though they cause cerebral infarction, their management is often quite different from that of the typical thrombotic or embolic arterial occlusion.

One of the key criteria for the diagnosis of stroke is the correspondence between the region of abnormality and a known vascular territory. If the region of altered attenuation and mass effect does not correspond to such distributions as the MCA, ACA, or PCA, some other process should be suspected, such as venous obstruction or global ischemia. In the latter case, edema and subsequent encephalomalacia may be seen bilaterally in so-called watershed regions between vascular territories, such as between the MCA and ACA, or the MCA and PCA. Moreover, arterial occlusion should produce a wedge-shaped configuration that extends out to the surface of the brain, involving the gray matter, whereas other stroke mimics may not.

Hemorrhagic versus Nonhemorrhagic Stroke Broadly speaking, there are two ways of classifying strokes: thrombotic versus embolic, and nonhemorrhagic versus hemorrhagic. Each has different management implications. Approximately two thirds of strokes are thrombotic in origin, and one third are embolic. The principal source of emboli causing stroke is the heart, with mural thrombi arising in myocardial infarction, valvular disease, and atrial fibrillation (where the combination of chamber dilatation and poor emptying is thrombogenic). The carotid arteries are another important source. Both the heart and the carotid arteries can be well evaluated by ultrasound, which noninvasively demonstrates atherosclerotic plaques and thrombi and can be used to assess the degree of vascular stenosis. MR angiography plays an important role in evaluation of the carotid and cerebral arteries; however, the gold standard remains contrast arteriography (**Fig. 9–42**).

Even if it were clinically possible to determine with certainty which patients were suffering from stroke, imaging would still play an important role in almost every case (**Fig. 9–43**). To manage patients optimally, it is necessary to know not only that they are suffering a stroke, but what kind of stroke they are suffering. From the standpoint of acute management, the distinction between thrombotic and embolic strokes is rarely critical. The crucial distinction to be drawn is that between hemorrhagic and nonhemorrhagic strokes. Hemorrhagic strokes may result from a hemorrhagic infarction, either thrombotic or embolic, in which the blood vessels themselves are so damaged by ischemia that they rupture, or from anatomic processes, such as aneurysms (**Fig. 9–44**). It is estimated that ~20% of strokes are hemorrhagic, and of these slightly over one half reflect hemorrhagic infarction. The remainder result from ruptured aneurysms and vascular malformations.

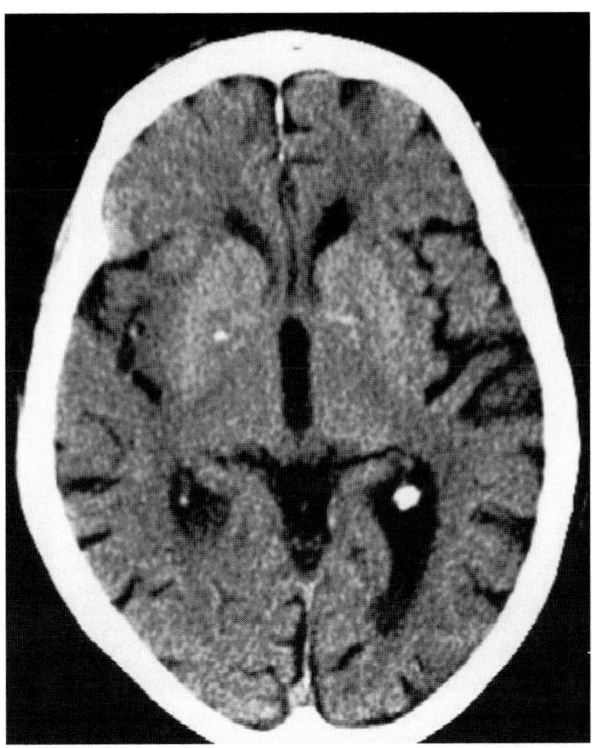

Figure 9–43 An elderly patient presented with acute left-sided weakness. This CT image demonstrates a so-called insular ribbon sign, with loss of the normal gray matter–white matter interface of the insular cortex on the right (compare with the preserved gray matter–white matter interface on the left). This represented an acute right middle cerebral artery infarction. Note also the generalized atrophy and calcification of the choroid plexus.

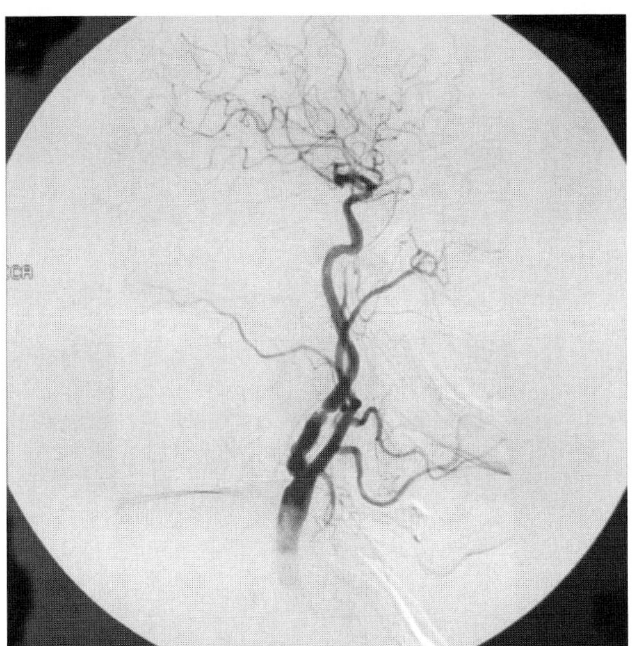

Figure 9–42 A 73-year-old man with diabetes, hypertension, and a long history of cigarette smoking presented with loss of vision in his left eye, with two episodes in the last week. This digital subtraction carotid arteriogram demonstrates an ~90% stenosis of the proximal left internal carotid artery. The atherosclerotic plaque was the source of the emboli that caused the patient's transient ischemic attacks (TIAs).

The clinician needs to know if the stroke is hemorrhagic because the therapeutic regimen for stroke may include thrombolysis, which could be catastrophic in a patient with intracranial bleeding. If instituted within 3 hours, thrombolytic therapy improves the odds of recovery. The phrase "Time is brain" reflects the fact that the earlier therapy is begun, the better the outcome. In an effort to reduce the average 13 hours that elapse between onset of symptoms and presentation for care, stroke centers frequently refer to strokes as "brain attacks," hoping that patients will take action sooner (**Fig. 9–45**).

Anticoagulation, once a mainstay of stroke management, has proven to be of no benefit in most situations, and is contraindicated in large infarctions. Anticoagulation may play a role in cases where the heart is a suspected source of emboli, and where there is documented large vessel stenosis. Aspirin administration appears to improve outcomes, thanks to its antiplatelet action.

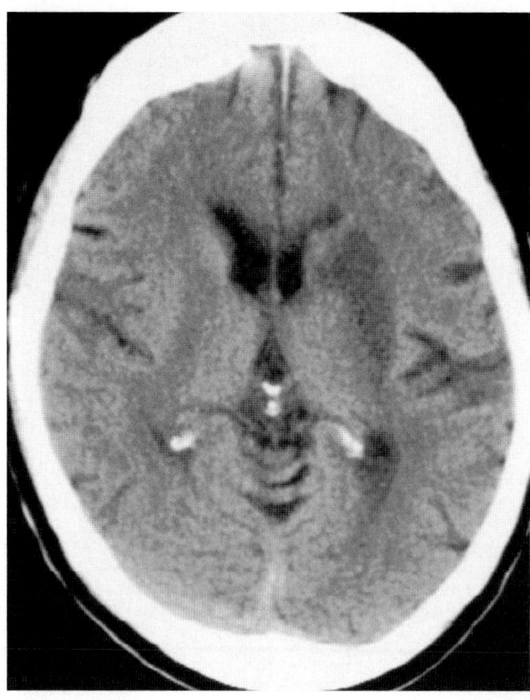

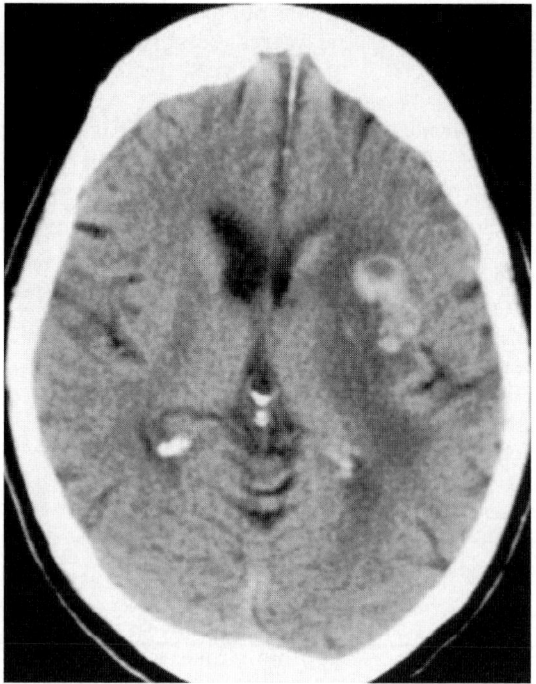

Figure 9–44 **(A)** This noncontrast CT image demonstrates hypodensity in the left middle cerebral artery distribution, indicating an acute stroke. **(B)** The next day, after further deterioration in neurologic status, a follow-up CT demonstrates new high-density blood in the same area, indicating hemorrhagic transformation.

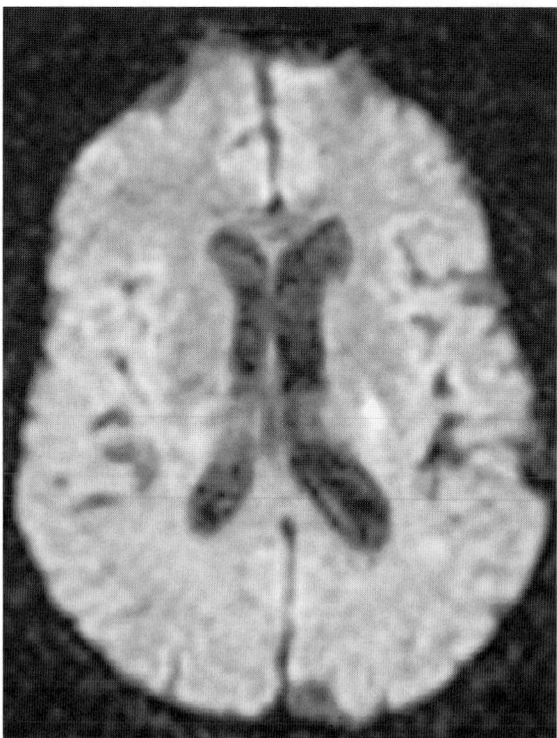

Figure 9–45 This axial diffusion-weighted MR image demonstrates a hyperintense focus in the basal ganglia on the left, representing an acute infarction from small vessel disease. Such a lesion would be occult on CT.

Acute cerebral hemorrhage is best detected by CT scan, which demonstrates fresh blood as high attenuation (bright) material, as compared with the low-density CSF and the isodense brain parenchyma. The blood may be confined to a portion of the parenchyma, or may rupture into the subarachnoid, subdural, or ventricular spaces. Aside from excluding hemorrhage, imaging also plays a role in defining the extent of the ischemic process and demonstrating arterial occlusions that may guide therapy. CT is excellent for excluding the hemorrhage, but it does not perform as well as MRI at these latter two tasks.

In addition to parenchymal hemorrhages, blood may be found in the subarachnoid space. The most common etiology of subarachnoid hemorrhage is trauma (**Fig. 9–46**). In the nontraumatic setting, subarachnoid hemorrhage usually results from rupture of an aneurysm, which occurs in ~30,000 patients per year. Sudden, severe headache is a common presentation, and patients complaining of the "worst headache of their life" must be evaluated for this possibility.

Most patients with nontraumatic subarachnoid hemorrhage have so-called berry aneurysms (saccular aneurysms) around the circle of Willis (**Fig. 9–47**). Common locations include the anterior communicating artery, the MCA, and the posterior communicating artery. Slightly more than half of patients with subarachnoid hemorrhage from a berry aneurysm are hypertensive smokers.

The presence of blood in the subarachnoid space can be confirmed with lumbar puncture; however, blood in the

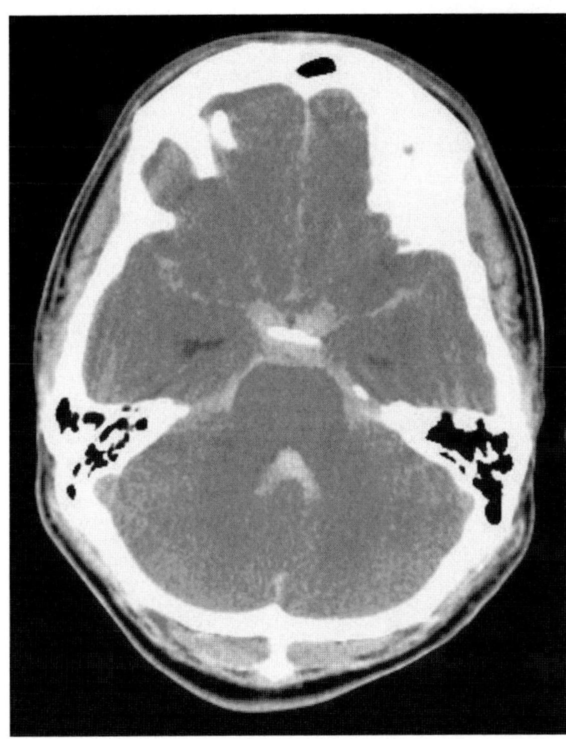

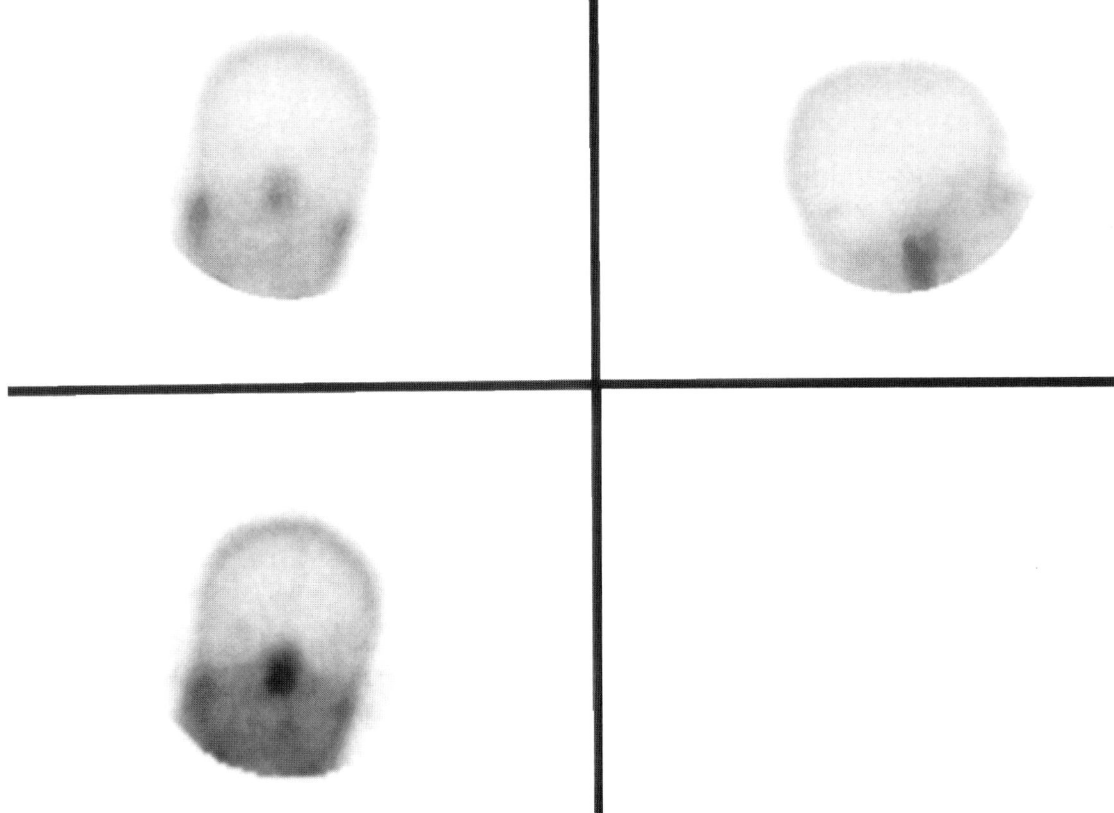

Figure 9–46 **(A)** This young man was struck in the head by a baseball. A noncontrast CT image at the level of the basal cisterns demonstrates extensive subarachnoid hemorrhage in the basal cisterns, sylvian fissure, and posterior fossa. **(B)** This nuclear medicine technetium-(Tc-) 99m hexamethylpropyleneamine oxime (HMPAO) brain death study, including frontal and lateral images, demonstrates absence of intracranial perfusion, indicating brain death.

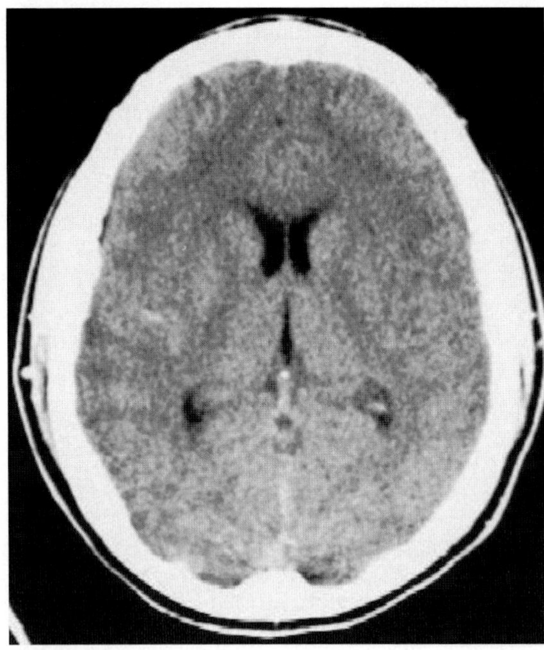

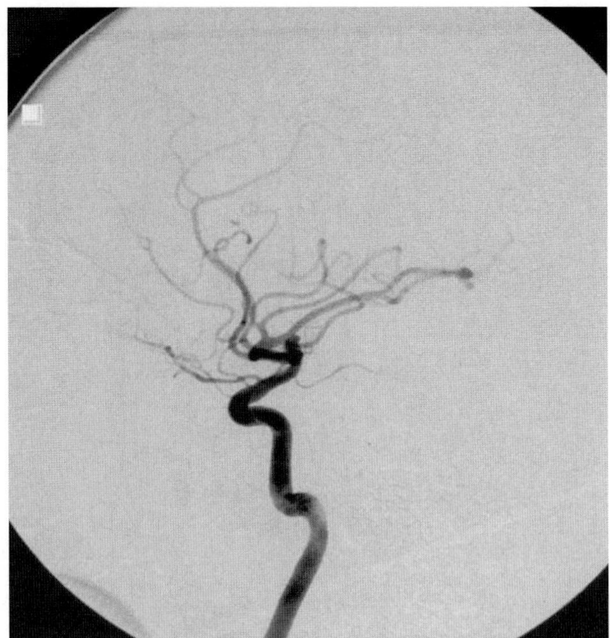

Figure 9–47 (A) This noncontrast head CT demonstrates subtle increased density in the right sylvian fissure in this young man with the "worst headache of his life." **(B)** A digital subtraction right carotid arteriogram demonstrates a 5 mm aneurysm at the bifurcation of the internal carotid artery. This represented subarachnoid hemorrhage from a berry aneurysm.

subarachnoid space does not always stem from a ruptured aneurysm, and may instead reflect a parenchymal hemorrhage that has extended into the ventricles or subarachnoid space. Patients with suspected aneurysm should be evaluated by cerebral angiography, in part to characterize the exact site and nature of the aneurysm in preparation for neurosurgical correction and in part to rule out the presence of other aneurysms (which are multiple in 20% of patients). Patients at increased risk for cerebral aneurysms include those with autosomal dominant polycystic kidney disease (10–30% of patients) and family histories of the disorder.

Primary parenchymal hemorrhages are usually seen in patients with a history of chronic hypertension, often with a more immediate acute exacerbation. For example, cocaine and amphetamine abusers are at increased risk, secondary to the acute increase in blood pressure that accompanies the use of these vasoactive drugs. Especially in a young patient, the possibility of an underlying vascular malformation, which may be surgically correctable, must be ruled out, although they account for only 1 in 20 parenchymal hemorrhages (**Fig. 9–48**). Other risk factors for parenchymal hemorrhage include anticoagulant therapy (which increases the risk 5 to 10 times) and amyloid angiopathy, which is seen in the elderly. Neoplasm also warrants consideration, and the most prevalent primary neoplasm to hemorrhage is glioblastoma. Relatively common hemorrhagic metastases include lung, thyroid, and renal cell carcinomas, as well as melanoma. Factors contributing to tumor hemorrhage include neovascularity, vascular invasion, and tumor necrosis, as the growth of malignant cells outstrips the local blood supply.

Contrast versus Non-Contrast Study A common question in the imaging of suspected stroke is whether to administer intravenous contrast material. In the acute setting, the answer is no. For one thing, the use of contrast infusion in CT may render the detection of small regions of bleeding more difficult, because both acute blood and contrast appear bright. Administering contrast after the nonenhanced study would add to the CT evaluation, but probably only on a case-by-case basis, with the non-contrast study proving adequate in the vast majority of cases. If the case can be monitored while the patient is in the scanner, the findings on the nonenhanced study will in some cases warrant contrast infusion, such as when the findings are suspicious for underlying tumor or abscess, which will be better characterized with enhancement. There is another at least theoretical basis for withholding iodinated contrast material in patients with typical strokes: contrast material that penetrates the disrupted blood–brain barrier may irritate cerebral tissues, increasing the risk of seizures, and increasing edema and associated mass effect. This does not appear to be a problem with the gadolinium-based contrast agents used in MRI, although contrast infusion is generally unnecessary to characterize a stroke by MRI.

Natural History of Stroke Although the brain is exquisitely dependent on a minute-to-minute basis for the oxygen and glucose necessary to sustain its neurons (it contains no myoglobin, glycogen, or fat), the imaging findings of neuronal death do not typically appear for hours or even a full day. The first cells to go are the neurons themselves, which consume 3 to 4 times as much energy as the glial cells of the white matter and are therefore more sensitive to a diminution of supply. As cells die, their membranes cease to maintain the usual balance between intra- and extracellular solutes, with the result that water begins to accumulate in the region of infarction. Both CT, which may show no significant change up to

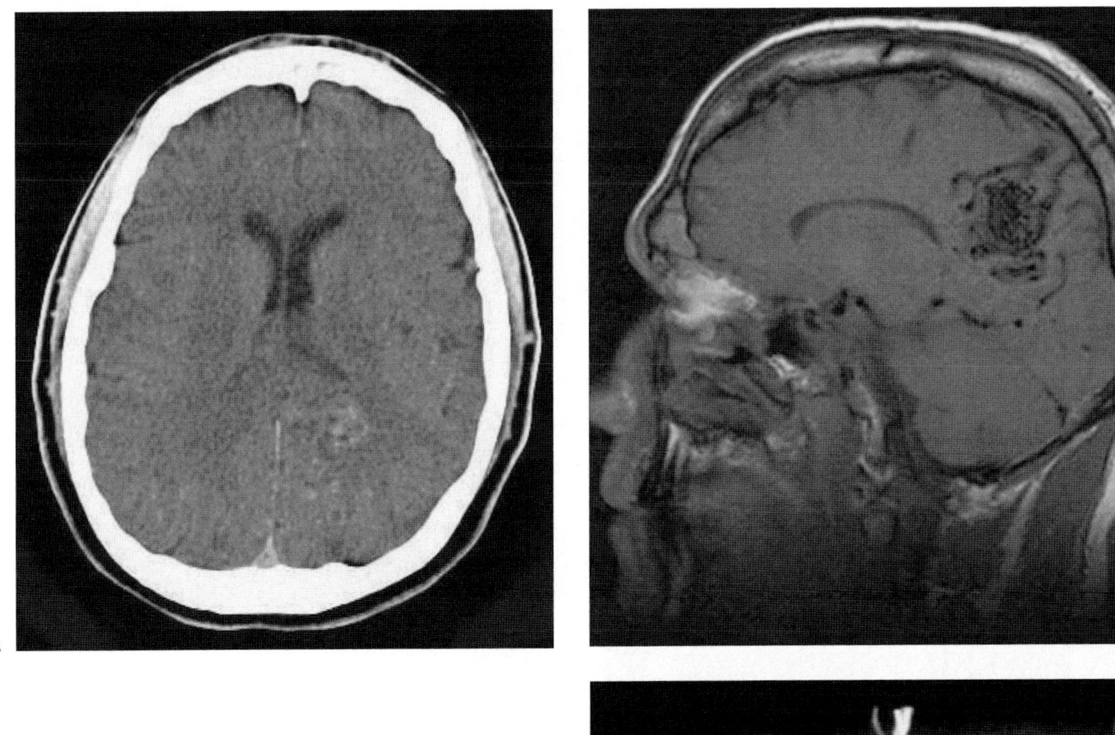

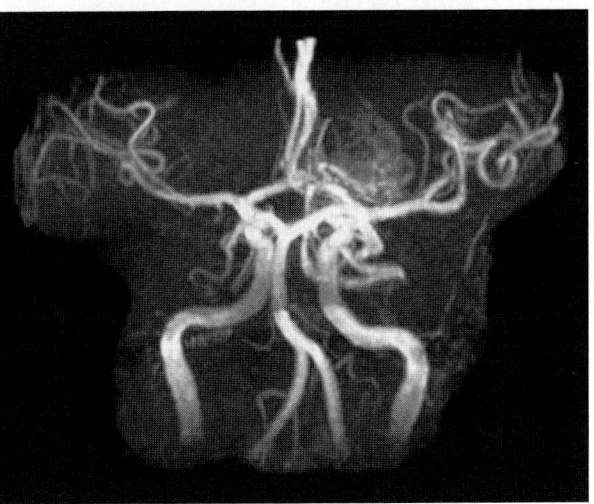

Figure 9–48 This young man presented with chronic headaches that had worsened over the past few hours. **(A)** A noncontrast CT demonstrates an area of increased attenuation (density) in the posterior aspect of the left cerebral hemisphere. **(B)** This sagittal T1-weighted MR image demonstrates serpiginous low signal, consistent with an arteriovenous malformation. **(C)** Magnetic resonance angiography using bright-blood technique demonstrates that the arterial supply is from branches of the left anterior and posterior cerebral arteries.

24 hours after infarction, and MRI, which can show changes within minutes, typically depend on the local increase in brain water to demonstrate acute stroke. In many centers, as long as the infarction is nonhemorrhagic and no other mimics of conventional stroke are involved, it does not matter clinically speaking whether the CT scan elucidates the stroke, because the patient's management will remain the same in either case. In some centers where thrombolysis is routinely employed, emergent MRI is performed, to ensure that only patients likely to benefit receive the treatment. If MRI does not demonstrate a stroke, no thrombolytics are given.

Both CT and MRI may demonstrate stroke within minutes of its occurrence. On CT the actual thrombus or embolus may be seen within a vessel, such as the MCA, as a hyperintense area of attenuation within the vessel lumen ("hyperdense MCA sign"). Another sign appearing within hours is a loss of the usually sharp gray matter–white matter demarcation and effacement of sulci, due to edema (**Fig. 9–49A,B**). MRI may demonstrate a lack of normal "flow void" within the affected vessel, when normally high-velocity blood is replaced by stationary clot. Newer diffusion-weighted MRI techniques are the most sensitive means available for detecting acutely ischemic brain tissue and require only about a minute of scan time.

As the infarction develops, edema begins to produce mass effect. This may range from increasing sulcal effacement to

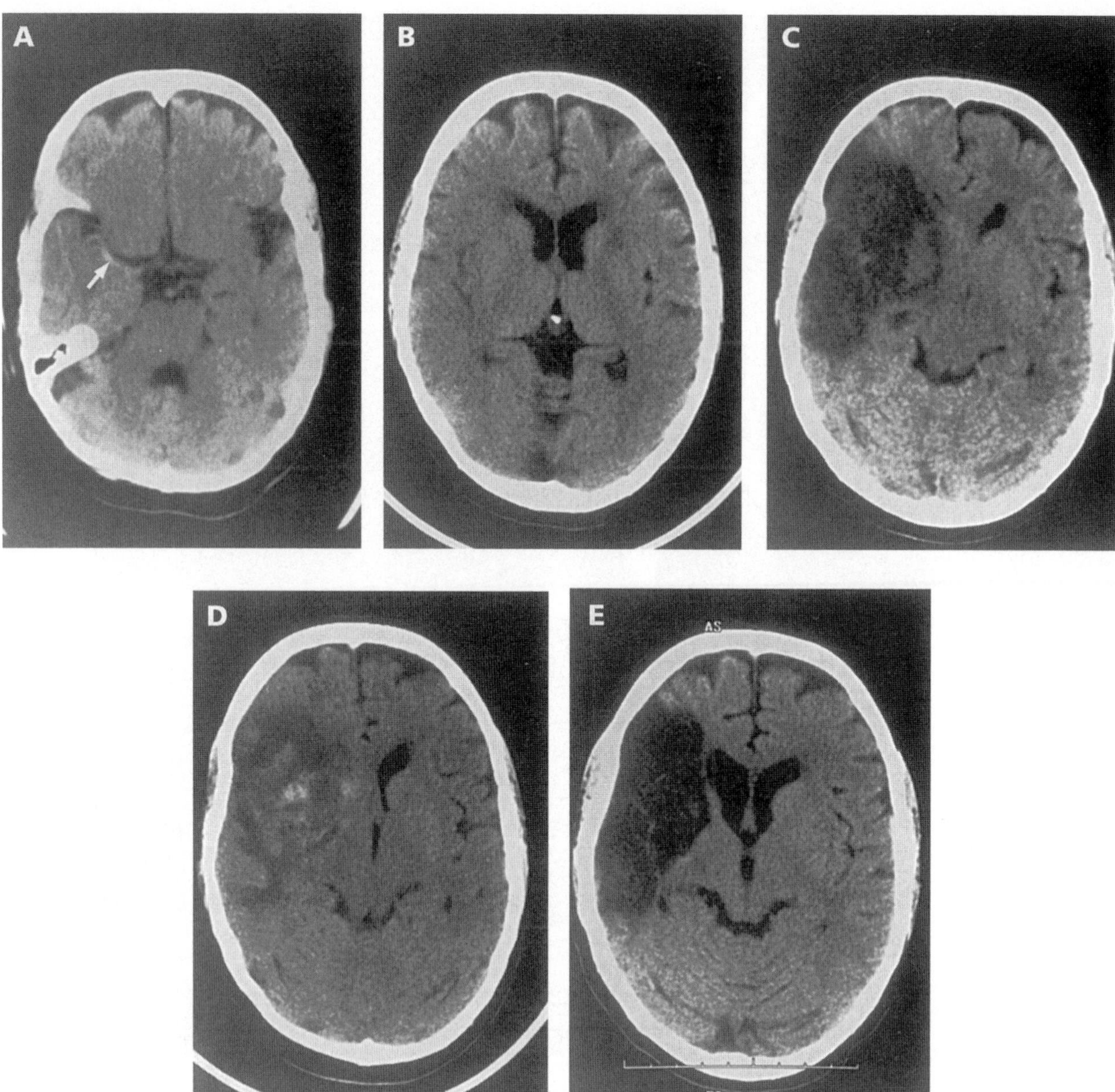

Figure 9–49 A 60-year-old woman presented with an 8-hour history of left hemiparesis and facial droop. **(A)** An axial image from a noncontrast CT scan at the level of the basilar cisterns demonstrates a subtle finding sometimes seen in early stroke; namely, a hyperdense cerebral artery—in this case, the right middle cerebral artery (MCA; arrow). This so-called hyperdense artery sign is due to the presence of in situ or embolic thrombus within the vessel lumen. Its equivalent on magnetic resonance imaging would be the absence of the expected flow void within the vessel. **(B)** Another image from the same study, near the level of the foramen of Monro, demonstrates subtle loss of gray matter–white matter demarcation and effacement of sulci in the right cerebral hemisphere as compared with those on the left. **(C)** An axial image from a scan several days later demonstrates prominent cerebral edema in the territory of the right MCA. The edema is causing mass effect on the frontal horn of the right lateral ventricle, as well as a shift of midline structures such as the third ventricle to the left. **(D)** An axial CT image obtained 10 days postevent demonstrates continued edema and mass effect in the right MCA distribution, but there has been interval appearance of high-density regions, indicating hemorrhage. **(E)** An axial CT image 14 weeks postevent reveals that the right-sided edema has completely subsided, and that the infarcted brain parenchyma has been almost completely replaced by CSF density fluid. The frontal horn of the right lateral ventricle is now larger than its left counterpart, a phenomenon called ex vacuo dilation.

more severe manifestations such as subfalcine or uncal herniation. In general, the larger the region of brain infarcted, the greater the peak mass effect observed during the third through seventh days postevent (**Fig. 9–49C**). In an effort to combat acute cerebral swelling, mannitol (which increases intravascular oncotic pressure, and therefore tends to draw water back into the intravascular space) and hyperventilation (which causes arteriolar smooth muscle contraction, and therefore decreases intravascular hydrostatic pressure) may be employed. Between ~3 to 10 days postevent, the risk of so-called reperfusion hemorrhage is increased (**Fig. 9–49D**). At ~1 week, the brain begins to soften, producing encephalomalacia. Encephalomalacia is seen as decreased attenuation on CT and as increased T2-weighted signal on MRI, in both cases secondary to the relative increase in water content. Eventually, the softened brain parenchyma is replaced by CSF, and the adjacent ventricular system dilates to fill the vacated space, a process referred to as ex vacuo dilation (**Fig. 9–49E**).

One or more lacunar infarcts are frequently found on CNS imaging, especially in hypertensive patients and the elderly. These measure less than 1.5 cm in diameter and are caused by the occlusion of small, penetrating arteries supplying the basal ganglia and internal capsule. Such strokes are suspected when the patient presents with pure motor or pure sensory deficits, or with syndromes such as dysarthria and clumsiness of the hands.

Low Back Pain

◇ Epidemiology

Low back pain is an extremely common problem in the United States, and it is estimated that 80% of Americans suffer from it at some point in their lives. It is second only to the common cold as the condition for which patients most often seek medical care, and it is the single most expensive medical condition afflicting Americans between the ages of 20 and 50. years. At this time, ~5 million Americans are disabled by low back pain. Although symptoms resolve in the majority of patients, they recur in 60 to 85%. Risk factors for low back pain include obesity, pregnancy, cigarette smoking, and psychosocial factors, such as lower educational status, which is positively correlated with both increased incidence of low back pain and poorer outcome. Imaging reveals the cause of continued pain and functional incapacitation in ~20% of cases.

Of conservatively treated patients, 50% experience resolution of symptoms within 1 week, and 90% have complete resolution within 12 weeks. Conservative treatment consists of bed rest and the use of nonsteroidal anti-inflammatory drugs. Weight reduction, smoking cessation, and regular exercise are effective long-term strategies to reduce the frequency and severity of recurrence. Surgical therapy is generally reserved for patients with definitive radiological evidence of an anatomic etiology, a corresponding pain syndrome and associated neurologic deficits, and failure to respond to 1 to 2 months of conservative therapy. Approximately 1 to 2% of Americans have undergone lumbar spine surgery to correct low back pain.

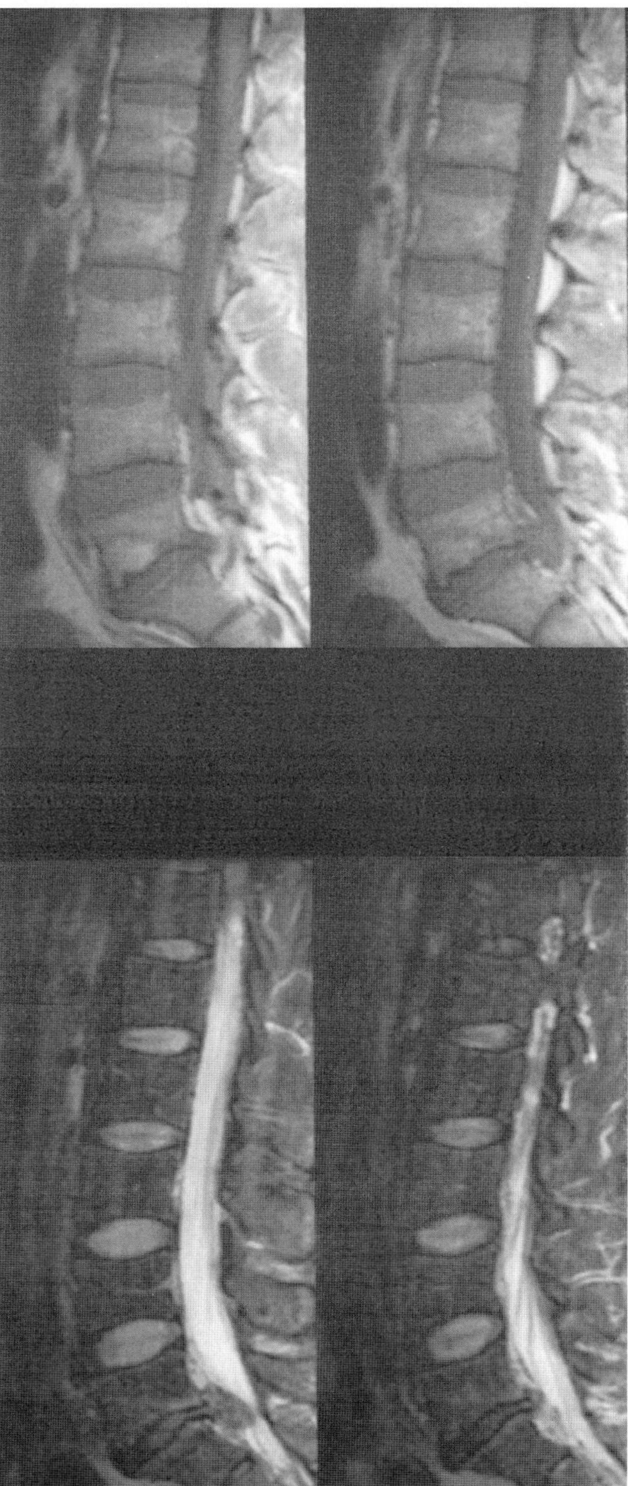

Figure 9–50 These T1 (top row) and T2 (bottom row) sagittal MR images of the lumbar spine demonstrate a disk herniation at the L5–S1 level, with protrusion of disk material into the vertebral canal and compression of nerve roots, which explained the patient's symptoms.

◇ Pathophysiology

There are several anatomic causes of low back pain, one of the most common being disk herniation (**Fig. 9–50**). The intervertebral disk is composed of a soft, fibrous center, the nucleus pulposus, surrounded by a tough outer covering, the annulus fibrosus. A disc herniation occurs when a portion of the nucleus pulposus ruptures through a tear in the annulus fibrosus. Beginning in the second decade of life, the intervertebral discs degenerate, exhibiting a decrease in water content and proteoglycans, with an increase in collagen. This is accompanied by a decrease in signal intensity within the disc on T2-weighted images, often referred to as desiccation. With time, there is loss of intervertebral disc height and bulging of the disk material against the anulus fibrosus. If the anulus remains intact, there can be no herniation, but with time, fissures and frank tears may form in the anulus, permitting the disk material to protrude beyond the column of the vertebral bodies, where it may impinge on the spinal cord or nerve roots. The pain of a herniated disk is thought to result from the impingement of the disk material on the receptors of the anulus fibrosus or posterior longitudinal ligament, which runs along the posterior margin of the vertebral bodies.

In the lumbar spine, a disk herniation may impinge on any nerve root still within the neural canal at that level (recalling that the cord itself generally terminates between T11 and L1). In the typical case, a disk herniation will cause symptoms one level below the disk, so that an L4–L5 herniation will cause an L5 radiculopathy (from the same Latin root as the word *radical*, meaning "root"). A typical presentation would be a history of back pain with more recent unilateral pain radiating down the leg in the distribution of the sciatic nerve, called sciatica. Physical examination reveals the level, with the L4 root responsible for the knee jerk, whereas the ankle jerk is at S1. More than 90% of lumbar disk herniations occur at the L4–L5 or L5–S1 levels.

The distinction between a posterior disk herniation and a lateral disk herniation is often difficult or impossible to make on purely clinical grounds. Only ~1 in 20 disk herniations is lateral, but failure to diagnose a lateral disk on imaging could cause the surgeon to operate at the wrong level. Consider, for example, a patient with clinical symptoms referable to the L4–L5 level. By far the most common etiology of such symptoms would be a posterior disk herniation causing compression of the L5 nerve root; however, a lateral disk at the L5–S1 level could cause identical symptoms and result in failed back surgery if the surgeon were to operate based on clinical criteria alone. In other words, a lateral L5–S1 disk herniation may produce clinical signs and symptoms identical to a posterior L4–L5 herniation.

The second major offender in low back pain is spondylosis, also referred to as degenerative disease or osteoarthritis of the spine (although the latter is a misnomer and should be reserved for degenerative change at the apophyseal joints only). It is more common than herniated disk; although approximately one third of asymptomatic individuals have at least one herniated disk, virtually every person has some degree of spondylosis by their later years. The back pain of spondylosis is usually of an aching nature and is exacerbated by prolonged standing or walking. Plain films may be used to diagnose lumbar spondylosis, but myelography, CT, or MRI is necessary to assess the degree of spinal stenosis and nerve root compression.

◇ Imaging

MRI has dramatically enhanced spine imaging, due to its superior tissue resolution, multiplanar imaging capabilities, noninvasive nature, and freedom from the artifact produced by bone in CT. T1-weighted images provide the best information about spinal anatomy, including the cord, whereas T2-weighted images (in which CSF is bright) provide a myelographic effect that is excellent for assessing both cord and nerve root compression and intrinsic cord lesions. A good search pattern for assessing the spine begins with sagittal sequences. Standard parameters, such as vertebral body and disk space height and vertebral alignment, should be assessed, as well as the signal of the bone marrow (which should be bright on T1 due to fat). The cord itself should be inspected for abnormalities in caliber or signal, and to ensure that it ends at or about the usual L1 level. On both sagittal and axial images, the neural foramina should be examined to rule out encroachment by osteophytes or disk material on the nerve roots.

Two types of disk abnormalities are seen on imaging, annular bulges and herniations (**Fig. 9–51**). An annular bulge is a broad extension of the disk beyond the vertebral end plate. This is a prominent finding in patients older than age 20 and is most often asymptomatic. A herniation is a focal protrusion of the disk material through the anulus fibrosus, which may extend into the vertebral canal, the neural foramen, or even extraforaminally, a so-called far-lateral herniation. When the herniated fragment of disk material becomes detached from the disk, it is referred to as a free fragment, which, if it migrates superiorly or inferiorly, may cause misleading clinical signs at a level above or below the actual herniation (**Fig. 9–52**).

Spondylosis manifests radiographically as osteophyte formation at the vertebral end plates and facet joints, which may encroach on both the vertebral canal, causing cord impingement, and the neural foramina, causing radiculopathy. Additional factors in a spondylosis syndrome include hypertrophy and ossification of the posterior longitudinal ligament and ligamentum flavum, which tend to compress the thecal sac in an anteroposterior dimension, and congenital spinal stenosis, or "short pedicle syndrome," which makes the canal narrower to begin with and therefore decreases neurologic tolerance for any degree of compromise. Spinal stenosis is a component of achondroplasia, the most common form of dwarfism.

In some cases, low back pain and radiculopathy may be traced to spondylolysis, a congenital or acquired defect in the pars interarticularis of the vertebral body, which appears on oblique radiographs as a break in the neck of the "Scottie dog" discussed below. Spondylolysis is often compounded by spondylolisthesis, which frequently occurs at the L5–S1 level, and represents the displacement of one vertebral body on another (**Fig. 9–53**). Such slippage tends to compromise the vertebral canal and is usually treated with a combination of posterior decompression laminectomy and posterior vertebral fusion.

Failed back surgery occurs in 10 to 40% of patients. Common causes of failed back surgery syndromes include recurrent or residual herniation, arachnoiditis, and spinal stenosis. Postoperative imaging plays an important role in patients with recurrent or residual symptoms. For example, either disk material or scar tissue may impress on the thecal sac or nerve roots. If the compression is due to disk material, the patient is often reoperated. Scar is generally not reoperated. The two can be distinguished based on their imaging charac-

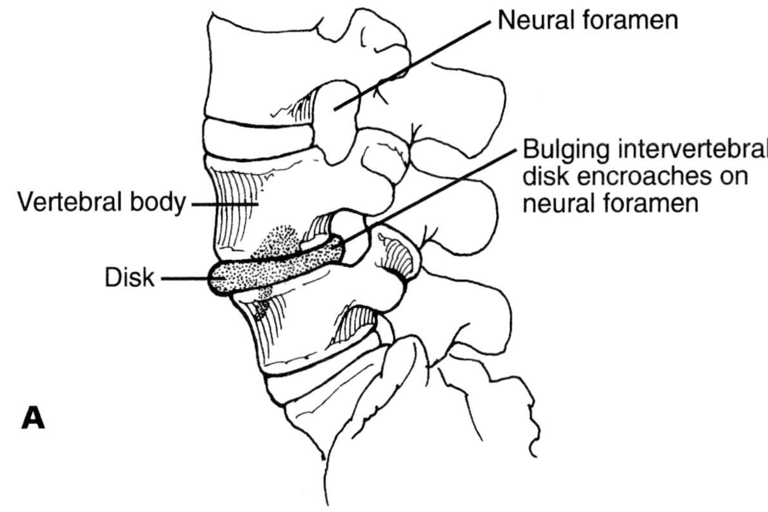

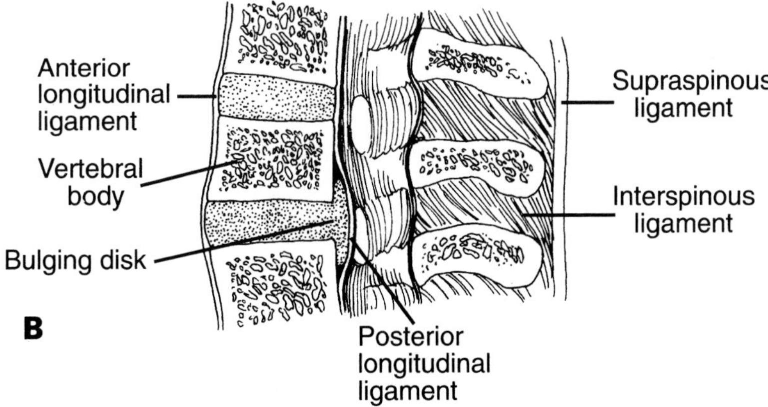

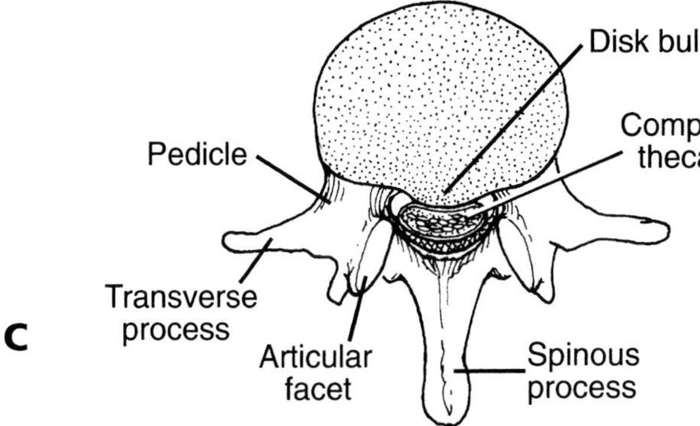

Figure 9–51 **(A)** The lumbar spine as seen in a lateral view demonstrates how a posteriorly bulging intervertebral disk might encroach on a neural foramen and compress an exiting lumbar nerve root. **(B)** A view through the midline of the spine shows how the bulging disk causes posterior displacement of the posterior longitudinal ligament. **(C)** An axial view shows the typical appearance of a disk bulge or herniation compressing the thecal sac, and potentially the nerve roots it contains.

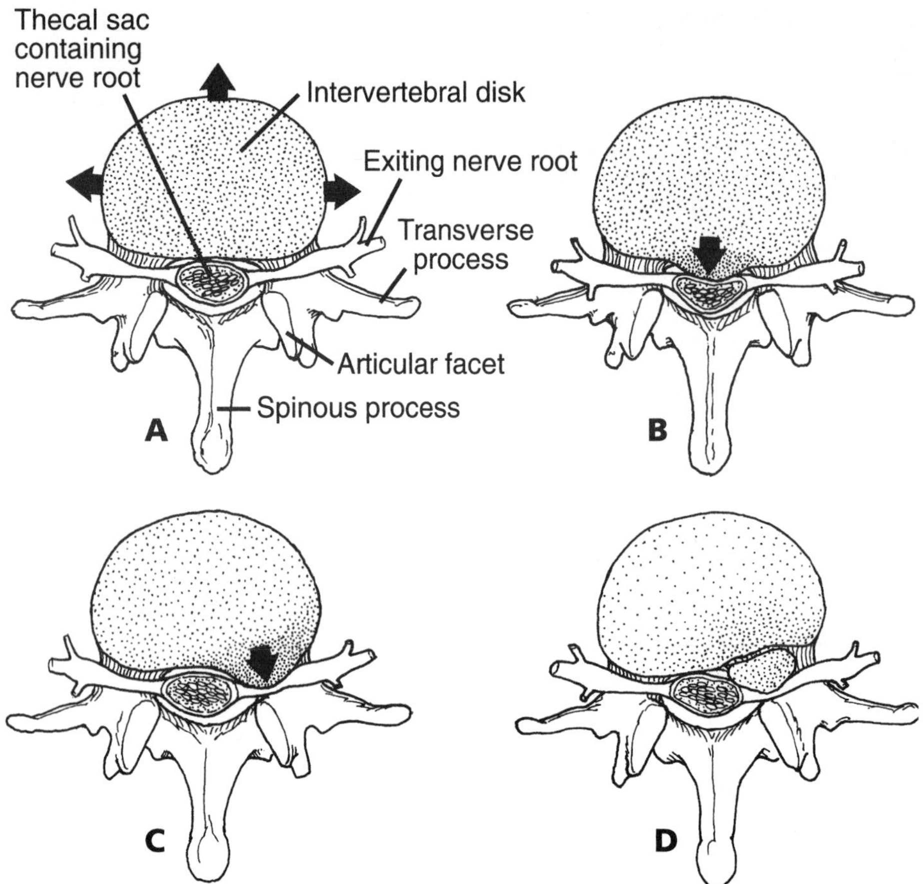

Figure 9–52 Intervertebral disk abnormalities illustrate the variety of ways in which nerve root compression may result. **(A)** There is a diffuse disk bulge extending anteriorly and laterally (arrows), but not affecting the thecal sac or exiting nerve roots. **(B)** A focal posterior disk bulge impinges on the thecal sac (arrow). **(C)** A lateral disk bulge compresses an exiting left nerve root (arrow). **(D)** A free fragment of herniated disk material, which may have migrated from another level, compresses an exiting nerve root.

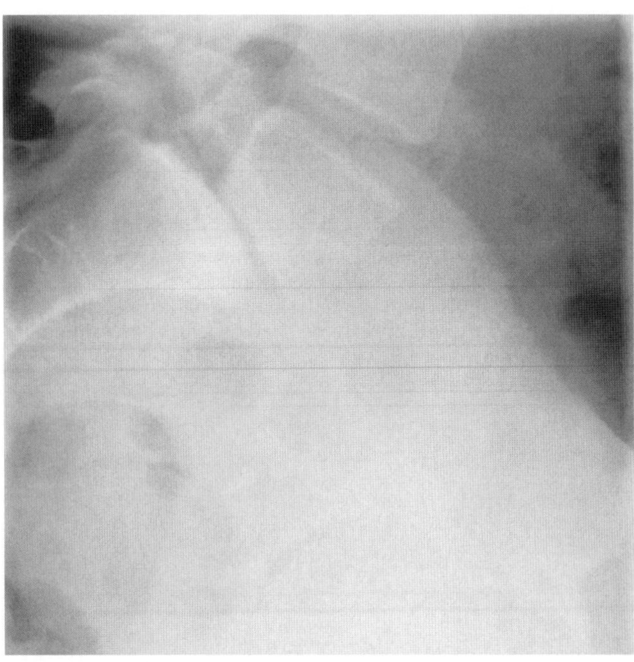

Figure 9–53 This lateral spine radiograph demonstrates anterior displacement (anterolisthesis) of L5 on S1.

teristics: scar, which is vascularized, will enhance with contrast administration; disk material, which is avascular, will not enhance (**Fig. 9–54**).

Cervical Disk Disease and Spondylosis

Principles similar to those in the low back apply to the neck as well. Patients with herniated cervical disks often complain of a dull, aching pain that radiates to the shoulder. When nerve root compression occurs, radicular symptoms result, including pain radiating into the arm, weakness, and loss of sensation in a specific nerve distribution. A lesion at C5–C6 commonly causes loss of the biceps reflex, whereas the triceps reflex is impaired by lesions at C6–C7. The most common level of cervical disk herniation is C6–C7, with approximately two thirds of herniations at this level, and the majority of the remainder at C5–C6. Cervical spondylosis occurs most frequently at the C5–C6 interspace and presents with a more insidious onset of symptoms than is seen in acute disk herniation. The encroachment of osteophytes on the neural foramina is well evaluated on oblique views of the cervical spine, although MRI is of course much more sensitive for the detection of noncalcified disk material (**Fig. 9–55**).

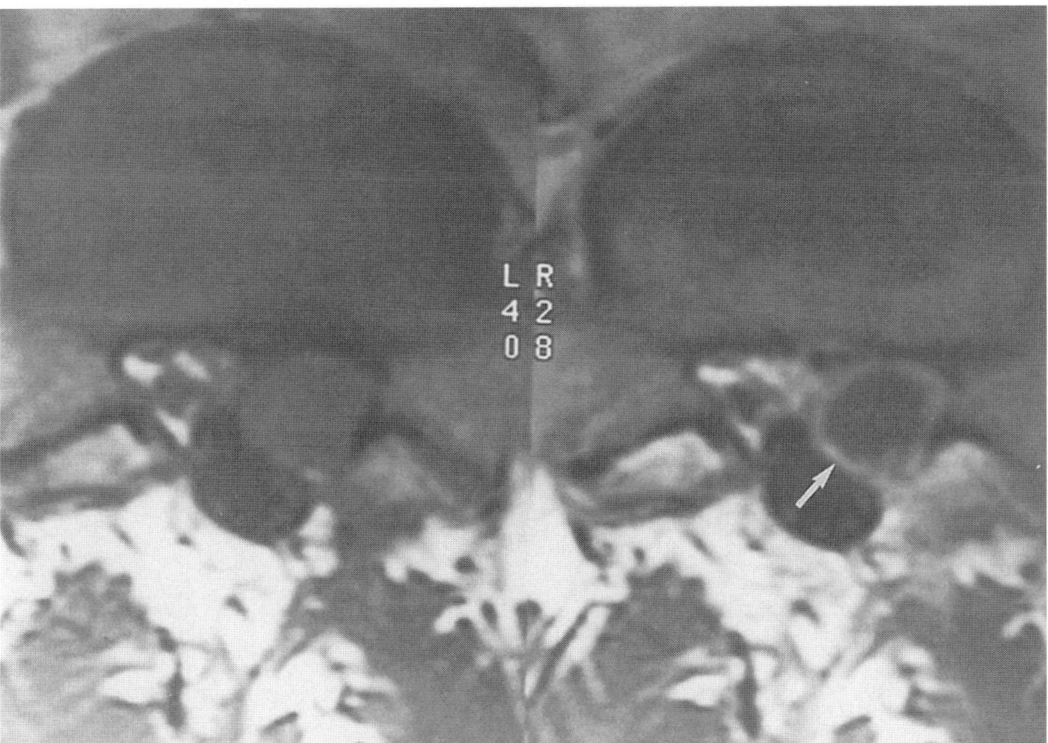

Figure 9–54 This middle-aged man with a history of L5–S1 diskectomy presents with left leg pain. The precontrast (left) and postcontrast (right) T1-weighted MR images demonstrate a soft tissue mass protruding posteriorly in the vertebral canal on the left, compressing the thecal sac. Note that on the postcontrast image, the mass shows peripheral enhancement (arrow), indicating that it is associated with granulation tissue or scar.

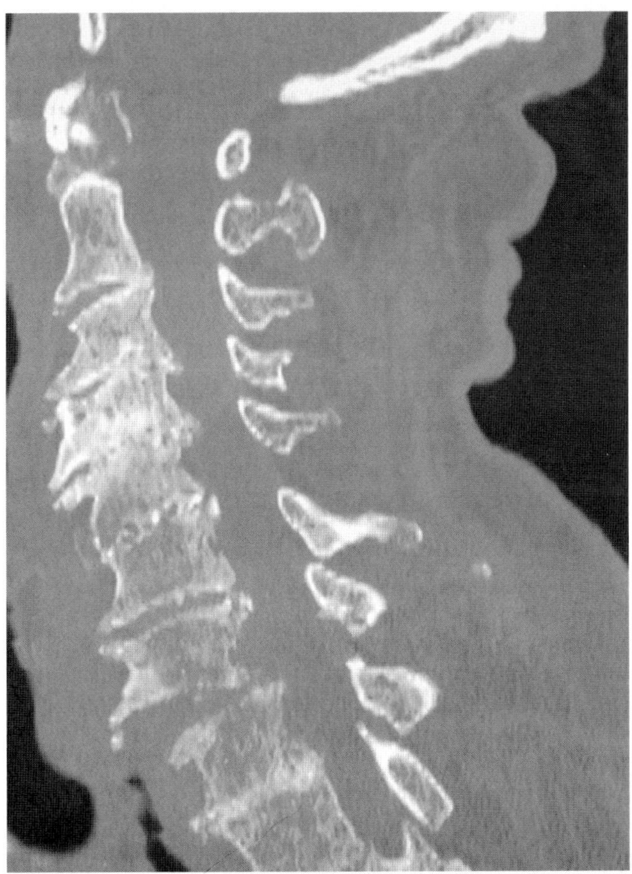

Figure 9–55 This sagittal reformat of axially acquired CT data of the cervical spine in a patient with recent neck trauma demonstrates severe degenerative changes with disk space narrowing and osteophytosis, as well as a fracture of the C7 vertebral body and anterolisthesis of C7 on T1.

10

Pediatric Radiology

The purpose of this chapter is not to survey all of pediatric radiology, but to explore some of the most common or illustrative pediatric medical and surgical pathologies, and to review some of the principal anatomic, physiologic, and pathologic differences between children and adults. Perhaps the most critical lesson of pediatrics is that children are poorly served if treated as miniature adults—a principle that applies in every area of pediatric imaging.

◆ Imaging

Several special characteristics of pediatric patients create special challenges and opportunities in pediatric imaging. One of the most important challenges is the need to prevent avoidable exposure to ionizing radiation. Although there is no definite evidence that the low levels of radiation exposure associated with diagnostic imaging produce adverse genetic or somatic effects, both experience with populations exposed to relatively high levels of radiation (Hiroshima and Nagasaki, Japan) and theoretical models of deoxyribonucleic acid (DNA) damage would suggest that the hazards of radiation exposure are greater at earlier ages. In practical terms, limiting exposure means reducing x-ray tube current, utilizing intermittent rather than continuous fluoroscopic monitoring, shielding radiosensitive tissues such as the gonads and breasts, and, whenever possible, choosing imaging modalities that do not involve ionizing radiation.

Another challenge faced by pediatric imaging is the need to immobilize the patient. Infants and young children typically cannot understand or comply with instructions to remain still, and they may be frightened and upset by the unfamiliar environment of the radiology department and its equipment. Not only lengthier examinations such as nuclear medicine, magnetic resonance imaging, and computed tomography, but even relatively quick procedures such as chest and bone radiographs require that the patient be still during data acquisition. In the case of a chest radiograph, the exposure may last only a split second, whereas nuclear medicine and MRI procedures may in some cases require 1 hour or more. When the procedure is brief, a parent can often restrain the child by holding the arms and/or legs. In addition, immobilization devices such as boards or "papoose" wraps may be used. When the examination requires more time, sedation may be necessary. Generally, children younger than several months of age are immobilized, and those between several months and 4 to 5 years require sedation for longer examinations. Children at risk for airway obstruction or with central nervous system disorders may not be eligible for conscious sedation and instead require general anesthesia and mechanical ventilation.

An imaging modality particularly well suited to infants and young children is ultrasound, which exhibits several important advantages. First, ultrasound involves no ionizing radiation, and there are no known risks to health associated with diagnostic sonography. Second, patients are often small enough that a surprisingly great extent of the body is accessible to sonographic imaging. The fact that the infantile calvarium is not completely closed renders ultrasound a key neuroimaging modality early in life. Third, although patients may occasionally complain that the ultrasound transducer "tickles," sonography involves no pain and can be comfortably performed in real time, thus making patient restraint and sedation generally unnecessary. Of course, several structures such as aerated lung and subcortical bone remain inaccessible to ultrasound, as in the adult.

◆ Pathology

Circulatory System

Congenital Heart Disease

◇ Epidemiology

Congenital heart disease is found in 1% of newborns. The two most common forms are bicuspid aortic valve and mitral valve prolapse (discussed in Chapter 2). These are generally asymptomatic in the pediatric patient.

◇ Pathophysiology

Fetal circulatory patterns differ markedly from those seen after birth (**Fig. 10–1**). The principal difference stems from the fact that the fetus is not breathing air, but acquires all of its oxygen and disposes of all of its carbon dioxide through the placenta and the maternal circulation. Two bypasses in the fetal circulation—the foramen ovale, an opening in the interatrial septum, and the ductus arteriosus, which connects the left pulmonary artery to the proximal descending aorta—serve to redirect blood flow away from the fetal lungs. During in utero life, the collapsed lungs manifest a high resistance to flow, and right heart pressures are higher than left heart pressures. As a result, blood is shunted through both these bypasses into the systemic circulation, where it either supplies systemic tissues or enters the umbilical artery and returns to the placenta. Beginning at birth, the combination of lung expansion and ventilation causes pulmonary vascular resistance to fall; once it falls lower than systemic resistance, shunts resulting from such lesions as a patent ductus arteriosus, atrial septal defect, or ventricular septal defect will shift from right to left to left to right.

◇ Clinical Presentation

A critical clinical discriminator in congenital heart disease is cyanosis (from the Greek *kyanos*, "blue"). Acyanotic disease implies that there is a left-to-right shunt, with oxygen-saturated blood being shunted back to the lungs. Cyanosis implies a right-to-left shunt or admixture lesion (e.g., a truncus arteriosus, in which the right and left ventricles empty into a single vessel), in which desaturated blood is entering the systemic circulation. Lesions that commonly present in the first few weeks of life include hypoplastic left heart syndrome and transposition of the great arteries. Hypoplastic left heart syndrome presents within a few days of birth with congestive heart failure (CHF), and closure of the ductus arteriosus during the first week commonly results in cardiogenic shock and death. Transposition of the great arteries consists of origination of the aorta from the right ventricle and

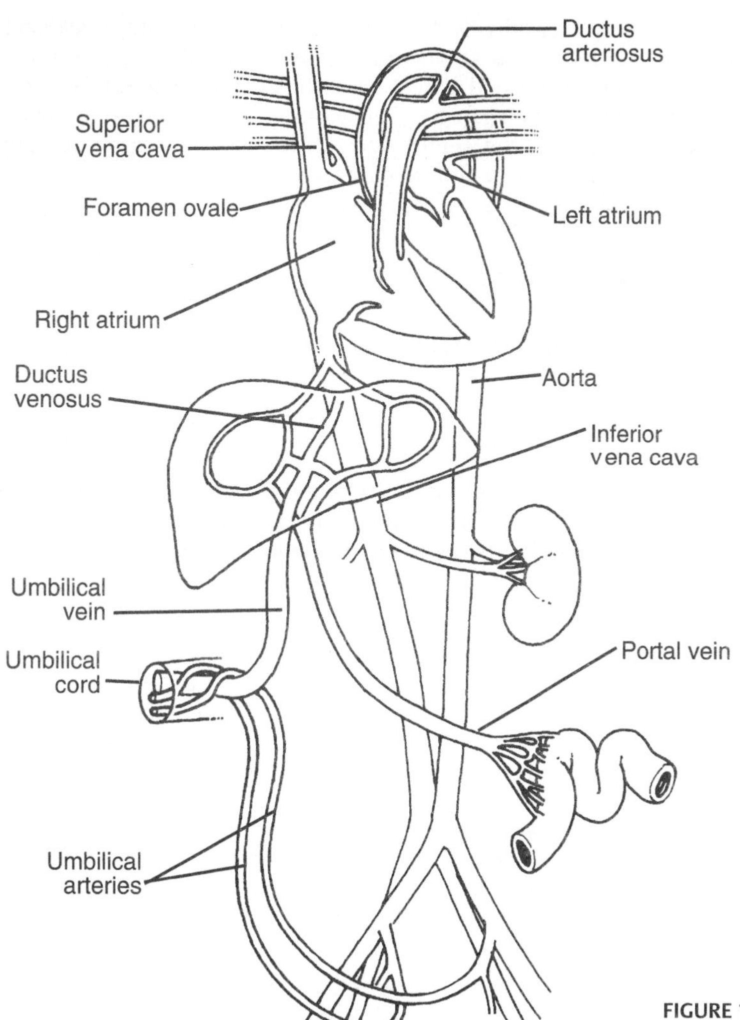

FIGURE 10–1 The major structures of the fetal circulation. Note that the foramen ovale and the ductus arteriosus represent major routes by which the pulmonary circulation is bypassed.

origination of the pulmonary artery from the left ventricle. This situation creates two separate circulations and is incompatible with life unless lesions such as atrial or ventricular septal defects permit mixing. This is the most common lesion to present with cyanosis in the first 24 hours of life.

◇ Imaging

Classically, cardiac catheterization represented the definitive means of diagnosing congenital heart disease. Today noninvasive modalities such as echocardiography and MRI are playing an increasing role. A key role of the radiologist is plain film diagnosis. Perhaps the single most important parameter in plain film diagnosis is pulmonary perfusion. Broadly speaking, pulmonary perfusion may be decreased, normal, or increased (**Fig. 10–2**). Other important features that can be employed in conjunction with pulmonary perfusion to arrive at a diagnosis include chamber enlargement, the appearance of the aorta and pulmonary vein, and soft tissue and bone changes (such as rib notching in coarctation of the aorta).

Decreased pulmonary perfusion, manifested by small pulmonary vessels and radiolucent lungs, generally implies an obstruction to right ventricular outflow. An important etiology is tetralogy of Fallot. This consists of an obstructed right ventricular outflow tract, right ventricular hypertrophy, a ventricular septal defect, and an aorta overriding the interventricular septum. It is associated with a right aortic arch in one quarter of cases, and the heart often exhibits a boot-shaped appearance, due to right ventricular enlargement. A less common but classic radiographic appearance is seen in Ebstein's anomaly, which is a form of right-sided cardiac obstruction associated with diminished pulmonary circulation and massive right atriomegaly, producing a "box-shaped" heart (**Fig. 10–3**).

Normal pulmonary vascularity often implies uncomplicated valvular disease or coarctation of the aorta. Types of valve disease include pulmonic stenosis and congenital aortic stenosis. Pulmonic stenosis may produce right ventricular hypertrophy and prominence of the main pulmonary artery; aortic stenosis generally causes left ventricular hypertrophy and CHF. Coarctation of the aorta is most often of the juxtaductal type, with narrowing of the aorta at or just below the ductus arteriosus, and generally does not present until later childhood. It is commonly associated with a bicuspid

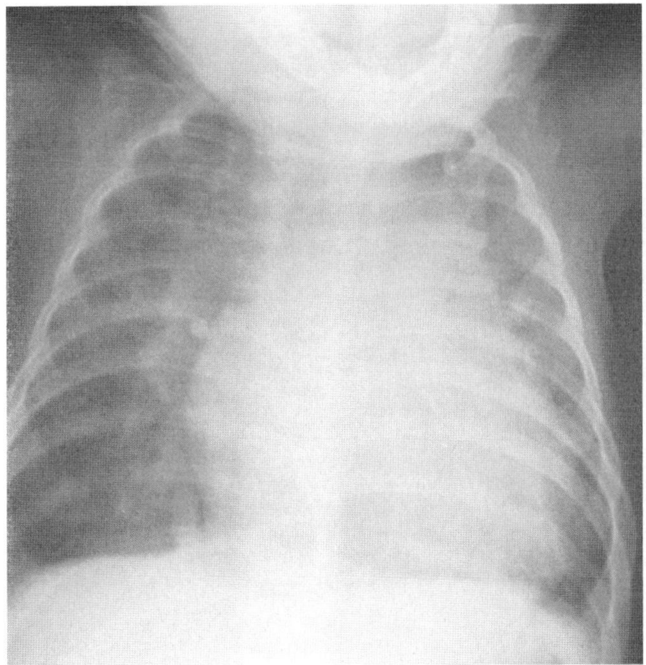

FIGURE 10–2 This infant's chest radiograph demonstrates cardiomegaly and a pulmonary vascular pattern consistent with left-to-right shunting, with enlarged pulmonary vessels and central air-space opacities typical of pulmonary edema. The patient was in mild respiratory distress but was not cyanotic. Echocardiography (not shown) revealed a large ventricular septal defect (VSD).

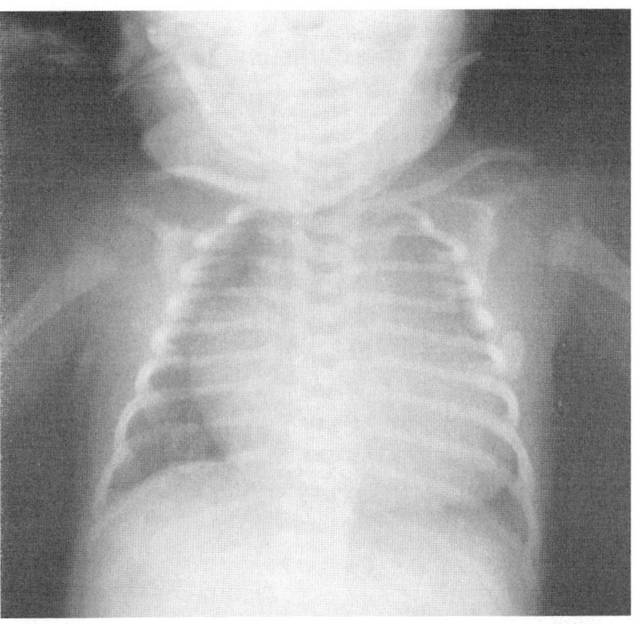

FIGURE 10–3 This infant was noted to be cyanotic shortly after birth. A frontal chest radiograph demonstrates marked cardiomegaly and decreased pulmonary perfusion. Echocardiography (not shown) revealed a massive right atrium and other findings of Ebstein's anomaly.

aortic valve. Important radiographic signs include a visible indentation in the aorta at the coarctation and inferior rib notching, which is produced when dilated intercostal arteries providing collaterals around the obstruction produce remodeling in the adjacent ribs (**Fig. 10–4**).

Increased pulmonary perfusion may represent either active or passive pulmonary overcirculation. Active pulmonary overcirculation implies a left-to-right shunt producing a right ventricular output at least 2 to 3 times that of the left ventricle. Common causes include atrial septal defect, ventricular septal defect, and patent ductus arteriosus. Atrial septal defect is a common symptomatic congenital cardiac anomaly. Due to low atrial pressures, it often does not present for decades, and is also the most prevalent congenital cardiac anomaly to present in adulthood (**Fig. 10–5**). Ventricular septal defect is the most common congenital cardiac anomaly, and if large may present with CHF in the second or third month of life. Fortunately, many lesions close spontaneously by the age of 10 years. The ductus arteriosus normally closes functionally at 48 hours. In patent ductus arteriosus, the fall in pulmonary vascular resistance with breathing produces a reversal of flow through the ductus, from the aorta and into the pulmonary arteries. Again, large lesions produce CHF at 2 to 3 months (**Fig. 10–6**).

Respiratory System

The neonatal chest differs from that of the older child and adult in several important respects. Anatomic differences include airways that are more flaccid, proportionately smaller peripheral airways, less developed collateral air circulation through the pores of Kohn and channels of Lambert, and greater mucus production. These factors mean that the lungs of neonates and infants are more susceptible to obstruction, either from airway collapse or blockage by secretions, than those of the adult. This obstruction, in turn, may result in either atelectasis (due to collapse of unaerated distal air spaces) or air trapping (due to increased residual volume in a check-valve type of airway obstruction). The following discussion concerns common or paradigmatic causes of neonatal respiratory distress.

Neonatal Respiratory Distress

The neonate in respiratory distress may exhibit a variety of nonspecific findings, including tachypnea, grunting, nasal flaring, chest wall retractions, cyanosis, or blood gas abnormalities. The conditions producing respiratory distress in the neonate may be divided somewhat arbitrarily into medical and surgical conditions. Surgical conditions are those that usually require urgent surgical intervention, whereas medical conditions usually respond to pharmacologic maneuvers and ventilatory support. Of course, this is not a hard-and-fast distinction, and in severe cases, conditions classified here as medical may also require surgical therapy, such as extracorporeal membrane oxygenation (ECMO) in patients with very severe pulmonary disease. The chest radiograph plays a

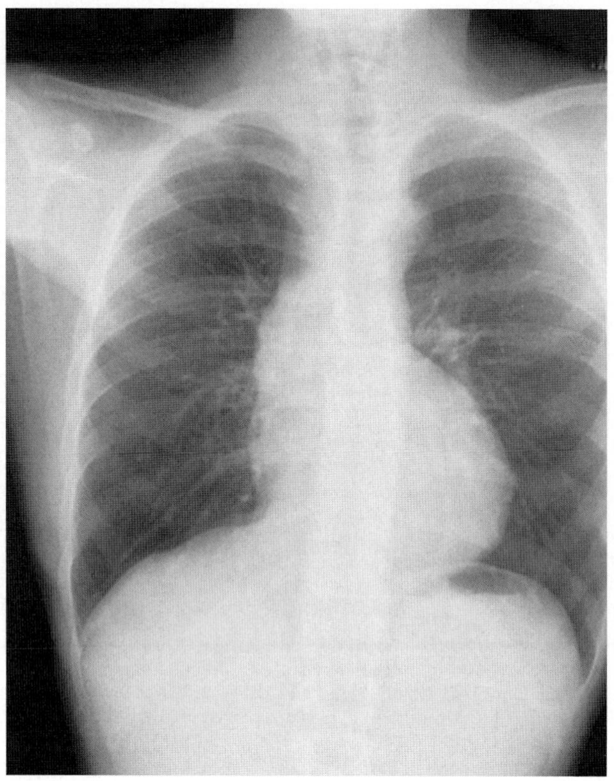

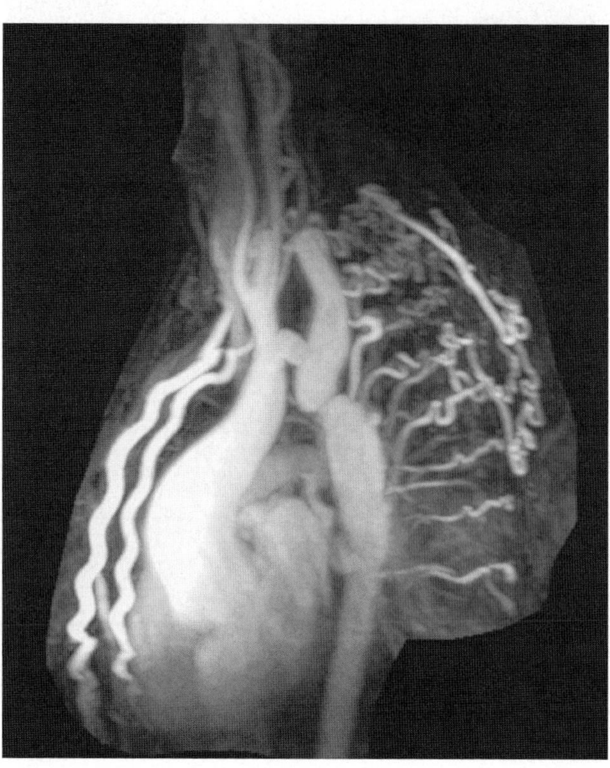

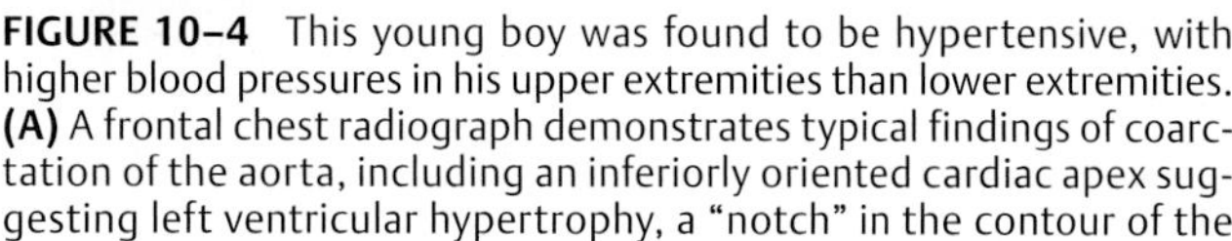

FIGURE 10–4 This young boy was found to be hypertensive, with higher blood pressures in his upper extremities than lower extremities. **(A)** A frontal chest radiograph demonstrates typical findings of coarctation of the aorta, including an inferiorly oriented cardiac apex suggesting left ventricular hypertrophy, a "notch" in the contour of the proximal descending thoracic aorta, and notching of the inferior borders of the posterior aspects of multiple ribs on each side. **(B)** A "bright blood" MR image clearly demonstrates the coarctation, as well as large collateral vessels attempting to bypass it, such as the internal mammary arteries.

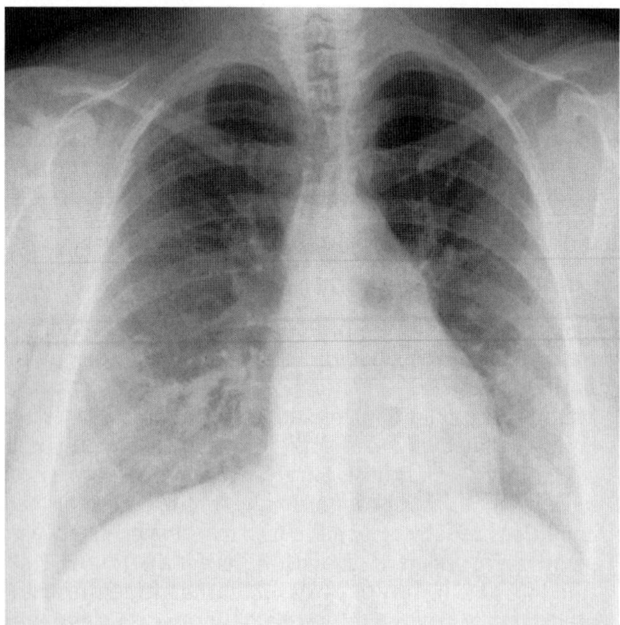

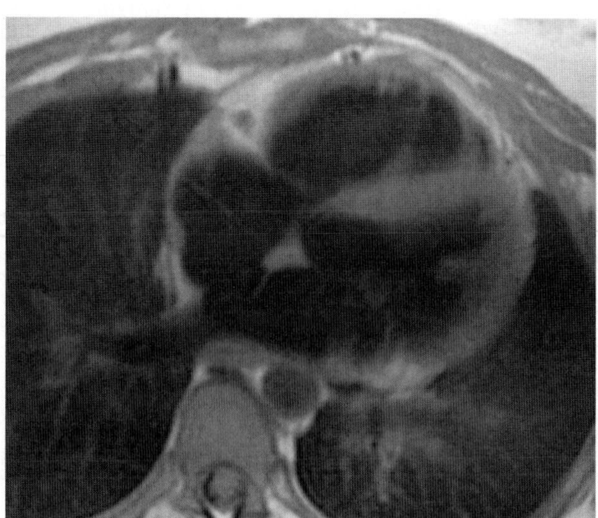

FIGURE 10–5 This young woman presented with pedal edema and shortness of breath. **(A)** Her frontal chest radiograph demonstrates enlarged pulmonary vessels, suggesting a left-to-right shunt. **(B)** An axial cardiac MR image demonstrates a large atrial septal defect (ASD).

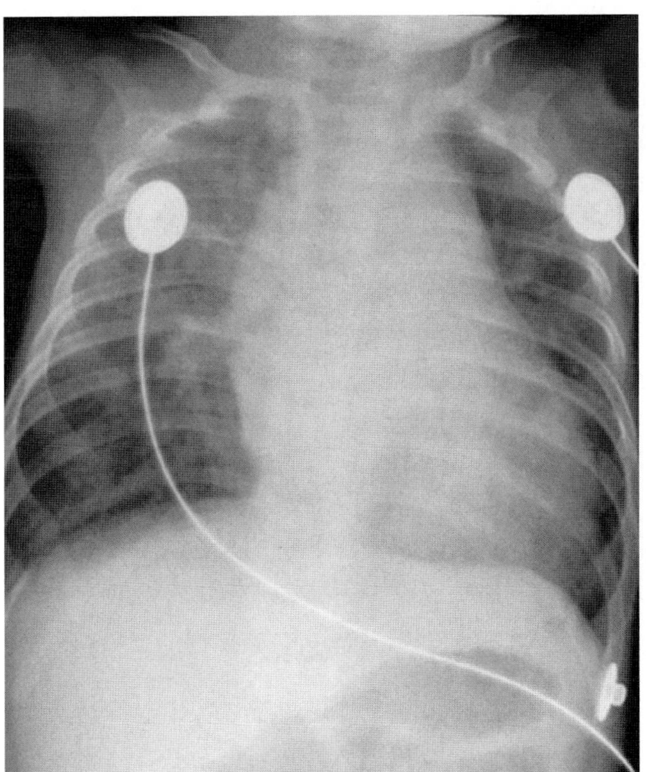

FIGURE 10–6 This infant presented with respiratory distress but was not cyanotic. A frontal chest radiograph demonstrates two electrocardiogram (ECG) leads and, more inferiorly, a metallic snap on the patient's clothing. More importantly, there is cardiomegaly, enlarged pulmonary vessels, and central air-space opacification consistent with pulmonary edema. The differential diagnosis would include VSD, ASD, and patent ductus arteriosus (PDA), among other possibilities. Echocardiography (not shown) demonstrated a PDA.

crucial role in differentiating between medical and surgical conditions. Moreover, it is vital in distinguishing between different disorders within each of these categories—a distinction that further powerfully influences therapy.

◇ Medical Condition: Surfactant Deficiency

Epidemiology Surfactant deficiency disease (SDD) is the most common cause of neonatal respiratory distress, seen in 30,000 to 50,000 infants per year in the United States. It nearly always occurs in premature infants, with a positive correlation between the degree of prematurity and the probability of developing SDD.

Pathophysiology The pathophysiology of SDD centers on a deficiency of pulmonary surfactant, which normally lowers the surface tension of the alveolar air sacs. Alveolar surface tension results from the fact that the water molecules lining the alveolar air sacs (without which the diffusion of gases could not occur) are more strongly attracted to one another than to the air above them in the alveolar sacs. This exerts a double effect: (1) the liquid layer resists any force that tends to increase its surface area, making the alveolus harder to inflate; and (2) the water molecules try to get as close together as possible, which tends to collapse the alveolus. As a result of these forces, the compliance of the lung, which is defined as the change in lung volume produced per unit force of inflation, decreases.

Surfactant is produced by type II pneumocytes, which can be differentiated microscopically from type I pneumocytes by their cuboidal shape and the fact that they contain lamellar inclusion bodies. Surfactant molecules are normally interposed between water molecules lining the alveoli. They lower the overall cohesive force between these molecules, because the attractive force between water molecules and surfactant molecules is very low. When surfactant supplies are deficient, alveolar surface tension is dramatically increased, with the result that the amount of muscular work required to snap them open at inspiration is considerably greater. Moreover, surfactant deficiency increases the recoil forces of the alveoli and promotes their tendency to collapse at expiration.

Unfortunately, alveolar atelectasis tends to set in motion a vicious cycle of alveolar hypoxia and decreased pulmonary perfusion. Atelectatic air spaces become hypoxic, which in turn leads to acidosis in the affected portion of the lung. This acidosis, in turn, leads to a reflex decrease in local pulmonary perfusion, which then exacerbates hypoxia and initiates another turn of the cycle; therefore, the short-term keys to maintaining adequate gas exchange are aerating collapsed air spaces and supplying supplementary oxygen.

The clinical result of surfactant deficiency is a neonate who is rapidly exhausted by the work of breathing. The child develops diffuse atelectasis, which in turn tips the balance of the Starling forces in favor of pulmonary edema. Proteinaceous material gradually builds up along the lining of the air sacs (hence the alternative name *hyaline membrane disease*) (**Fig. 10–7**). Because surfactant production, which is not necessary during in utero life, does not begin until ~24 weeks gestation, low birth weight infants are at higher risk, with nearly two thirds of those less than 1000 g developing some degree of SDD. Two thirds of affected neonates are male, who also are more often severely affected.

Clinical Presentation Clinically, neonates with SDD exhibit chest wall retractions, because the infant recruits accessory muscles of respiration in an effort to generate greater negative intrathoracic pressures; cyanosis, due to lower oxygen saturation; grunting, indicative of the increased work of breathing; tachypnea, which results from the attempt to maintain adequate ventilation in the face of lower tidal volumes; and expiratory grunting, the result of the effort to open up collapsed alveoli. Of course, such findings can be seen in a variety of pulmonary pathologies, and the chest radiograph is crucial in helping to establish the correct diagnosis of SDD. This is especially true in older premature neonates, for example, those weighing 1500 g, whose risk of developing SDD is only 16%. The probability of developing SDD can be assessed based on measurement of the lecithin–sphingomyelin ratio, which is decreased in infants at risk.

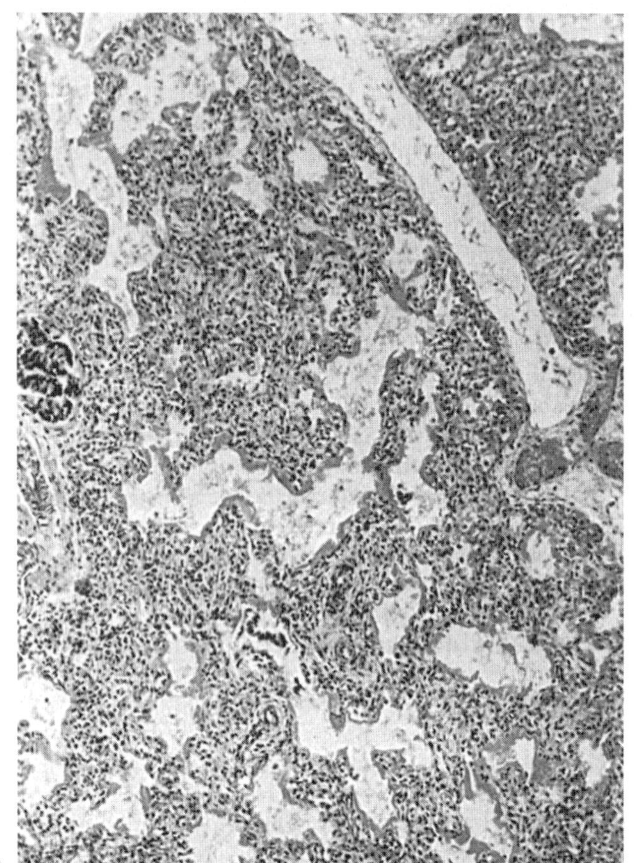

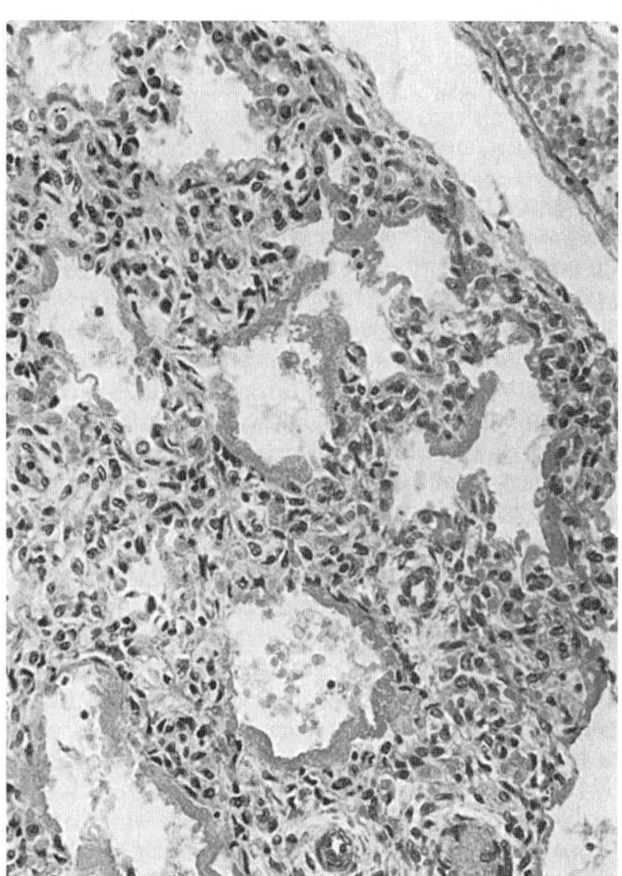

FIGURE 10–7 These light micrographs demonstrate the typical histologic appearance of hyaline membrane disease. **(A)** The distal air spaces are collapsed, and both proximal and distal air spaces are lined by hyaline membranes. **(B)** At higher power, the hyaline membranes lining the airways and larger air spaces are seen to better advantage. These membranes appear pink (eosinophilic) when viewed in color.

Imaging The radiographic findings of SDD are predictable. It is critical that the abnormalities are diffuse and bilateral, because surfactant is homogeneously deficient throughout the pulmonary parenchyma. Characteristic findings include low lung volumes, manifesting as a bell-shaped thorax; a diffuse, fine granular appearance to the lungs, due to accumulation of edema and proteinaceous secretions within the acini; and air bronchograms, because the conducting airways coursing through partially collapsed lung are both patent and overdistended, due to their high neonatal compliance (**Fig. 10–8**).

Recent advances in the treatment of SDD now save the lives of many premature infants who would have certainly died only a few decades ago. One such advance is the ability to prevent SDD in many cases of expected premature birth. Maturity of the surfactant system is normally induced by glucocorticoid secretion, and its development can be accelerated in utero by the administration of exogenous glucocorticoids. Another recent advance is the availability of exogenous pulmonary surfactant, which can be administered as an aerosol directly into the air spaces through the endotracheal tube.

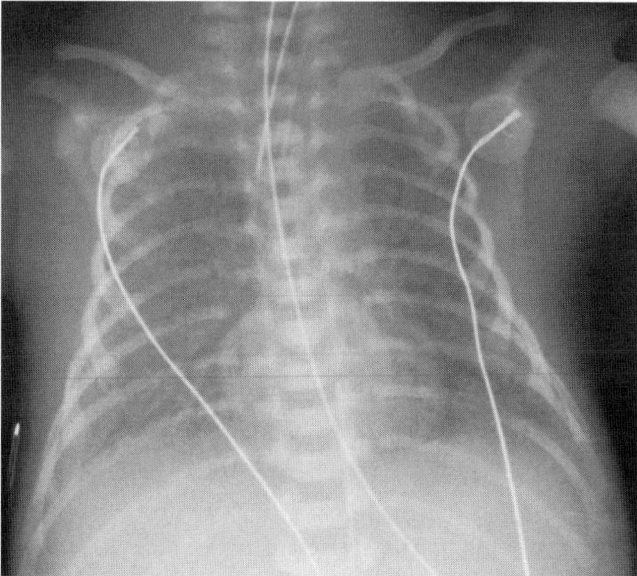

FIGURE 10–8 This premature newborn's portable chest radiograph demonstrates classic findings of surfactant deficiency disease, with diffuse bilateral, somewhat fine, granular air-space opacities. Note that the patient is intubated, with the endotracheal tube tip in the midthoracic trachea. An orogastric tube and umbilical arterial catheter, as well as ECG leads, are also in place.

Despite these advances, however, many neonates still require ventilatory support to inflate their stiff air spaces and to provide adequate levels of arterial oxygenation. Especially in this situation, imaging is helpful not only in diagnosing SDD but in assessing response to treatment and the development of complications. Mechanical ventilation involves insertion of an endotracheal tube and the use of positive airway pressures. Higher oxygen concentrations are employed to maintain an adequate level of tissue oxygenation. Umbilical vessel catheters may be inserted to administer medications and to monitor blood gases. Diuretics are often administered in an effort to counteract pulmonary edema, which decreases alveolar oxygen diffusion.

Unfortunately, each of these therapeutic maneuvers has potential adverse consequences, which are not peculiar to SDD, but may be seen in any condition requiring intensive monitoring and ventilatory support. Umbilical artery catheters (UACs) and umbilical vein catheters (UVCs) are favored routes of central venous access in neonates, because the vessels are relatively large and easy to cannulate. The UAC traverses the inferior epigastric artery, the internal iliac artery, the common iliac artery, and the abdominal aorta. Its tip should be positioned above or below the renal arteries to prevent the possibility of renal artery occlusion, either at the level of the 8th through 12th thoracic vertebral bodies or at the third or fourth lumbar vertebral body. The UVC is used primarily for blood draws (other than arterial blood gases) and for the administration of medications. It traverses the portal sinus (where the portal veins branch), the ductus venosus (which normally closes on the third or fourth day of life), the hepatic veins, and the inferior vena cava, with its tip coming to rest in the right atrium. Misplacement in the left atrium (through a patent foramen ovale) can cause systemic embolization from thrombi that may form on the tip, while placement of the tip into a portal or hepatic venous branch may cause complete vascular occlusion.

Ventilatory support has several potential complications. As in the older child and adult, tube malposition may give rise to several problems. If the tube is too high in the trachea, the lungs will not be properly ventilated. Alternatively, a tube that is positioned too low, such as in the right mainstem bronchus, may cause only the right lung to be ventilated, with collapse of the left lung.

A complication of SDD more peculiar to the intensive care nursery is pulmonary interstitial emphysema (PIE), which results from overdistention of poorly compliant air sacs, with buildup of gas in the pulmonary interstitium. The presence of PIE aggravates the difficulty of adequately ventilating the lungs, because the presence of air within the interstitium stiffens them and reduces pulmonary compliance. The intensivist managing a patient with SDD and PIE may feel caught in a vicious cycle. The increased airway pressures necessary to ventilate the stiff lungs of SDD may themselves result in stiffer lungs through the development of PIE, which in turn may necessitate higher airway pressures to maintain ventilation.

PIE is recognized radiographically when streaks or bubbles of air begin to appear in the lungs. These may be focal or diffuse, unilateral or bilateral (**Fig. 10–9**). The principal complications of PIE, which occur when air migrates centrally or peripherally through the lymphatics, are the development of pneumomediastinum and pneumothorax. Air reaches the pleural space through rupture of a subpleural bleb. Findings of barotrauma on chest radiography include not only pneumothorax and pneumomediastinum but also pneumopericardium, pneumoperitoneum, and venous air embolism, the presence of air in the heart and great vessels.

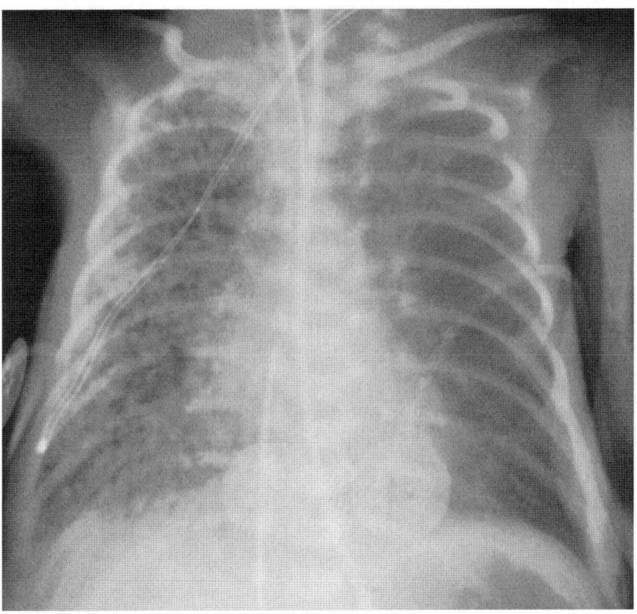

FIGURE 10–9 This premature neonate was becoming more difficult to ventilate. A portable chest radiograph demonstrates cylindrical and ovoid lucencies throughout the right lung, typical of pulmonary interstitial emphysema (PIE). Though typically bilateral and relatively symmetrical, PIE can be unilateral, as in this case. Note also a well-positioned endotracheal tube and orogastric tube, as well as an umbilical venous catheter positioned somewhat high in the right atrium. There are also three ECG leads.

Another complication of SDD is persistent patent ductus arteriosus. This occurs when the ductus remains physiologically open longer than the usual 48 hours after birth. It results from the effect of abnormally low arterial oxygen pressure on the ductus itself. The progressive fall in pulmonary vascular resistance that normally occurs after birth allows a left-to-right shunt to develop, manifesting as increased pulmonary vascularity and congestive heart failure (CHF). Treatment is with indomethacin, which blocks the synthesis of prostaglandin E1, which otherwise acts as a vasodilator and keeps the duct open. In the 40% of patients in whom indomethacin is not successful, the duct may be surgically ligated via a left thoracotomy.

An important complication of long-term ventilatory support is bronchopulmonary dysplasia (BPD), which occurs secondary to oxygen toxicity (likely mediated by highly chemically reactive superoxides) and barotrauma. Pathologically, BPD is characterized by destruction of type I pneumocytes and interstitial edema, followed by interstitital fibrosis and emphysema. These changes often result in long-term dependence on oxygen support. BPD in its later stages is recognized as bubbly, coarse interstitial opacities, with hyperaeration, and the lung often eventually acquires a honeycomb appearance. BPD is associated with an increased incidence of lower respiratory tract infections and reactive airways disease (asthma), likely because of scarred (and hence lower caliber) airways and less efficient clearance mechanisms.

Fortunately, with time many children can "grow out" of their BPD, because the lung continues to manufacture new alveoli through much of childhood. Only ~15 to 20% of the adult number of alveoli are present at birth.

◇ Medical Condition: Transient Tachypnea of the Newborn

The fetal lung is filled with fluid that is essential to normal lung development. Recall that oligohydramnios (as seen in such conditions as renal agenesis and in utero urinary tract obstruction) is associated with pulmonary hypoplasia. Transient tachypnea of the newborn (TTN) occurs when there is inadequate or delayed clearance of this fluid at birth, resulting in a "wet lung." Normally, fetal lung fluid is cleared during parturition by the squeezing action of the birth canal on the fetal thorax and by the resorptive capacity of the fetal lymphatics and pulmonary capillaries. Any condition that interferes with these normal mechanisms, including cesarean section, precipitous delivery, and lymphatic obstruction, predisposes to TTN. The characteristic radiographic appearance includes interstitial edema and hyperinflation (large lung volumes, as opposed to the low lung volumes of SDD). Some infants will also have small pleural effusions, indicating that the usual lymphatic drainage of the pleural space is, at least temporarily, inadequate. Even many normal newborns will have a TTN-like chest radiograph in the first minutes after birth, before clearance mechanisms have had an opportunity to take full effect. The natural history of TTN is complete resolution within 48 hours.

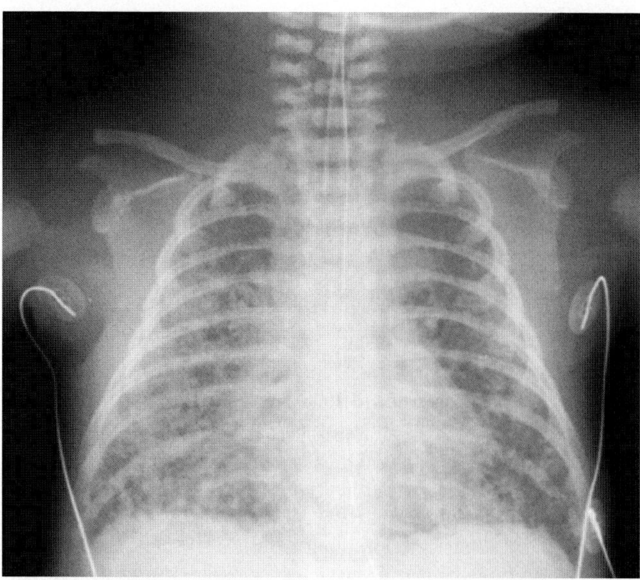

FIGURE 10–10 A frontal radiograph of a post-term neonate in whom meconium was suctioned from below the vocal cords demonstrates hyperinflated lungs with patchy bilateral nodular and linear opacities radiating outward from the hila. This is a typical appearance of meconium aspiration syndrome.

◇ Medical Condition: Meconium Aspiration

Meconium is the term for the normal neonatal bowel contents and is composed primarily of desquamated mucosal epithelial cells and bile salts. It usually has a greenish appearance and is evacuated within ~6 hours after birth; however, it may be evacuated in utero in response to perinatal stress, most likely as a vagal response. Approximately 20% of pregnancies have meconium-stained fluid, but only ~1 in 20 meconium-stained neonates develops meconium aspiration syndrome. The syndrome arises when meconium is aspirated below the level of the vocal cords, with predictable consequences. Meconium particles can produce mechanical airway obstruction. The tenacious character of meconium renders such airway plugs difficult for the neonate to clear. Bile acids and pancreatic enzymes in meconium can rapidly produce a chemical pneumonitis, due to direct toxicity on the epithelium of the airways and air spaces. Radiographic findings begin with disordered aeration, with areas of atelectasis due to complete airway obstruction and areas of hyperinflation due to a check-valve type of obstruction. Overall, the lungs are usually hyperinflated, with patchy areas of strandlike opacity (**Fig. 10–10**). Up to one quarter of patients will demonstrate a pneumothorax, most often as a complication of mechanically assisted ventilation.

◇ Medical Condition: Neonatal Pneumonia

Pneumonia complicates ~1 in 200 births. Risk factors for neonatal pneumonia include maternal sepsis and premature rupture of membranes, reflecting the two routes of infection: transplacental transmission in utero and perinatal transmission via an infected birth canal. The most common organism is β-hemolytic streptococci, acquired via the birth canal. Patients present with respiratory distress and metabolic acidosis that may progress to sepsis and shock. The latter complications make early recognition critical. The radiographic appearance of neonatal pneumonia is variable and may mimic that of SDD, with diffuse granularity, or TTN, with diffuse, streaky opacities. Pleural effusion, present in two thirds of cases of neonatal pneumonia, can be an important discriminating factor in this regard, as it is never found in pure SDD. The classic lobar infiltrates seen in older children and adults are only rarely seen in the neonate (**Fig. 10–11**).

◇ Surgical Condition: Diaphragmatic Hernia

Congenital diaphragmatic hernia (CDH) occurs in 1 in 2500 live births, with a high mortality rate, especially when the condition is not immediately recognized. In an increasing number of cases, the defect is detected via prenatal ultrasound. CDH-related morbidity stems from the presence of abdominal contents, including bowel or solid organs, within the thorax. The lack of space for lung development results in pulmonary hypoplasia. Hence, respiratory distress in the neonate with CDH has two causes: the presence of a mass within the thorax and a lack of a normal volume of lung tissue. The first cause is remediable through surgical repair, with reposition of the abdominal contents and repair of the hernia; however, the second is not, or at least only marginally so, as not only alveoli but also airways and associated vasculature are absent. Radiographic features of CDH include the presence of a soft tissue mass within the thorax and contralateral displacement of the

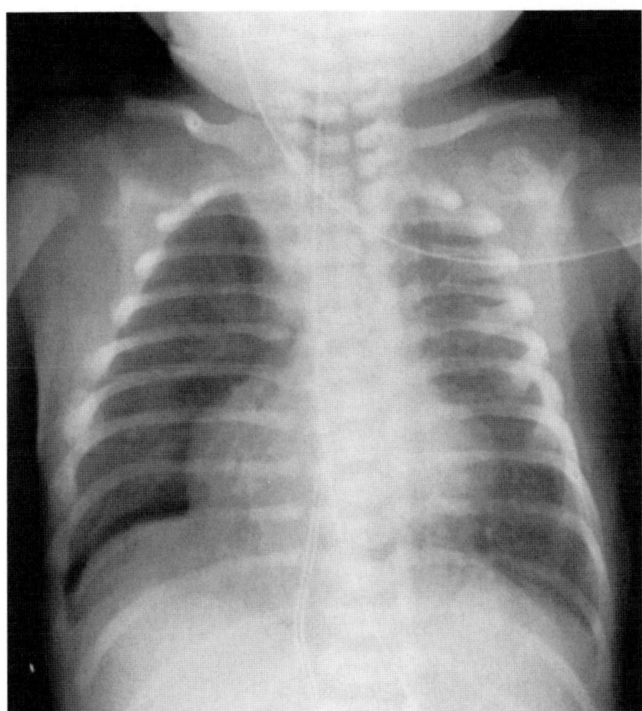

FIGURE 10–11 This neonate developed respiratory distress soon after birth. A portable chest radiograph demonstrates air-space opacification and volume loss in the right upper lobe, adjacent to which is an abnormal rim of lucency. This represented an atypical pattern of neonatal pneumonia, complicated by spontaneous pneumothorax. Note also an orogastric tube and an umbilical venous catheter tip at the level of the right atrium.

mediastinum (**Fig. 10–12**). Confirmatory tests include the passage of an orogastric tube, which may follow an abnormal course through the thorax; injection of air through the nasogastric tube, which will result in the development of cystic-appearing spaces within the intrathoracic soft tissue mass (representing air within bowel); the introduction of a small amount of contrast material through the nasogastric tube; and ultrasound, which will disclose the diaphragmatic defect and the presence of peristalsing bowel within the thorax. As expected, CDH is associated with other abnormalities, including malrotation of the bowel.

◇ Surgical Condition: Cystic Adenomatoid Malformation

A radiographic mimic of CDH is cystic adenomatoid malformation, which may also present with a multicystic appearing mass in the thorax. Abnormal growth of terminal respiratory structures leads to a hamartomatous mass of glandular tissue that may communicate with the airways, exhibiting air or air–fluid levels in the cysts (**Fig. 10–13**). Surgical resection of the abnormal lobe is curative.

◇ Surgical Condition: Congenital Lobar Emphysema

Congenital lobar emphysema results from progressive hyperinflation of one or more of the pulmonary lobes. At least half of all cases are idiopathic, but many result from central airway obstruction, with a check-valve mechanism that

A

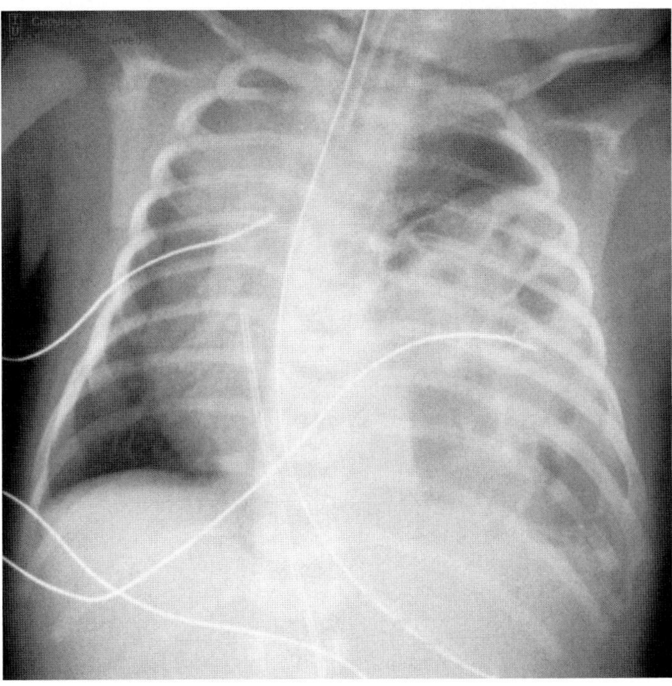

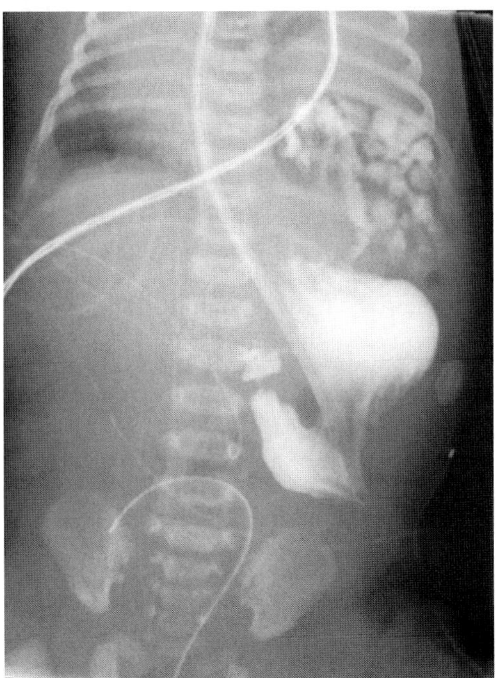

B

FIGURE 10–12 This neonate exhibited respiratory distress at birth. **(A)** A chest radiograph demonstrates multiple air-containing segments of bowel in the left hemithorax, diagnostic of congenital diaphragmatic hernia (CDH). Note the rightward shift of the mediastinum, including the umbilical venous catheter in the inferior vena cava (IVC) and right atrium, as well as the orogastric tube. Also seen is an endotracheal tube with its tip in the upper thoracic trachea, as well as three ECG wires. **(B)** Injection of low-osmolar contrast material through the orogastric tube in another patient with CDH demonstrates opacification of a normally positioned stomach as well as multiple segments of small bowel in the left hemithorax. There is a bladder catheter in the pelvis.

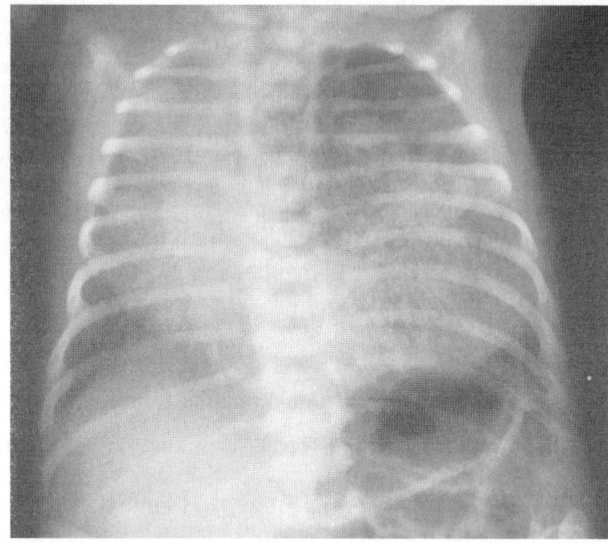

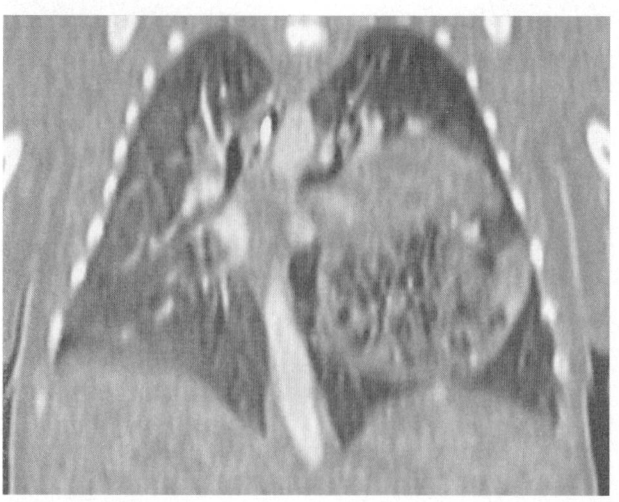

FIGURE 10–13 This newborn was diagnosed with a left lung mass. **(A)** A frontal chest radiograph demonstrates a large mixed cystic and solid left lung mass with rightward shift of the mediastinum. **(B)** The coronal reformat of axially acquired CT data again demonstrates the mixed cystic and solid character of the mass. At surgery, the pathologic findings confirmed cystic adenomatoid malformation.

allows the lobe to fill during inspiration but prevents emptying at expiration. In decreasing order of frequency, the most commonly affected lobes are the left upper lobe, the right middle lobe, and the right upper lobe. The lesion characteristically presents as an opacity in the first few days of life, due to impaired emptying of lung fluid; thereafter, it presents as a hyperlucent, hyperexpanded lobe, which causes contralateral shift of the mediastinum.

◇ Surgical Condition: Tracheoesophageal Fistula

Esophageal atresia (EA) and tracheoesophageal fistula (TEF) both represent anomalies in the development of the primitive foregut, which normally separates during the fifth week of life into the esophagus and trachea. These anomalies occur in ~1 in 2500 live births. EA may be suggested by a prenatal ultrasound showing polyhydramnios, secondary to the inability of the fetus to ingest normal quantities of amniotic fluid. EA and TEF are suggested postnatally by the development of coughing, choking, and cyanosis in the first day of life. Most commonly, attempted passage of a nasogastric tube and subsequent chest radiograph reveal the tube ending in a blind pouch in the upper chest. The presence of gas within the bowel proves that there is a distal esophageal-tracheal communication. Although many anatomic types are possible, the most common involves a blind esophageal pouch with a more distal fistula between the trachea and esophagus. A gasless abdomen indicates that the second most prevalent anatomic type is likely present, with no communication between the trachea and esophagus (pure EA). In a small percentage of cases, the esophagus is patent, but there is a fistula connecting it to the trachea (**Fig. 10–14**).

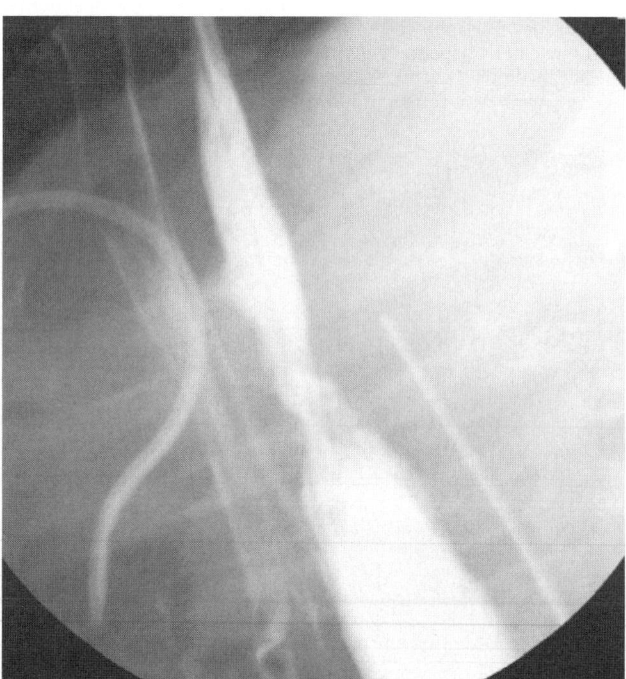

FIGURE 10–14 This patient developed recurrent choking with feedings after surgical repair of an esophageal atresia with tracheoesophageal fistula. The right lateral fluoroscopic spot image of the upper mediastinum was obtained after injection of barium contrast material into the esophagus through an oroesophageal tube. Above the level of the esophageal anastomosis, which demonstrates some narrowing and irregularity, there is opacification of a recurrent tracheoesophageal fistula, as well as the trachea itself, which is seen in double-contrast view. The line overlying the trachea is a central venous catheter. Which direction is the patient facing? Because the trachea is anterior to the esophagus, the patient is facing the viewer's left.

Childhood Respiratory Distress

Many of the conditions that cause respiratory distress in the adult manifest similarly in children. These include such common disorders as asthma and pneumonia; however, there are three common, community-acquired childhood respiratory conditions that deserve special mention. These are foreign body aspiration, croup, and epiglottitis.

◇ Foreign Body Aspiration

Airway foreign bodies represent a common cause of respiratory distress, particularly between ages 6 months and 4 years, when children characteristically put objects in their mouths. In contrast to croup and epiglottitis, there is generally no history of antecedent infectious symptoms, and the child presents with acute stridor, wheezing, and cough. As expected, foreign bodies follow the path of least resistance through the tracheobronchial tree, and most lodge in the right mainstem bronchus or its branches. Foreign bodies that are not removed may result in long-term complications such as recurrent pneumonias, hemoptysis, and bronchial stenosis, and bronchoscopic removal is generally indicated. Most aspirated foreign bodies are not radiopaque. Common radiographic findings include unilateral air trapping and hyperinflation due to a check-valve type of obstruction, and less commonly, atelectasis from complete obstruction (**Fig. 10–15**). It is uncommon to visualize the foreign body directly, because most are radiolucent. By obtaining inspiratory and expiratory films, or by observation of breathing under fluoroscopy, it is possible to increase diagnostic confidence. The nonobstructed lung will be able to empty normally, whereas the obstructed lung will not. Therefore, on an expiratory film the mediastinum will shift away from the side of the foreign body.

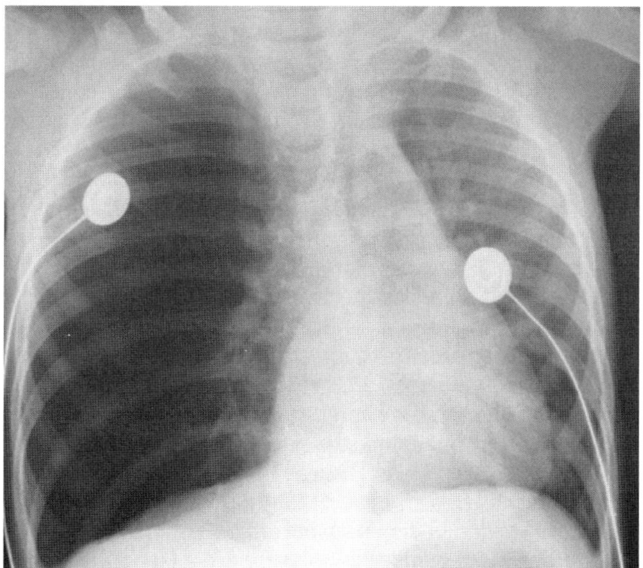

FIGURE 10–15 This young child presented with abrupt onset respiratory distress. A frontal chest radiograph (with ECG leads in place) demonstrates severe hyperinflation of the right lung with leftward shift of the mediastinum. This is highly suggestive of a right bronchial foreign body, although none is seen. At bronchoscopy, a piece of apple was removed from the right mainstem bronchus.

◇ Croup

Croup, more descriptively referred to as acute laryngotracheobronchitis, represents the most common cause of upper airway obstruction in children. It is most commonly seen in the 6-month-to-3-year age group. The principal infectious organisms in croup include parainfluenza virus and respiratory syncytial virus. Although it involves the entire upper airway, the critical zone of airway narrowing is the immediate subglottic region, ~1 cm below the larynx, due to the fact that loose mucosal attachment in this region permits excessive edematous narrowing. Patients present with a barky cough and stridor. The classic finding on a frontal radiograph is a tapered narrowing of the trachea in the subglottic region, producing a "V" configuration of airway narrowing (**Fig. 10–16**). The critical reason for obtaining radiographs is not to diagnose croup, which is generally a self-limited process of several days' duration, but to exclude other more worrisome entities such as foreign body aspiration and epiglottitis.

◇ Epiglottitis

Epiglottitis represents an acutely life-threatening condition, because it may result in sudden and complete airway obstruction with asphyxiation. Children suspected of suffering from this condition should not be moved, and no maneuvers that might compromise breathing should be performed until personnel and equipment capable of airway intervention and management are present. If it is necessary to obtain radiographs, a portable unit should be used. Epiglottitis most commonly occurs between 3 and 6 years of age and is most often due to *Haemophilus influenzae*, although widespread immunization against *H. flu* is altering this. Patients present with a history of fever, dysphagia, drooling, and sore throat.

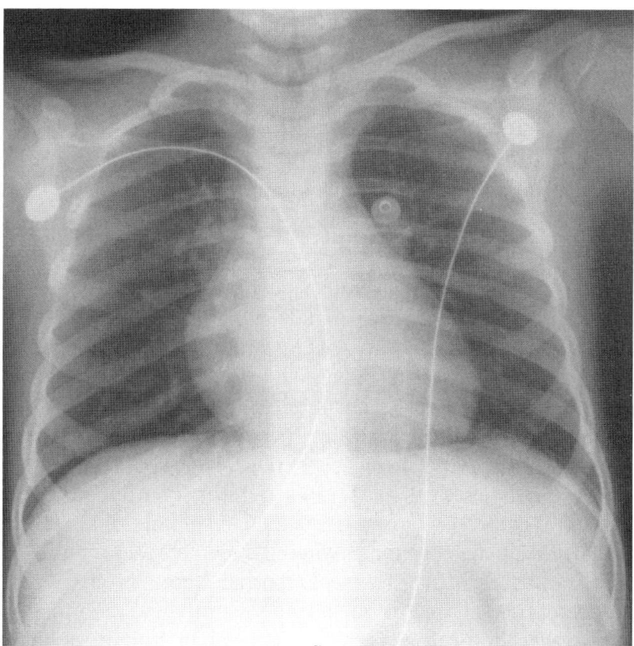

FIGURE 10–16 This young child presented with respiratory distress. A frontal radiograph demonstrates no pneumonia, but there is a gradually tapering of the subglottic trachea, producing the so-called steeple sign of croup.

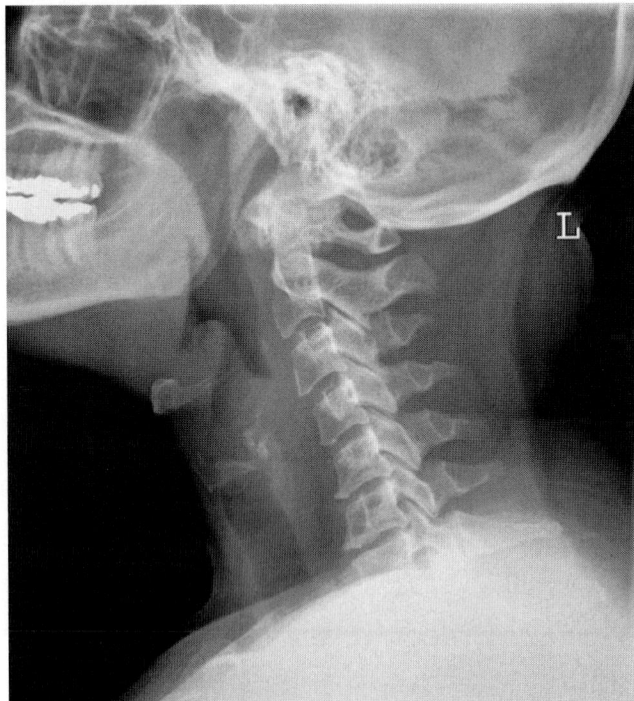

FIGURE 10–17 Though typically a pediatric diagnosis, epiglottitis can be seen even in adults. This middle-aged woman presented with severe odynophagia (painful swallowing) and high fever. A lateral soft tissue radiograph of the neck demonstrates the classic "thumb sign" of epiglottic swelling.

The classic radiographic and pathologic finding is thickening of the aryepiglottic folds, which manifests as a thumblike thickening of the epiglottis on lateral views of the neck soft tissues (**Fig. 10–17**).

Nervous System

Neonatal Intracranial Hemorrhage

◇ Epidemiology

Infants born prior to 32 weeks' gestation suffer a markedly increased risk of intracranial hemorrhage and ischemia. Twenty-five percent of infants less than 1500 g develop intracranial hemorrhage, and it develops to some degree in up to two thirds of infants at 28 to 32 weeks' gestation. Such events can prove catastrophic, because infants so affected may suffer permanent and severe neurologic sequelae.

The occurrence of intracranial hemorrhage is linked to several risk factors. Antepartum factors include the medical condition of the mother, involving such risk factors as toxemia, diabetes, heart disease, and other factors predisposing to premature birth. The most effective medical response to intracranial hemorrhage is the prevention of premature birth. Intrapartum factors include abnormal fetal presentation and prolonged labor. Postpartum events associated with increased risk include respiratory distress, cardiopulmonary abnormalities, infection, and hemolysis.

◇ Pathophysiology

To understand why premature infants are at risk for intracranial hemorrhage, it is necessary to understand the special developmental neuroanatomy of neonates. As one would predict, the areas of the brain most vulnerable to ischemic insult are the zones with the highest metabolic rate. In the neonate, these include the zones characterized by the highest rates of neural proliferation, maturation, and myelination, including the cerebellum, the basal ganglia, and the periventricular white matter. An area of special risk is the germinal matrix, located near the head of the caudate nucleus (**Fig. 10–18**). The germinal matrix is the subventricular and ventricular area of proliferation of neuronal and glial precursors. Cells migrate from this subependymal location out into the cortex. Of special note is the fact that this area is richly vascularized and has little supporting stroma; thus, any microscopic interruption of vascular integrity would tend not to be well contained and likely to develop into macroscopic hemorrhage. Germinal matrix hemorrhage is more prevalent in very premature infants and rare in those of 40 weeks' gestation, because the germinal matrix becomes less and less prominent over the last 12 weeks of gestation and virtually disappears by term.

The pathophysiology of the condition centers on the autoregulation of cerebral blood flow. This autoregulation is disrupted in the premature newborn, who is less adept than a full-term infant at maintaining constant cerebral perfusion pressure in the face of changing arterial pressure. Moderate to severe asphyxia is the disrupting factor, rendering cerebral blood flow pressure-passive. This "pressure passivity" is the key to understanding the apparently paradoxical development of both ischemic and hemorrhagic injury, and in experimental models predicts the later development of ultrasonographically detectable hemorrhage. In normal infants, cerebral blood flow is independent of arterial pressure over a wide pressure range. When arterial pressure is reduced, flow can be maintained by lowering cerebrovascular resistance. When hypertension obtains, arteriolar constriction is induced. In the distressed newborn, small decreases in arterial pressure lead to a significant decrease in cerebral blood flow, which, if sustained, eventuates in ischemic injury. This situation is further aggravated by hypoxemia. In hypertension, increased pressure is transmitted unimpeded to the walls of the capillary bed, with an associated increased risk of hemorrhage. Thus, the key pathophysiologic factor is a change in blood pressure, and management focuses on reducing distress and maintaining stable pressures.

Several other factors are critical to understanding why intracranial hemorrhage constitutes such a thorny problem. The prevention of asphyxia is a key strategy, yet the birth process itself can be likened to an asphyxial insult. Asphyxia normally leads first to hypertension, then later to hypotension, perhaps due to depletion of cardiac carbohydrate stores. Abrupt increases in arterial pressure are a fact of life in the first few days, accompanying even handling, feeding, and other routine activities. A second such factor is arterial $PaCO_2$ (partial pressure of carbon dioxide in arterial blood), which is a major regulator of intracranial vascular resistance at all stages of life. High $PaCO_2$ causes vasodilation and is associated with increased incidence of germinal matrix

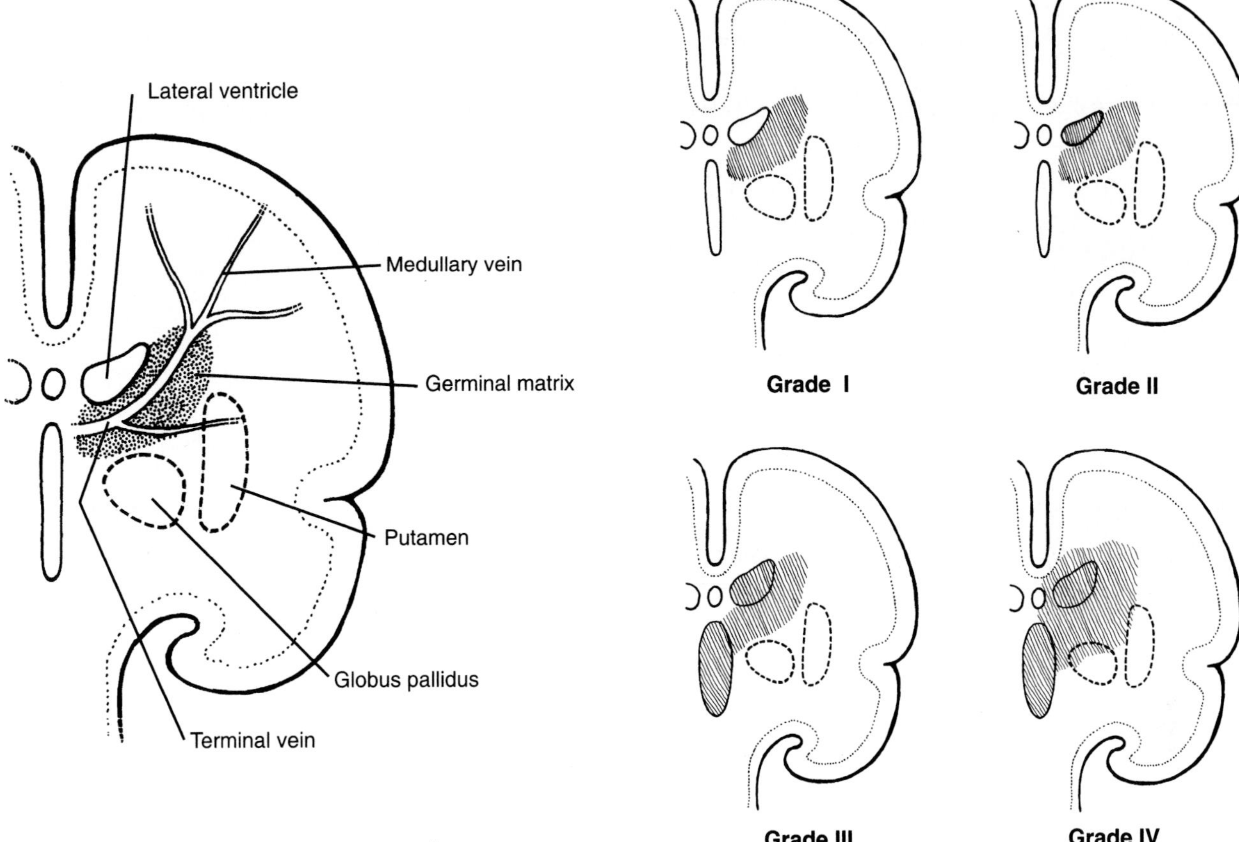

FIGURE 10–18 The normal position of the germinal matrix adjacent to the head of the caudate nucleus, as well as the different grades of germinal matrix hemorrhage (coronal view).

hemorrhage, while hyperventilation (blowing off carbon dioxide) at birth seems to suppress the development of hemorrhage. A third such factor is the blood–brain barrier, which is compromised in asphyxia through the combined effects of hypertension and vasodilation. This helps to explain why asphyxiated infants are at higher risk for kernicterus (hyperbilirubinemia-mediated brain damage), even with only moderate hyperbilirubinemia. The fourth factor is ischemic injury. Arterial hypoxemia and hypercarbia result from decreased placental and/or alveolar gas exchange. Depletion of myocardial glycogen leads to decreased blood pressure. Cerebral edema (from lactic acid accumulation, tissue injury, and compromised blood–brain barrier) and/or intraventricular hemorrhage may further decrease perfusion pressure. Finally, cerebral ischemia itself predisposes to further injury by delaying the restoration of autoregulation.

◇ Clinical Presentation

Intracranial hemorrhage most commonly presents in the first several days of neonatal life. Classic signs include obtundation, hypotonia, and a drop in the hematocrit. It is also associated with intractable metabolic acidosis; however, most cases detected by sonography are clinically silent, indicating the importance of sonographic screening in premature neonates at risk.

◇ Imaging

The key imaging modality in this setting is ultrasound, which can be performed quickly and efficiently in the neonatal intensive care unit and involves no exposure to ionizing radiation. Because the anterior fontanelle has not yet closed in these infants, it provides an excellent acoustic window on the brain. Head ultrasound is routinely performed in infants less than 32 weeks' gestation, generally around postnatal day 4 to 7, by which time 90% of hemorrhages will have occurred. Clinical indications for earlier screening include an abnormal neurologic examination and a drop in hematocrit with no known source of bleeding. Another important setting is infants who will require anticoagulation for ECMO, in whom the presence of intracranial hemorrhage must first be ruled out.

Intracranial hemorrhage is graded on a scale of I to IV. Grade I is confined to the subependymal germinal matrix. The classic ultrasound finding in germinal matrix hemorrhage is echogenic foci immediately posterior to the caudothalamic groove. Grade II adds to this extension of blood into the ventricles, seen as echogenic intraventricular material, without ventriculomegaly. Grade III includes both ventricular extension and ventriculomegaly (**Fig. 10–19**). Grade IV includes intracerebral hemorrhage as well. Prognosis declines with increasing grade, and grades III and IV are

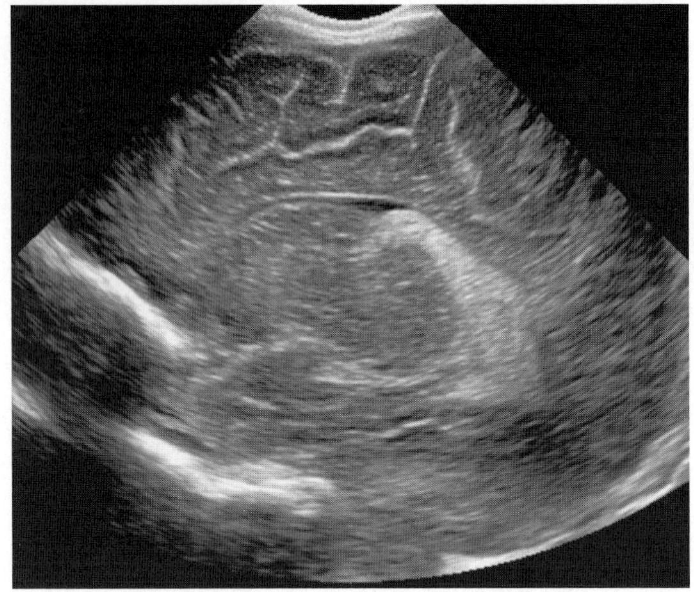

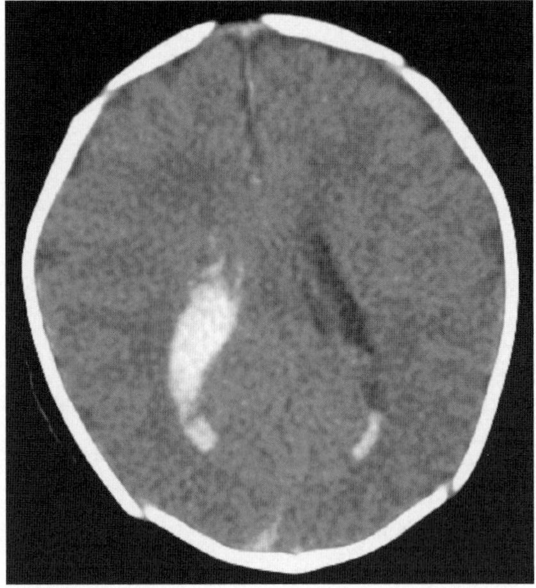

FIGURE 10–19 This near full-term neonate suffered an unexplained drop in hematocrit. **(A)** A sagittal sonogram of the right cerebral hemisphere demonstrates echogenic hematoma in the posterior portion of the lateral ventricle. **(B)** An axial CT image demonstrates bulky acute hematoma in the right lateral ventricle, as well as some acute blood layering out in the posterior horn on the left. This represents a Grade III germinal matrix hemorrhage.

associated with large increases in morbidity and mortality. Between 40 and 50% of infants with grade IV hemorrhage suffer severe neurologic impairment, and more than three quarters of infants with grades I and II hemorrhage develop only mild or no neurologic impairment.

Periventricular leukomalacia is another common finding in ischemic injury, which results from ischemic damage to the deep white matter of the hemispheres. It manifests initially as areas of edema or hemorrhage, followed eventually by cystic lesions (porencephaly), giving the brain an appearance that may resemble Swiss cheese (**Fig. 10–20**).

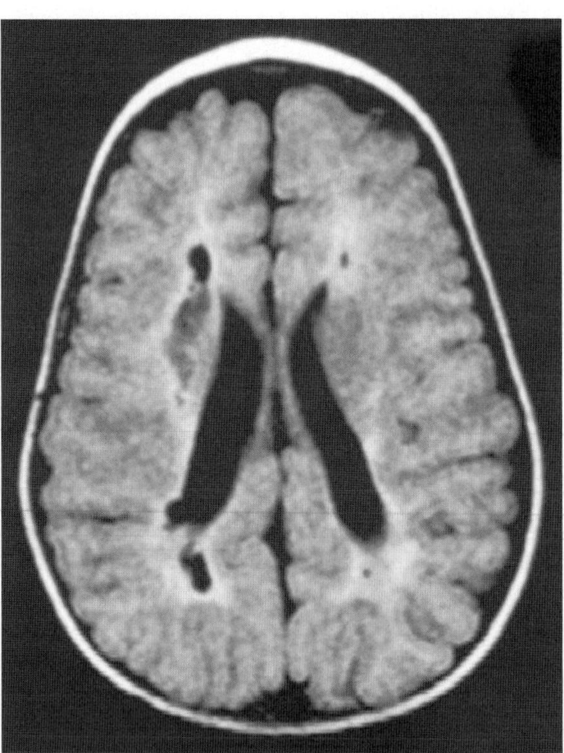

FIGURE 10–20 This now 15-month-old child was born at 30 weeks' gestation. The axial fluid-attenuation inversion recovery (FLAIR) MR image demonstrates bilateral hemispheric atrophy and periventricular cystic changes typical of periventricular leukomalacia.

Abdomen

Acute Abdomen

Several acute abdominal processes are unique to the pediatric population, or at least occur predominantly in infants and children. To determine which process is involved in a particular patient, several extraradiologic factors are critical. First is the patient's age. Pediatric patients are predisposed to certain conditions at certain points in their development. For example, conditions such as necrotizing enterocolitis (NEC), meconium ileus, and bowel atresias will present in the first few days of extrauterine life, while hypertrophic pyloric stenosis presents around the age of 1 month, and it would be somewhat unusual to see intussusception in the first few months of life. Additional factors include whether the patient is infected (fever, leukocytosis), the appearance of the vomitus (bilious vomiting implies obstruction distal to the ampulla of Vater), and history of previous surgery (in which case adhesions constitute one of the most important etiologies of obstruction throughout life).

In terms of radiologic workup, plain radiographs can be used to evaluate for obstruction. If bowel obstruction is proximal, there will be relatively little intestinal air, although the stomach and duodenum may be dilated (as in the classic "double bubble" of duodenal atresia, with air in the stomach and duodenal bulb); more distal obstruction will often be accompanied by numerous distended segments (**Fig. 10–21**). If obstruction is high, upper gastrointestinal (GI) contrast studies will often be indicated, while a pattern of distal obstruction warrants contrast enema. The plain radiograph can also rule out free intraperitoneal air, although a view allowing air to be seen in tangent in the nondependent portion of the abdomen should be used, such as an upright or left-side-down decubitus film. Ultrasound is used primarily to assess for appendicitis and hypertrophic pyloric stenosis, and to rule out masses. CT is seldom necessary in the acute, nontraumatic setting.

It is sometimes said that if a clinician can order only one radiograph in children with acute abdominal presentations, it should be the upright chest radiograph. The reasoning behind this dictum is that apparent acute abdominal presentations often turn out to stem from extra-abdominal pathology. A classic example is the child with abdominal pain and fever who is discovered on chest radiography to have a lower lobe pneumonia. Occasionally, the pulmonary infiltrate will be detected on the abdominal radiograph as increased opacity in the otherwise overpenetrated lung base, which is only detectable if the physician remembers to look at the corners of the image. Even when an abdominal plain film has been obtained and reveals nothing more than a nonspecific ileus pattern, a chest radiograph will sometimes hold the key to the diagnosis.

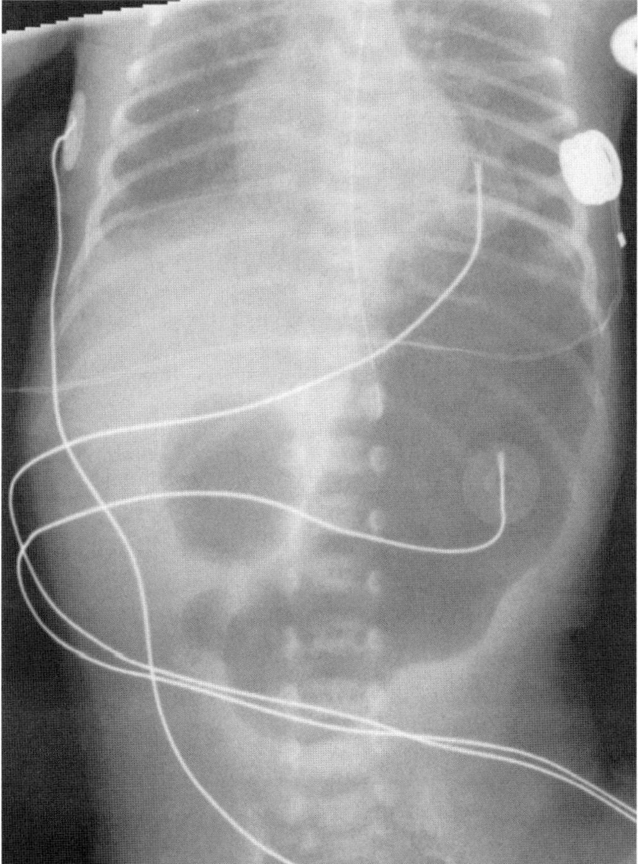

FIGURE 10–21 This newborn vomited after every feeding. A plain radiograph of the abdomen demonstrates a classic "double bubble" pattern, with a gas-filled gastric lumen and duodenal bulb, and no distal bowel gas. At surgery, the diagnosis of duodenal atresia was confirmed.

◇ The Neonate

NEC occurs primarily in premature neonates exposed to hypoxic stress. Such infants have immature guts that exhibit poor peristalsis and impaired immune function, and are therefore at risk for infection. Clinicians note onset of vomiting, blood in the stools, metabolic acidosis, and episodes of apnea and bradycardia in the first week of life. It is important to recognize NEC so that feedings may be halted, as the continued introduction of hyperosmolar feeds into the gut markedly exacerbates the mucosal injury and bacterial superinfection. The usual radiologic examination is the plain radiograph, which may demonstrate bowel distention, an abnormally dilated, fixed loop of bowel, and free air within the peritoneal cavity (indicating bowel perforation). Two highly specific findings in the appropriate clinical setting are pneumatosis intestinalis (thin collections of air within the bowel wall, secondary to disruption of the mucosa) (**Fig. 10–22**) and portal venous gas (branching collections of air in the right upper quadrant produced by passage of intraluminal air into

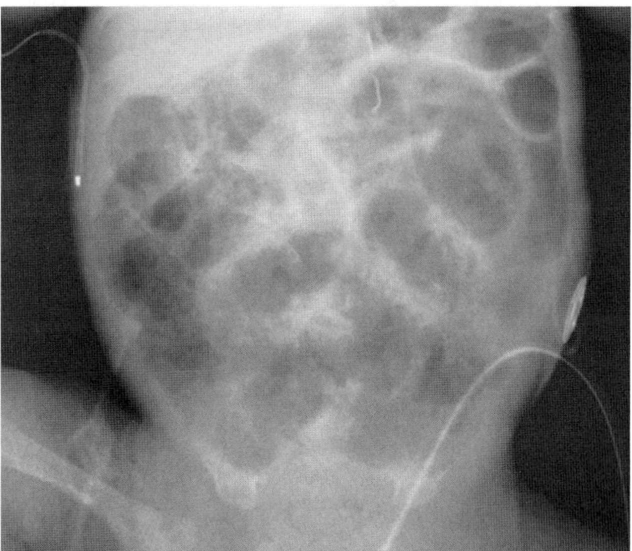

FIGURE 10–22 This premature neonate developed abdominal distention and feeding intolerance at 2 weeks of life. A portable abdominal radiograph demonstrates tubular, dilated bowel and many linear and bubbly lucencies scattered throughout the abdomen. These lucencies represent pneumatosis intestinalis, a classic finding in necrotizing enterocolitis. Note also an orogastric tube tip overlying the stomach.

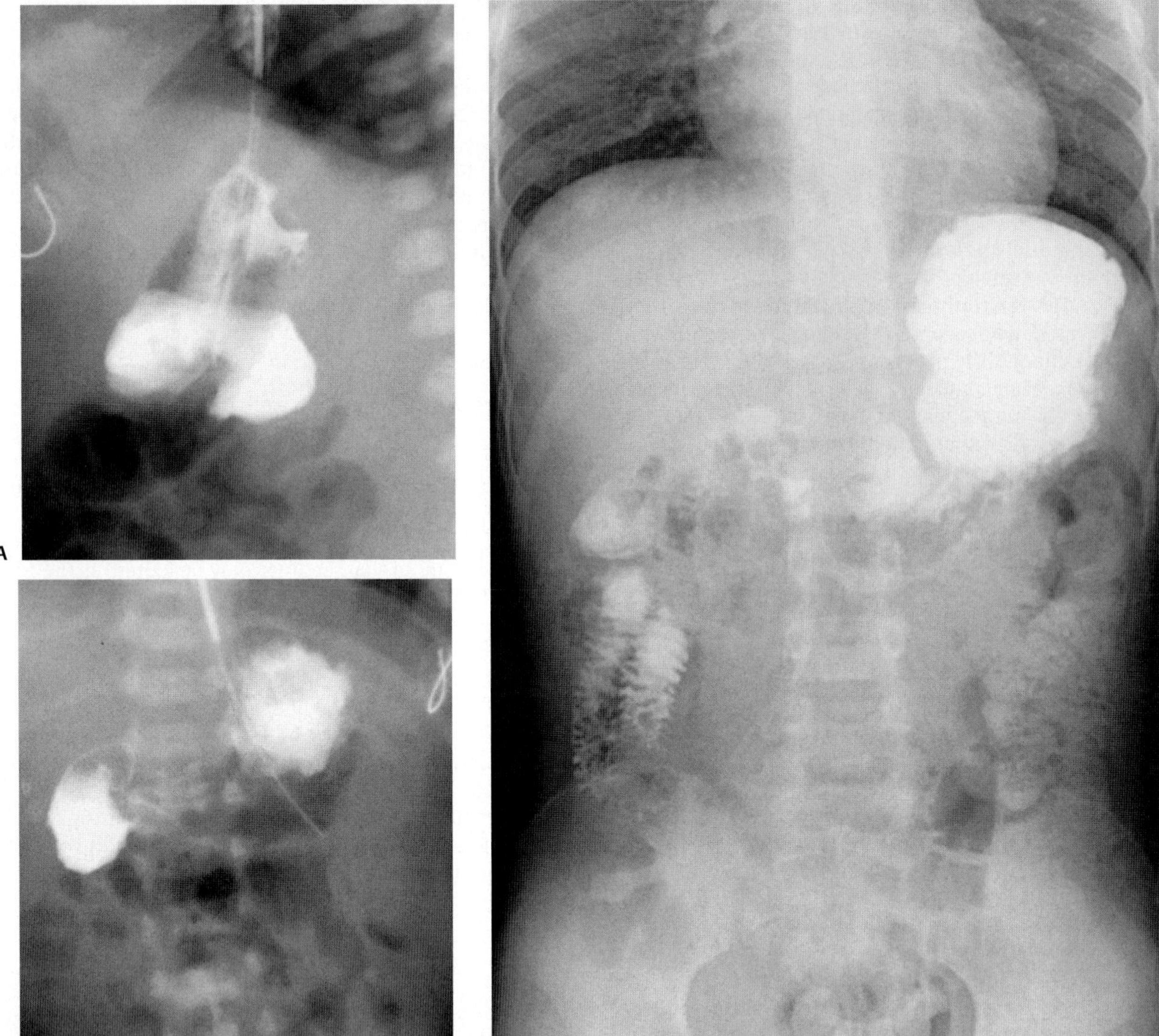

FIGURE 10–23 This neonate presented with bilious vomiting. Two spot images **(A,B)** from a barium upper gastrointestinal (GI) exam demonstrate a complete obstruction of the descending duodenum without much dilation of the duodenal bulb, which tends to suggest acute obstruction. At surgery, there was malrotation with midgut volvulus, with the twisting of the bowel causing the obstruction. **(C)** This abdominal radiograph from a barium upper GI exam in an older child with a history of episodic abdominal pain demonstrates that the duodenum and proximal jejunum are located in the right upper quadrant, indicating malrotation. The duodenal-jejunal junction should be fixated by the ligament of Treitz in the left upper quadrant, usually just to the left of the first lumbar vertebra.

the portal venous system). Once NEC is diagnosed, continued radiographic follow-up is important to detect pneumoperitoneum, which suggests that NEC has led to bowel necrosis and perforation, and warrants surgical intervention.

Midgut volvulus (from the Latin *volvere*, "to roll") may present at any age, but is typically seen in term infants within the first several days of life. It constitutes a surgical emergency, because it may result in infarction and necrosis of bowel. To occur, it requires the presence of malrotation, with an abnormally short mesentery and defective fixation of bowel due to failure of normal intestinal rotation and fixation during the sixth week of intrauterine life. Volvulus occurs when the malrotated proximal small intestine twists around its abnormally short mesentery. This in turn may twist the superior mesenteric artery (SMA), compromising its flow and potentially infarcting all of the bowel supplied by it (extending from the proximal jejunum at the ligament of Treitz to the splenic flexure of the colon). A neonate who develops bilious vomiting, abdominal pain and distention, and blood-tinged stools should undergo an upper GI barium study to rule out midgut volvulus. If volvulus is present, there will be obstruction at the duodenal "C" loop, often with a "corkscrew appearance" as the barium traces out the helical pattern of the twisted bowel (**Fig. 10–23**).

Even if volvulus is not present at the time of examination, malrotation will be evidenced by abnormal location of the duodenal-jejunal junction, which is normally positioned to the left of the spine at the level of the duodenal bulb. Alternatively, if no malrotation is present, the duodenal "C" loop will have a normal appearance, and the duodenal-jejunal junction will be identified to the left of the L1 vertebral body, the expected location of the ligament of Treitz.

Other neonatal conditions merit brief discussion. Bowel atresia, probably reflecting an in utero ischemic insult, involves the distal small bowel more often than the proximal and presents in the first few hours of life with vomiting and obstruction (**Fig. 10–24**). Meconium ileus is seen almost exclusively in newborn patients with cystic fibrosis, whose viscous meconium may "plug up" the bowel, most commonly the ileum, with resultant evidence of obstruction. The radiologist may both diagnose and treat this condition, if it is not complicated by an atresia, volvulus, or stenosis. Refluxing contrast through the colon may loosen the thick viscous meconium in these infants and relieve the obstruction.

◇ The Infant and Child

Hypertrophic pyloric stenosis involves idiopathic hypertrophy of the circular muscle surrounding the pyloric channel connecting the stomach and duodenum. It occurs in 1 of every 500 children around the age of 1 month, most frequently in boys. It presents as nonbilious vomiting and dehydration, with laboratory tests indicating a hypochloremic metabolic alkalosis due to the loss of gastric hydrochloric acid (HCl). It is best diagnosed clinically with palpation of an "olive" in the right upper quadrant. In equivocal cases, ultrasound can confirm the diagnosis by revealing increased muscular thickness and length of the pyloric channel (**Fig. 10–25**). On barium upper GI exams, there is fixed elongation and narrowing of the pyloric lumen. Because the patient can be stabilized via intravenous hydration, it does not constitute a surgical emergency.

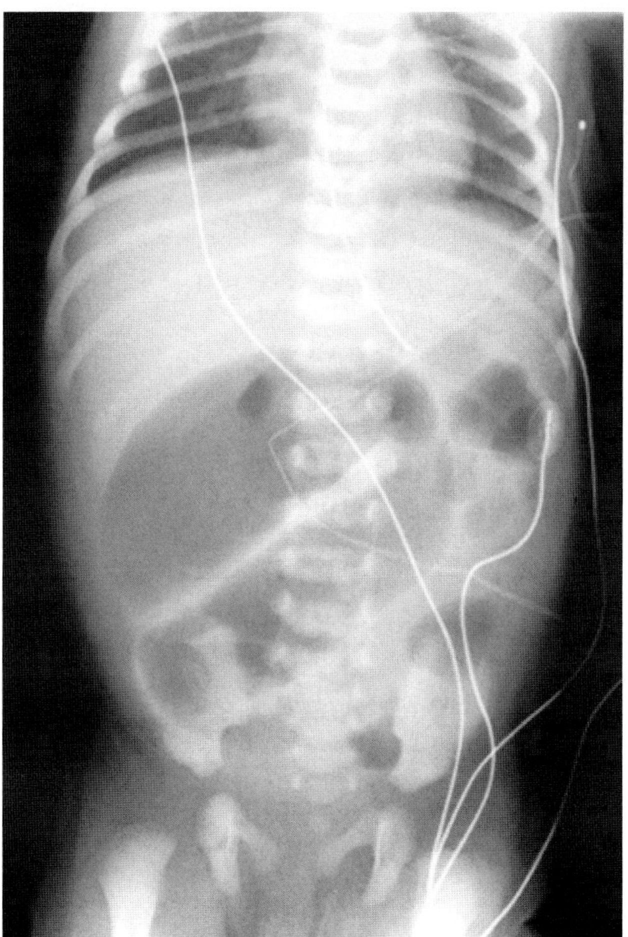

FIGURE 10–24 This neonate failed to pass meconium, vomited feedings, and had a distended abdomen. An abdominal radiograph demonstrates marked distention of the distal bowel. The surgical diagnosis was ileal atresia.

The most common cause of intestinal obstruction in infants older than 1 week of age is inguinal hernia, 90% of which occur in males. Patency of the processus vaginalis, the canal through which the testis descends into the scrotum, allows abdominal contents to slide into the inguinal canal, in some cases extending down into the scrotum, where a mass can be palpated. Eighty percent of inguinal hernias are right sided. The typical patient presents with abdominal distention, vomiting, and irritability. Plain film findings include small bowel obstruction, thickening of the inguinal fold on the affected side, and air-filled bowel in the inguinal canal or scrotum (**Fig. 10–26**). Ultrasound may show a peristalsing mass in the same regions.

Appendicitis is the principal cause of emergency surgery in children. Stasis within the appendix, often caused by an obstructing appendicolith, allows bacterial overgrowth, inflammation, vascular compromise, and eventual perforation, which may result in fatal peritonitis. A calcified appendicolith is visible on plain film in only 15% of patients. Other plain film findings include evidence of small bowel obstruction, a soft tissue mass in the right lower quadrant, focal right lower quadrant ileus, and free intraperitoneal air. Barium enema may demonstrate mass effect on the cecum and failure to fill the entire appendix; however, the appendix may fail to fill in up to 10% of normal patients. Ultrasound and CT are excellent imaging options in suspected appendicitis. Findings on ultrasound include a noncompressible appendix with a total diameter of more than 6 mm. Both CT and ultrasound may demonstrate a dilated, fluid-filled appendix, an appendicolith, or a complex periappendiceal fluid collection if the appendix has ruptured (**Fig. 10–27**).

Another condition the radiologist may be called on not only to diagnose but also to treat is intussusception, the telescoping of a more proximal segment of bowel into a more distal segment, typically involving the downstream displacement of a segment of ileum (the intussusceptum) into the right colon (the intussuscepiens) (**Fig. 10–28**). Ninety percent of cases occur in the first 2 years of life. It is thought that most cases of intussusception in children stem from virally induced intestinal lymphoid hyperplasia, which acts as a lead point. On plain radiography, the abdomen may demonstrate signs of intestinal obstruction, a right-sided soft tissue mass, or even the head of the intussusceptum within air-filled colon. Ultrasound may demonstrate an oval soft tissue mass on longitudinal view and a round mass on the cross-sectional view, both often demonstrating concentric rings of bowel. Retrograde contrast examination of the bowel will demonstrate the head

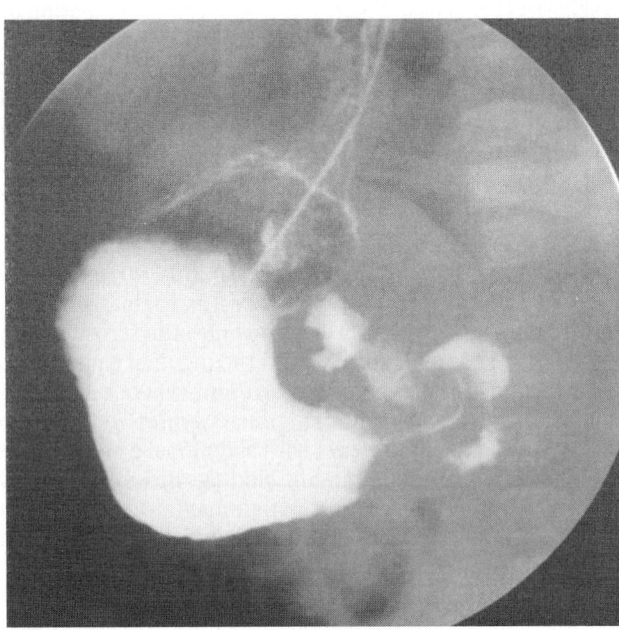

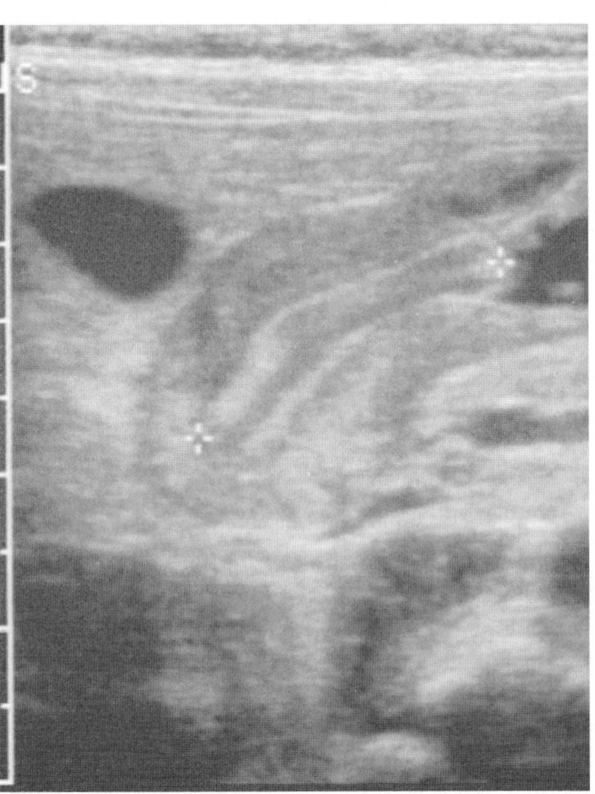

FIGURE 10–25 This 4-week-old infant presented with projectile nonbilious vomiting and dehydration. **(A)** A spot fluoroscopic image from a barium upper GI exam demonstrates marked elongation and narrowing of the pyloric channel. **(B)** A longitudinal sonographic view demonstrates elongation of the pyloric channel (measured at 20 mm between the cursors), as well as marked thickening of the pyloric wall. These findings are diagnostic of hypertrophic pyloric stenosis.

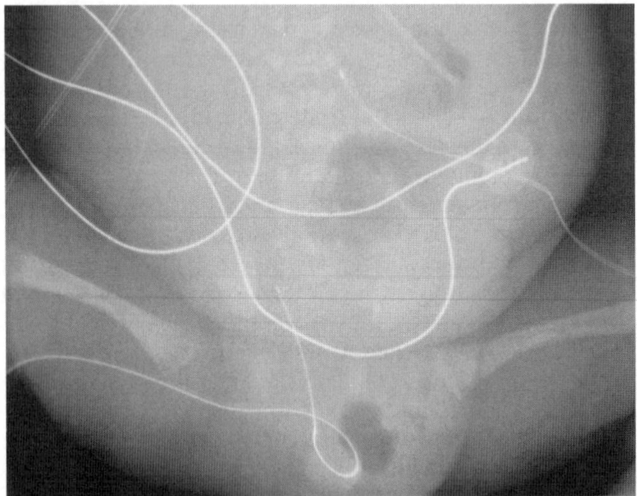

FIGURE 10–26 This 5-week-old infant presented with intermittent vomiting and abdominal distention. An abdominal radiograph demonstrates an abnormally dilated segment of bowel in the lower abdomen, but more importantly, a gas collection in the scrotum. This was due to an inguinal hernia, with gas-containing bowel in the scrotum. Note that nasogastric and transurethral bladder catheters are in place.

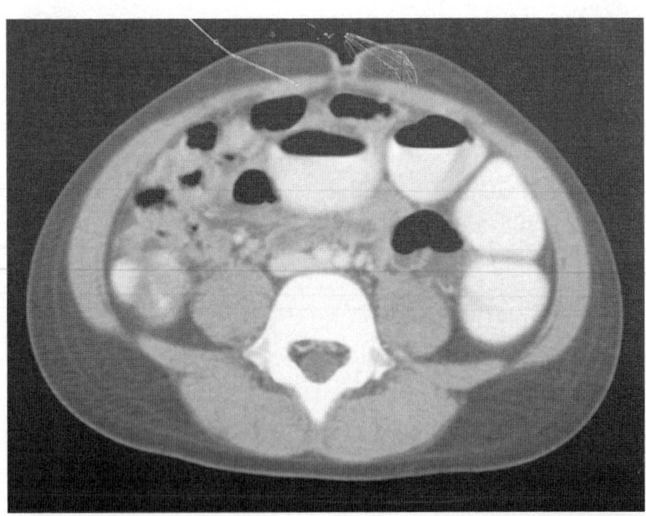

FIGURE 10–27 This young boy presented with abdominal pain and low-grade fever. An axial CT image of the abdomen after intravenous (IV) and oral contrast demonstrates the dilated, fluid-filled appendix just anterior to the IVC and iliac arteries. Surgery confirmed acute appendicitis.

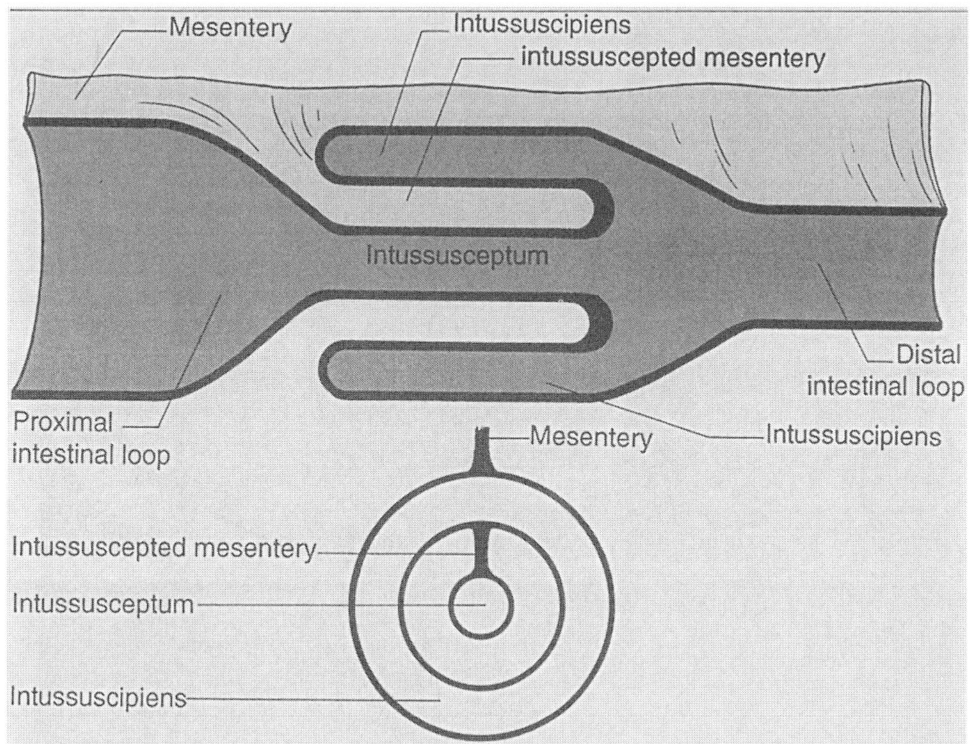

FIGURE 10–28 Anatomy of intussusception. The lower cross-sectional diagram explains the "target" sign of intussusception by ultrasound.

of the intussusceptum as a filling defect within the intussuscepiens. In addition to diagnosis, pressure from retrograde flow of contrast or air will often reduce the intussusception (**Fig. 10–29**). There is a 5% risk of recurrence. The only contraindications to radiologic reduction are signs of perforation, such as free air, and symptoms of peritonitis.

Masses

◇ Wilms' Tumor

Epidemiology The most prevalent solid abdominal mass of childhood, which is also the most common renal cancer of childhood, is Wilms' tumor, of which ~400 cases per year are reported in the United States. It also represents the fourth most common childhood malignancy, after leukemia, central nervous system neoplasms, and neuroblastoma. The mean age of presentation in Wilms' tumor is 3 years, and 85% of cases present before the age of 6 years.

Pathophysiology Also known as nephroblastoma, Wilms' tumor arises from the primitive metanephric blastema and is typically centered in the renal cortex, sparing the collecting system. Roughly 1 in 10 tumors presents bilaterally, which seems to be associated with a better prognosis. Another important prognostic factor is the histology of the tumor, with 85% of tumors exhibiting a favorable triphasic pattern (consisting of primitive blastema, stroma, and epithelial cells), while 15% of tumors are anaplastic, an unfavorable pattern. Wilms' tumor is associated with several syndromes, including sporadic aniridia, hemihypertrophy, Beckwith-Wiedemann syndrome (macroglossia, organomegaly, and omphalocele), and Drash syndrome (pseudohermaphroditism, glomerulonephritis, and nephrotic syndrome). In addition, it appears with increased frequency in horseshoe and fused kidneys.

Clinical Presentation Presenting complaints typically consist of a rapidly enlarging, painless abdominal mass, without systemic symptoms. A minority of patients demonstrate microscopic hematuria.

Imaging Ultrasound constitutes the first line of imaging, because it provides quick and reliable detection as well as the best assessment of the degree of vascular invasion. Many Wilms' tumors will involve the renal vein and inferior vena cava, some actually extending into the heart. Sonography usually reveals a large mass, with internal areas of necrosis and hemorrhage, arising from the kidney and displacing adjacent abdominal structures. CT typically demonstrates a well-defined, low-attenuation mass with heterogeneous enhancement (**Fig. 10–30**). Only ~15% of Wilms' tumors demonstrate calcifications. Treatment usually consists of surgery and chemotherapy, with radiation therapy reserved for more advanced tumors that are not totally resectable or have metastasized hematogenously. Despite the rapid growth of Wilms' tumor, the prognosis is generally favorable, with overall survival approaching 90%.

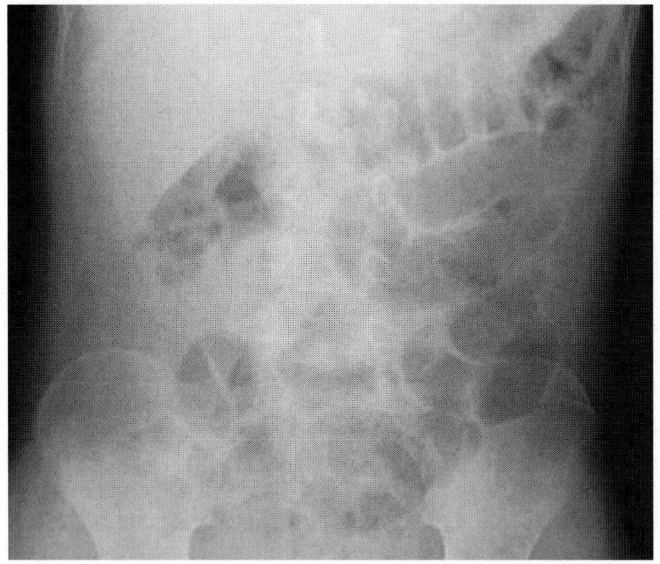

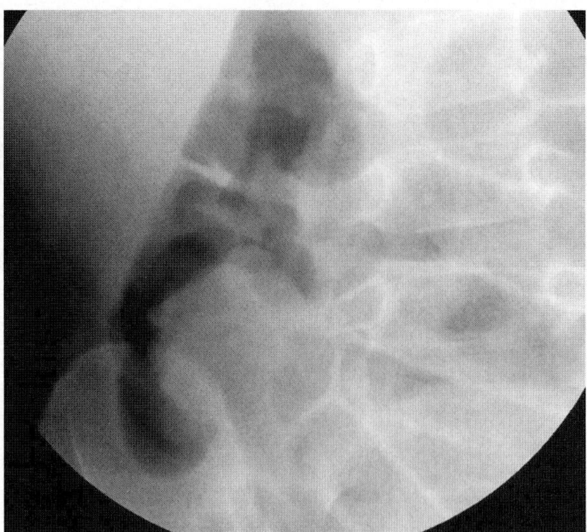

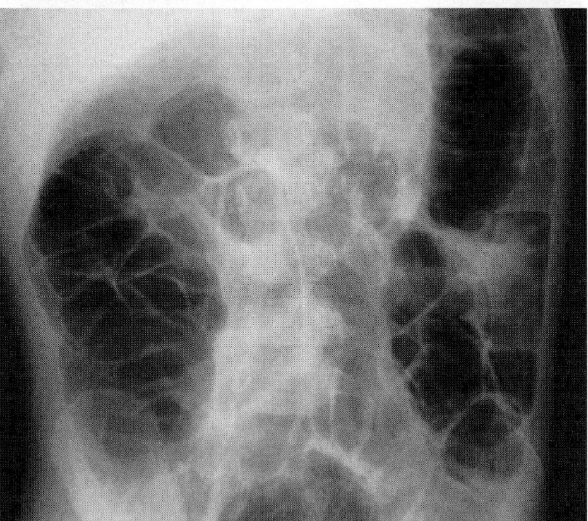

FIGURE 10–29 This 2-year-old boy presented with intermittent abdominal pain over several days, now with bloody stools. **(A)** The abdominal radiograph shows a possible partial small bowel obstruction with a soft tissue mass in the right lower quadrant. An air-contrast enema was performed to assess for intussusception. **(B)** A fluoroscopic spot view of the right lower quadrant demonstrates a soft tissue filling defect in the cecum, typical for an ileocolic intussusception. **(C)** After successful air reduction, the filling defect has disappeared, and there is free reflux of air into the small bowel.

◇ Neuroblastoma

Epidemiology Neuroblastoma is the second most common intra-abdominal malignancy of childhood. Approximately 70% of neuroblastomas arise in the abdomen, with over 40% originating in the adrenal gland, while the chest, neck, and pelvis represent other sites. At 2 years, the mean age of this neoplasm is slightly lower than that of Wilms' tumor, and three quarters of patients present before age 5 years.

Pathophysiology The tumor arises from neural crest tissue either in the adrenal gland or somewhere along the sympathetic chain. Neuroblastoma is at the malignant end of a spectrum of tumors ranging to the intermediate grade ganglioneuroblastoma and the benign ganglioneuroma. Some neuroblastomas spontaneously differentiate into these more mature forms. They also occasionally exhibit the extraordinary property of undergoing spontaneous regression, even in very advanced disease. In contrast to Wilms' tumor, neuroblastoma has fewer and less syndromic associations; however, it does sometimes exhibit certain clinical constellations of metastatic spread. Orbital ecchymosis and proptosis so-called raccoon eyes, often occur in combination with a primary adrenal tumor and extensive skeletal involvement, especially the skull, which is called Hutchinson's syndrome. The "blueberry muffin" syndrome is associated with multiple skin metastases.

Clinical Presentation Patients typically present with large abdominal masses and metastatic disease. In addition, 70% will have systemic symptoms, including hypertension, hyperglycemia, tachycardia, and other signs of increased catecholamine production. Hence, laboratory analysis usually reveals increased urine levels of vanillylmandelic acid or homovanillic acid. A minority of patients will present with paraneoplastic effects, including the so-called dancing eyes and dancing feet syndrome.

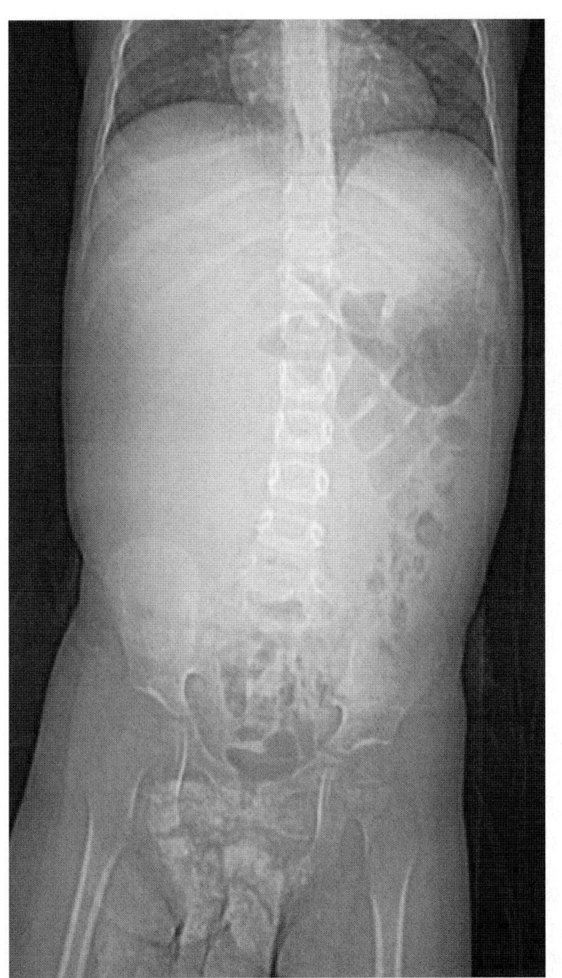

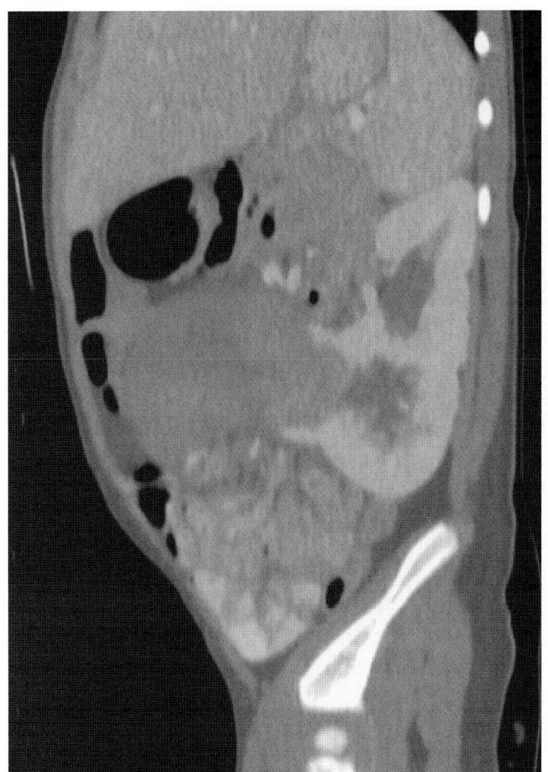

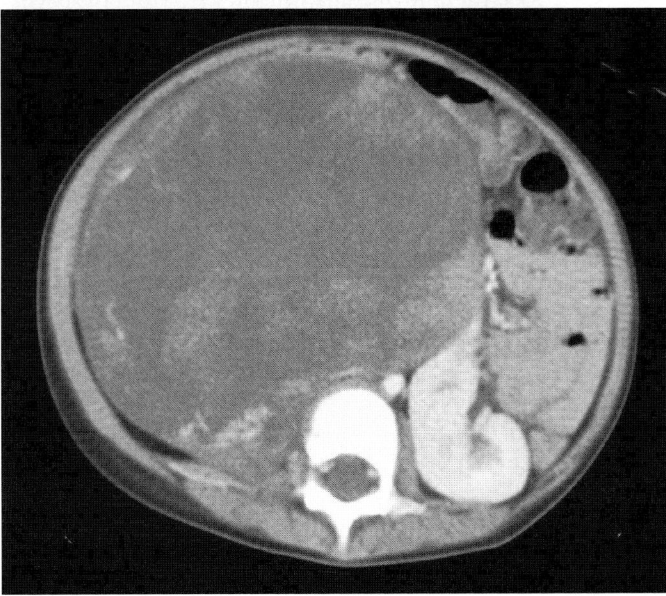

FIGURE 10–30 This 3-year-old presented with anemia and was found to have an abdominal mass. **(A)** A scout image from an abdominal CT exam with IV and oral contrast demonstrates a right-sided soft tissue mass. **(B)** An axial CT image shows a huge heterogeneous mass originating on the right. **(C)** An oblique coronal reconstruction confirms that the mass, a Wilms' tumor, arose on the right side of a horseshoe kidney.

Imaging The imaging of neuroblastoma contrasts with that of Wilms' tumor in several respects. Whereas Wilms' tumor seldom calcifies, 50% of neuroblastomas demonstrate calcifications on plain radiography, and 90% are calcified on CT. In contrast to Wilms' tumor, neuroblastoma tends to be a poorly marginated mass that insinuates itself around and engulfs other abdominal structures. It often extends across the midline and even into the thorax. Ultrasound usually demonstrates a large mass with

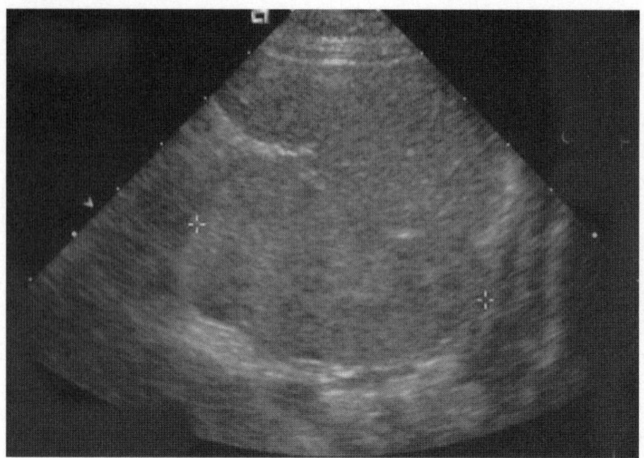

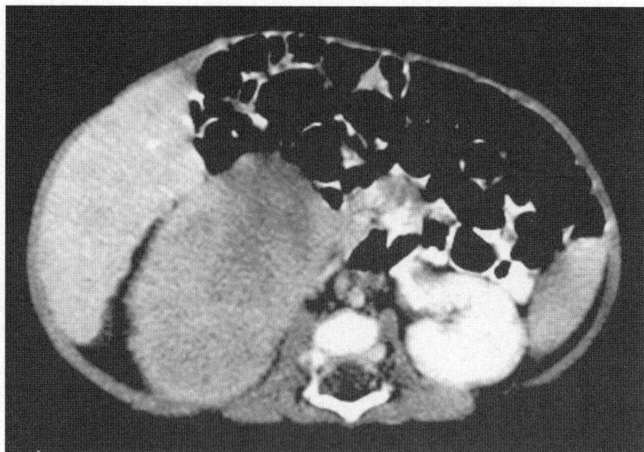

FIGURE 10–31 This 10-week-old male was referred for imaging with a diagnosis of "hepatosplenomegaly." **(A)** A transverse sonographic view of the right upper quadrant demonstrates a large soft tissue mass (between cursors) behind the liver. **(B)** An axial CT image shows a large heterogeneous mass, likely arising from the right adrenal gland. This was a neuroblastoma.

heterogeneous and echogenic echotexture. As an extrarenal mass, it often displaces the axis of the kidney. In addition to demonstrating calcifications, CT is used to detect metastatic disease, which most often involves the liver and lymph nodes (**Fig. 10–31**). Bone marrow involvement, which is common, is typically assessed by bone scintigraphy. MRI is often used in patients with neurologic symptoms, in whom intraspinal involvement must be ruled out. Prognosis is best for younger patients and those with a nonabdominal primary tumor.

Musculoskeletal System

Developmental Dysplasia of the Hip

◇ Epidemiology

Once referred to as congenital hip dislocation, developmental dysplasia of the hip (DDH) is seen most frequently in white infants and exhibits a female to male ratio of 5:1. It can also be associated with neuromuscular diseases, such as myelomeningocele. The incidence is estimated at 1 per 1000 births.

◇ Pathophysiology

In most cases, DDH is thought to be secondary to hormonally induced laxity of the capsular ligaments, compounded by in utero positions that stress the hip, such as a restricted intrauterine space due to oligohydramnios. It more commonly involves the left hip than the right, which is thought to be due to the fact that fetuses tend to lie with their backs to the maternal left side, with their left hips against the maternal sacrum. If uncorrected, DDH can lead to early secondary osteoarthritic changes, with deformity of both the acetabulum and femoral head. Treatment includes casting in a frog-leg position if the hip is relocatable or surgery in cases of irreducibility or failed conservative therapy.

◇ Clinical Presentation

DDH is suspected clinically in newborns with a breech presentation, who have a 25% risk, because the hips are extended during birth. Findings on clinical examination include asymmetry of the normal skinfolds around the hip, shortening of the thigh, and a "click" during the Ortolani reduction test (performed by flexing the hip and gently abducting).

◇ Imaging

Imaging plays a critical role in the diagnosis of DDH. The essential parameter in the imaging evaluation is the relationship of the femur to the acetabulum. The finding of a well-seated and nondislocatable femoral head on stress views excludes the diagnosis. A variety of measurements have been described that provide quantifiable criteria of dysplasia and dislocation. Formerly, plain films represented the mainstay of imaging diagnosis, but currently ultrasound represents the best modality. Ultrasound shows the cartilaginous femoral head and acetabulum without ionizing radiation or the administration of contrast material, requires no sedation, and can evaluate the dynamic function of the hip joint in real time (**Fig. 10–32**); however, ultrasound is optimal only up to 6 months of age; after that point, ossification of the hip structures interferes with adequate beam penetration. One of the disadvantages of ultrasound as compared with other modalities such as CT and MRI is the fact that it is extremely operator dependent.

Trauma

Musculoskeletal trauma in children differs from that in adults in several important respects. First, children generate smaller forces and are situated closer to the ground than adults, which tends to protect their skeletons from fracture; however, the bones of children are different from adult bones in ways that make them more liable to fracture. Pediatric bones are shorter and thinner than those in adults, and they are also less dense, containing proportionately more water. Children's bones are therefore not as resistant to bending, torquing, and axial loading forces. Yet this also means that the bone of a child will often bend to a remarkable degree before it develops the frank fracture one would expect in an adult.

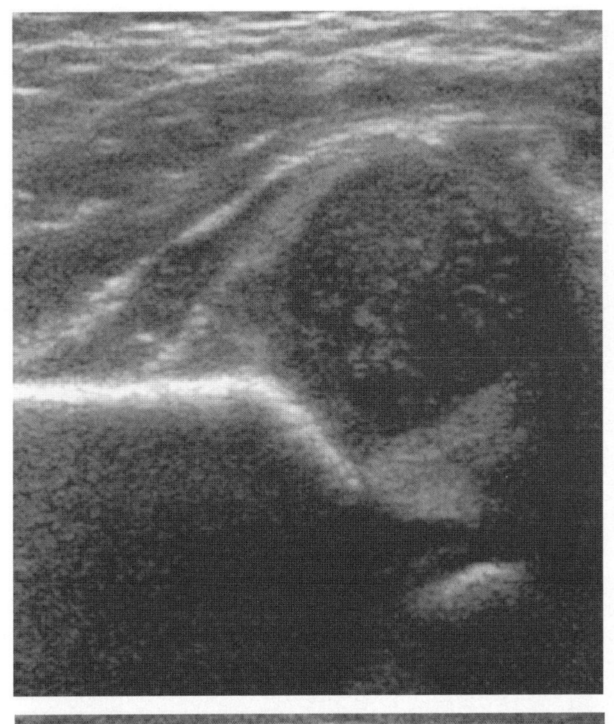

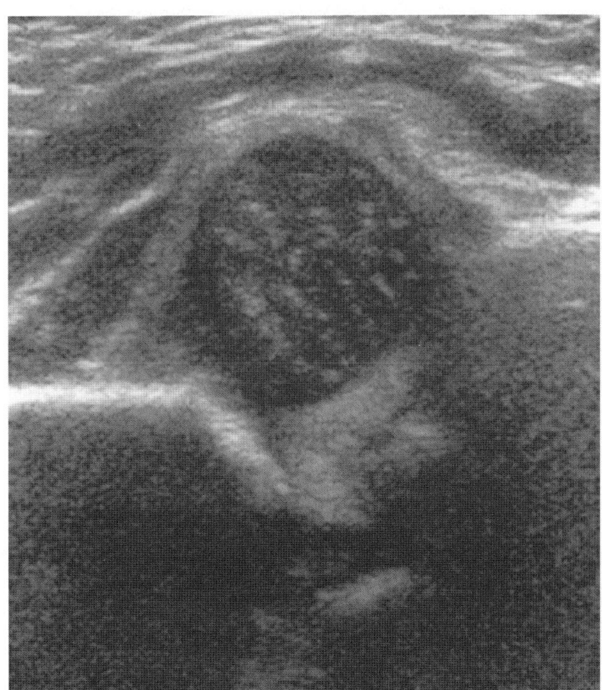

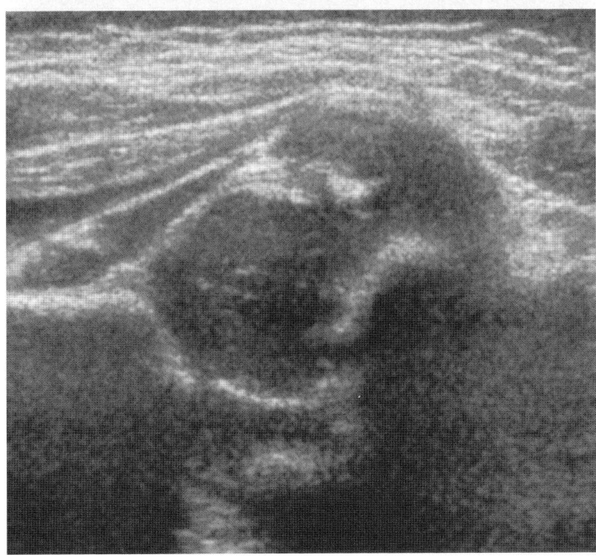

FIGURE 10–32 **(A)** This longitudinal sonogram of the right hip in a 1-month-old infant demonstrates that most of the femoral head is lateral to the acetabulum. **(B)** With stress, the femoral head subluxes even further. **(C)** A normal longitudinal hip sonogram for comparison.

One result of the greater flexibility of children's bones is the occurrence of several types of fractures that do not occur in adults. One such peculiarly pediatric fracture is the so-called greenstick fracture, so named because the injury resembles the effect sometimes produced by bending a green stick until it breaks: one side of the shaft fractures, but the other merely bends. A variant is the bending fracture, in which neither side of the cortex appears to be disrupted, but the bone is clearly bent. It should be noted that in both cases, the apparent bending in fact represents multiple microfractures that are not seen radiographically; however, the distinction is real, because the adult bone would fracture completely through. Another special pediatric type of fracture is the torus fracture, which manifests as a bulge in the cortex on one or both sides, secondary to axial loading forces and buckling of the bone (**Fig. 10–33**).

A third difference between the pediatric and adult musculoskeletal systems is the differing strength of ligaments and bones in the two groups. The bones of a young adult are typically stronger than the ligaments holding them together, meaning that sprains are quite common. In the later decades of life, osteoporosis tends to weaken the bones, and fractures occur more easily. In a child, however, the bones are usually not as strong as the ligaments, and a fracture is more likely than a ligamentous injury to result from trauma to such joints as the ankle, elbow, and wrist. Typically, the apophyses at which ligaments attach to the bone are weaker than the ligaments themselves; hence the increased incidence of avulsion injuries (**Fig. 10–34**). So common are fractures and avulsion injuries, and so uncommon are the dislocations that often occur in strong-boned adults, that anytime a dislocation is suspected in a child, an

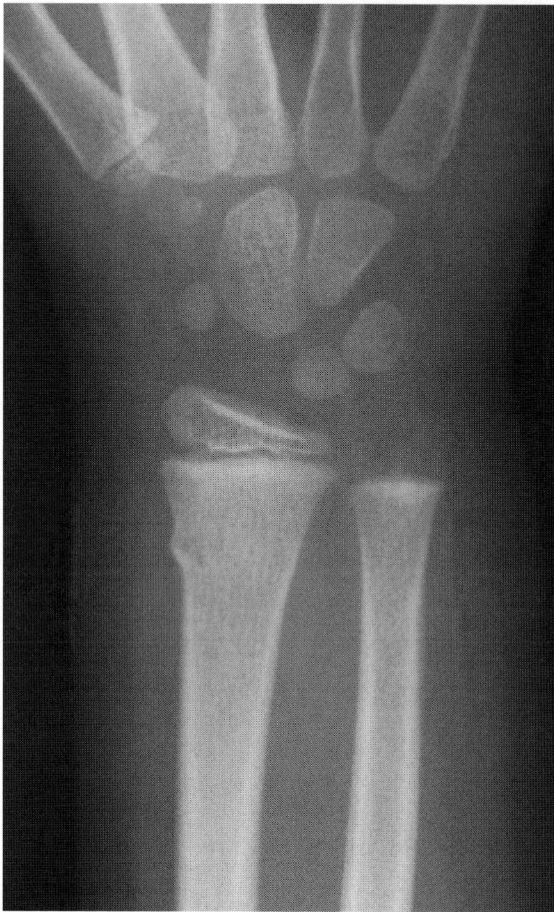

FIGURE 10–33 A wrist radiograph of a child who fell on his hand demonstrates a bulge along the radial aspect of the distal radial metaphysis, a classic torus or buckle fracture.

FIGURE 10–34 This 16-year-old athlete presented with severe right upper thigh and hip pain after lifting weights. **(A)** A frontal pelvis radiograph demonstrates a possible avulsion of the right ischeal tuberosity apophysis. **(B)** Coronal reconstruction of axially acquired CT data clearly shows the minimally displaced avulsion, due to traction from the knee flexor muscles.

additional search should probably be made for an occult fracture.

Perhaps the most important anatomic difference between adult fractures and pediatric fractures is the presence in the child's bones of growth plates (physes) between the epiphyses and metaphyses of the long bones (and elsewhere). The growth plate is the weakest part of the bone and is involved in many pediatric fractures. Approximately 80% of these injuries are due to shearing forces, and 20% to axial loading. The site involved in one half of growth plate injuries is the distal radius. The Salter-Harris classification is widely used to categorize growth plate injuries (**Fig. 10–35**). A Salter-Harris type I injury represents a slip of the epiphysis due to shearing forces and hence involves only the growth plate. A type II injury extends at least partially through the growth plate, but with metaphyseal extension. A type III injury involves the growth plate and the epiphysis (**Fig. 10–36**). A type IV injury extends through the epiphysis, growth plate, and metaphysis. A type V injury represents a crush injury to the growth plate, which often appears radiographically normal. The prognosis for normal growth is good in types I and II injuries, fair for type III injuries, and poor for type IV and particularly type V injuries.

To understand why the prognosis varies according to fracture type, it is necessary to review the structure of the growth plate. At the epiphyseal end are both the germinal zone of proliferating cartilage cells, without which growth cannot occur, and the epiphyseal blood vessels that nourish them. On the metaphyseal side are the centers of ossification and the blood vessels supplying them, which are easily replaced in case of injury. The most serious injuries are those that disrupt the epiphyseal aspect of the growth plate, as the loss of cells in the germinal zone, either through direct trauma or vascular compromise, is irreversible, at least if it involves more than a short segment of the physis. Hence, injury to the epiphyseal side of the growth plate may produce partial or complete growth arrest, most likely when the entire physis has been destroyed in the type V crush injury. The restoration of normal alignment is also critical. If the growth plate is not properly realigned, a bony bar may form across a portion of it, which can cause the bone to become angulated and deformed, as the intact remainder of the growth plate continues to grow. The younger the patient (and the more growth remaining to be completed), the greater the potential damage of a growth plate injury.

Because fracture lines in children may be particularly subtle, one secondary sign of fracture frequently sought by pediatric radiologists is evidence of a joint effusion or hemarthrosis. If of sufficient magnitude, these are frequently manifest by the elevation or even obliteration of fat pads around joints,

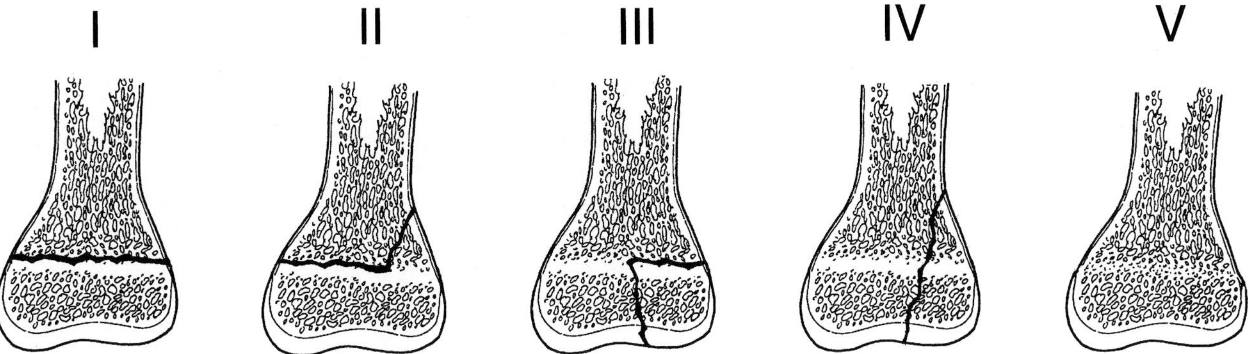

FIGURE 10–35 The Salter-Harris classification of growth plate injuries, as described in the text.

particularly the elbow on a lateral radiograph. In a child, elevation of the anterior humeral fat pad or appearance of the posterior humeral fat pad (which is not normally visible, being hidden by the olecranon fossa) is considered presumptive evidence of a supracondylar humeral fracture. The patient is usually splinted or casted and brought back in 10 days for repeat imaging, by which time osteoclastic lysis along the fracture line or periosteal reaction should be present.

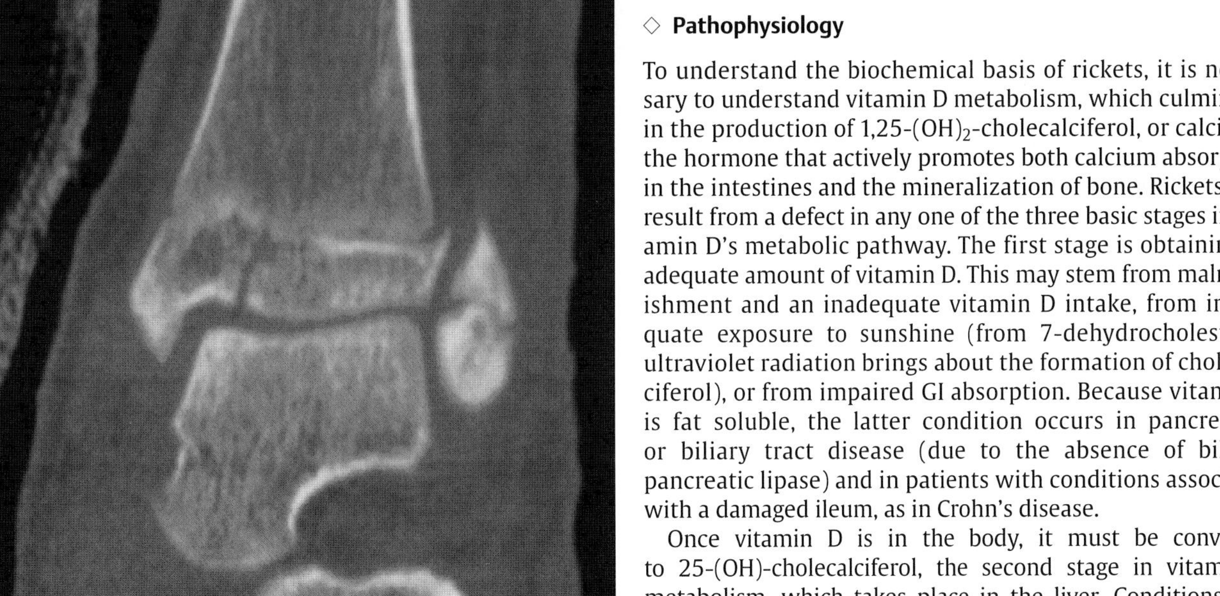

FIGURE 10–36 This teenager complained of ankle pain after a fall. A CT scan was performed with the ankle in a plastic cast. Coronal reconstruction of axial data demonstrates a Salter-Harris type III fracture involving the lateral aspect of the distal tibial growth plate and extending perpendicularly through the epiphysis. This is a so-called juvenile Tillaux fracture, which occurs at an age when the medial aspect of the physis has begun to fuse.

Rickets

◇ Epidemiology

Rickets is an example of osteomalacia, the inadequate mineralization of osteoid, which in the immature skeleton of a growing child tends to manifest itself at the physis, or growth plate, of long bones. Although the majority of children in many large metropolitan areas appear to have suffered some degree of rickets at the turn of the 20th century, the disorder is not commonly seen today, due in large part to the supplementation of milk with vitamin D.

◇ Pathophysiology

To understand the biochemical basis of rickets, it is necessary to understand vitamin D metabolism, which culminates in the production of 1,25-$(OH)_2$-cholecalciferol, or calcitriol, the hormone that actively promotes both calcium absorption in the intestines and the mineralization of bone. Rickets may result from a defect in any one of the three basic stages in vitamin D's metabolic pathway. The first stage is obtaining an adequate amount of vitamin D. This may stem from malnourishment and an inadequate vitamin D intake, from inadequate exposure to sunshine (from 7-dehydrocholesterol, ultraviolet radiation brings about the formation of cholecalciferol), or from impaired GI absorption. Because vitamin D is fat soluble, the latter condition occurs in pancreatitis or biliary tract disease (due to the absence of bile or pancreatic lipase) and in patients with conditions associated with a damaged ileum, as in Crohn's disease.

Once vitamin D is in the body, it must be converted to 25-(OH)-cholecalciferol, the second stage in vitamin D metabolism, which takes place in the liver. Conditions that interfere with this process include a variety of hepatic parenchymal diseases, as well as anticonvulsant therapy. Anticonvulsants induce hepatic microsomal enzymes and thereby hasten the degradation of biologically active vitamin D metabolites.

The third stage in vitamin D metabolism is the conversion of 25-(OH)-vitamin D to 1,25-$(OH)_2$-vitamin D in the kidney. A variety of conditions may interfere with this step, including chronic renal failure and a variety of renal tubular disorders.

Although a combination of insufficient sun exposure and malnutrition was responsible for most cases of rickets in the past, renal osteodystrophy is now the most common cause.

Because bone mineralization also requires an adequate supply of phosphate and calcium, a deficiency of either of these may also cause osteomalacia. Lack of calcium may result from insufficient dietary intake or malabsorption. Defective phosphate metabolism has a variety of causes, including simple phosphate deficiency and numerous disorders of renal tubular reabsorption of phosphate, such as Fanconi's syndrome. Hypophosphatasia is a rare disorder associated with low levels of the enzyme alkaline phosphatase, which is required by osteoblasts to create the locally high concentrations of phosphate necessary for bone mineralization, and often presents with many of the radiographic features of rickets.

◇ Clinical Presentation

Children with long-standing rickets present with bowing of weight-bearing bones such as the femur and tibia and have an increased incidence of fractures due to weakening of the bones.

◇ Imaging

The radiographic findings in rickets stem from the production of defective bone, particularly at the growth plate. As one would predict, the most severely affected bones will be those undergoing the most rapid growth, such as the distal femur, the proximal tibia, the proximal humerus, and the distal radius and ulna. Aside from generalized osteopenia and retarded growth, rickets demonstrates widening of the growth plate, flaring and cupping of the metaphyses, and eventually, bowing and deformity of the bones due to bone softening (**Fig. 10–37**). Once skeletal deformity results, surgical correction may be required. Although rickets is not as common as in years past, it is a disease the radiologist cannot afford to miss, because simple vitamin supplementation may prevent the development of severe skeletal deformity.

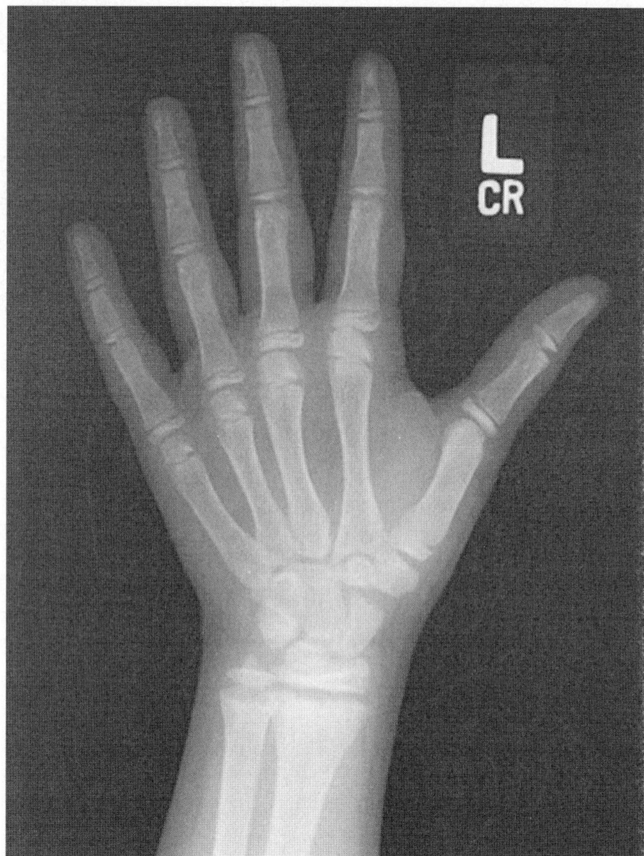

FIGURE 10–37 A hand radiograph of a child with hypophosphatasia demonstrates classic changes of rickets at the wrist, including cupping and fraying of the distal radial and ulnar metaphyses, and widening of the growth plates. The cupping is most prominent in the ulna.

Child Abuse

◇ Epidemiology

The term *abuse* is subject to variable interpretation and may encompass intentional physical injury, sexual assault, neglect, and varying degrees of psychological trauma. Between 1 and 2 million cases of abuse occur every year in the United States.

◇ Pathophysiology

Children who have suffered one episode of undetected abuse have a 15% risk of repeat abuse, which carries a mortality rate of up to 10%. In other words, 1 to 2% of children who suffer undetected abuse will die as a result. Many others will suffer permanent disability. A failure to detect child abuse therefore carries a high risk of mortality. For this reason, mandatory reporting statutes have been adopted in all 50 states, and health care providers have been granted immunity for reports made in good faith.

◇ Clinical Presentation

Two thirds of abuse takes place before the age of 6 years, at which stage it may be difficult for children to provide a history; however, a host of clinical clues applicable even at these young ages should increase suspicion of abuse. These include a history that does not correspond to the child's injury, an inconsistent or conflicting history, inappropriate parental concern, failure to seek parental sympathy and support, evidence of poor hygiene or nutrition, and an unreasonable delay in seeking care. Examples include a 2-month-old who supposedly rolled off the changing table and fell onto the floor (the ability to roll over is acquired around the age of 5 months) and a child who supposedly sat down in scalding water (pain in the feet would prevent the child from sitting down). As a general rule, no child who is too young to move independently can cause itself significant injury.

◇ Imaging

If the definition of abuse is restricted to physical injury, it is estimated that up to two thirds of cases are radiologically detectable, meaning that radiologists play a critical role in making the diagnosis of abuse. Often, the radiologist detects evidence of abuse in a child in whom the diagnosis was not even suspected. Findings of child abuse on radiologic examination include skeletal injuries, intracranial injuries, and injuries to the abdominal viscera. Although any form of skeletal injury may result, certain patterns of injury are relatively specific for abuse. These include metaphyseal fractures, such as the so-called corner or bucket handle fractures at the chondro-osseous junction, which are commonly bilateral and involve the tibia, femur, and humerus (**Fig. 10–38**). When the child is squeezed in the anteroposterior axis, posterior rib fractures near the costovertebral junction may result. The finding of multiple fractures of various ages should set off alarm bells, although other disorders such as osteogenesis imperfecta must be considered. A classic sign of fracture is periosteal reaction secondary to subperiosteal hemorrhage, which lifts the infant's loosely bound periosteum off the shaft and is followed by subperiosteal mineralization within 1 to 2 weeks.

Intracranial injury carries a high risk of mortality and developmental delay. The most specific finding is an interhemispheric subdural hematoma, usually as part of the "shaken baby" syndrome, although skull fractures, subarachnoid hemorrhage, cerebral edema, and atrophy may also be seen. The retinas should be closely inspected in every case, because the vast majority of "shaken babies" will exhibit retinal hemorrhages. Visceral injuries typically involve the liver, spleen, or kidneys, and the presence of visceral trauma in children younger than 5 years old (absent a history of motor vehicle accident or the like) should raise high suspicion of abuse.

What constitutes an appropriate imaging strategy for the suspected abuse victim? The mainstay of diagnosis is a plain radiographic skeletal survey, with tightly coned views of each anatomic region. Clinicians and radiologists must resist the temptation to reduce the child's radiation dose by obtaining as few radiographs as necessary to image the whole skeleton. The findings of abuse are often subtle and can only be detected with tightly coned views of each anatomic region (anteroposterior and lateral skull, anteroposterior and lateral chest with bone technique, humeri, forearms, femurs, tibias, and perhaps the hands and feet). Some investigators suggest the use of bone scintigraphy as a screening procedure, due to its high sensitivity and ability to encompass the entire skeleton. If neurologic findings are present, a noncontrast head CT is warranted, which should be followed up with MRI if the CT is negative and clinical suspicion is high. Body CT is indicated only in the presence of clinical findings such as abdominal distention and tenderness or to better evaluate skeletal injuries.

Urinary Tract

Infection

◇ Epidemiology

Urinary tract infections are a relatively common problem in children, constituting the second most prevalent infection in the pediatric age group (after respiratory tract infections) and the most common problem of the urinary tract. It is estimated that up to 10% of girls experience a urinary tract infection. In children with urinary tract infections, reflux of urine from the bladder into the ureters and/or renal collecting systems is seen in one quarter to one half of patients.

◇ Pathophysiology

Pathophysiologically, most urinary tract infections are thought to stem from the ascent of bacteria from the perineum up through the urethra. Girls are thought to be at especially high risk, due to their relatively short urethras. The close proximity of the female urethral orifice and the anus may be another factor. This latter suggestion is supported by the fact that the most common organism, responsible for up to three quarters of cases, is the enteric commensal, *Escherichia coli*. There are several normal barriers to bacterial growth and migration. First, the low pH of the vagina and perineum exerts a bacteriostatic effect. Second, any bacteria that reach the bladder are normally flushed out with voiding. Third, the ureterovesical junction exhibits an antireflux valve flap action. Factors that interfere with these protective mechanisms include an alteration in normal vaginal/perineal flora, urinary stasis, and immaturity or deformity of the ureterovesical junction.

Vesicoureteral reflux tends to resolve spontaneously with time, as the distance traveled by the distal ureter in the submucosa of the bladder increases with age. The longer the submucosal ureter, the more effective the ureterovesical junction's intrinsic antireflux mechanism. Contraction of the smooth muscle within the bladder wall at voiding increases intravesical pressure and tends to produce reflux if the ureterovesical junction valve mechanism is incompetent. Aside from primary valve incompetence, other structural lesions that predispose to vesicoureteral reflux include a periureteral diverticulum (an outpouching of the bladder wall), a ureterocele (protrusion of the distal ureter into the bladder lumen), and a ureteral duplication. Moreover, any form of bladder outlet obstruction will lead to abnormally increased intravesical pressures during voiding, with a further increase in the probability of reflux. Complications of ascending infection due to reflux include pyelonephritis, renal scarring, hypertension, and renal failure.

◇ Clinical Presentation

A urinary tract infection is defined as the presence of more than 100,000 organisms in a clean-catch urine specimen. The presence of any bacteria in a specimen obtained by catheterization or suprapubic puncture is also abnormal. The younger the child, the less likely that the clinical presentation will be specific. Anorexia, fever, lethargy, and failure to thrive are the most frequently noted findings in the young patient. More classic symptoms of frequency, dysuria, flank pain, and fever are seen in older children.

◇ Imaging

The imaging of urinary tract infection in children is focused on answering two critical questions. First, is there a structural abnormality of the urinary tract that would predispose to infection, such as a urethral outlet obstruction or a

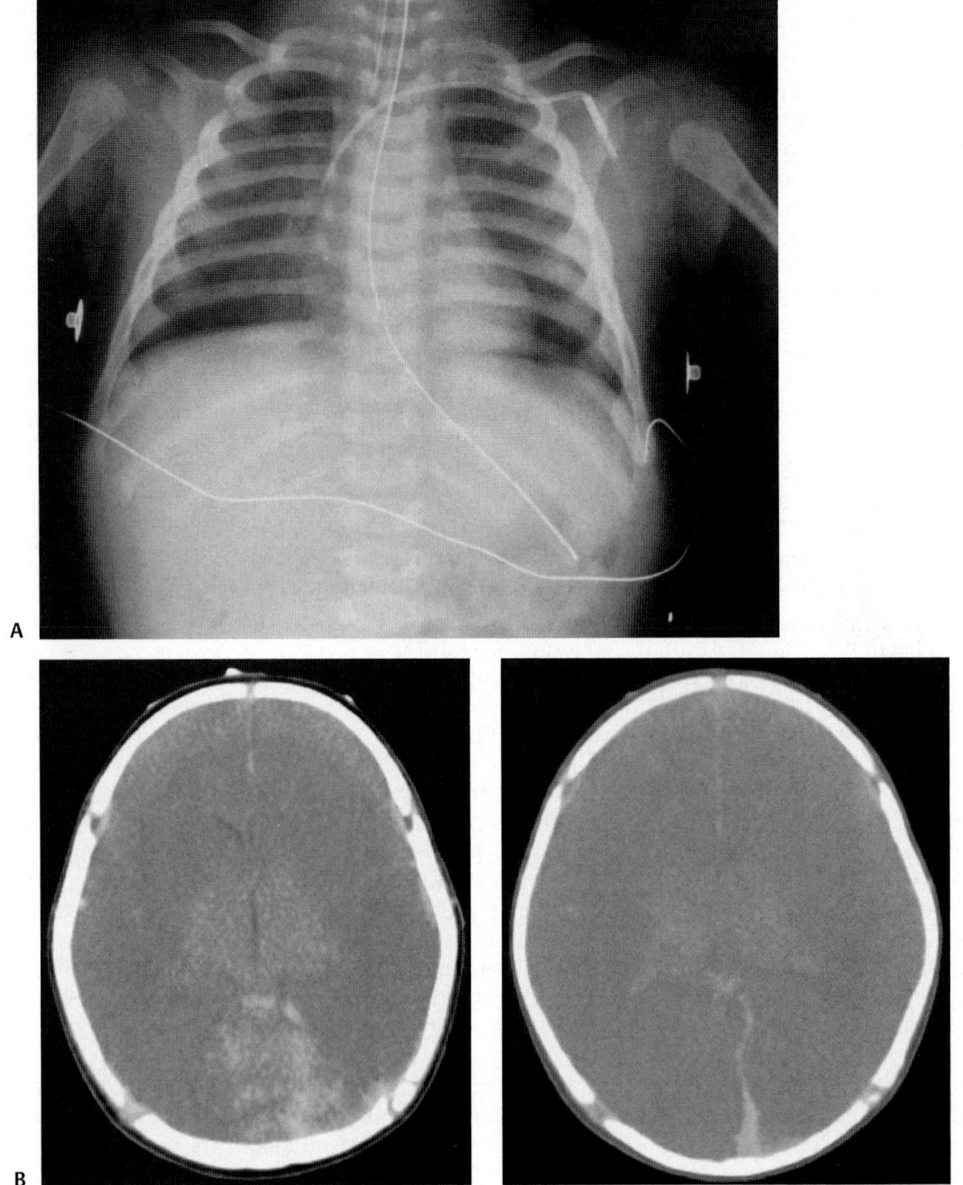

FIGURE 10–38 This 1-year-old boy was brought to the emergency room unconscious. **(A)** The chest radiograph demonstrates an acute fracture of the left 5th rib, as well as healing fractures with callus formation of both left 9th and 10th ribs. **(B,C)** Noncontrast head CT at "blood windows" demonstrates diffuse edema of the brain parenchyma as well as acute subdural hemorrhage involving the tentorium and the posterior aspect of the falx cerebri.

(*Continued*)

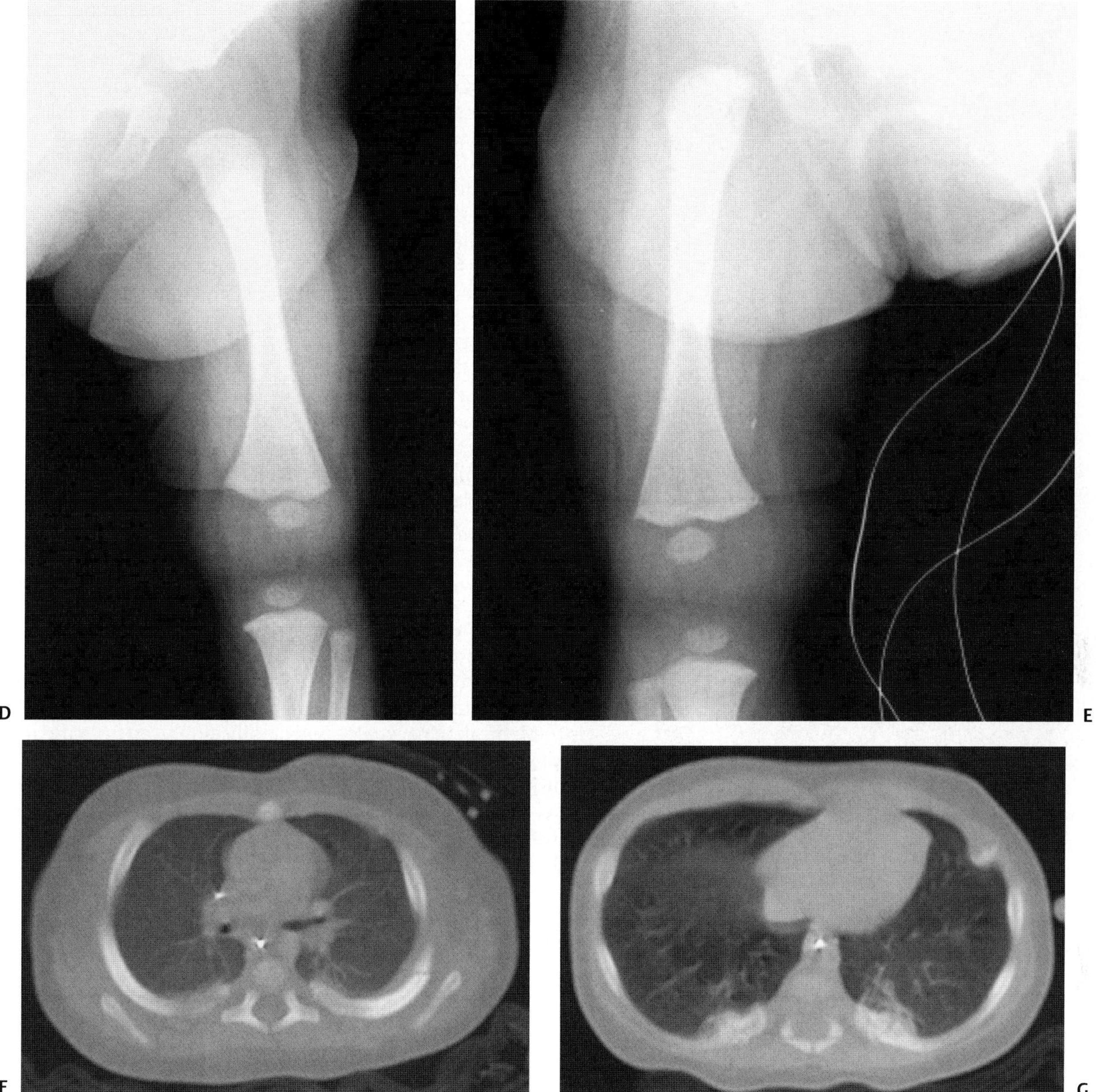

Figure 10–38 (*Continued*) **(D,E)** Images of the knees from a skeletal survey demonstrate bucket handle fractures of the distal femurs. **(F,G)** Bone-window CT images more clearly demonstrate the acute (no callus) and chronic (callus formation) rib fractures with subperiosteal hemorrhages at the site of the acute fracture. Fundoscopic exam also revealed retinal hemorrhages. Eighteen months after the child's death from the injuries, a parent was convicted of reckless homicide.

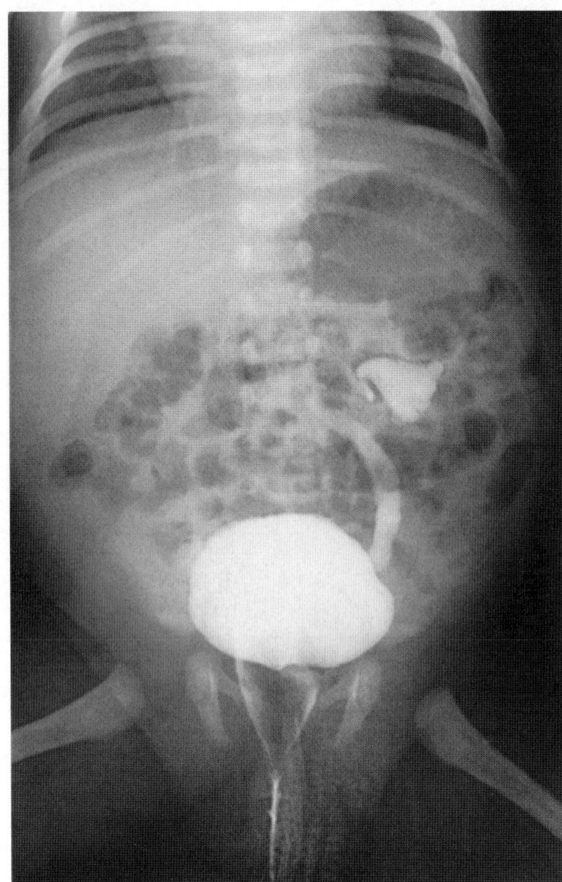

FIGURE 10–39 This infant girl underwent voiding cystourethrography after a urinary tract infection. An abdominal radiograph at the conclusion of voiding shows large postvoid residual volume in the bladder, as well as vesicoureteral reflux into the lower pole of the left renal collecting system. The upper pole was obstructed and hydronephrotic due to a ureterocele, which causes downward displacement of the lower pole, the so-called drooping lily sign.

bladder diverticulum producing urinary stasis? Second, is there vesicoureteral reflux? Although a first urinary tract infection in a girl may be treated empirically, it is generally agreed that any recurrent urinary tract infection in a girl or the first urinary tract infection in a boy warrants imaging evaluation. Some clinicians recommend that any child younger than 4 years of age with a urinary tract infection undergo imaging.

Key studies include the voiding cystourethrogram, the nuclear medicine cystogram, and ultrasound of the upper urinary tract. The voiding cystourethrogram provides the best anatomic evaluation of the bladder and urethra, and is also quite sensitive in the detection of vesicoureteral reflux (**Fig. 10–39**). It is performed by the transurethral insertion of a bladder catheter, followed by the instillation of iodinated contrast under fluoroscopic monitoring. The nuclear medicine cystogram involves the transurethral introduction of a radiotracer into the bladder. Although radionuclide cystography provides a poorer anatomic evaluation of the urinary tract than voiding cystourethrogram, it possesses the advantage that its radiation dose is lower, and it is equally sensitive in the detection of reflux. Ultrasound is employed primarily to evaluate for renal size, the presence of renal parenchymal scarring, and hydronephrosis (**Fig. 10–40**). The imaging study with the best sensitivity in the diagnosis of pyelonephritis is renal cortical scintigraphy, which can also be used to evaluate function and parenchymal scarring.

Medical management is generally employed for more mild degrees of vesicoureteral reflux, the theory being that if the urine can be kept sterile, no complications of reflux are likely to arise, and meantime, most children will outgrow their reflux. When reflux is more severe and associated with dilatation of the upper urinary tract (hydronephrosis), surgical intervention may be indicated.

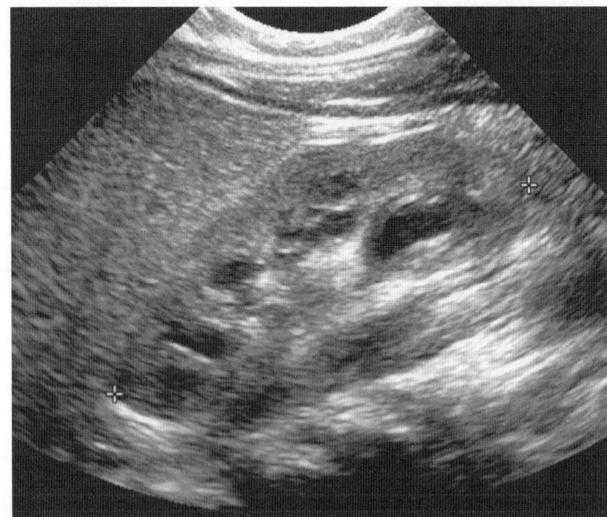

A

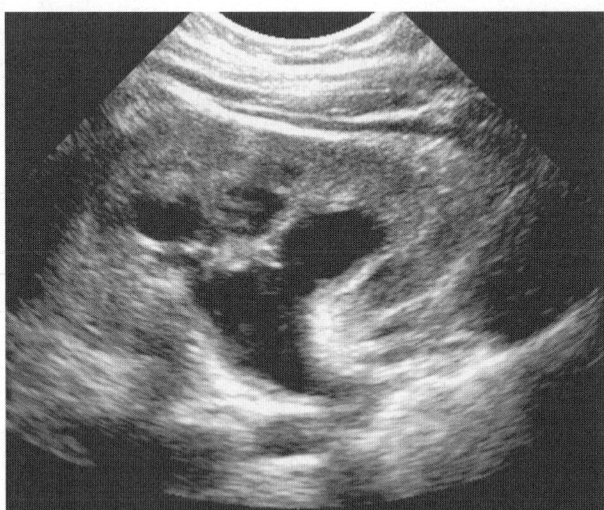

B

FIGURE 10–40 This child was being evaluated for a urinary tract infection. **(A)** A longitudinal ultrasound image of the right kidney demonstrates dilation of the calices. **(B)** Minutes later, the degree of hydronephrosis increases, with greater caliectases and new pelviectasis (distention of the renal pelvis). These findings indicate that the hydronephrosis is likely secondary to vesicoureteral reflux, which may wax and wane.

Appendix

Normal Cross-Sectional Anatomy

Chest Anatomy

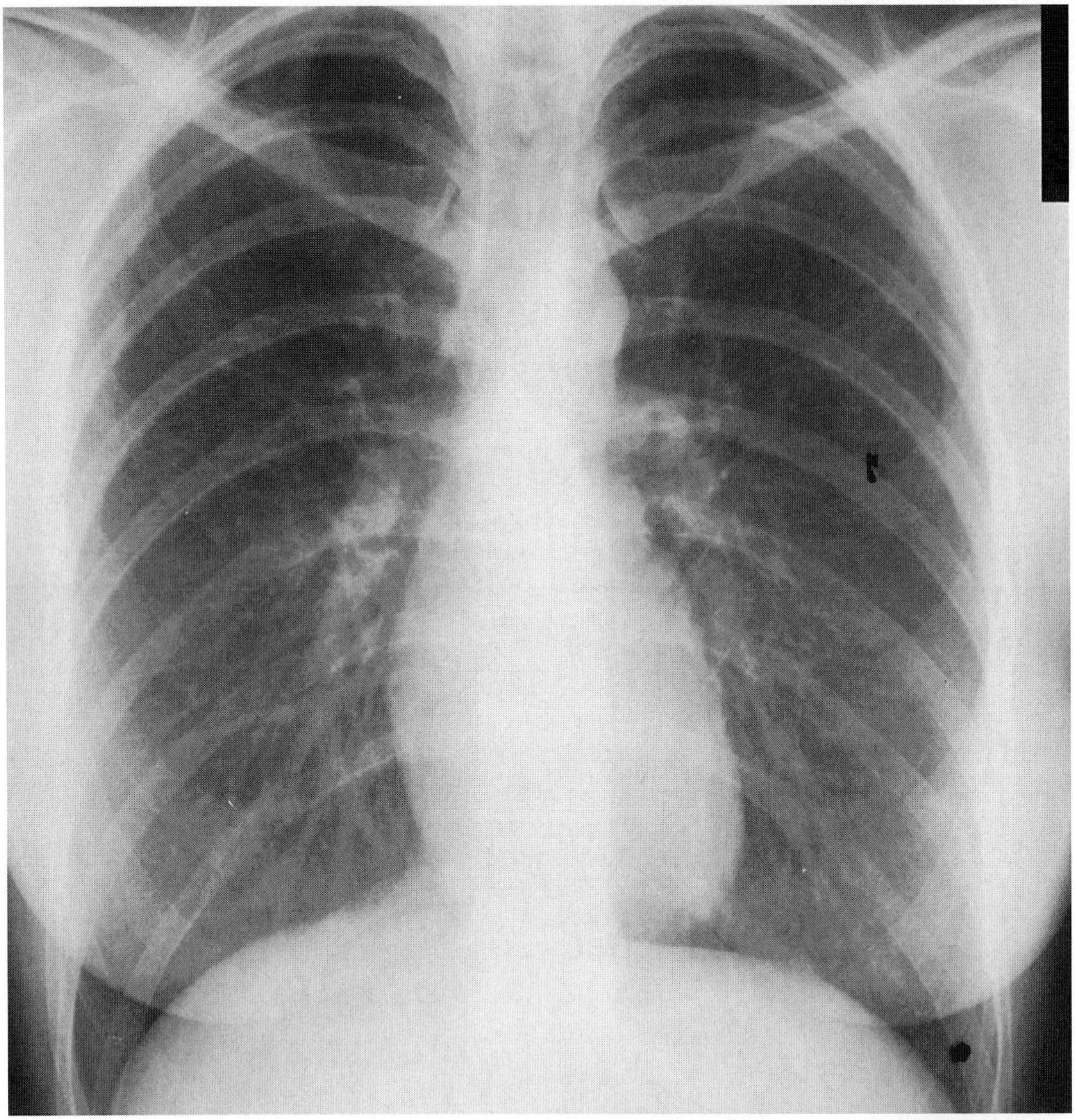

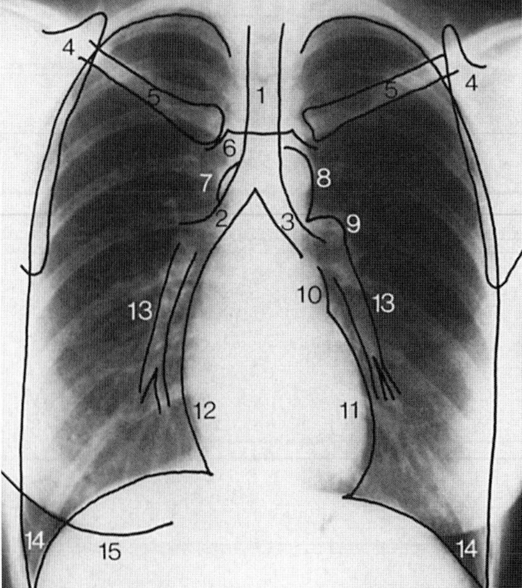

Figure 1 Frontal chest radiograph.

1. Trachea
2. Right main bronchus
3. Left main bronchus
4. Scapula
5. Clavicle
6. Manubrium sterni
7. Azygous vein
8. Aortic arch
9. Left pulmonary artery
10. Left atrial appendage
11. Ventricular curve of left heart
12. Right atrium
13. Lower lobe pulmonary artery
14. Lateral costophrenic sulcus
15. Breast shadow

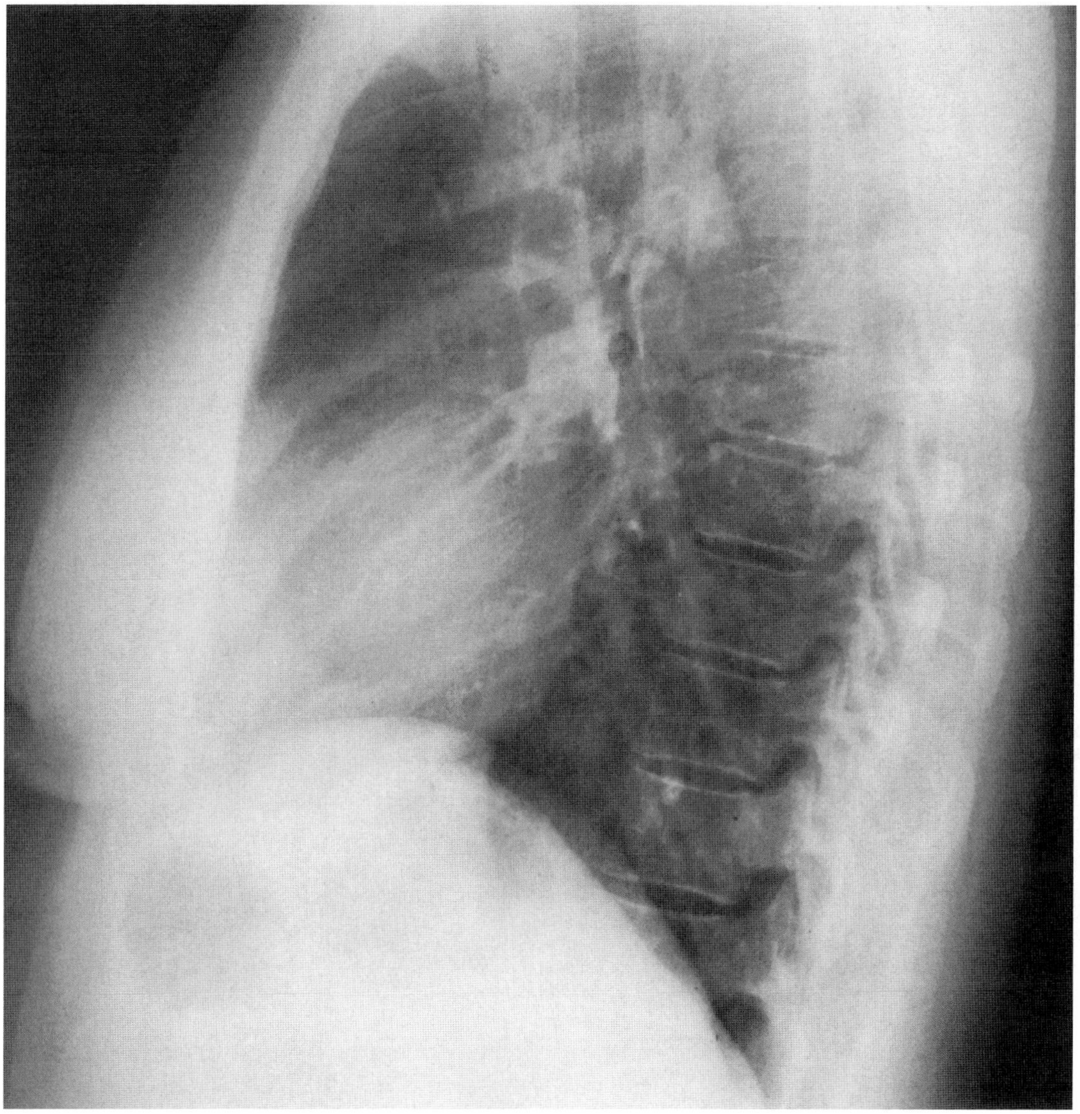

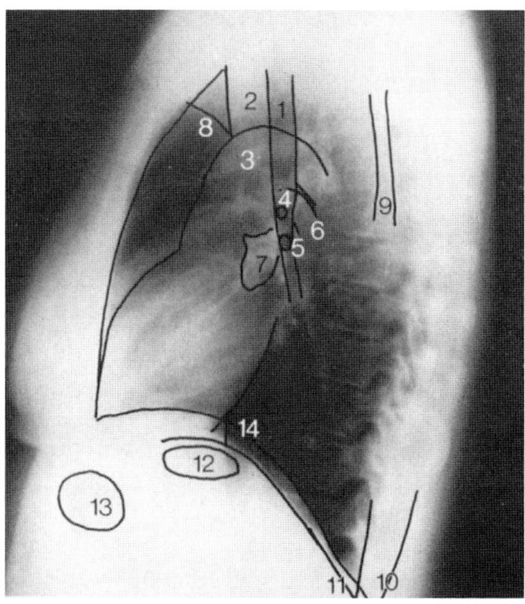

Figure 2 Lateral chest radiograph.

1. Trachea
2. Pretracheal vascular bundle
3. Aortic arch
4. Right upper lobe bronchus
5. Left upper lobe bronchus
6. Left pulmonary artery
7. Right pulmonary artery in pretracheal vascular oval
8. Axillary fold
9. Scapula
10. Right posterior costophrenic sulcus (right hemidiaphragm with complete contour to sternum)
11. Left dorsal costophrenic sinus (left hemidiaphragm with incomplete contour to sternum)
12. Stomach bubble
13. Transverse colon
14. Inferior vena cava

Neuroanatomy

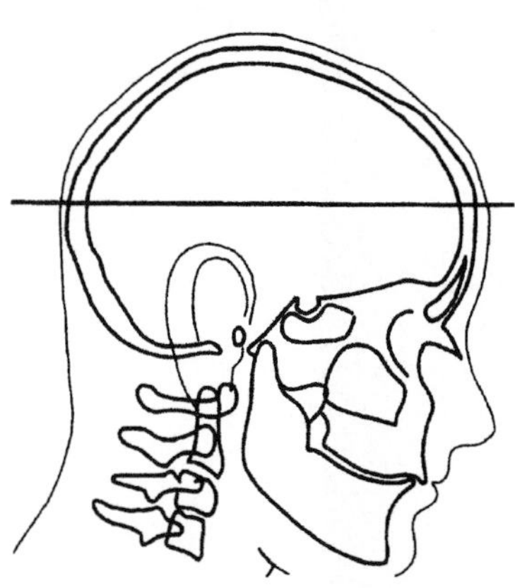

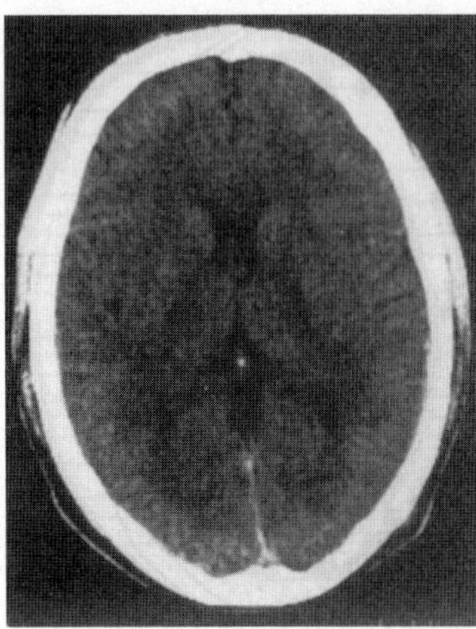

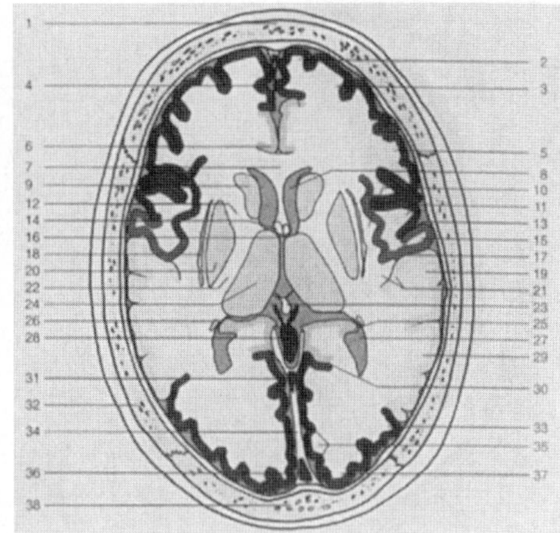

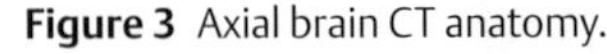

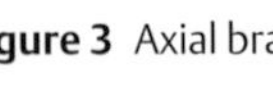

Figure 3 Axial brain CT anatomy.

1. frontal bone
2. superior frontal gyrus
3. middle frontal gyrus
4. falx of cerebrum
5. inferior frontal gyrus
6. cingulate gyrus
7. corpus callosum
8. lateral ventricle (anterior horn)
9. caudate nucleus (head
10. insular lobe
11. precentral gyrus
12. internal capsule (anterior crus)
13. central sulcus
14. fornix
15. postcentral gyrus
16. interventricular foramen (of Monro)
17. lateral sulcus
18. claustrum
19. superior temporal gyrus
20. putamen
21. transverse temporal gyri (Heschl's convolution)
22. internal capsule (posterior crus)
23. pineal body
24. thalamus
25. hippocampus
26. caudate nucleus (tail)
27. lateral ventricle (posterior horn)
28. vermis of cerebellum
29. middle temporal gyrus
30. parietooccipital sulcus
31. straight sinus
32. parietal bone
33. parietal bone
33. occipital gyri
34. falx of cerebrum
35. striate cortex
36. superior sagittal sinus
37. occipital pole
38. occipital bone

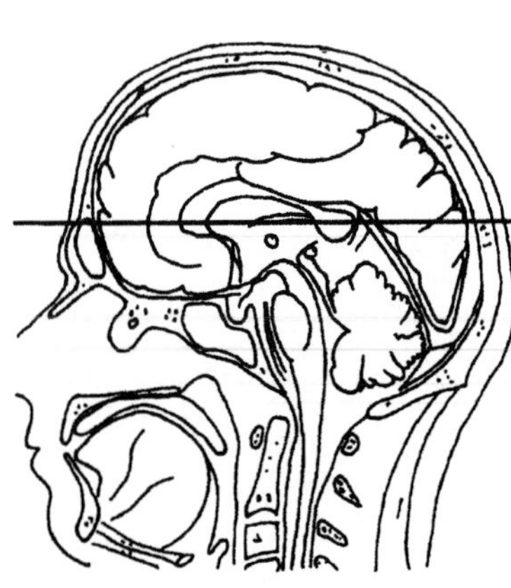

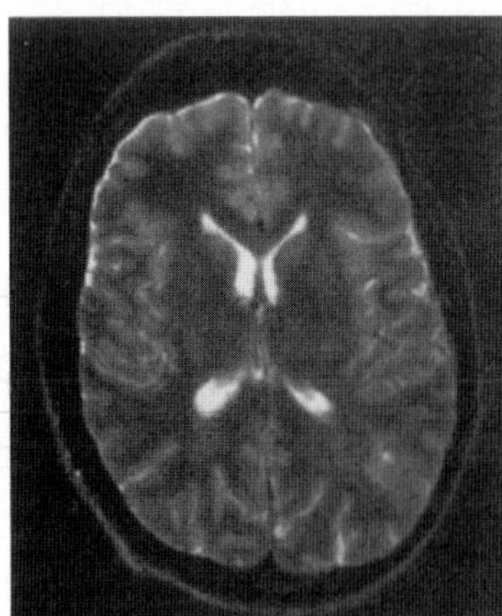

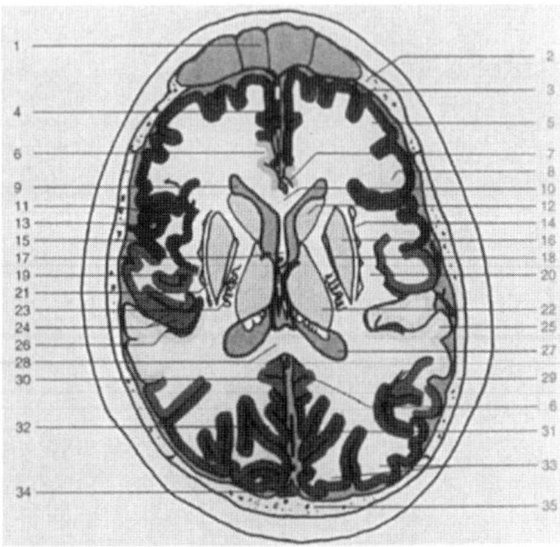

Figure 4 Axial brain MRI anatomy.

1. frontal sinus
2. forntal bone
3. superior frontal gyrus
4. falx of cerebrum (interhemispheric fissure)
5. middle frontal gyrus
6. cingulate gyrus
7. pericallosal artery
8. inferior frontal gyrus
9. lateral ventricle (anterior horn)
10. corpus callosum (genu)
11. precentral gyrus
12. caudate nucleus (head)
13. central sulcus

14. claustrum
15. postcentral gyrus
16. putamen
17. pellucid septum
18. globus pallidus
19. extreme capsule
20. insular lobe
21. external capsule
22. thalamus
23. internal capsule
24. transverse temporal gyri (Heschl's convolutions)
25. superior temporal gyrus
26. lateral sulcus
27. lateral ventricle (posterior horn)
28. corpus callosum (splenium)
29. parietal bone
30. parietooccipital sulcus
31. straight sinus
32. cuneus
33. occipital gyri
34. superior sagittal sinus
35. occipital bone

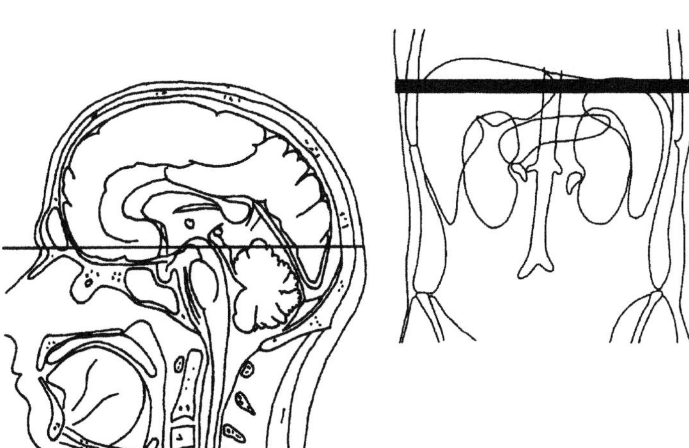

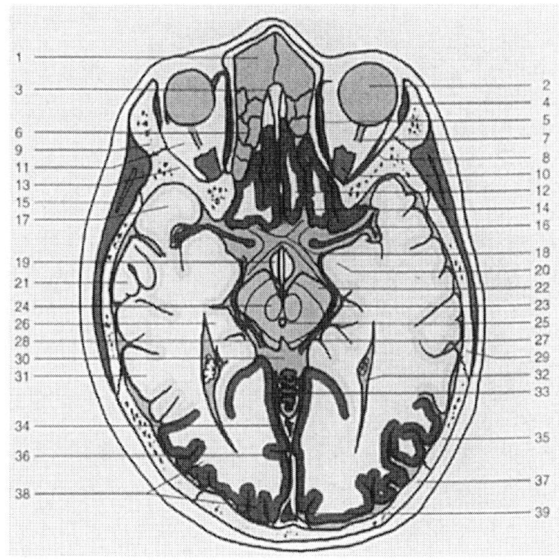

Figure 5 Axial brain MRI anatomy.

1. frontal sinus
2. ocular bulb
3. crista galli
4. lacrimal gland
5. superior oblique muscle
6. ethmoid labyrinth
7. optic nerve
8. lateral rectus muscle
9. zygomatic bone
10. superior rectus muscle
11. orbit
12. gyrus
13. sphenoid bone
14. anterior cerebral artery
15. temporal muscle
16. middle cerebral artery
17. superior temporal gyrus
18. optic chiasm
19. hypothalamus
20. uncus
21. middle temporal gyrus
22. cerebral peduncle
23. posterior cerabral artery
24. red nucleus
25. aqueduct
26. hippocampus
27. cranial colliculus
28. ambient cistern
29. temporal bone
30. Bichat's canal (cisterna venae magnae cerebri)
31. inferior temporal gyrus
32. lateral ventricle (temporal horn)
33. cranial lobe of cerebellum
34. straight sinus
35. parietal bone
36. calcarine sulcus
37. occipital bone
38. superior sagittal sinus

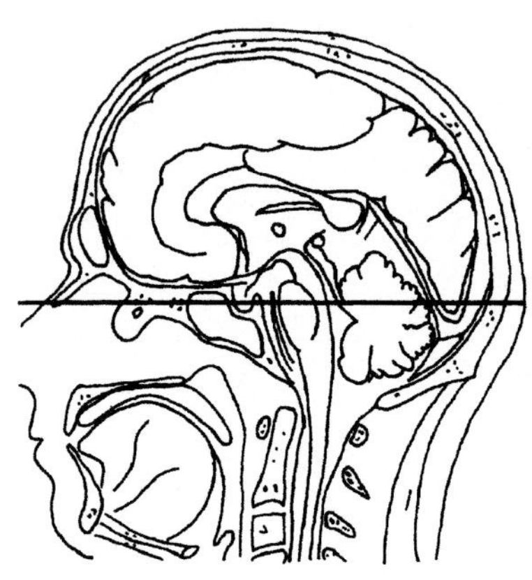

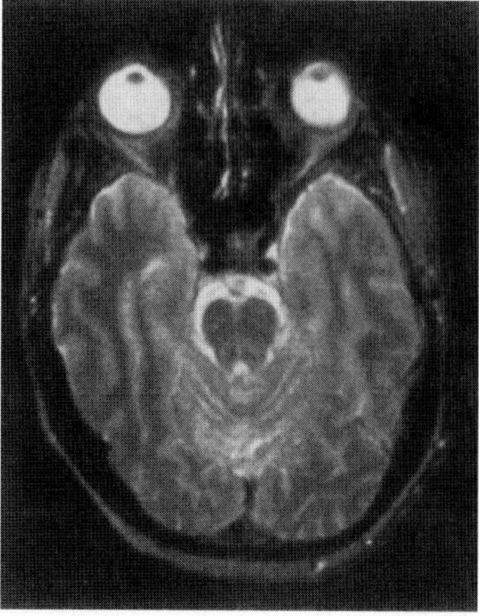

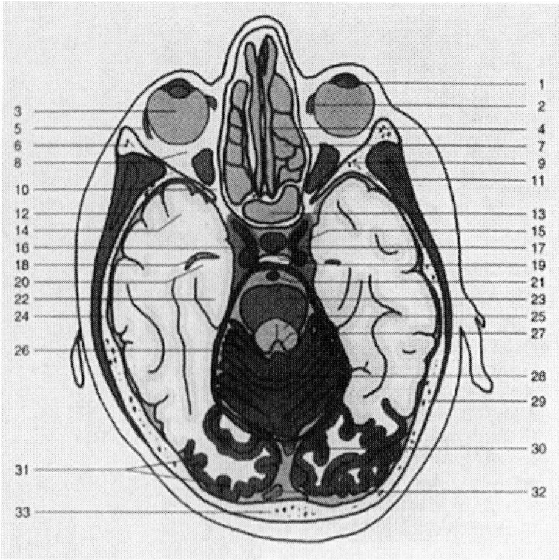

Figure 6 Axial brain MRI anatomy.

1. lens
2. medial rectus muscle
3. ocular bulb
4. nasal septum
5. lateral rectus muscle
6. zygomatic bone
7. ethmoid labyrinth
8. orbit
9. inferior rectus muscle
10. superior orbital fissure
11. sphenoid bone
12. temporal muscle
13. sphenoid sinus
14. temporal lobe
15. cavernous sinus
16. internal carotid artery
17. pituitary gland
18. lateral ventricle (temporal horn)
19. dorsum sellae
20. hippocampus
21. basilar artery
22. parahippocampal gyrus
23. pons
24. termporal bone
25. reticular formation
26. tentorium of cerebellum
27. fourth ventricle
28. cranial lobe of cerebellum
29. parietal bone
30. straight sinus
31. occipital gyri
32. superior sagittal sinus
33. occipital bone

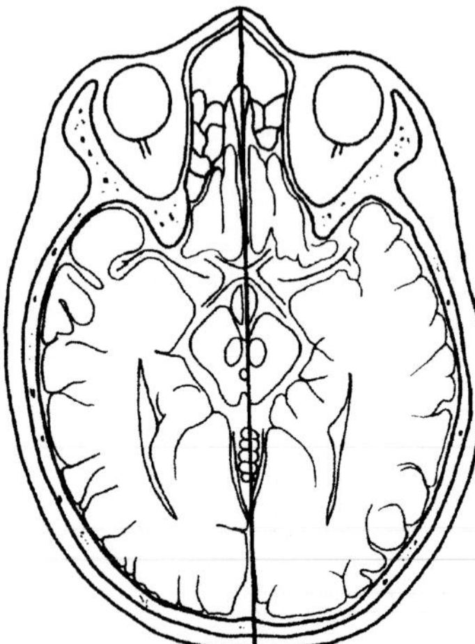

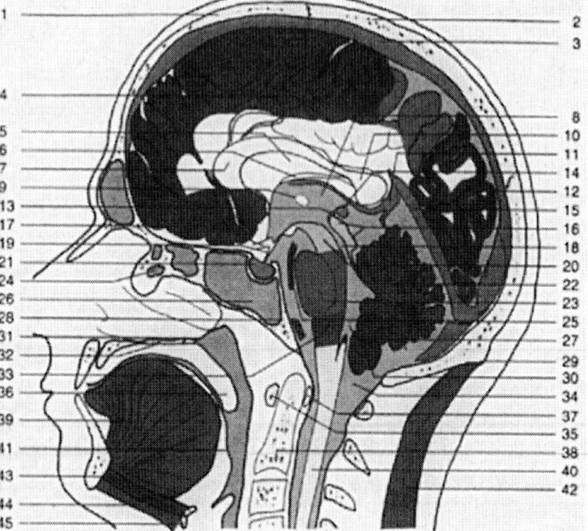

Figure 7 Sagittal MRI brain anatomy.

1. frontal bone
2. parietal bone
3. superior sagittal sinus
4. cingulate sulcus
5. pellucid septum
6. internal cerebral vein
7. corpus callosum (genu)
8. third ventricle
9. intermediate mass
10. corpus callosum (splenium)
11. great vein of Galen
12. parietooccipital sulcus
13. anterior and posterior commissures
14. pineal body
15. straight sinus
16. cranial and caudal colliculi
17. optic nerve
18. aqueduct
19. infundibulum
20. mesencephalic tegmentum

21. pituitary gland
22. cerebellum' 23. pons
24. ethmoid labyrinth
25. basilar artery
26. sphenoid sinus
27. fourth ventricle
28. clivus
29. occipital bone (external occipital protuberance)
30. uvula vermis
31. nasopharynx
32. hard palate
33. medulla oblongata
34. cerebellomedullary cistern
35. atlas (arch)
36. uvula
37. transverse ligament of atlas
38. Odontoid process of axis
39. genioglossus muscle
40. spinal cord
41. oropharynx
42. semispinalis capitis muscle
43. geniohyoid muscle
44. mylohyoid muscle
45. hyoid bone

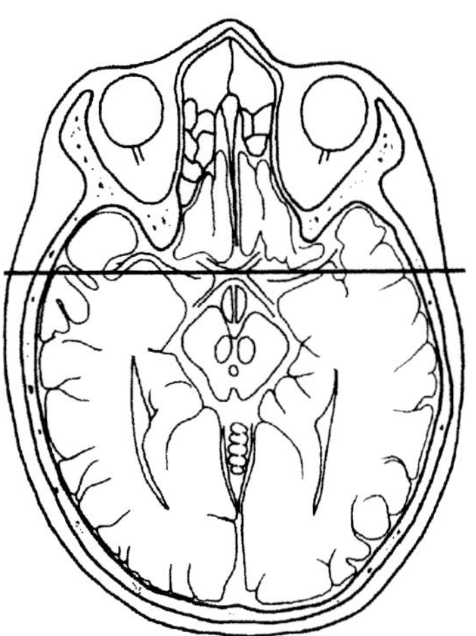

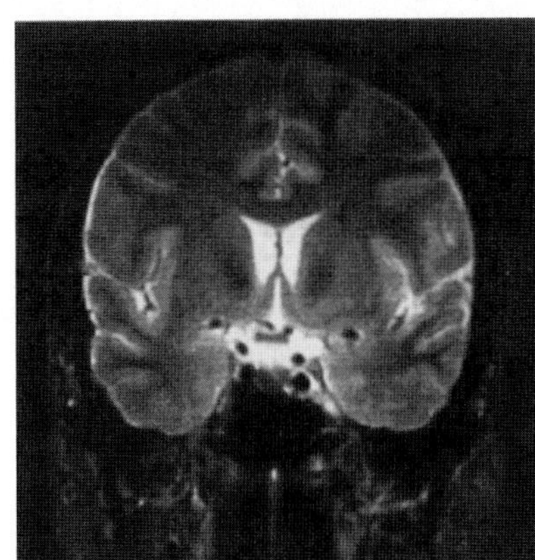

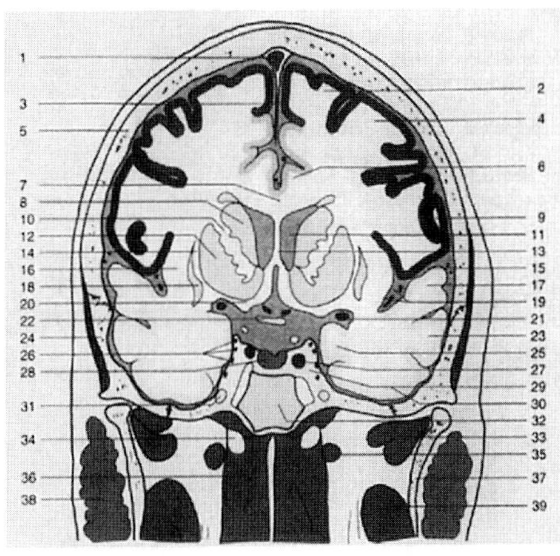

Figure 8 Coronal MRI brain anatomy.

1. superior sagittal sinus
2. superior frontal gyrus
3. falx of cerebrum
4. middle frontal gyrus
5. parietal bone
6. cingulate sulcus
7. corpus callosum (body)
8. caudate nucleus (head)
9. inferior frontal gyrus
10. internal capsule (anterior crus)
11. lateral ventricle (anterior horn)
12. putamen
13. pellucid septum
14. external capsule
15. lateral sulcus
16. extreme capsule
17. superior termporal gyrus
18. claustrum
19. insular lobe and insular cistern
20. roof of chiasmatic cisten
21. middle cerebral artery
22. optic chiasm
23. middle temporal gyrus
24. temporal bone
25. parahippocampal gyrus
26. oculomotor (CN II), trochlear (CN), and abducens (CN VI) nerves
27. internal carotid artery
28. pituitary gland
29. cavernous sinus
30. lateral occipitotemporal gyrus
31. trigeminal ganglion
32. sphenoid sinus
33. lateral pterygoid muscle
34. auditory tube
35. levator veli palatini muscle
36. nasopharynx (constrictor muscle)
37. mandible (ramus)
38. parotid gland
39. medial pterygoid muscle

Thoracic Anatomy

A

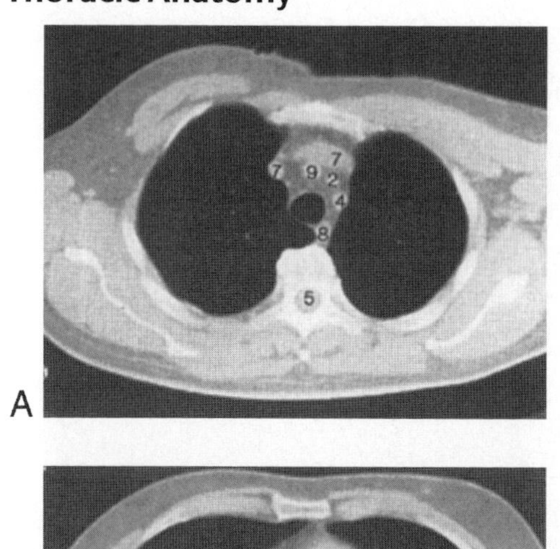

B

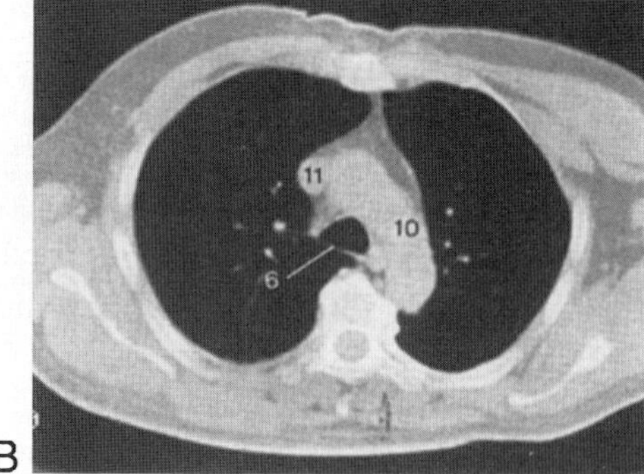

C

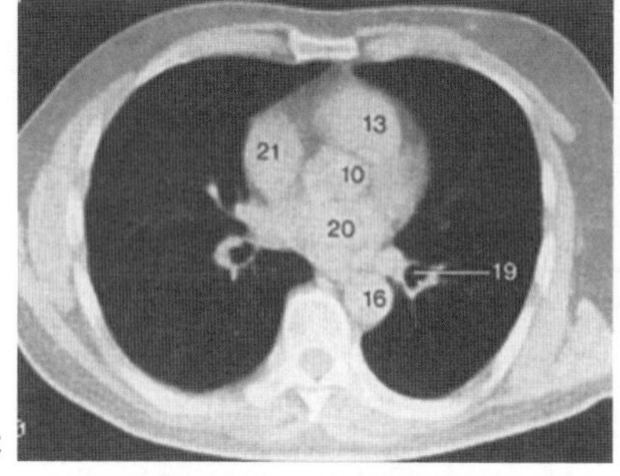

D

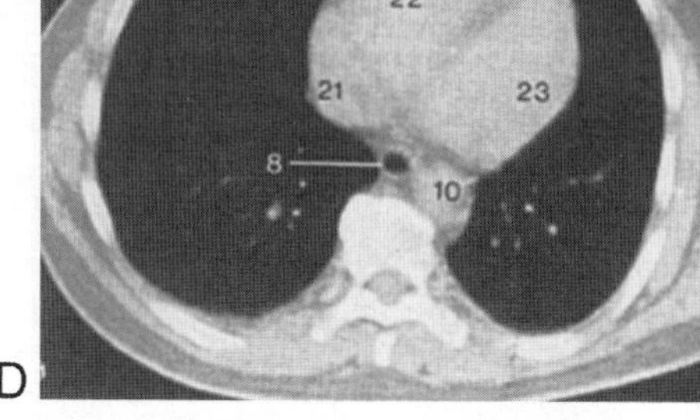

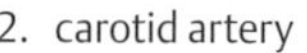

Figure 9 Axial thoracic CT anatomy.

2. carotid artery
4. subclavian artery
5. vertebra
6. trachea
7. subclavian vein
8. esophagus
9. brachiocephalic artery
10. aorta
11. vena cava
13. main pulmonary artery
16. ascending aorta
19. lower lobe artery and vein
20. left atrium
21. right atrium
22. right ventricle
23. left venticle

A

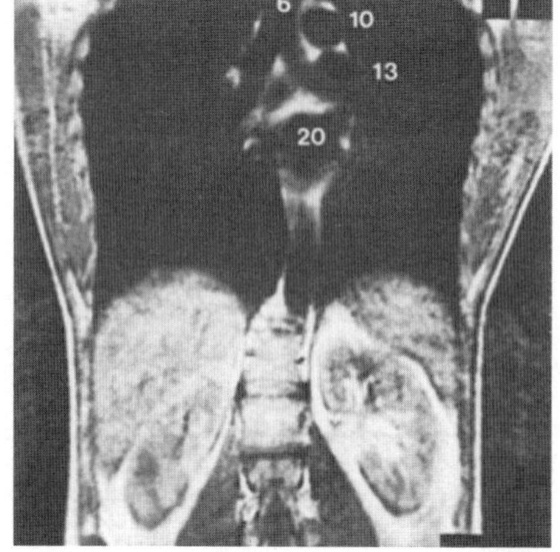

B

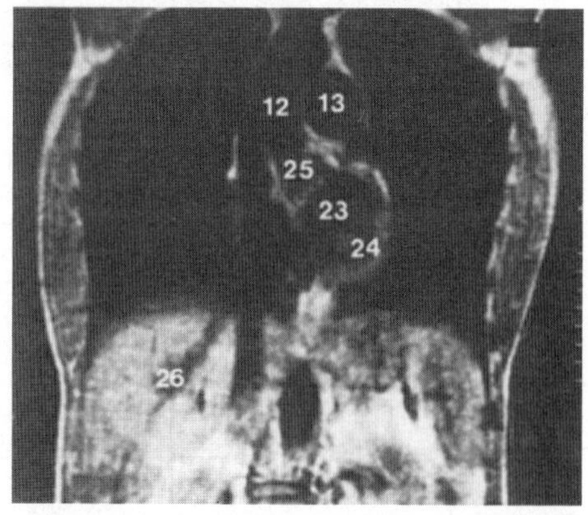

C

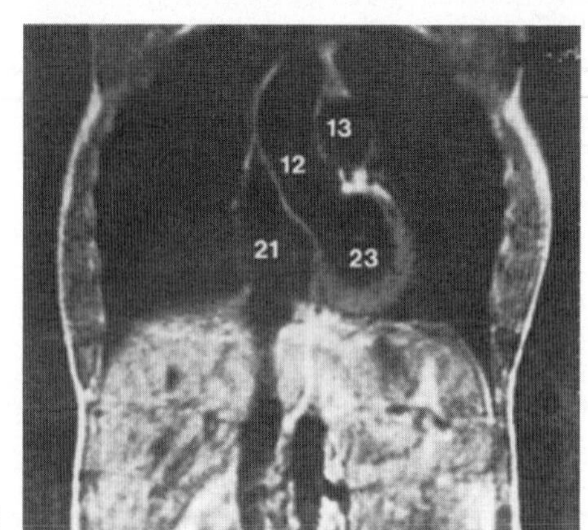

D

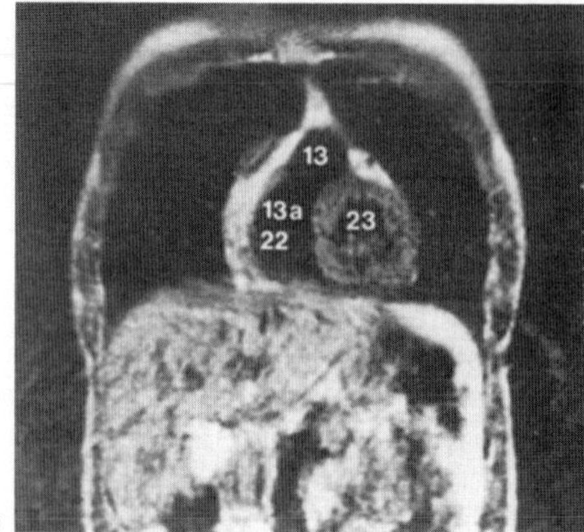

Figure 10 Coronal thoracic MRI anatomy.

6. trachea
10. aorta
12. ascending aorta
13. main pulmonic valve
20. left atrium
21. right atrium
22. right ventricle
23. left ventricle
24. papillary muscle
25. aortic valve
26. hepatic vein

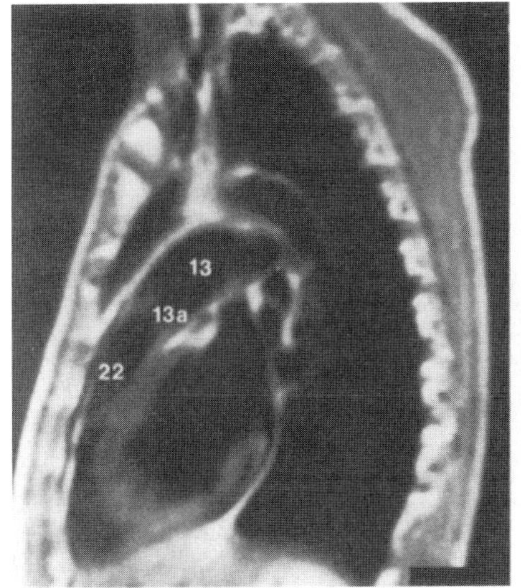

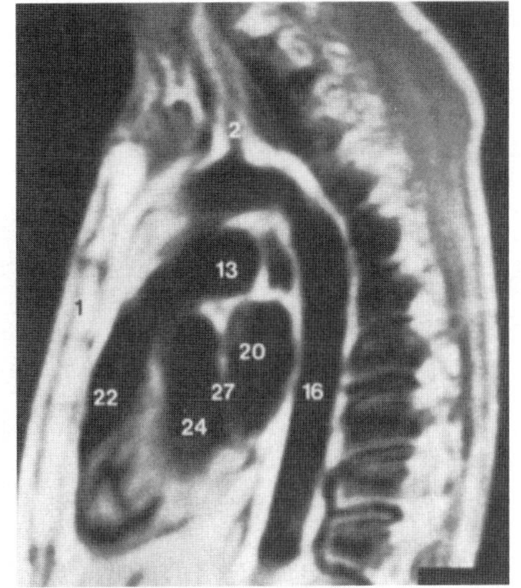

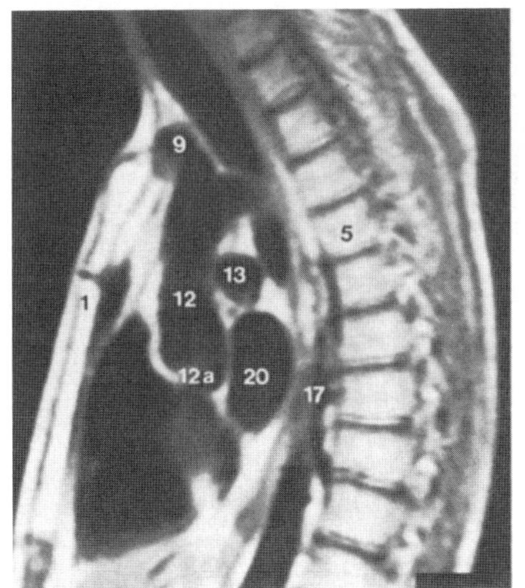

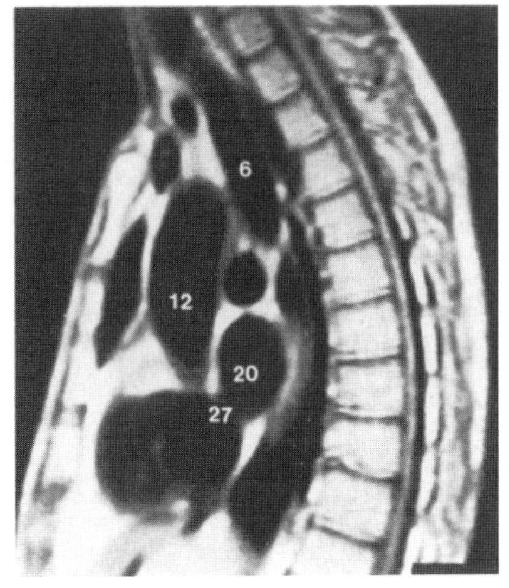

Figure 11 Sagittal thoracic MRI anatomy.

2. carotid artery
5. vertebra
6. trachea
9. brachiocephalic artery
12. ascending aorta
12a. aortic valve
13. main pulmonary artery
13a. pulmonic valve
16. descending aorta
17. azygos vein
20. left atrium
22. right ventricle
24. papillarly muscle
27. mitral valve

Abdominal Pelvic Anatomy

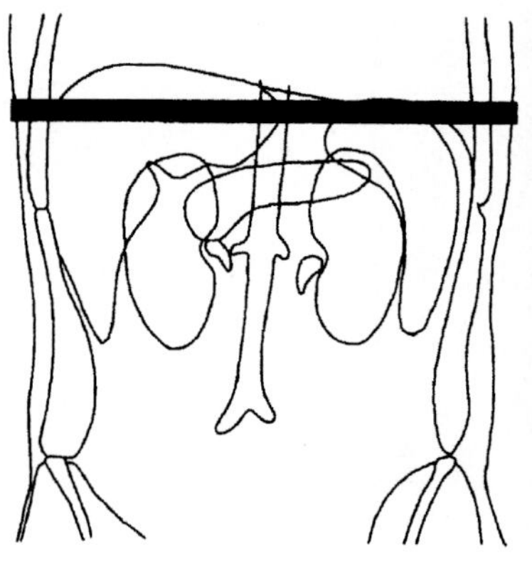

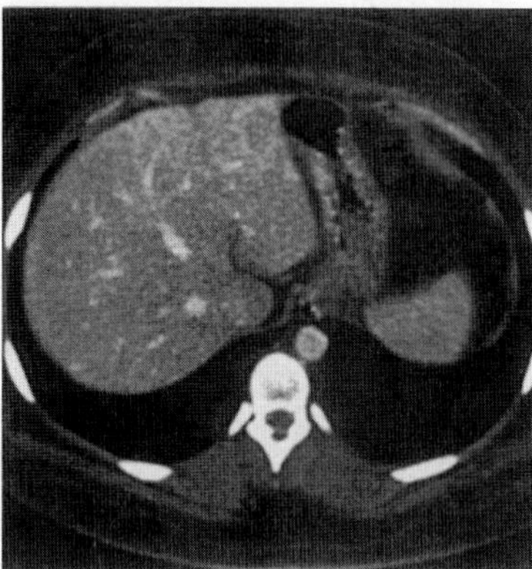

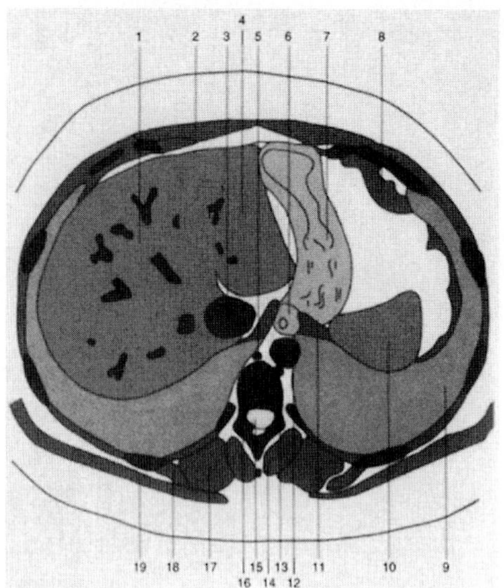

Figure 12 Axial abdomen and pelvis CT anatomy.

1. liver
2. rectus abdominis muscle
3. inferior vena cava
4. liver (left lobe)
5. azygos vein
6. esophagus
7. stomach
8. diaphragm
9. left lung
10. spleen
11. diaphragm (lumbar part)
12. abdominal aorta
13. hemiazygos vein
14. spinalis muscle
15. spinal canal
16. thoracic vertebra 9
17. longissimus thoracis muscle
18. illiocostalis lumborum muscle
19. latissimus dorsi muscle

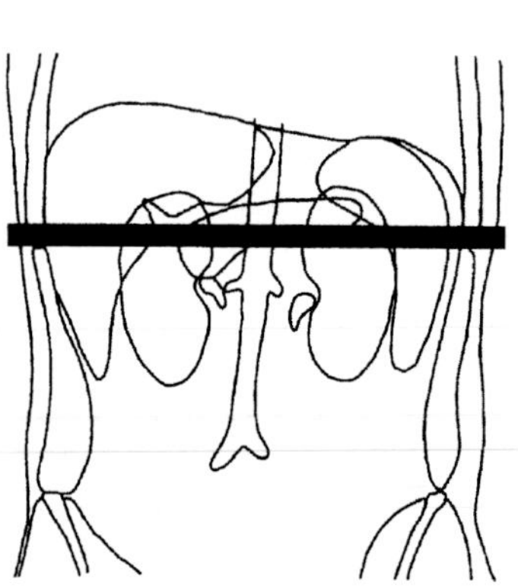

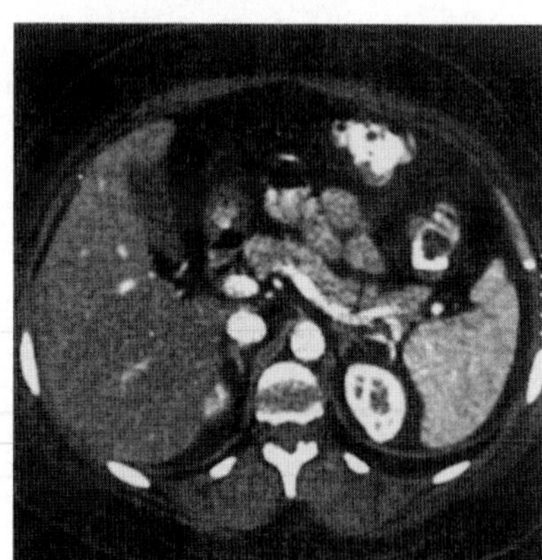

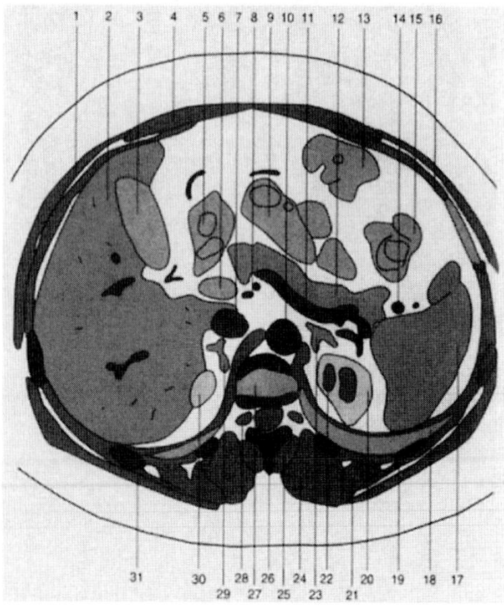

Figure 13 Axial abdomen and pelvis CT anatomy.

1. external oblique muscle
2. liver
3. gall bladder
4. rectus abdominis muscle
5. ampulla of duodenum
6. duodenum
7. inferior vena cava
8. left gastric artery and vein
9. jejunum
10. abdominal aorta
11. splenic vein
12. pancreas
13. transverse colon
14. splenic artery
15. descending colon
16. internal oblique muscle
17. spleen

18. left lung (costodiaphragmatic recess)
19. inferior posterior serratus anterior muscle
20. left renal cortex
21. iliocostalis thoracis muscle
22. renal medulla
23. left adrenal gland
24. longissimus thoracis muscle
25. spinalis muscle
26. spinal canal
27. thoracis vertebra 11
28. spinal nerve root T 11
29. right adrenal gland
30. right kidney
31. latissimus dorsi muscle

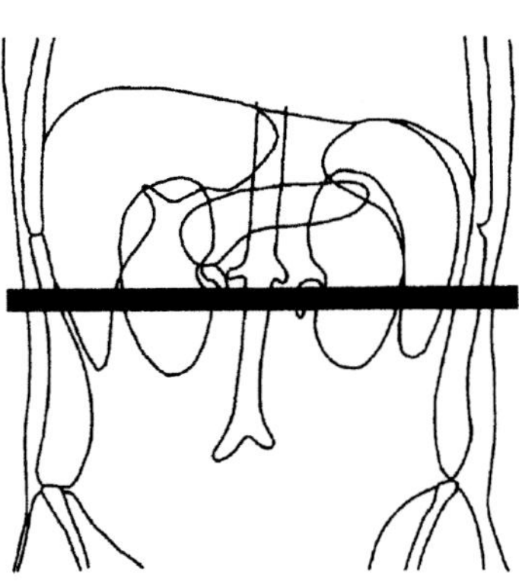

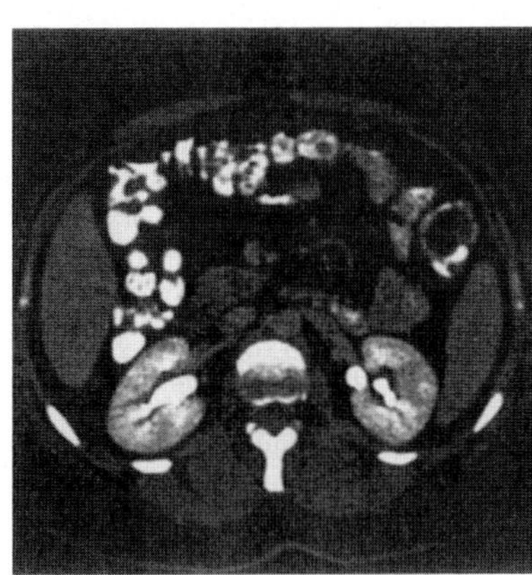

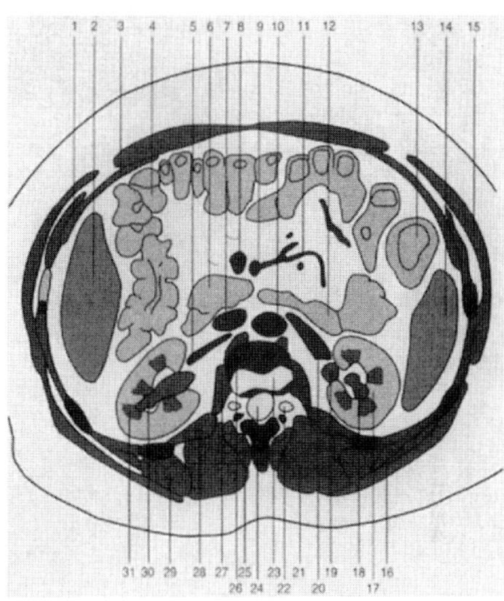

Figure 14 Axial adbomen and pelvis CT anatomy.

1. internal oblique muscle
2. liver
3. transversus abdominis muscle
4. transverse colon
5. right renal artery
6. duodenum
7. inferior vena cava
8. superior mesenteric vein
9. superior mesenteric artery
10. abdominal aorta
11. middle colic artery
12. duodenum (inferior horizontal part)
13. descending colon
14. spleen
15. external oblique muscle
16. inferior posterior serratus anterior muscle
17. left kidney
18. renal calix
19. ureter
20. left renal vein
21. longissimus thoracis muscle
22. spinal nerve root
23. lumbar vertebra 1
24. spinal canal
25. spinalis muscle
26. diaphragm
27. psoas muscle
28. quadratus lumborum muscle
29. iliocostalis lumborum muscle
30. renal pelvis
31. renal pyramid

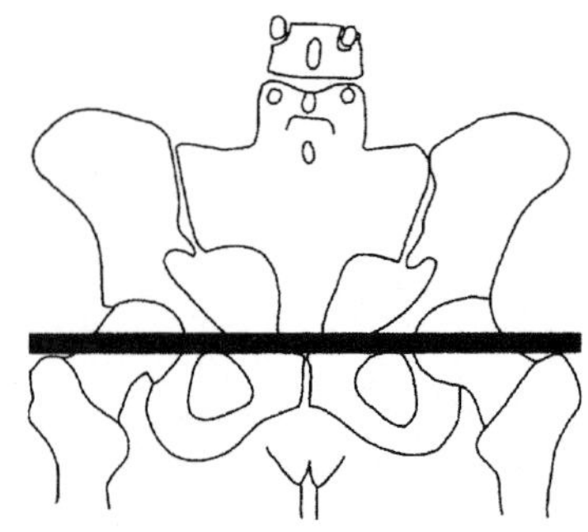

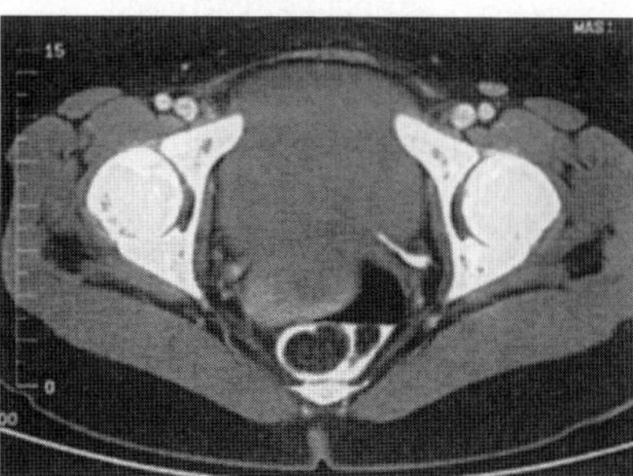

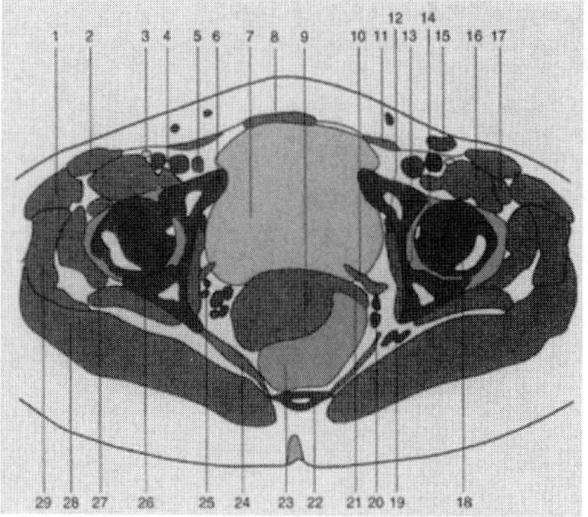

Figure 15 Axial abdomen and pelvis CT anatomy.

1. tensor fasciae latae muscle
2. sartorius muscle
3. femoral nerve
4. external iliac artery and vein
5. medial external iliac lymph node
6. pubic bone
7. urinary blader
8. rectus abdominis muscle
9. uterus
10. ureter
11. internal oblique muscle
12. obturator artery
13. internal obturator muscle
14. fovea of head of femur
15. superficial inguinal lymph nodes
16. iliopsoas muscle
17. rectus femoris muscle
18. head of femur
19. inferior gluteal artery and vein
20. inferior vesical artery and vein
21. fallopian tube
22. coccyx
23. rectum
24. sacrospinal ligament
25. internal pudendal artery and vein
26. ischium
27. gluteus minimus muscle
28. gluteus maximus muscle
29. gluteus medius muscle

Index

Page numbers followed by f indicate figures.